HANDBOOK OF SELF-REGULATION

HANDBOOK OF
SELF-REGULATION
Research, Theory, and Applications

SECOND EDITION

EDITED BY
Kathleen D. Vohs
Roy F. Baumeister

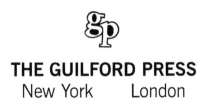

THE GUILFORD PRESS
New York   London

© 2011 The Guilford Press
A Division of Guilford Publications, Inc.
72 Spring Street, New York, NY 10012
www.guilford.com

Printed in the United States of America

This book is printed on acid-free paper.

Last digit is print number: 9   8   7   6   5   4   3   2

Library of Congress Cataloging-in-Publication Data

Handbook of self-regulation : research, theory, and applications / edited by Kathleen D.
Vohs, Roy F. Baumeister.–2nd ed.
   p. cm.
   Includes bibliographical references and index.
   ISBN 978-1-60623-948-3 (hardcover); ISBN 978-1-4625-0951-5 (paperback)
   1. Self-control.   2. Self-management (Psychology)   I. Vohs, Kathleen
D.   II. Baumeister, Roy F.
   BF632.H262 2011
   153.8—dc22
                                         2010009381

To Lauren
—*K. D. V.*

To Athena
—*R. F. B.*

About the Editors

Kathleen D. Vohs, PhD, is Associate Professor of Marketing at the Carlson School of Management at the University of Minnesota. She holds a McKnight Presidential Fellowship and has recently been named the Board of Overseers Professor of Marketing. Dr. Vohs has more than 120 professional publications, including six books. Her research is concerned with self-regulation, particularly in regard to impulsive spending and eating, decision making, self-esteem, the fear and feeling of being duped, self-escape behaviors, and the psychology of money.

Roy F. Baumeister, PhD, holds the Eppes Professorship in the Department of Psychology at Florida State University. He also has taught and conducted research at the University of California, Berkeley; Case Western Reserve University; the University of Texas; the University of Virginia; the Max-Planck Institute in Munich (Germany); and Stanford University's Center for Advanced Study in the Behavioral Sciences. Dr. Baumeister has written nearly 500 professional publications (including 27 books). His research on self-regulation addresses such topics as aggression, eating, sexuality, emotion, limited resources, addiction, free will, physiology, and task performance.

Contributors

Henk Aarts, PhD, Department of Psychology, Utrecht University, Utrecht, The Netherlands

Ozlem Ayduk, PhD, Department of Psychology, University of California, Berkeley, Berkeley, California

Alan D. Baddeley, PhD, Department of Psychology, University of York, York, United Kingdom

Austin S. Baldwin, PhD, Department of Psychology, Southern Methodist University, Dallas, Texas

Russell A. Barkley, PhD, Department of Psychiatry, SUNY Upstate Medical University, Syracuse, New York

Isabelle M. Bauer, PhD, Department of Psychology, Florida State University, Tallahassee, Florida

Roy F. Baumeister, PhD, Department of Psychology, Florida State University, Tallahassee, Florida

Clancy Blair, PhD, Department of Applied Psychology, Steinhardt School of Culture, Education, and Human Development, New York University, New York, New York

Susan D. Calkins, PhD, Department of Human Development and Family Studies and Department of Psychology, University of North Carolina at Greensboro, Greensboro, North Carolina

Evan C. Carter, MS, Department of Psychology, University of Miami, Coral Gables, Florida

Charles S. Carver, PhD, Department of Psychology, University of Miami, Coral Gables, Florida

Daniel Cervone, PhD, Department of Psychology, University of Illinois at Chicago, Chicago, Illinois

Benjamin A. Converse, PhD, Department of Psychology, University of Virginia, Charlottesville, Virginia

Colin G. DeYoung, PhD, Department of Psychology, University of Minnesota, Minneapolis, Minnesota

Nancy Eisenberg, PhD, Department of Psychology, Arizona State University, Tempe, Arizona

Lesa K. Ellis, PhD, Department of Psychology, Westminster College, Salt Lake City, Utah

Ronald J. Faber, PhD, School of Journalism and Mass Communication, University of Minnesota, Minneapolis, Minnesota

Eli J. Finkel, PhD, Department of Psychology, Northwestern University, Evanston, Illinois

Ayelet Fishbach, PhD, Booth School of Business, University of Chicago, Chicago, Illinois

Gráinne M. Fitzsimons, PhD, Department of Psychology, University of Waterloo, Waterloo, Ontario, Canada

Malte Friese, PhD, Institute of Psychology, University of Basel, Basel, Switzerland

Paul T. Fuglestad, PhD, Department of Psychology, University of Minnesota, Minneapolis, Minnesota

Peter M. Gollwitzer, PhD, Department of Psychology, New York University, New York, New York, and Faculty of Psychology, University of Konstanz, Konstanz, Germany

Kasey M. Griffin, MS, Department of Psychology, University of Pittsburgh, Pittsburgh, Pennsylvania

James J. Gross, PhD, Department of Psychology, Stanford University, Stanford, California

Jennifer Guadagno, BA, Department of Psychology and Neuroscience, Duke University, Durham, North Carolina

Todd F. Heatherton, PhD, Department of Psychological and Brain Sciences, Dartmouth College, Hanover, New Hampshire

Julie D. Henry, PhD, School of Psychology, University of New South Wales, Sydney, New South Wales, Australia

C. Peter Herman, PhD, Department of Psychology, University of Toronto, Toronto, Ontario, Canada

Andrew W. Hertel, PhD, Department of Psychology, University of Minnesota, Minneapolis, Minnesota

E. Tory Higgins, PhD, Department of Psychology, Columbia University, New York, New York

Wilhelm Hofmann, PhD, Center for Decision Research, University of Chicago, Chicago, Illinois

Sander L. Koole, PhD, Faculty of Psychology and Education, VU University Amsterdam, Amsterdam, The Netherlands

Mark R. Leary, PhD, Department of Psychology and Neuroscience, Duke University, Durham, North Carolina

Alison Ledgerwood, PhD, Department of Psychology, University of California, Davis, Davis, California

Esther M. Leerkes, PhD, Department of Human Development and Family Studies, University of North Carolina at Greensboro, Greensboro, North Carolina

Michael E. McCullough, PhD, Department of Psychology, University of Miami, Coral Gables, Florida

Kateri McRae, PhD, Department of Psychology, University of Denver, Denver, Colorado

Walter Mischel, PhD, Department of Psychology, Columbia University, New York, New York

Nilly Mor, PhD, School of Education, Hebrew University of Jerusalem, Jerusalem, Israel

Kevin N. Ochsner, PhD, Department of Psychology, Columbia University, New York, New York

Gabriele Oettingen, PhD, Department of Psychology, New York University, New York, New York, and Faculty of Psychology, University of Hamburg, Hamburg, Germany

Heather Orom, PhD, Department of Health Behavior, School of Public Health and Health Professions, University at Buffalo, Buffalo, New York

Esther K. Papies, PhD, Department of Psychology, Utrecht University, Utrecht, The Netherlands

Janet Polivy, PhD, Department of Psychology, University of Toronto, Mississauga, Ontario, Canada

Michael I. Posner, PhD, Department of Psychology, University of Oregon, Eugene, Oregon

Catherine D. Rawn, PhD, Department of Psychology, University of British Columbia, Vancouver, British Columbia, Canada

Mary K. Rothbart, PhD, Department of Psychology, University of Oregon, Eugene, Oregon

Alexander J. Rothman, PhD, Department of Psychology, University of Minnesota, Minneapolis, Minnesota

M. Rosario Rueda, PhD, Department of Experimental Psychology, University of Granada, Granada, Spain

Michael A. Sayette, PhD, Department of Psychology, University of Pittsburgh, Pittsburgh, Pennsylvania

Michael F. Scheier, PhD, Department of Psychology, Carnegie Mellon University, Pittsburgh, Pennsylvania

Brandon J. Schmeichel, PhD, Department of Psychology, Texas A&M University, College Station, Texas

Abigail A. Scholer, PhD, Department of Psychology, Gettysburg College, Gettysburg, Pennsylvania

Walter D. Scott, PhD, Department of Psychology, University of Wyoming, Laramie, Wyoming

William G. Shadel, PhD, Department of Psychology, University of Pittsburgh, Pittsburgh, Pennsylvania

Gal Sheppes, PhD, Department of Psychology, Stanford University, Stanford, California

Cynthia L. Smith, PhD, Department of Human Development, Virginia Polytechnic Institute and State University, Blacksburg, Virginia

Tracy L. Spinrad, PhD, Department of Family and Human Development, Arizona State University, Tempe, Arizona

Yaacov Trope, PhD, Department of Psychology, New York University, New York, New York

Alexandra Ursache, MA, Department of Applied Psychology, Steinhardt School of Culture, Education, and Human Development, New York University, New York, New York

Lotte F. van Dillen, PhD, Department of Social and Organizational Psychology, Utrecht University, Utrecht, The Netherlands

Kathleen D. Vohs, PhD, Department of Marketing, Carlson School of Management, University of Minnesota, Minneapolis, Minnesota

William von Hippel, PhD, School of Psychology, University of Queensland, St. Lucia, Queensland, Australia

Dylan D. Wagner, BA, Department of Psychological and Brain Sciences, Dartmouth College, Hanover, New Hampshire

Preface

Self-regulation has emerged from obscurity and uncertain beginnings to become one of the most centrally important concepts in all of psychology. The first edition of the *Handbook of Self-Regulation* was created to reflect self-regulation's place in understanding human behavior, and it was a great success. Yet the continuing spread of influence of self-regulation has rendered the first edition obsolete, much more rapidly than would happen for many topics. Hence, we have reconvened most of our original authors and an impressive lineup of additional ones to produce the second edition of the *Handbook of Self-Regulation*. No chapter has remained the same from the first to the second edition. Still, the amount of change inevitably varies from one chapter to another. Some authors have updated their coverage with the latest findings, whereas others have made fundamental changes based on new research and directions in the area.

Undoubtedly the most dramatic changes from the first to the second edition are to be found in the new topics and chapters. There is a chapter on automaticity to reflect the growing awareness that not all self-regulation is confined to controlled processes. Another exciting new chapter links self-regulation to working memory, thereby merging two literatures that grew up somewhat independently but increasingly dealt with many of the same issues and concerns. We are pleased with the chapter linking self-regulation to construal level, which follows recent developments that connected the level of abstraction of thought to processes of self-regulation. A new chapter on counteractive self-control explores the complementary processes of reducing temptations and strengthening goals. We also have added a pair of exciting chapters on development across the lifespan. One provides views on the role of executive functioning in children's growth, and the other is on similar processes in older adults.

A new focus for this edition is strong coverage of the social basis of self-regulation in Part IV. One chapter argues that people often subjugate personal well-being for interpersonal acceptance, such that what looks like self-regulation failure might be self-regulation aimed at social acceptance. Twin chapters discuss the bidirectional influences of interpersonal relationships and self-regulation. The influence of religion on self-regulation rounds out the section by addressing culture's institutional forces in the service of promoting self-regulation.

Another recent trend in self-regulation is the growing importance of individual differences. Our new chapter on impulsivity (including the Big Five) demonstrates the wide variation in chronic tendencies to engage in regulated responding.

In this Preface we have highlighted new chapters, but all the chapters have been revised, some of them quite extensively. Our goal is for this volume to be an even more comprehensive and valuable resource to the researchers and practitioners scattered across myriad fields who want to understand this basic key to human nature and social life.

This project thrived with the support of some key people. We are grateful once again for the encouragement we received from Seymour Weingarten, our insightful and good-natured editor at The Guilford Press. Carolyn Graham at Guilford was helpful at crucial points. Finally, we thank Jessica Alquist for preparing the book's indexes.

Enjoy!

KATHLEEN D. VOHS
ROY F. BAUMEISTER

Contents

PART III. DEVELOPMENT OF SELF-REGULATION

PART IV. SOCIAL DIMENSION OF SELF-REGULATION

PART I

BASIC REGULATORY PROCESSES

CHAPTER 1

Self-Regulation of Action and Affect

CHARLES S. CARVER
MICHAEL F. SCHEIER

This chapter outlines the fundamentals of a viewpoint on self-regulation in which behavior is seen as reflecting processes of feedback control. Indeed, we propose that two layers of control manage two different aspects of behavior, jointly situating behavior in time as well as space. We suggest further that this arrangement helps people handle multiple tasks in their life space. More specifically, it helps transform simultaneous concerns with many different goals into a stream of actions that shifts repeatedly from one goal to another over time.

The view described here has been identified with the term *self-regulation* for a long time (e.g., Carver & Scheier, 1981, 1990, 1998, 1999a, 1999b). This term, however, means different things to different people. Many authors in this book use this term as roughly equivalent to *self-control*: overriding of one action tendency in order to attain another goal. We prefer to reserve the term *self-control* for such cases and use the term *self-regulation* more broadly. When we use the term *self-regulation*, we intend to convey the sense of purposive processes, the sense that self-corrective adjustments are taking place as needed to stay on track for the purpose being served (whether this entails overriding another impulse or simply reacting to perturbations from other sources), and the sense that the corrective adjustments originate within the person. These points converge in the view that behavior is a continual process of moving toward (and sometimes away from) goal representations. We also believe that this process embodies characteristics of feedback control. Additional points are made in this chapter, but these ideas lie at its heart.

The ideas presented in this chapter are broad strokes, as much meta-theory as theory. We describe a viewpoint on the structure of behavior that accommodates diverse ways of thinking about what qualities of behavior matter and why. For this reason, we believe this viewpoint complements a wide variety of other ideas about what goes on in human self-regulation.

BEHAVIOR AS GOAL DIRECTED AND FEEDBACK CONTROLLED

In describing this viewpoint, the easiest place to start is with another concept altogether: goals. The goal construct is quite prominent in today's psychology (Austin & Vancouver, 1996; Elliott, 2008), under a wide variety of names. The concept is broad enough to cover both long-term aspirations (e.g., creating and maintaining a good impression among colleagues) and the end points of very short-term acts (e.g., pulling one's car squarely into a parking space). Goals generally can be reached in diverse ways, leading to the potential for vast complexity in the organization of action. People who think about behavior in terms of goals tend to assume that understanding a person means understanding that person's goals—indeed, that the substance of the self consists partly of the person's goals and the organization among them (cf. Mischel & Shoda, 1995).

Feedback Loops

We actually are less concerned here with the goals themselves than with the process of attaining them. We have long subscribed to the view that movement toward a goal reflects the functioning of a negative, or discrepancy-reducing, feedback loop (MacKay, 1966; Miller, Galanter, & Pribram, 1960; Powers, 1973; Wiener, 1948). Such a loop involves a sensing of some present condition, which is compared to a desired or intended condition (as a reference value). If the two are identical, nothing more happens. If there is a discrepancy between the two, the discrepancy is countered by subsequent action to change the sensed condition. The overall effect of such an arrangement is to bring the sensed condition into conformity with the intended condition (Powers, 1973). If the intended condition is a goal, the overall effect is to bring the person's behavior into conformity with the goal—thus, goal attainment.

There also are discrepancy-enlarging loops, in which deviations from the comparison point are increased rather than decreased. The value in this case is a threat, an "anti-goal." Effects of discrepancy-enlarging processes in living systems are typically constrained by discrepancy-reducing processes. Thus, for example, acts of avoidance often segue into other acts of approach. Put differently, sometimes people are able to avoid something they find aversive by the very act of approaching something else. Such dual influence occurs in instances of what is called *active avoidance*: An organism fleeing a threat spots a relatively safe location and approaches it.

Given the preceding description, people sometimes infer that feedback loops act only to create and maintain steady states, and are therefore irrelevant to behavior. Some reference values (and goals) *are* static. But others are dynamic (e.g., taking a vacation across Europe, raising children to be good citizens). In such cases, the goal is the process of traversing the changing trajectory of the activity, not just the arrival at the end point. The principle of feedback control applies readily to moving targets (Beer, 1995).

We started here with the goal construct. Many people write about goal-directed behavior. What we have brought to the conversation about goals (and though we were not the first, we are probably the most persistent) is the notion that goal seeking (human behavior) involves feedback control. Why feedback control? Why not just goals and goal attainment? Good question.

Many people view the feedback loop as an engineering concept (and engineers do use it), but the concept has roots in physiology and other fields. *Homeostasis*, the processes by which the body self-regulates physical parameters such as temperature, blood sugar, and heart rate, is the prototypic feedback process (Cannon, 1932). The concept has been useful enough in diverse fields that sometimes it is even suggested that feedback processes are some of the fundamental building blocks of all complex systems.

We believe there is merit in the recognition of functional similarity between the systems underlying human behavior and other complex systems (cf. Ford, 1987; von Bertalanffy, 1968). Nature is a miser and a recycler. It seems likely that an organization that works in one complex system recurs over and over in nature. For the same reason, it seems likely that principles embodied in physical movement control (which also rely in part on principles of feedback) have more than just a little in common with principles embodied in higher mental functions (Rosenbaum, Carlson, & Gilmore, 2001). For these reasons, we have continued to use the principle of feedback control as a conceptual heuristic over the years.

Levels of Abstraction

Goals exist at many levels of abstraction. One can have the goal of being a good citizen, one can also have the goal of conserving resources—a narrower goal that contributes to being a good citizen. One way to conserve resources is recycling. Recycling entails other, more-concrete goals: placing newspapers and empty bottles into containers and moving them to a pickup location. All of these are goals, values to be approached, but at varying levels of abstraction.

It is often said that people's goals form a hierarchy (Powers, 1973; Vallacher & Wegner, 1987), in which abstract goals are attained by attaining the concrete goals that help define them. Lower-level goals are attained by briefer sequences of action (formed from subcomponents of motor control; e.g., Rosenbaum, Meulenbroek, Vaughan, & Jansen, 2001). Some sequences of action have a self-contained quality, in that they run off fairly autonomously once triggered.

Viewed from the other direction, sequences can be organized into programs of action (Powers, 1973). Programs are more planful than sequences and require choices at various points. Programs, in turn, are sometimes (though not always) enacted in the service of principles. Principles are abstractions that provide a basis for making decisions within programs and suggest undertaking or refraining from certain programs. What Powers called *principles* are roughly equivalent to values (Schwartz & Bilsky, 1990; Schwartz & Rubel, 2005). Even that is not the end of potential complexity. Patterns of values can coalesce to form a very abstract sense of desired (and undesired) self, or a sense of desired (and undesired) community.

All these classes of goals, from very concrete to very abstract, can be reference points for self-regulation. When self-regulation is undertaken regarding a goal at one level, presumably self-regulation is simultaneously being invoked at all levels of abstraction below that one. We return to this diversity among potential superordinate goals later in the chapter.

Other Phenomena of Personality–Social Psychology and Feedback Control

The goal concept, in its various forms, is one place in which the constructs of personality and social psychology intersect with the logic of the feedback loop. Before moving on, we note briefly that the intersection is actually broader. The notion of reducing sensed discrepancies has a long history in social psychology, in topics such as behavioral conformity to norms (Asch, 1955) and cognitive consistency (Festinger, 1957; Heider, 1946; Lecky, 1945). The self-regulatory feedback loop, in effect, constitutes a meta-theory for such effects.

FEEDBACK PROCESSES AND AFFECT

Thus far we have considered behavior—getting from here to there. Another important part of experience is feelings, or *affect*. Two fundamental questions about affect are what it consists of and where it comes from. Affect pertains to one's desires and whether they are being met (e.g., Clore, 1994; Frijda, 1986, 1988; Ortony, Clore, & Collins, 1988). But what exactly is the internal mechanism by which it arises?

The answer we posed to this question (Carver & Scheier, 1990, 1998, 1999a, 1999b) focuses on some of the functional properties that affect seems to display in the behaving person. We used feedback control again as an organizing principle. We suggested that feelings are a consequence of a feedback process that runs automatically, simultaneously with and in parallel to the behavior-guiding process. Perhaps the easiest way to convey what this second process is doing is to say that it is checking on how well the first process (the behavior loop) is doing at reducing *its* discrepancies (we focus first on approach loops). Thus, the input for this second loop is some representation of the *rate of discrepancy reduction in the action system over time*.

An analogy may be useful. Action implies change between states. Thus, behavior is analogous to distance. If the action loop controls distance, and if the affect loop assesses the progress of the action loop, then the affect loop is dealing with the psychological analogue of velocity, the first derivative of distance over time. To the extent that this analogy is meaningful, the perceptual input to the affect loop should be the first derivative over time of the input used by the action loop.

Input per se does not create affect (a given rate of progress has different affective implications in different circumstances). We believe that, as in any feedback system, this input is compared to a reference value (cf. Frijda, 1986, 1988). In this case, the reference is an acceptable or desired rate of behavioral discrepancy reduction. As in other feedback loops, the comparison checks for deviation from the standard. If there is one, the output function changes.

We suggest that the error signal from the comparison in this loop (the representation of a discrepancy) is manifest subjectively as affect, positive or negative valence. If the rate of progress is below the criterion, negative affect arises. If the rate is high enough to exceed the criterion, positive affect arises. If the rate is not distinguishable from the criterion, no affect arises.

In essence, the argument is that feelings with a positive valence mean you are doing better at something than you need to, and that feelings with a negative valence mean you are doing worse than you need to (for more detail, see Carver & Scheier, 1998, chaps. 8 and 9). One implication of this line of thought is that, for any given action domain, affective valence should potentially form a bipolar dimension; that is, for a given action, affect can be positive, neutral, or negative, depending on how well or poorly the action is going.

What determines the criterion for this loop? The criterion is probably quite flexible when the activity is unfamiliar. If the activity is familiar, the criterion is likely to reflect the person's accumulated experience, in the form of an expected rate (the more experience you have, the more you know what is reasonable to expect). Whether "desired" or "expected" or "needed" most accurately depicts the criterion may depend greatly on the context.

The criterion can also change. The less experience the person has in a domain, the more fluid the criterion; in a familiar domain, change is slower. Still, repeated overshoot of the criterion automatically yields an upward drift of the criterion (e.g., Eidelman & Biernat, 2007); repeated undershoots yield a downward drift. Thus, the system recalibrates over repeated experience in such a way that the criterion stays within the range of those experiences (Carver & Scheier, 2000). An ironic effect of recalibration would be to keep the balance of a person's affective experience (positive to negative) relatively similar, even when the rate criterion changes considerably.

Two Kinds of Behavioral Loops, Two Dimensions of Affect

Now consider discrepancy-enlarging loops. The view just outlined rests on the idea that positive feeling results when a behavioral system is making rapid progress in *doing what it is organized to do*. The systems considered thus far are organized to reduce discrepancies. There is no obvious reason, though, why the principle should not apply as well to systems organized to enlarge discrepancies. If that kind of a system is making rapid progress doing what it is organized to do, there should be positive affect. If it is doing poorly, there should be negative affect.

The idea that affects of both valences can occur would seem comparable across both approach and avoidance systems; that is, both approach and avoidance have the potential to induce positive feelings (by doing well), and both have the potential to induce negative feelings (by doing poorly). But doing well at moving *toward an incentive* is not quite the same as doing well at moving *away from a threat*. Thus, the two positives may not be quite the same, nor may the two negatives.

Based on this line of thought, and drawing on insights from Higgins (e.g., 1987, 1996) and his collaborators (see Scholer & Higgins, Chapter 8, this volume), we assume two sets of affects, one relating to approach, the other to avoidance (Carver & Scheier, 1998). Approach activities lead to such positive affects as elation, eagerness, and excitement, and such negative affects as frustration, anger, and sadness (Carver, 2004; Carver & Harmon-Jones, 2009b). Avoidance activities lead to such positive affects as relief and contentment (Carver, 2009), and such negative affects as fear, guilt, and anxiety.

Merging Affect and Action

The two-layered viewpoint described in the preceding sections implies a natural link between affect and action. If the input function of the affect loop is a sensed rate of progress in action, the output function must be a change in rate of that action. Thus, the affect loop has a direct influence on what occurs in the action loop.

Some changes in rate output are straightforward. If you are lagging behind, you push harder. Sometimes the changes are less straightforward. The rates of many "behaviors" are defined not by a pace of physical action but by choices among actions or entire programs of action. For example, increasing your rate of progress on a project at work may mean choosing to spend a weekend working rather than skiing. Increasing your rate of being kind means choosing to do an action that reflects that value when an opportunity arises. Thus, adjustment in rate must often be translated into other terms, such as concentration, or reallocation of time and effort.

The idea of two feedback systems functioning in concert with one another is something we more or less stumbled into. It turns out, however, that such an arrangement is quite common in control engineering (e.g., Clark, 1996). Engineers have long recognized that having two feedback systems functioning together—one controlling position, the other controlling velocity—permits the device in which they are embedded to respond in a way that is both quick and stable, without overshoots and oscillations.

The combination of quickness and stability is valuable in the kinds of electromechanical devices with which engineers deal, but its value is not limited to such devices. A person with strongly reactive emotions is prone to overreact and to oscillate behaviorally. A person who is emotionally nonreactive is slow to respond, even to urgent events. A person whose reactions are between the two extremes responds quickly but without undue overreaction and oscillation.

For biological entities, being able to respond quickly yet accurately confers a clear adaptive advantage. We believe this combination of quick and stable responding is a consequence of having both behavior-managing and affect-managing control systems. Affect causes people's responses to be quicker (because this control system is time-sensitive) and, provided that the affective system is not overresponsive, the responses are also stable.

Our focus here is on how affects influence behavior, emphasizing the extent to which they are interwoven. Note, however, that the behavioral responses related to the affects also lead to *reduction of the affects*. Thus, in a very basic sense, the affect system is self-regulating. Certainly people also make voluntary efforts to regulate emotions (Gross, 2007), but the affect system does a good deal of that self-regulation on its own. Indeed, if the system is optimally responsive, then affective arousal is generally minimized over the long term because the relevant deviations are countered before they become intense (cf. Baumeister, Vohs, DeWall, & Zhang, 2007).

AFFECT ISSUES

This theoretical model differs from others in several ways. At least two of the differences appear to have interesting and important implications.

Divergent Views of Dimensionality Underlying Affect

One difference concerns how affects are organized. A number of theories conceptualize affects as aligned along dimensions (though not all theories do so). Our view fits this picture, in holding that affects related to approach and to avoidance both have the potential to be either positive or negative, thus forming a bipolarity for each motivational tendency.

Most dimensional models of affect, however, take a different form. For example, Gray (1990, 1994) held that one system is engaged by cues of punishment and cues of frustrative nonreward. It thus is responsible for negative feelings, whether those feelings relate to approach or to avoidance. Similarly, he held that another system is engaged by both cues of reward and cues of escape or avoidance of punishment. It thus is responsible for positive feelings, whether the feelings relate to avoidance or to approach.

In this view, each system is responsible for affect of one valence. This yields two unipolar dimensions, each linked to the functioning of a behavioral system. A similar position has been taken by Lang and colleagues (e.g., Lang, 1995; Lang, Bradley, & Cuthbert, 1990), Cacioppo and colleagues (e.g., Cacioppo & Berntson, 1994; Cacioppo, Gardner, & Berntson, 1999), and Watson, Wiese, Vaidya, and Tellegen (1999).

What does the evidence say? There is not a wealth of information from studies targeting the issue, but there is some. Least studied is "doing well" in threat avoidance. Higgins, Shah, and Friedman (1997, Study 4) found that having an avoidance orientation to a task (instructions to avoid failing) plus a good outcome led to elevations in reports of calmness. Calmness was not affected, however, with an approach orientation (instructions to succeed). Thus, calmness was linked to doing well at avoidance, not to doing well at approach. Other research asked people to respond to hypothetical scenarios introducing, then removing, a threat (Carver, 2009). Reports of relief related principally to individual differences in threat sensitivity.

A larger accumulation of evidence links certain negative affects to "doing poorly" in approaching incentives; just a few are noted here (see Carver & Harmon-Jones, 2009b, for details). In the study by Higgins and colleagues (1997) we just described, people with an approach orientation who experienced failure reported elevated sadness. This did not occur with an avoidance orientation. This suggests a link between sadness and doing poorly at approach.

The broader literature of self-discrepancy theory also makes a similar point. Many studies have shown that sadness relates uniquely (controlling for anxiety) to discrepancies between actual selves and ideal selves (for reviews, see Higgins, 1987, 1996). Ideals are qualities the person intrinsically desires: aspirations, hopes, positive images for the self. There is evidence that pursuing an ideal is an approach process (Higgins, 1996). Thus, this literature also suggests that sadness stems from a failure of approach.

Another study examined the situation of frustrative nonreward. Participants were led to believe they could obtain a reward if they performed well on a task (Carver, 2004). All were told they had done poorly, however, and got no reward. Sadness and discouragement at that point related to sensitivity of the approach system, but not sensitivity of the avoidance system.

There is also a good deal of evidence linking the approach system to anger (e.g., Carver & Harmon-Jones, 2009b). As one example, Harmon-Jones and Sigelman (2001) induced anger in some persons but not others, then examined cortical activity. They found elevated left anterior activity, which previous research (e.g., Davidson, 1992) had linked to activation of the approach system. In other studies (Carver, 2004), people reported the feelings they experienced in response to hypothetical events (Study 2) and after the destruction of the World Trade Center (Study 3). Reports of anger related to sensitivity of the approach system, whereas reports of anxiety related to the avoidance system.

There is also, however, an accumulation of evidence that contradicts this position, instead placing all negative affects on one dimension and all positive affects on another dimension. This evidence, briefly summarized by Watson (2009), consists primarily of a large number of studies in which people reported their moods at a particular time or across a particular span of time. As Carver and Harmon-Jones (2009a) pointed out, however, an affective response to a particular event differs in important ways from a mood, which may aggregate experiences over multiple events. It seems likely that different sets of influences come into play in the creation or maintenance of moods than underlie specific, focused affective responses to events.

We have devoted a good deal of space to this issue. Why? It is an important issue because it has implications in the search for a conceptual mechanism underlying affect. Theories postulating two unipolar dimensions appear to equate greater activation of a system to more intense affect of that valence. If the approach system actually relates to feelings of both valences, such a mechanism is not tenable. A conceptual mechanism is needed that addresses both positive and negative feelings within the approach function (and, separately, the avoidance function). The mechanism described here does so.

One more word about dimensionality. Our viewpoint is dimensional in the sense that it is predicated on a dimension of system functioning (from very well to very poorly). However, the affects that fall on that dimension do not themselves form a dimension, apart from the fact that they represent both valences. For example, depression (when things are going extremely poorly) is not simply a more intense state of frustration (when things are going less poorly). The affects themselves appear to be nonlinear consequences of linear variation in system functioning. Anger and depression are both potential consequences of approach going poorly; which one emerges appears to depend on whether the goal seems lost or not (see also Rolls, 1999, 2005).

Coasting

Another potentially important issue also differentiates this model from most other viewpoints on the meaning and consequences of affect (Carver, 2003). Return to the argument that affect reflects the error signal in a feedback loop. Affect thus would be a signal to adjust progress—whether rate is above the criterion or below it. This is intuitive for negative feelings, but not positive feelings.

Here theory becomes counterintuitive. In this model, positive feelings arise when things are going better than they need to. But the feelings still reflect a discrepancy, and the function of a negative feedback loop is to minimize discrepancies. Such a system "wants" to see neither negative nor positive affect. Either one would represent an "error" and lead to changes in output that eventually would reduce it (see also Izard, 1977).

This model argues that people who exceed the criterion rate of progress (and who thus have positive feelings) automatically tend to reduce effort in this domain. They "coast" a little—don't stop, but ease back, such that subsequent rate of progress returns to the criterion. The impact on affect would be that the positive feeling itself is not sustained for very long. It begins to fade.

Expending effort to catch up when behind and coasting when ahead are both presumed to be specific to the goal to which the affect is linked. Usually (though not always) this is the goal from which the affect arises in the first place. We should also be clear about time frames. This view pertains to the current, ongoing episode. This is *not* an argument that positive affect makes people less likely to do the behavior again later on.

A system of this sort would operate in the same way as a car's cruise control. If progress is too slow, negative affect arises. The person responds by increasing effort, trying to speed up. If progress is better than needed, positive affect arises, leading to coasting. A car's cruise control is similar. A hill slows you down; the cruise control feeds the engine more fuel, speeding back up. If you come across the crest of a hill and roll downward too fast, the system cuts back on fuel and the speed drags back down.

The analogy is intriguing partly because both sides are asymmetrical in the consequences of deviation from the criterion. In both cases, addressing the problem of going too slow requires adding resources. Addressing the problem of going too fast entails only cutting back. The cruise control does not apply the brakes, but only reduces fuel. The car coasts back to the velocity set point. The effect of the cruise control on a high rate of speed thus depends partly on external circumstances. If the hill is steep, the car may exceed the cruise control's set point all the way to the valley below. In the same fashion, people usually do not respond to positive affect by trying to dampen the feeling. They only ease back a little on resources devoted to the domain in which the affect has arisen. The feelings may be sustained for a long time (depending on circumstances) as the person coasts down the subjective hill. Eventually, though, the reduced resources would cause the positive affect to fade. Generally, then, the system would act to prevent great amounts of pleasure, as well as great amounts of pain (Carver, 2003; Carver & Scheier, 1998).

Does positive affect (or making greater than expected progress) lead to coasting? To test this idea, a study must assess coasting with respect to the goal underlying the affect (or the unexpectedly high progress). Many studies have created positive affect in one context and assessed its influence elsewhere (e.g., Isen, 1987, 2000; Schwarz & Bohner, 1996), but that does not test this question.

A few studies have satisfied these criteria. Mizruchi (1991) found that professional basketball teams in playoffs tend to lose after winning. It is unclear, however, whether the prior winner slacked off, the loser tried harder, or both. Louro, Pieters, and Zeelenberg (2007) explicitly examined the role of positive feelings from surging ahead in the context of multiple-goal pursuit. In three studies they found that when people were relatively close to a goal, positive feelings prompted decrease in effort toward that goal and a shift of effort to an alternate goal. They also found a boundary on this effect (it occurred only when people were relatively close to their goal). Another, more recent study using an intensive experience sampling procedure across a 2-week period similarly found that greater than expected progress toward a goal was followed by reduction in effort toward that goal (Fulford, Johnson, Llabre, & Carver, in press).

Coasting and Multiple Concerns

The idea that positive affect leads to coasting, which would eventually result in reduction of the positive affect, strikes some people as unlikely. On the surface it is hard to see why a process could possibly be built in that limits positive feelings—indeed, that reduces them. After all, a truism of life is that people supposedly are organized to seek pleasure and avoid pain.

There are at least two potential bases for this tendency. One is that it is adaptive for organisms not to spend energy needlessly. Coasting prevents that. A second stems from the fact that people have multiple simultaneous concerns (Atkinson & Birch, 1970; Carver, 2003; Carver & Scheier, 1998; Frijda, 1994). Given multiple concerns, people do not optimize performance on any one of them but rather *satisfice* (Simon, 1953)—do a good-enough job to deal with each concern satisfactorily. This permits handling of many concerns adequately, rather than just one (see also Fitzsimons, Friesen, Orehek, & Kruglanski, 2009).

A tendency to coast would virtually define satisficing regarding that particular goal; that is, reducing effort would prevent attainment of the best possible outcome. A tendency to coast would also promote satisficing regarding a broader array of goals; that is, if progress toward goal attainment in one domain exceeds current needs, then a tendency to coast in that particular domain (*satisficing*) would make it easy to devote energy to another domain. This would help to ensure satisfactory goal attainment in the other domain and, ultimately, across multiple domains.

PRIORITY MANAGEMENT AS A CORE ISSUE IN SELF-REGULATION

The line of argument just outlined begins to implicate positive feelings in a broad function within the organism that deserves much further consideration. This function is the shifting from one goal to another as focal in behavior (Dreisbach & Goschke, 2004; Shallice, 1978; Shin & Rosenbaum, 2002). This basic and very important function is often overlooked. Let's consider it more closely. Humans usually pursue many goals simultaneously, but only one can have top priority at a given moment. People manage their many goals by shifting among them. This means there are changes over time in which goal has the top priority. How are those changes managed?

One view of priority management among goals was proposed many years ago by Simon (1967). He noted that although goals with less than top priority are largely out of awareness, ongoing events still can be relevant to them. Sometimes events that occur during the pursuit of the top-priority goal create problems for a goal with a lower priority. Indeed, the mere passing of time can sometimes create a problem for the second goal because passing of time may make its attainment less likely. If the second goal is also important, an emerging problem for its attainment needs to be taken into account. If there arises a serious threat to the second goal, a mechanism is needed for changing priorities, so that the second goal replaces the first one as focal.

Feelings and Reprioritization

Simon (1967) reasoned that emotions are calls for reprioritization. He suggested that emotion arising with respect to a goal that is outside awareness eventually induces people to interrupt what they are doing and give that goal a higher priority than it had. The stronger the emotion, the stronger is the claim being made that the unattended goal should have higher priority than the current focal goal. Simon did not address negative affect that arises with respect to a currently focal goal, but the same principle seems to apply. In that case, negative affect seems to be a call for an even greater investment of resources and effort in that focal goal than is now being made.

Simon's analysis applies easily to negative feelings, cases in which a nonfocal goal demands a higher priority and *intrudes* on awareness. However, there is another way in which priority ordering can shift: The currently focal goal can *relinquish its place*. Simon acknowledged this possibility obliquely, noting that goal completion terminates pursuit of that goal. However, he did not address the possibility that an as-yet-unattained goal might also yield its place in line.

Carver (2003) expanded on that possibility, suggesting that positive feelings are a cue to *reduce* the priority of the goal to which the feeling pertains. This possibility appears consistent with the sense of Simon's analysis, but suggests that the prioritizing function of affect pertains to affects of both valences. Positive affect regarding an avoidance act (relief or tranquility) indicates that a threat has dissipated, no longer requires as much attention as it did, and can now assume a lower priority. Positive affect regarding approach (happiness, joy) indicates that an incentive is being attained. Even if it is not yet attained, the affect is a signal that you could temporarily put this goal aside because you are doing so well.

If a focal goal diminishes in priority, what follows? In principle, this situation is less directive than when a nonfocal goal demands higher priority. What happens next in this case depends partly on what else is waiting in line and whether the context has changed in important ways while you were busy with the focal goal. Opportunities to attain incentives sometimes appear unexpectedly, and people put aside their plans to take advantage of such unanticipated opportunities (Hayes-Roth & Hayes-Roth, 1979; Payton, 1990). It seems reasonable that people experiencing positive affect should be most prone to shift goals at this point if something else needs fixing or doing (regarding a next-in-line goal or a newly emergent goal), or if an unanticipated opportunity for gain has appeared.

On the other hand, sometimes neither of these conditions exists. In such a case, no change in goal would occur because the downgrade in priority of the now-focal goal does not render it lower in priority than the alternatives. Thus, positive feeling does not *require* that there be a change in direction. It simply sets the stage for such a change to be more likely.

Apart from evidence of coasting per se, there is also evidence consistent with the idea that positive affect tends to promote shifting of focus to other things that need attention (for broader discussion, see Carver, 2003). As an example, Trope and Neter (1994) induced a positive mood in some people but not others, gave them all a social sensitivity test, then told them that they had performed well on two parts of the test but poorly on a third. Subjects then indicated their interest in reading more about their performances on the various parts of the test. Positive mood participants showed more interest in the part they had failed than did controls, suggesting that they were inclined to shift focus to an area that needed their attention. This effect has been conceptually replicated by Trope and Pomerantz (1998) and Reed and Aspinwall (1998).

Phenomena such as these have contributed to the emergence of the view that positive feelings represent psychological resources (see also Aspinwall, 1998; Fredrickson, 1998; Isen, 2000; Tesser, Crepaz, Collins, Cornell, & Beach, 2000). The idea that positive affect serves as a resource for exploration resembles the idea that positive feelings open people up to noticing and turning to emergent opportunities, to being distracted into enticing alternatives—to opportunistic behavior. Some evidence also fits this idea (Kahn & Isen, 1993).

Priority Management and Depressed Affect

One more aspect of priority management should be addressed here concerning the idea that, in some circumstances, goals are not attainable and are better abandoned. Sufficient doubt about goal attainment results in an impetus to disengage from efforts to reach the goal, and even to abandon the goal itself (Carver & Scheier, 1998, 1999a, 1999b). Abandonment is clearly a decrease in priority for that goal. How does this sort of reprioritization fit into the picture sketched earlier?

At first glance, this seems to contradict Simon's (1967) position that negative affect is a call for higher priority. However, there is an important distinction between two approach-related negative affects, which elaborates on Simon's thinking. Some negative affects pertaining to approach coalesce around frustration and anger. Others coalesce around sadness, depression, and dejection. The former demand increase in priority, the latter promote decrease in priority.

As noted earlier, our view on affect rests on a dimension from doing well to doing poorly, but the affects themselves do not simply flow in a continuum (Figure 1.1). In theory, inadequate movement forward (or no movement, or loss of ground) gives rise at first to frustration, irritation, and anger. These feelings (or the mechanism that underlies them) engage effort more completely, to overcome obstacles and enhance current progress. This case fits the priority management model of Simon (1967).

Sometimes, however, continued efforts do not produce adequate movement forward. Indeed, if the situation involves loss, movement forward is precluded because the incentive is gone. When failure seems (or is) assured, the feelings are sadness, depression, despondency, grief, and hopelessness (cf. Finlay-Jones & Brown, 1981). Behaviorally, the person tends to disengage from—give up on—further effort toward the incentive (Klinger, 1975; Lewis, Sullivan, Ramsay, & Allessandri, 1992; Mikulincer, 1988; Wortman & Brehm, 1975).

As noted, negative feelings in these two kinds of situations parallel two divergent effects on action. Both effects have adaptive properties. In the first situation, when the person falls behind but the goal is not seen as lost, feelings of frustration and anger accompany increase in effort, a struggle to gain the incentive despite setbacks (Figure 1.1). This struggle is adaptive (thus, the affect is adaptive) because the struggle fosters goal attainment.

In the second situation, when effort appears futile, feelings of sadness and depression accompany *reduction* of effort (Figure 1.1). Sadness and despondency imply that things cannot be set right, that effort is pointless. Reducing effort in this circumstance

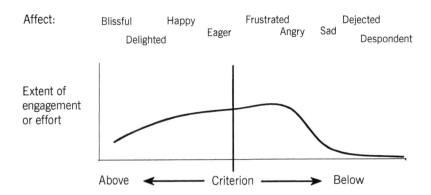

FIGURE 1.1. Hypothesized approach-related affects as a function of doing well versus doing poorly compared to a criterion velocity. A second (vertical) dimension indicates the degree of behavioral engagement posited to be associated with affects at different degrees of departure from neutral. From Carver (2004). Copyright 2004 by the American Psychological Association. Adapted by permission.

can also be adaptive (Carver & Scheier, 2003; Wrosch, Scheier, Carver, & Schulz, 2003; Wrosch, Scheier, Miller, Schulz, & Carver, 2003). It conserves energy rather than waste it in pursuit of the unattainable (Nesse, 2000). If reducing effort also helps to diminish commitment to the goal (Klinger, 1975), then it eventually readies the person to take up other incentives in place of this one.

TWO-MODE MODELS OF FUNCTIONING

One more topic that we would like to mention briefly is the idea that human behavior reflects two modes of functioning, an idea that has acquired a good deal of popularity over the past decade or so. Epstein (1985, 1990, 1994) has advocated this view for quite a long time. What he called the *rational* system operates mostly consciously, uses logical rules, is verbal and deliberative, and thus is fairly slow. What he called the *experiential* system is intuitive and associative. It relies on salient information and uses shortcuts and heuristics. It functions automatically, nonverbally, and quickly, even impulsively. Both systems are always at work. What behavior occurs depends on which system is presently dominant, which can be influenced by both situational constraints and individual differences.

A great many others have since made arguments that resemble these in broad strokes (see Carver, 2005; Carver, Johnson, & Joormann, 2008; Hofmann, Friese, & Strack, 2009). Perhaps most widely noted in social psychology is that of Strack and Deutsch (2004). What they called a *reflective* system anticipates future conditions, makes decisions from those anticipations, and forms intentions. It is planful and wide-ranging in its search for information. What they called an *impulsive* system acts spontaneously when its schemas or production systems are sufficiently activated, without consideration for broader consequences of the action.

Dual-process thinking has also been influential in developmental psychology. Rothbart and others (e.g., Rothbart, Ahadi, & Evans, 2000; Rothbart, Ellis, Rueda, & Posner, 2003; see also Kochanska & Knaack, 2003; Nigg, 2000) propose three temperament systems: *approach, avoidance*, and *effortful control*. Effortful control is superordinate to approach and avoidance temperaments (e.g., Ahadi & Rothbart, 1994). It concerns attentional management and *inhibitory control* (the ability to suppress an approach behavior when it is situationally inappropriate). The label *effortful* conveys the sense that this is an executive, planful activity, resembling depictions of the deliberative mode of the models just outlined.

Another Look at Hierarchical Organization

Various theorists' depictions of the characteristics of these two modes of functioning have some resemblance to depictions made earlier in the chapter between two levels of abstraction in action control. Specifically, the deliberative mode of functioning has some similarity to what was earlier described as *program control*, and the impulsive mode of functioning has some similarity to what was earlier described as *sequence control*.

We said earlier that programs require decisions and reflect intentions. They seem to be managed top-down, using effortful processing. Planfulness, characteristic of programs, is also characteristic of behavior managed by a deliberative system. In contrast, sequences occur in a relatively automatic stream once triggered, and they may be triggered simply by associations in memory. This resembles the more basic mode of functioning in the dual-process view.

Also of interest is evidence that different brain areas manage effortful and automatic versions of the same behavior (Casey, Tottenham, & Fossella, 2002; Lieberman, Gaunt, Gilbert, & Trope, 2002; Posner & DiGirolamo, 2000). This in itself hints that there may be an important boundary between action control that is deliberative versus action sequences that are organized enough to be spontaneous once cued. Other evidence also supports the idea that intention-based and stimulus-based actions involve different process of action initiation (Keller et al., 2006).

In previous discussions (e.g., Carver & Scheier, 1998, 1999a) we frequently noted that what level of control is functionally superordinate can vary with the situation (and across persons); that is, a person can presently be behaving according to a principle (e.g., a moral or ethical value) and the same person may be behaving according to a more concrete program. One can also imagine cases, though, in which the person is behaving impulsively and spontaneously, without regard to either principle or plan. In the past, we noted this point and how different the behaviors are. Now we find ourselves wondering whether this division maps onto the two modes of processing that have been postulated by others.

Self-Control: Impulse and Constraint

Finally, we come to self-control per se. The idea that both spontaneous and planful goals can come into conflict with each other is also part of the literature on self-control and self-control failure (Baumeister & Heatherton, 1996; Baumeister, Heatherton, & Tice, 1994). This literature focuses on cases in which a person is both motivated to act in some particular way and also motivated to restrain that action.

Literature on self-control failure tends to portray these cases as involving a relatively automatic tendency to act in one way, opposed by a planful and effortful tendency to restrain that act. The action that is being inhibited is often characterized as an *impulse*, a desire that will automatically be translated into action unless it is controlled (perhaps in part because this action is habitual, perhaps in part because it is more primal). The restraint is typically presumed to be effortful and to depend on limited resources. If the planful part of the mind is able to attend to the conflict, the person may be able to resist the impulse. If not, the impulse is more likely to be expressed.

This portrayal seems consonant with two-mode models of functioning (Hofmann et al., 2009). This raises an interesting question. Do all cases of self-control map onto the two-mode view? If we understand better what makes the two modes of functioning distinct from each other, will we have gained an important key to understanding self-control and self-control failure? This seems a particularly interesting question for further exploration. We look forward to seeing what these explorations reveal in the years to come.

ACKNOWLEDGMENT

Preparation of this chapter was facilitated by support from the National Cancer Institute (Grant No. CA64710) and the National Science Foundation (Grant No. BCS0544617).

REFERENCES

Ahadi, S. A., & Rothbart, M. K. (1994). Temperament, development and the Big Five. In C. F. Halverson, Jr., G. A. Kohnstamm, & R. P. Martin (Eds.), *The developing structure of temperament and personality from infancy to adulthood* (pp. 189–207). Hillsdale, NJ: Erlbaum.

Asch, S. E. (1955). Opinions and social pressure. *Scientific American, 193*, 31–35.

Aspinwall, L. G. (1998). Rethinking the role of positive affect in self-regulation. *Motivation and Emotion, 22*, 1–32.

Atkinson, J. W., & Birch, D. (1970). *The dynamics of action.* New York: Wiley.

Austin, J. T., & Vancouver, J. B. (1996). Goal constructs in psychology: Structure, process, and content. *Psychological Bulletin, 120*, 338–375.

Baumeister, R. F., & Heatherton, T. F. (1996). Self-regulation failure: An overview. *Psychological Inquiry, 7*, 1–15.

Baumeister, R. F., Heatherton, T. F., & Tice, D. M. (1994). *Losing control: Why people fail at self-regulation.* San Diego, CA: Academic Press.

Baumeister, R. F., Vohs, K. D., DeWall, C. N., & Zhang, L. (2007). How emotion shapes behavior: Feedback, anticipation, and reflection, rather than direct causation. *Personality and Social Psychology Review, 11*, 167–203.

Beer, R. D. (1995). A dynamical systems perspective on agent–environment interaction. *Artificial Intelligence, 72*, 173–215.

Cacioppo, J. T., & Berntson, G. G. (1994). Relationship between attitudes and evaluative space: A critical review, with emphasis on the separability of positive and negative substrates. *Psychological Bulletin, 115*, 401–423.

Cacioppo, J. T., Gardner, W. L., & Berntson, G. G. (1999). The affect system has parallel and integrative processing components: Form follows function. *Journal of Personality and Social Psychology, 76*, 839–855.

Cannon, W. B. (1932). *The wisdom of the body.* New York: Norton.

Carver, C. S. (2003). Pleasure as a sign you can attend to something else: Placing positive feelings within a general model of affect. *Cognition and Emotion, 17*, 241–261.

Carver, C. S. (2004). Negative affects deriving from the behavioral approach system. *Emotion, 4*, 3–22.

Carver, C. S. (2005). Impulse and constraint: Perspectives from personality psychology, convergence with theory in other areas, and potential for integration. *Personality and Social Psychology Review, 9*, 312–333.

Carver, C. S. (2009). Threat sensitivity, incentive sensitivity, and the experience of relief. *Journal of Personality, 77*, 125–138.

Carver, C. S., & Harmon-Jones, E. (2009a). Anger and approach: Reply to Watson (2009) and Tomarken and Zald (2009). *Psychological Bulletin, 135*, 215–217.

Carver, C. S., & Harmon-Jones, E. (2009b). Anger is an approach-related affect: Evidence and implications. *Psychological Bulletin, 135*, 183–204.

Carver, C. S., Johnson, S. L., & Joormann, J. (2008). Serotonergic function, two-mode models of self-regulation, and vulnerability to depression: What depression has in common with impulsive aggression. *Psychological Bulletin, 134*, 912–943.

Carver, C. S., & Scheier, M. F. (1981). *Attention and self-regulation: A control-theory approach to human behavior.* New York: Springer-Verlag.

Carver, C. S., & Scheier, M. F. (1990). Origins and functions of positive and negative affect: A control-process view. *Psychological Review, 97*, 19–35.

Carver, C. S., & Scheier, M. F. (1998). *On the self-regulation of behavior.* New York: Cambridge University Press.

Carver, C. S., & Scheier, M. F. (1999a). Several more themes, a lot more issues: Commentary on the commentaries. In R. S. Wyer, Jr. (Ed.), *Advances in social cognition* (Vol. 12, pp. 261–302). Mahwah, NJ: Erlbaum.

Carver, C. S., & Scheier, M. F. (1999b). Themes and issues in the self-regulation of behavior. In R. S. Wyer, Jr. (Ed.), *Advances in social cognition* (Vol. 12, pp. 1–105). Mahwah, NJ: Erlbaum.

Carver, C. S., & Scheier, M. F. (2000). Scaling back goals and recalibration of the affect system are processes in normal adaptive self-regulation: Understanding "response shift" phenomena. *Social Science and Medicine, 50,* 1715–1722.

Carver, C. S., & Scheier, M. F. (2003). Three human strengths. In L. G. Aspinwall & U. M. Staudinger (Eds.), *A psychology of human strengths: Fundamental questions and future directions for a positive psychology* (pp. 87–102). Washington, DC: American Psychological Association.

Casey, B. J., Tottenham, N., & Fossella, J. (2002). Clinical, imaging, lesion and genetic approaches toward a model of cognitive control. *Developmental Psychobiology, 40,* 237–254.

Clark, R. N. (1996). *Control system dynamics.* New York: Cambridge University Press.

Clore, G. C. (1994). Why emotions are felt. In P. Ekman & R. J. Davidson (Eds.), *The nature of emotion: Fundamental questions* (pp. 103–111). New York: Oxford University Press.

Davidson, R. J. (1992). Anterior cerebral asymmetry and the nature of emotion. *Brain and Cognition, 20,* 125–151.

Dreisbach, G., & Goschke, T. (2004). How positive affect modulates cognitive control: Reduced perseveration at the cost of increased distractibility. *Journal of Experimental Psychology: Learning, Memory, and Cognition, 30,* 343–353.

Eidelman, S., & Biernat, M. (2007). Getting more from success: Standard raising as esteem maintenance. *Journal of Personality and Social Psychology, 92,* 759–774.

Elliot, A. J. (Ed.). (2008). *Handbook of approach and avoidance motivation.* Mahwah, NJ: Erlbaum.

Epstein, S. (1985). The implications of cognitive–experiential self theory for research in social psychology and personality. *Journal for the Theory of Social Behavior, 15,* 283–310.

Epstein, S. (1990). Cognitive–experiential self theory. In L. Pervin (Ed.), *Handbook of personality: Theory and research* (pp. 165–192). New York: Guilford Press.

Epstein, S. (1994). Integration of the cognitive and the psychodynamic unconscious. *American Psychologist, 49,* 709–724.

Festinger, L. (1957). *A theory of cognitive dissonance.* Evanston, IL: Row, Peterson.

Finlay-Jones, R., & Brown, G. W. (1981). Types of stressful life event and the onset of anxiety and depressive disorders. *Psychological Medicine, 11,* 803–815.

Fitzsimons, G. M., Friesen, J., Orehek, E., & Kruglanski, A. W. (2009). Progress-induced goal shifting as a self-regulatory strategy. In J. P. Forgas, R. F. Baumeister, & D. Tice (Eds.), *The psychology of self-regulation* (pp. 109–126). New York: Psychology Press.

Ford, D. H. (1987). *Humans as self-constructing living systems: A developmental perspective on behavior and personality.* Hillsdale, NJ: Erlbaum.

Fredrickson, B. L. (1998). What good are positive emotions? *Review of General Psychology, 2,* 300–319.

Frijda, N. H. (1986). *The emotions.* Cambridge, UK: Cambridge University Press.

Frijda, N. H. (1988). The laws of emotion. *American Psychologist, 43,* 349–358.

Frijda, N. H. (1994). Emotions are functional, most of the time. In P. Ekman & R. J. Davidson (Eds.), *The nature of emotion: Fundamental questions* (pp. 112–126). New York: Oxford University Press.

Fulford, D., Johnson, J. L., Llabre, M. M., & Carver, C. S. (in press). Pushing and coasting in dynamic goal pursuit: Coasting is attenuated in bipolar disorder. *Psychological Science.*

Gray, J. A. (1990). Brain systems that mediate both emotion and cognition. *Cognition and Emotion, 4,* 269–288.

Gray, J. A. (1994). Three fundamental emotion systems. In P. Ekman & R. J. Davidson (Eds.), *The nature of emotion: Fundamental questions* (pp. 243–247). New York: Oxford University Press.

Gross, J. J. (Ed.). (2007). *Handbook of emotion regulation.* New York: Guilford Press.

Harmon-Jones, E., & Sigelman, J. D. (2001). State anger and prefrontal brain activity: Evidence that insult-related relative left-prefrontal activation is associated with experienced anger and aggression. *Journal of Personality and Social Psychology, 80,* 797–803.

Hayes-Roth, B., & Hayes-Roth, F. (1979). A cognitive model of planning. *Cognitive Science, 3,* 275–310.

Heider, F. (1946). Attitudes and cognitive organization. *Journal of Psychology, 21,* 107–112.

Higgins, E. T. (1987). Self-discrepancy: A theory relating self and affect. *Psychological Review, 94,* 319–340.

Higgins, E. T. (1996). Ideals, oughts, and regulatory focus: Affect and motivation from distinct pains and pleasures. In P. M. Gollwitzer & J. A. Bargh (Eds.), *The psychology of action: Linking cognition and motivation to behavior* (pp. 91–114). New York: Guilford Press.

Higgins, E. T., Shah, J., & Friedman, R. (1997). Emotional responses to goal attainment: Strength of regulatory focus as moderator. *Journal of Personality and Social Psychology, 72,* 515–525.

Hofmann, W., Friese, M., & Strack, F. (2009). Impulse and self-control from a dual-systems perspective. *Perspectives on Psychological Science, 4,* 162–176.

Isen, A. M. (1987). Positive affect, cognitive processes, and social behavior. In L. Berkowitz (Ed.), *Advances in experimental social psychology* (Vol. 20, pp. 203–252). San Diego, CA: Academic Press.

Isen, A. M. (2000). Positive affect and decision making. In M. Lewis & J. M. Haviland-Jones (Eds.), *Handbook of emotions* (2nd ed., pp. 417–435). New York: Guilford Press.

Izard, C. E. (1977). *Human emotions.* New York: Plenum Press.

Kahn, B. E., & Isen, A. M. (1993). The influence of positive affect on variety-seeking among safe, enjoyable products. *Journal of Consumer Research, 20,* 257–270.

Keller, P. E., Wascher, E., Prinz, W., Waszak, F., Koch, I., & Rosenbaum, D. A. (2006). Differences between intention-based and stimulus-based actions. *Journal of Psychophysiology, 20,* 9–20.

Klinger, E. (1975). Consequences of commitment to and disengagement from incentives. *Psychological Review, 82,* 1–25.

Kochanska, G., & Knaack, A. (2003). Effortful control as a personality characteristic of young children: Antecedents, correlates, and consequences. *Journal of Personality, 71,* 1087–1112.

Lang, P. J. (1995). The emotion probe: Studies of motivation and attention. *American Psychologist, 50,* 372–385.

Lang, P. J., Bradley, M. M., & Cuthbert, B. N. (1990). Emotion, attention, and the startle reflex. *Psychological Review, 97,* 377–395.

Lecky, P. (1945). *Self-consistency: A theory of personality.* New York: Island Press.

Lewis, M., Sullivan, M. W., Ramsay, D. S., & Allessandri, S. M. (1992). Individual differences in anger and sad expressions during extinction: Antecedents and consequences. *Infant Behavior and Development, 15,* 443–452.

Lieberman, M. D., Gaunt, R., Gilbert, D. T., & Trope, Y. (2002). Reflection and reflexion: A social cognitive neuroscience approach to attributional inference. In M. Zanna (Ed.), *Advances in experimental social psychology* (Vol. 34, pp. 199–249). San Diego, CA: Academic Press.

Louro, M. J., Pieters, R., & Zeelenberg, M. (2007). Dynamics of multiple-goal pursuit. *Journal of Personality and Social Psychology, 93,* 174–193.

MacKay, D. M. (1966). Cerebral organization and the conscious control of action. In J. C. Eccles (Ed.), *Brain and conscious experience* (pp. 422–445). Berlin: Springer-Verlag.

Mikulincer, M. (1988). Reactance and helplessness following exposure to learned helplessness following exposure to unsolvable problems: The effects of attributional style. *Journal of Personality and Social Psychology, 54*, 679–686.

Miller, G. A., Galanter, E., & Pribram, K. H. (1960). *Plans and the structure of behavior.* New York: Holt, Rinehart & Winston.

Mischel, W., & Shoda, Y. (1995). A cognitive-affective system theory of personality: Reconceptualizing the invariances in personality and the role of situations. *Psychological Review, 102*, 246–268.

Mizruchi, M. S. (1991). Urgency, motivation, and group performance: The effect of prior success on current success among professional basketball teams. *Social Psychology Quarterly, 54*, 181–189.

Nesse, R. M. (2000). Is depression an adaptation? *Archives of General Psychiatry, 57*, 14–20.

Nigg, J. T. (2000). On inhibition/disinhibition in developmental psychopathology: Views from cognitive and personality psychology as a working inhibition taxonomy. *Psychological Bulletin, 126*, 220–246.

Ortony, A., Clore, G. L., & Collins, A. (1988). *The cognitive structure of emotions.* New York: Cambridge University Press.

Payton, D. W. (1990). Internalized plans: A representation for action resources. In P. Maes (Ed.), *Designing autonomous agents: Theory and practice from biology to engineering and back* (pp. 89–103). Cambridge, MA: MIT Press.

Posner, M. I., & DiGirolamo, G. J. (2000). Cognitive neuroscience: Origins and promise. *Psychological Bulletin, 126*, 873–889.

Powers, W. T. (1973). *Behavior: The control of perception.* Chicago: Aldine.

Reed, M. B., & Aspinwall, L. G. (1998). Self-affirmation reduces biased processing of health-risk information. *Motivation and Emotion, 22*, 99–132.

Rolls, E. T. (1999). *The brain and emotion.* Oxford, UK: Oxford University Press.

Rolls, E. T. (2005). *Emotion explained.* Oxford, UK: Oxford University Press.

Rosenbaum, D. A., Carlson, R. A., & Gilmore, R. O. (2001). Acquisition of intellectual and perceptual–motor skills. *Annual Review of Psychology, 52*, 453–470.

Rosenbaum, D. A., Meulenbroek, R. G. J., Vaughan, J., & Jansen, C. (2001). Posture-based motion planning: Applications to grasping. *Psychological Review, 108*, 709–734.

Rothbart, M. K., Ahadi, S. A., & Evans, D. E. (2000). Temperament and personality: Origins and outcomes. *Journal of Personality and Social Psychology, 78*, 122–135.

Rothbart, M. K., Ellis, L. K., Rueda M. R., & Posner, M. I. (2003). Developing mechanisms of temperamental effortful control. *Journal of Personality, 71*, 1113–1143.

Schwartz, S. H., & Bilsky, W. (1990). Toward a theory of the universal content and structure of values: Extensions and cross-cultural replications. *Journal of Personality and Social Psychology, 58*, 878–891.

Schwartz, S. H., & Rubel, T. (2005). Sex differences in value priorities: Cross-cultural and multimethod studies. *Journal of Personality and Social Psychology, 89*, 1010–1028.

Schwarz, N., & Bohner, G. (1996). Feelings and their motivational implications: Moods and the action sequence. In P. M. Gollwitzer & J. A. Bargh (Eds.), *The psychology of action: Linking cognition and motivation to behavior* (pp. 119–145). New York: Guilford Press.

Shallice, T. (1978). The dominant action system: An information-processing approach to consciousness. In K. S. Pope & J. L. Singer (Eds.), *The stream of consciousness: Scientific investigations into the flow of human experience* (pp. 117–157). New York: Wiley.

Shin, J. C., & Rosenbaum, D. A. (2002). Reaching while calculating: Scheduling of cognitive and perceptual–motor processes. *Journal of Experimental Psychology: General, 131*, 206–219.

Simon, H. A. (1953). *Models of man.* New York: Wiley.

Simon, H. A. (1967). Motivational and emotional controls of cognition. *Psychology Review, 74*, 29–39.

Strack, F., & Deutsch, R. (2004). Reflective and impulsive determinants of social behavior. *Personality and Social Psychology Review, 8*, 220–247.

Tesser, A., Crepaz, N., Collins, J. C., Cornell, D., & Beach, S. R. H. (2000). Confluence of self-esteem regulation mechanisms: On integrating the self-zoo. *Personality and Social Psychology Bulletin, 26*, 1476–1489.

Trope, Y., & Neter, E. (1994). Reconciling competing motives in self-evaluation: The role of self-control in feedback seeking. *Journal of Personality and Social Psychology, 66*, 646–657.

Trope, Y., & Pomerantz, E. M. (1998). Resolving conflicts among self-evaluative motives: Positive experiences as a resource for overcoming defensiveness. *Motivation and Emotion, 22*, 53–72.

Vallacher, R. R., & Wegner, D. M. (1987). What do people think they're doing?: Action identification and human behavior. *Psychological Review, 94*, 3–15.

von Bertalanffy, L. (1968). *General systems theory.* New York: Braziller.

Watson, D. (2009). Locating anger in the hierarchical structure of affect: Comment on Carver and Harmon-Jones (2009). *Psychological Bulletin, 135*, 205–208.

Watson, D., Wiese, D., Vaidya, J., & Tellegen, A. (1999). The two general activation systems of affect: Structural findings, evolutionary considerations, and psychobiological evidence. *Journal of Personality and Social Psychology, 76*, 820–838.

Wiener, N. (1948). *Cybernetics: Control and communication in the animal and the machine.* Cambridge, MA: MIT Press.

Wortman, C. B., & Brehm, J. W. (1975). Responses to uncontrollable outcomes: An integration of reactance theory and the learned helplessness model. In L. Berkowitz (Ed.), *Advances in experimental social psychology* (Vol. 8, pp. 277–336). New York: Academic Press.

Wrosch, C., Scheier, M. F., Carver, C. S., & Schulz, R. (2003). The importance of goal disengagement in adaptive self-regulation: When giving up is beneficial. *Self and Identity, 2*, 1–20.

Wrosch, C., Scheier, M. F., Miller, G. E., Schulz, R., & Carver, C. S. (2003). Adaptive self-regulation of unattainable goals: Goal disengagement, goal re-engagement, and subjective well-being. *Personality and Social Psychology Bulletin, 29*, 1494–1508.

CHAPTER 2

The Self-Regulation of Emotion

SANDER L. KOOLE
LOTTE F. VAN DILLEN
GAL SHEPPES

A teenager goes off on an eating binge whenever she feels lonely or depressed. A bank manager runs for hours each morning to take his mind off his impending divorce. A politician is struggling to hide her joy over a rival's downfall during a press conference. A CEO practices yoga to handle the stress of her demanding work life. A student works through a childhood trauma by keeping a diary on his innermost feelings.

In these and in many other situations in everyday life, people are at once engaged in the self-regulation of action (briefly, *self-regulation*) and the self-regulation of emotion (briefly, *emotion regulation*). Self-regulation and emotion regulation are often so intertwined that it is hard to say where one ends and the other begins. Over the past few decades, both types of regulation have become the focus of considerable theoretical and empirical research (for reviews, see Baumeister, Schmeichel, & Vohs, 2007; Koole, 2009; for comprehensive overviews, see Gross, 2007; this volume). Nevertheless, the interface between self-regulation and emotion regulation has only recently received systematic attention. Learning how self-regulation interfaces with emotion regulation is likely to generate important new insights into both processes. Among other things, self-regulation research may illuminate how people function as active agents in managing their emotional lives. Conversely, emotion regulation research may illuminate how people direct their actions in emotion-arousing contexts.

In this chapter, we contribute to the ongoing integration between self-regulation and emotion regulation research by reviewing contemporary research on the self-regulation of emotion. Our plan in this chapter is fourfold. First, we consider the *emotion* part of emotion regulation by discussing the kinds of responses that people may target in the emotion regulation process. Second, we turn to the *regulation* part of emotion regulation by discussing the control processes that may underlie emotion regulation. Here, we review models that emphasize effortful control processes (Erber & Erber, 2000; Ochsner & Gross, 2008; McRae, Ochsner, & Gross, Chapter 10, this volume), as well as models that touch upon more intuitive aspects of emotion regulation (Koole, 2009). Third, we consider the emerging literature on training self- and emotion-regulatory skills and how it may be informed by recent models of emotion regulation. Finally, we provide a summary of our main conclusions regarding the self-regulation of emotion.

THE "EMOTION" IN EMOTION REGULATION

In emotion regulation, people seek to redirect the spontaneous flow of their emotions. Emotions are understood here as people's valenced (positive or negative) reactions to events that they perceive as relevant to their ongoing concerns. Emotions in the present conception consist of multiple components that include specific thoughts and feelings, along with behavioral and physiological responses (Cacioppo, Berntson, & Klein, 1992; Frijda, 2006; Mauss, Levenson, McCarter, Wilhelm, & Gross, 2005). Inevitably, there is overlap between emotion regulation and related constructs such as mood regulation, coping with stress, and affect regulation. Our definition of *emotion regulation* is therefore broad and inclusive, and subsumes the regulation of specific emotions such as anger or fear, along with global mood states, stress, and all kinds of affective responses.

Virtually any stimulus or activity that can cause changes in people's emotional states may be recruited in emotion regulation. Thus, people can draw from a very large pool of different strategies in managing their emotional lives. Yet underneath this diversity, some broad patterns can be discerned in the kinds of emotion responses targeted in emotion regulation. Some researchers have sought to uncover these broad patterns through data-driven methods such as factor analysis (Thayer, Newman, & McClain, 1994) or rational sorting (Parkinson & Totterdell, 1999). These approaches have generally failed to produce a replicable and readily interpretable set of dimensions, and have been plagued by difficulties in ensuring the comprehensiveness of the investigated set of emotion regulation strategies (Skinner, Edge, Altman, & Sherwood, 2003). Consequently, it seems more productive to begin by developing a coherent theoretical logic for analyzing the basic processes that underlie various kinds of emotion regulatory activities.

What's Special about Emotion Regulation?

A first way to understand which types of emotion processes are targeted in emotion regulation is to ask whether there is something special about emotion regulation relative to other types of emotion processing. As noted by the late emotion theorist Larazus (1991), who made some insightful observations with regard to this issue, people's primary emotional response to a situation can be qualitatively different from their secondary emotional response. The *primary* emotional response relates to people's immediate, raw response to emotion-relevant events. The *secondary* response relates to people's ability to cope with their primary emotional response (Baumann, Kaschel, & Kuhl, 2007). Lazarus's observations thus help to delineate how emotion regulation differs from other emotion processes. People's primary emotional response represents their immediate, unregulated emotional response. This primary response is succeeded by a secondary emotional response, which is driven by emotion regulation. The transition from primary to secondary emotional responding may occur so fast that people hardly notice it. As such, it can be challenging empirically to separate people's primary emotional response from their subsequent emotion regulation processes.

At a conceptual level, however, the distinction between primary emotion generation and subsequent emotion regulation is straightforward. To illustrate this distinction, Figure 2.1 displays how a prototypical emotional response unfolds in time. To keep things simple, we focus on a single emotional response with a single maximum strength. People's primary emotional response is represented by the entry gradient, or steepness, with which the emotional response reaches its full force. This primary response can be thought of as emotional sensitivity, or the ease with which people get into a specific emotional state. Emotional sensitivity is determined by any variable that influences people's initial emotional response to the situation, including qualities of the stimuli that people encounter (e.g., highly arousing stimuli are likely to trigger emotions more rapidly than mildly arousing stimuli), person characteristics (e.g., highly neurotic individuals may enter negative states more quickly than less neurotic individuals), and the broader situation (e.g., during an economic crisis, threatening thoughts may spring to mind more easily).

The offset of the emotional response is depicted in Figure 2.1 as the exit gradient, or steepness with which the emotional response returns to a neutral baseline. This return to baseline may occur without any conscious regulatory effort, in a process known as *habituation* (Rankin, 2009). Habituation is a very basic form of psychological adaptation that occurs at different levels in the nervous system. Rudimentary forms of habituation can already be observed in animals such as sea slugs, who possess only a few hundred neurons (LeDoux, 2002). Although habituation can apparently occur without any higher-order processing, it nevertheless exerts an important influence on the exit gradient of emotional responding. As such, habituation may be one of the most rudimentary processes that people may recruit in emotion regulation. When more complex self-regulatory strategies fail, people may still be capable of leaving unwanted emotional states by resorting to elementary habituation processes.

Over the course of evolution, humans eventually acquired the capacity for more cognitively sophisticated forms of emotion regulation. Presumably, these more sophisticated processes increase the efficiency and flexibility of emotion regulation. Similar to

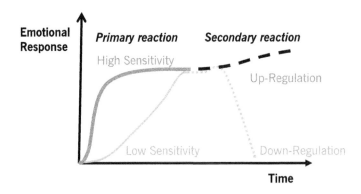

FIGURE 2.1. Hypothetical model of emotional sensitivity versus emotion regulation. From Koole (2009). Copyright 2009 by Taylor & Francis Group. Reprinted by permission.

emotional sensitivity, emotion regulation is determined by qualities of the stimuli that the person encounters (e.g., stimuli that appear at irregular intervals may be harder to adjust to than stimuli that appear at regular intervals), characteristics of the person (e.g., ruminators may dwell on negative experiences more than nonruminators), and the broader situation (e.g., when at home and among friends, people may down-regulate emotional distress more quickly than when they are alone in a foreign country).

Although emotion regulation refers to the ease with which people exit a given emotional state, this should not be taken to mean that emotion regulation always serves to speed up this exiting process. Indeed, whereas some forms of emotion regulation are aimed at decreasing the intensity of an emotional response (down-regulation), other forms of emotion regulation involve the up-regulation or maintenance of an emotional response. In the latter cases emotion regulation is aimed at increasing the intensity of an emotional response (up-regulation) or at keeping the intensity of an emotional response stable over time (maintenance). Common to all instances of emotion regulation, however, is that they alter the steepness of the exit gradient, and thus determine how long (or short) the activation of an emotional response persists over time.

The Process Model of Emotion Regulation

A second way to understand which emotion processes are targeted in emotion regulation is to ask how emotion regulation intervenes in specific components of emotional responding. The latter approach has been advanced by the *process model* of emotion regulation (Gross, 1998, 2001). The process model assumes that emotions are generated in a sequence of stages. In the first stage, people encounter a situation with features that can potentially trigger an emotional response. In the second stage, people may or not attend to the emotion-relevant features of the situation. In the third stage, people generate cognitive appraisals of the situation that may or not give rise to an emotional response. In the fourth and final stage, people express their emotions in their behavior. According to the process model, each of the four stages of emotion generation may be targeted for regulation. For our present exposition, the discussion concentrates on situations in which people want to down-regulate an unwanted emotion.

First, whenever people foresee that a given situation may give rise to unwanted emotional outcomes, they may engage in situation selection. In this strategy, people move to a different situation that is less likely to give rise to the unwanted emotion. A closely related strategy in which people may engage is *situation modification*, taking actions that reduce the odds of ending up in a situation with undesirable emotional outcomes. In these two proactive forms of emotion regulation, the regulatory activity subjectively precedes the onset of emotion. However, merely anticipating an emotional experience already leads to a partial (often unconscious) simulation of that emotion, which triggers emotion systems similar to those that become activated during online emotion generation (Niedenthal, Barsalou, Winkielman, Krauth-Gruber, & Ric, 2005). Thus, in anticipatory strategies, emotion regulation succeeds a primary emotional response triggered by the anticipation of unwanted emotional outcomes.

If an emotion-eliciting situation cannot be avoided, a second type of emotion regulation strategy that people may use is *attentional deployment*. In this strategy, people seek to direct their attention away from stimuli that give rise to undesirable emotion. For instance, people may bury themselves in work to forget about a romantic breakup, or they may engage in vigorous physical exercise to take their minds of work-related stress. Consistent with this, research has shown that positive and negative emotions become down-regulated when people perform a cognitively demanding task during or after an encounter with an emotional event (Erber & Tesser, 1992; van Dillen & Koole, 2007, 2009). By diverting their attention elsewhere, people may prevent full processing of the emotional aspects of a stimulus. As such, the emotional impact of the stimulus may be reduced.

When people are forced to pay attention to a stimulus that may arouse unwanted emotions, they may engage in a third type of strategy that involves *cognitive change*, in which people attempt to change their cognitive appraisals to reduce the emotional impact of the situation. For instance, people may reinterpret a potentially upsetting situation as being innocuous or assume the position of a detached observer (Ochsner & Gross, 2008).

Finally, when the aforementioned strategies are not applicable, people may engage in a fourth type of strategy that involves *response modulation*. In this type of emotion regulation, people directly manipulate the physiological, experiential, or behavioral expressions of their emotions. For instance, people may inhibit their spontaneous emotional expressions (Gross, 1998), exaggerate their responses to an emotional stimulus (Schmeichel, Demaree, Robinson, & Pu, 2006), or intentionally direct their emotional impulses toward a substitute object (Bushman, 2002). Other forms of response modulation are controlled breathing (Philippot, Chapelle, & Blairy, 2002) and progressive muscle relaxation (Pawlow & Jones, 2002).

The process model has made several major contributions to the understanding of emotion regulation. First, the process model identifies key response systems that may be targeted in emotion regulation. Second, the model provides a comprehensive descriptive framework for classifying different emotion regulation strategies (Gross, 2001). Third, the process model explains why some emotion regulation strategies may be more effective than others. Specifically, the process model proposes that emotion regulation strategies are likely to be more successful and less effortful when they are applied earlier rather than later in the emotion generation process (Gross, 2001). This prediction has received initial support from studies that compared the effects of cognitive reappraisal with the effects of expressive suppression (e.g., Gross, 1998). In line with the process model, cognitive reappraisal has been found to be more effective than expressive suppression in down-regulating negative emotion (e.g., Gross, 1998). Moreover, cognitive reappraisal appears to be less cognitively effortful than expressive suppression (Richards & Gross, 2000).

Though these previous results are important, the operationalizations of cognitive reappraisal and expressive suppression in relevant studies differed in at least two respects. First, the target of the strategies differed given that whereas reappraisal aims to bring about cognitive change, suppression aims to achieve response modulation. Second, there were temporal differences between the investigated strategies given that reappraisal intervened earlier than suppression in the emotion-generative process. Unconfounding these two aspects would require manipulating the temporal difference, while holding the target of emotion regulation constant. A recent study took an important step in this direction by comparing the effectiveness of distraction and reappraisal early and late in the emotion-generative process (Sheppes & Meiran, 2007). As predicted by the process model, late reappraisal was less effective than early reappraisal. However, distraction was effective regardless of its timing (i.e., whether it was initiated early or late). These results suggest

unsure

that the link between the effectiveness and timing of emotion regulation strategies is contingent on additional cognitive and physiological parameters (Sheppes, Catran, & Meiran, 2009; Sheppes & Meiran, 2008).

Other studies raise doubts about the notion that emotion regulation through cognitive change strategies (which are assumed to target early emotion responses) is inherently more effective than response modulation strategies (which are assumed to target late emotional responses). At least in some instances, response modulation strategies may be quite effective. For instance, studies have demonstrated emotion regulatory effects of controlled breathing, a technique in which people are asked to produce patterns that fit with specific emotional states (Philippot et al., 2002). Likewise, progressive muscle relaxation, a technique in which people successively tense and relax specific muscle groups, has been shown to down-regulate emotional stress effectively (Pawlow & Jones, 2002). Conversely, some cognitive change strategies may be maladaptive. For instance, rumination, a cognitive emotion regulation strategy, has been found to be ineffective in dealing with negative emotions (Nolen-Hoeksema, Wisco, & Lyubomirsky, 2008).

A further complication is that emotion generation may be messier than the process model assumes. For instance, bodily movements may directly activate emotional experiences (Niedenthal et al., 2005), and affective stimuli may directly trigger behavioral tendencies associated with emotional responding (e.g., R. Neumann, Förster, & Strack, 2003). Different components of emotional responding may thus become activated in a highly variable order. Consequently, it seems questionable to assume a priori that the target of an emotion regulation strategy determines its timing within the emotion generation process. An emotion regulation strategy such as cognitive reappraisal might intervene early or late in the emotion generation process, depending on the circumstances. The same applies to any other emotion regulation strategy. Thus, the role of timing in determining the effectiveness of emotion regulation strategies cannot be inferred from the targets of emotion regulation. To reach firm conclusions, the timing of a given emotion regulation strategy must be established independently, through measurement or manipulation (e.g., Sheppes & Meiran, 2007).

Taken together, the link between the targets of emotion regulation strategies and their effectiveness seems more complex than the process model (Gross, 2001) assumes. Perhaps this conclusion is not all that surprising given the process model's exclusive focus on the *emotion* part of emotion regulation. The *regulation* part of emotion regulation is not systematically considered by the process model. Nevertheless, it seems plausible that the effectiveness of emotion regulation depends at least partly on how well people are able to monitor whether a given situation calls for emotion regulation and how capable they are of implementing a particular emotion regulation strategy. The latter processes are central to control models of emotion regulation, which have addressed the *regulation* in emotion regulation.

THE "REGULATION" IN EMOTION REGULATION

Emotion regulation is by definition a control process. As such, emotion regulation belongs to a larger family of processes whereby people exert control over their own behavior. Indeed, modern emotion regulation research has drawn considerable inspiration from theories of human self-regulation and cognitive control (Carver & Scheier, 1998; Chapter

1, this volume; Kuhl, 2000; Posner & Snyder, 1975; Rueda, Posner, & Rothbart, Chapter 15, this volume). Building on these theories, researchers have proposed several models of the control processes that mediate emotion regulation.

Goal-Oriented Models of Emotion Regulation

Social and personality psychologists have suggested that emotion regulation may be understood as a form of effortful self-regulation (Erber & Erber, 2000; Larsen, 2000; Tice & Bratslavsky, 2000). Self-regulation is conceived as a cybernetic control process that consists of two main components. First, there is a monitoring process, which compares the individual's current state with a desired state. Second, there is an operating system that reduces any discrepancies between these two states (Carver & Scheier, 1998). Thus, when people engage in emotion regulation, they may compare their current emotional state to a desired emotional state and take appropriate steps to bring their current emotional state closer to the desired emotional state. Self-regulatory systems of this sort are typically hierarchically ordered (Carver & Scheier, 1998), with lower-order goals geared toward concrete behavior control, and higher-order goals oriented toward more abstract principles. Accordingly, emotion regulation processes may range from the control of concrete behavior (e.g., "Take a deep breath and count to 10") to abstract goals (e.g., "I want to be in control of my emotions").

A related approach has proposed that emotion regulation is governed by cognitive control processes. *Cognitive control* is a superordinate control process that allows people to override strongly activated but situation-inappropriate action tendencies (Posner & Snyder, 1975). Cognitive control may be applied to emotional responses whenever hot, emotion-driven response tendencies threaten to interfere with cool, more cognitively driven response tendencies (McClure, Botvinick, Yeung, Greene, & Cohen, 2007; Ochsner & Gross, 2008; Schmeichel, 2007). Cognitive control involves two major processes associated with distinct neural structures (Botvinick, Braver, Barch, Carter, & Cohen, 2001). The first is a conflict-monitoring process, which constantly, efficiently, and nonconsciously scans for the presence of conflicts between alternative response tendencies. Whenever such conflicts are detected, the effortful regulatory process engaged to override the unwanted response tendency is proportional to the level of response conflict.

The link between emotion regulation and cognitive control has been confirmed by neuroimaging studies, which have demonstrated a close correspondence between the neurological systems involved in both types of control. For instance, reappraisal of emotions, which consists of actively reinterpreting the meaning of a stimulus to lessen its emotional impact, leads to increased activation in the dorsal anterior cingulate cortex and prefrontal cortex, areas that also support other forms of cognitive control (Botvinick et al., 2001; Miller & Cohen, 2001). Importantly, activation of these control systems leads to corresponding changes in the activity of regions such as the amygdala and/or insula, which are important for assessing the emotional relevance of a stimulus (e.g., Beauregard, Levesque, & Bourgouin, 2001; Ochsner, Bunge, Gross, & Gabrieli, 2002; for a review, see Ochsner & Gross, 2008). Such findings support the view that emotion regulation may rely on cognitive control processes.

Self-regulation and cognitive control models have been highly influential in shaping modern thinking about emotion regulation. Both models converge on key points about the nature of goal-directed control processes (Robinson, Schmeichel, & Inzlicht, 2010). Moreover, self-regulation and cognitive control models agree in their characterization of emotion regulation as an effortful top-down control process guided by goals (i.e., largely conscious verbal/symbolic representations of desired outcomes and intended actions). We therefore refer to self-regulation and cognitive control models jointly as goal-oriented models of emotion regulation.

There are two main ways in which goal-oriented emotion regulation may operate. First, people often hold beliefs about the utility of particular emotional states. These beliefs may be derived from verbal instructions about the desirability of certain emotional states (e.g., Achtziger, Gollwitzer, & Sheeran, 2008; Gross, 1998), implicit or explicit beliefs about the utility of particular emotional states (Tamir, Chiu, & Gross, 2007), or more abstract theories that people hold about emotion regulation (Tamir, John, Srivastava, & Gross, 2007). When people believe that the utility of other emotional states is higher than the utility of their present emotional state, this may give rise to goal-oriented emotion regulation.

Second, an ongoing goal, task, or norm may change the relevance of emotionally charged information. Emotionally charged information that is (potentially) relevant to the ongoing task is likely to be maintained, whereas irrelevant emotionally charged information is likely to be ignored or down-regulated (van Dillen & Koole, 2007, 2009). Because goals, norms, or tasks may favor various types of emotional outcomes, goal-oriented emotion regulation may either promote or inhibit emotional states that are hedonically rewarding.

Beyond Goals: Need- and Person-Oriented Emotion Regulation

Goal-oriented models capture important aspects of the emotion regulation process. Nevertheless, some forms of emotion regulation fit less well with the goal-oriented model. For instance, certain emotion regulation processes unfold in the absence of explicit goals and display many aspects of automatic processing (Koole & Jostmann, 2004; Mauss, Bunge, & Gross, 2007). Likewise, some forms of emotion regulation do not involve any explicit attempts to control one's emotion states, and even involve efforts to stay away from goal-directed control processes (Brown, Ryan, & Creswell, 2007). As such, it seems useful to consider how goal-oriented models of emotion regulation may be complemented by other types of emotion regulatory processes.

Need-Oriented Emotion Regulation

A first extension of the goal-oriented model relates to basic hedonic needs to seek pleasure and avoid pain. The far-ranging psychological significance of hedonic needs was first elaborated by Freud (1920/1961), when he proposed his classic pleasure principle. Freud regarded the pleasure principle as the prime directive of the *id*, an impulsive, child-like aspect of personality. Although Freud's personality theory soon fell into disrepute, the importance of hedonic needs continues to be recognized by modern theories of emotion regulation (e.g., Larsen, 2000; Westen, 1994).

Consistent with the notion of need-oriented emotion regulation, developmental psychologists have observed that children display early forms of self-soothing, such as sucking or turning away from angry faces, within 3 months after birth (Calkins & Leerkes,

Chapter 19, this volume; Kopp, 1989; Rothbart, Ziaie, & O'Boyle, 1992). These hedonic behaviors emerge regardless of caregiver intervention and well before children are capable of forming linguistic representations that can support abstract goals. It thus appears that need-oriented emotion regulation is driven by elementary, sublinguistic processes. The elementary nature of hedonic needs is bolstered by findings that, among adult participants, tendencies to approach positive affective stimuli and to avoid negative affective stimuli can be triggered automatically and without conscious intent (Chen & Bargh, 1999; R. Neumann et al., 2003). Moreover, hedonic biases in information processing display important aspects of automaticity (Paulhus & Levitt, 1987; Roese & Olson, 2007; Tesser, 2000). These and related findings suggest that basic hedonic tendencies may remain ingrained in the human psyche throughout people's lives.

Although hedonic needs are grounded in prelinguistic processes, they may acquire the capacity to bias conscious reasoning processes (Kunda, 1990), as evidenced by numerous ego-defensive biases (Baumeister & Newman, 1994; Pyszczynski & Greenberg, 1987; Tesser, 2000). For instance, people may engage in selective criticism of threatening information (Liberman & Chaiken, 1992), or make self-serving attributions (Campbell & Sedikides, 1999) or downward social comparison (Taylor & Lobel, 1989). Notably, defensive bias is associated with neural activity in regions such as the ventromedial prefrontal cortex, which have been implicated in emotion regulation (Westen, Kilts, Blagov, Harenski, & Hamann, 2006). At the same time, defensive bias is not associated with activation in brain regions that support effortful self-regulation (Ochsner & Gross, 2008; van Dillen, Heslenfeld, & Koole, 2009), suggesting that defensive bias is mediated by different processes than goal-oriented emotion regulation.

Need-oriented emotion regulation is narrow in its aims, in that hedonic needs are invariably oriented toward a positive hedonic balance in the immediate present. Because people's goals typically have a broader temporal horizon, conflicts may arise between need-oriented emotion regulation and self-regulatory efforts geared toward long-term goals. Indeed, a provocative series of experiments found that emotional distress may cause need-oriented emotion regulation to take precedence over goal-directed forms of self-regulation (Tice, Bratslavsky, & Baumeister, 2001). Relatedly, field studies indicate that harmful activities that people may use in need-oriented emotion regulation, such as binge eating or excessive alcohol intake, are more prevalent in people with high levels of emotional distress (Greeno & Wing, 1994; Mohr, Brannan, Mohr, Armeli, & Tennen, 2008).

Despite the potential for conflict with broader self-regulation processes, need-oriented emotion regulation is likely to have important benefits. Enduring negative emotional states invoke considerable psychological costs because such states mobilize many mental and physical resources within the individual (Sapolsky, 2007). By shortening the duration of negative emotional states, need-oriented emotion regulation may allow people to preserve important resources. Moreover, even though need-oriented emotion regulation is rigid in its aims, there may be considerable flexibility in the means by which people attain hedonically favorable outcomes (Tesser, 2000).

Person-Oriented Emotion Regulation

A second extension of the goal-oriented model of emotion regulation derives from existential/humanistic approaches to personality (e.g., Frankl, 1975; Maslow, 1968), and has roots in Asian philosophy (Cahn & Polich, 2006; Tang & Posner, 2009) and many religious traditions (Koole, McCullough, Kuhl, & Roelofsma, 2010). These seemingly disparate paradigms have converged on notions of self-regulatory process that go beyond fragments of the self (e.g., goals or hedonic needs), and rather encompass the functioning of the whole person. In person-oriented emotion regulation, the person's functioning is coordinated by integrating as many subsystems and processes as possible for supporting a chosen course of action. Person-oriented emotion regulation thus supports an "inner democracy" (Kuhl, 2000) by regulating people's actions in harmony with the totality of their inner needs, motives, and autobiographical experiences. These integrated networks of personality systems are closely connected with the autonomic nervous system. Person-oriented emotion regulation is not mediated by explicit intentions, but rather by integrated feelings or intuitions about appropriate courses of action (Baumann & Kuhl, 2002).

There are two main ways in which emotion regulation may coordinate the functioning of the whole person. First, person-oriented emotion regulation may prevent people from becoming trapped in specific motivational–emotional states, thus promoting flexibility in global personality functioning (Rothermund, Voss, & Wentura, 2008). Second, by facilitating emotional changes, emotion regulation may promote coherence in personality functioning and personal growth (Baumann, Kaschel, & Kuhl, 2005).

Flexibility in emotional functioning may be promoted by counterregulation (Rothermund et al., 2008), a process whereby people switch their attention toward emotional states that are opposite in valence to emotional states that are momentarily activated. Counterregulation has emerged as a distinct pattern in various attentional biases toward positive or negative information (Derryberry, 1993; Rothermund et al., 2008; Tugade & Frederickson, 2004). Depending on the valence of the emotion that predominates in a given context, counterregulation may inhibit either positive or negative emotion (Rothermund et al., 2008). If counterregulation supports flexible self-regulation, then the pattern should be especially apparent among individuals who display high levels of self-regulatory efficiency. Consistent with this, counterregulation is markedly stronger among individuals disposed toward flexible action control (Jostmann, Koole, Van der Wulp, & Fockenberg, 2005; Koole & Coenen, 2007; Koole & Jostmann, 2004), and markedly weaker among individuals suffering from chronic anxiety, phobia, or dysphoria (Mathews & MacLeod, 2005).

Integration and personal growth may be promoted by emotion regulation strategies that foster deep cognitive processing of people's emotional experiences. For instance, expressive writing, which can turn initially disturbing emotional experiences into coherent narratives (Pennebaker & Chung, 2007), down-regulates emotional distress and promotes self-insight (Klein & Boals, 2001). After a painful experience has been integrated into more extended cognitive networks, people may subsequently deal more effectively with similar emotional experiences. Indeed, individuals with more differentiated knowledge of self and emotion show greater efficiency in emotion regulation (Barrett, Gross, Conner, & Benvenuto, 2001; Rafaeli-Mor & Steinberg, 2002).

Person-oriented emotion regulation seeks to bridge the duality between mind and body. Indeed, bodily activities are typically integrated in emotion-regulatory activities such as meditation or mindfulness exercises. Research indicates that bodily activities, such as controlled breathing or progressive muscle relaxation, have a distinct influence on emotion regulation that cannot be reduced to attentional or appraisal processes (Boiten,

Frijda, & Wientjes, 1994; Esch, Fricchione, & Stefano, 2003; Philippot et al., 2002; Rausch, Gramling, & Auerbach, 2006).

ENHANCING THE CAPACITY FOR EMOTION REGULATION THROUGH TRAINING

Given the important role that emotion regulation plays in self-regulatory functioning, it is important to learn about ways to enhance people's emotion regulatory abilities. In recent years, a growing number of studies have shown that people's competencies at emotion regulation can be enhanced through training (for reviews, see Baumeister, Gailliot, DeWall, & Oaten, 2006; MacLeod, Koster, & Fox, 2009; Tang & Posner, 2009). This evidence could have far-ranging implications by contributing to the development of more effective therapies and interventions aimed at overcoming self- and emotion regulatory deficits. In addition, studying the effects of training may provide a new paradigm for unravelling the causal mechanisms that underlie emotion regulation. As such, there is great interest in the effects of training on the capacity for emotion regulation.

Studies examining the effects of training on emotion regulation have so far been guided by "inspired guesswork" (MacLeod et al., 2009, p. 95) rather than a systematic analysis of the underlying causal mechanisms. Nevertheless, a systematic theoretical analysis is necessary to obtain a scientific understanding of how emotion regulatory abilities may be altered and enhanced through training. In this regard, the models of the targets and control processes of emotion regulation discussed in previous sections of this chapter may serve as a preliminary framework for interpreting the effects of training on emotion regulation. As such, we rely on these models in considering which types of mechanism may be implicated in training emotion regulation abilities.

Which Emotion Responses Are Targeted in Training Studies?

A first question that arises is whether training has differential effects on emotional sensitivity (i.e., people's primary emotional response) and emotion regulation (i.e., people's secondary emotional response). Training studies have not systematically distinguished between these different components of emotion processing. However, developmental research indicates that emotional sensitivity follows an intrinsic path of development that is largely independent of environmental influences (McCrae et al., 2000; Terracciano, Costa, & McCrae, 2005), whereas competencies at emotion regulation are strongly influenced by the quality of children's social interactions with their caregivers (Mikulincer, Shaver, & Pereg, 2003; Southam-Gerow & Kendall, 2002) and continue to improve even into old age (Carstensen, Fung, & Charles, 2003; Gröpel, Kuhl, & Kazén, 2004; John & Gross, 2004). As such, there are grounds to suspect that emotion regulation is more susceptible to training than is emotional sensitivity.

A further question is which types of emotional responses may be enhanced through training. We are not aware of studies that have systematically addressed the effects of training on situation selection or situation modification, the first emotion regulatory strategies proposed by the process model (Gross, 2001). The remaining strategies proposed by the process model have received more empirical attention. Studies on cognitive bias modification have sought to change attentional or interpretive biases with regard to emotional information, typically by training attentional or interpretative procedures in a speeded response task (MacLeod et al., 2009). Both types of training have been found to facilitate more efficient disengagement from intrusive thoughts and negative emotional states (Dandeneau, Baldwin, Baccus, Sakellaropoulo, & Pruessner, 2007; MacLeod et al., 2009; see also a special section in the first issue of the *Journal of Abnormal Psychology*, 2009). In addition, a number of successful training programs include the regulation of bodily expressions of emotion, such as relaxation and breath adjustment (Tang & Posner, 2009). Taken together, research suggests that most of the major response systems that may be targeted in emotion regulation are implicated in programs designed to enhance emotion regulatory abilities.

Which Control Processes Can Be Trained?

Goal-oriented models of emotion regulation (Erber & Erber, 2000; Ochsner & Gross, 2008) propose a close correspondence between effortful self-regulation and goal-oriented emotion regulation. In line with this, a number of training studies have found that training effortful self-regulation may yield important benefits for emotion regulation. For instance, in one study, physical exercise led to significant reductions in participants' perceived stress and increases in self-reported ability to control their tempers (Oaten & Cheng, 2006a). Similar effects on emotion regulation were reported when people trained in other effortful self-regulatory behaviors, such as regular academic study (Oaten & Cheng, 2006b) or prudent money management (Oaten & Cheng, 2007). Goal-oriented models also may predict an effect in the opposite direction, such that practicing goal-oriented emotion regulation should improve people's capacity for effortful self-regulation of nonemotional behaviors. But as far as we know, the latter prediction has yet to be submitted to empirical testing.

Other training studies seem to involve need-oriented forms of emotion regulation. In particular, studies within the cognitive bias modification paradigm have often focused on changing processing biases in a more hedonically favorable direction (MacLeod et al., 2009). Notably, the cognitive bias modification paradigm originated in the study of attentional processes among individuals high in trait anxiety (Mathews & MacLeod, 2005). As such, it may be that anxiety problems are associated with abnormalities in need-oriented emotion regulation. Consistent with this, exaggerated forms of need-oriented emotion regulation are empirically associated with *repressive coping style* (Weinberger, Schwartz, & Davidson, 1979), a coping style that is characterized by latent anxiety (Derakshan, Eysenck, & Myers, 2007). The link between anxiety problems and deficits in need-oriented emotion regulation warrants more attention in future research.

Finally, several training programs seem aimed at cultivating person-oriented self-regulation and emotion regulation processes. In so-called *mindfulness meditation training*, people are encouraged to focus their attention on the present and to refrain from evaluating their ongoing experience (Kabat-Zinn, 1990). Mindfulness training has been found to reduce the symptoms of stress, depression, and anxiety among many different clinical populations (Bishop, 2002). Mindfulness training presumably fosters these broad emotion regulatory effects by reducing negative ruminations about the self (Ramel, Goldin, Carmona, & McQuaid, 2004) and by promoting integrative processes (Koole, Govorun, Cheng, & Gallucci, 2009). A related research program has examined the effects of integrated body–mind training (Tang & Posner, 2009). In the latter program, trainees are guided by a coach in body relaxation, breathing adjustment, mental imagery, music, and mindfulness training to achieve gradually a balanced state of relaxation and focused attention. Research indicates that integrated body–mind training fosters top-down attention control, lowers negative emotion and stress-related cortisol, and increases immune functioning (Tang et al., 2007). Moreover, integrated body–mind training has been found to increase coordination between attentional networks and the autonomic nervous system (Tang et al., 2009).

In summary, the effects of training in emotion regulatory abilities can be meaningfully related to existing models of emotion regulation. Although training research has not systematically pursued the distinction between emotional sensitivity and emotion regulation, developmental research suggests that emotion regulation may be particularly susceptible to training. Furthermore, training studies indicate that the regulation of various emotion response systems can be improved through training, including regulation of attention, cognitive appraisals, and expressive responses. Different training programs, furthermore, seem to invoke different control processes, with some programs emphasizing goal-oriented emotion regulation and others emphasizing need- or person-oriented emotion regulation.

SUMMARY AND CONCLUSIONS

When people self-regulate, they are frequently confronted with potentially emotion-arousing situations. Processes of self-regulation are therefore closely connected with processes of emotion regulation. This chapter has highlighted key aspects of the interface between self-regulation and emotion regulation by addressing some of the basic psychological processes that underlie the self-regulation of emotion.

In the first section, we considered the *emotion* in emotion regulation, or the targets of emotion regulation. We conceived of emotion regulation processes broadly, as processes whereby people regulate any type of affective or emotionally charged response, including attention, cognitive representations, and physical or behavioral responses. Emotion regulation targets the offset of emotional responding and is thus distinct from processes that involve the onset of emotional responding, or emotional sensitivity. The process model of emotion regulation has offered a comprehensive analysis of the various emotional response systems that people may target for regulation. The model suggests that people may regulate their emotions by selecting or altering emotion-eliciting situations, attentional deployment, cognitive change, or response modulation.

In the second section, we took a closer look at the *regulation* in emotion regulation by reviewing the types of control processes that people may use during emotion regulation. Control processes determine how people monitor whether emotion regulation is required and how they implement specific acts of emotion regulation. Goal-oriented models have portrayed emotion regulation as an effortful self-regulation or cognitive control process. Although goal-oriented models explain important aspects of emotion regulation, emotion regulation may also serve other types of regulatory functions. The extended functions of emotion regulation include the satisfaction of hedonic needs, facilitation of specific goals and tasks, and coordination of global personality functioning.

In the third section of this chapter we discussed emerging research on the effects of training on emotion regulatory abilities. In reviewing the training literature, we drew upon key concepts from the emotion regulation literature. Our brief review suggests that there exists considerable integrative potential between the two literatures. Emotion regulation researchers have much to gain from investigating how training studies afford new insights into the causal mechanisms of emotion regulation. Conversely, training researchers may benefit from paying closer attention to specific mechanisms and processes. In this regard, the emotion regulation literature offers a rich set of methods and concepts to develop a mechanistic understanding of how emotion regulatory abilities are shaped and altered by experience.

More generally, the study of emotion regulation has broad implications for psychologists' understanding of self-regulation processes. In recent years, psychological theories have predominantly emphasized goals as the core mental representation that drives human self-regulation (Austin & Vancouver, 1996; Baumeister et al., 2006; Carver & Scheier, 1998). However, as this chapter indicates, goals account for only a limited number of emotion regulation processes. Some forms of emotion regulation operate on levels that are more elementary than goals, and they appear to be driven by powerful hedonic needs. Other forms of emotion regulation transcend single goals and seek to forge a union between passion and reason, mind and body, and other dualities that may divide the human psyche. A complete understanding of human self-regulation thus extends beyond goals and includes the regulation of people's deep-seated emotional needs and overall personality functioning.

ACKNOWLEDGMENT

Preparation of this chapter was facilitated by a stay of Sander Koole at the Center for Advanced Study in the Behavioral Sciences, Stanford University.

REFERENCES

Achtziger, A., Gollwitzer, P. M., & Sheeran, P. (2008). Implementation intentions and shielding goal striving from unwanted thoughts and feelings. *Personality and Social Psychology Bulletin, 34*, 381–393.

Austin, J. T., & Vancouver, J. B. (1996). Goal constructs in psychology: Structure, process, and content. *Psychological Bulletin, 120*, 338–375.

Barrett, L. F., Gross, J. J., Conner, T., & Benvenuto, M. (2001). Knowing what you're feeling and knowing what to do about it: Mapping the relation between emotion differentiation and emotion regulation. *Cognition and Emotion, 15*, 713–724.

Baumann, N., Kaschel, R., & Kuhl, J. (2005). Striving for unwanted goals: Stress-dependent discrepancies between explicit and implicit achievement motives reduce subjective well-being and increase psychosomatic symptoms. *Journal of Personality and Social Psychology, 89*, 781–799.

Baumann, N., Kaschel, R., & Kuhl, J. (2007). Affect sensitivity and affect regulation in dealing with positive and negative affect. *Journal of Research in Personality, 41*, 239–248.

Baumann, N., & Kuhl, J. (2002). Intuition, affect, and personality: Unconscious coherence judgments and self-regulation of negative affect. *Journal of Personality and Social Psychology, 83*, 1213–1223.

Baumeister, R. F., Gailliot, M., DeWall, C. N., & Oaten, M. (2006). Self-regulation and personality: How interventions increase regulatory success, and how depletion moderates the effects of traits on behavior. *Journal of Personality, 74*, 1773–1801.

Baumeister, R. F., & Newman, L. S. (1994). Self-regulation of cognitive inference and decision processes. *Personality and Social Psychology Bulletin, 20,* 3–19.

Baumeister, R. F., Schmeichel, B. J., & Vohs, K. D. (2007). Self-regulation and the executive function: The self as controlling agent. In A. W. Kruglanski & E. T. Higgins (Eds.), *Social psychology: Handbook of basic principles* (2nd ed., pp. 516–539). New York: Guilford Press.

Beauregard, M., Levesque, J., & Bourgouin, P. (2001). Neural correlates of conscious self-regulation of emotion. *Journal of Neuroscience, 21,* 1–6.

Bishop, S. R. (2002). What do we really know about mindfulness-based stress reduction? *Psychosomatic Medicine, 64,* 71–84.

Boiten, F. A., Frijda, N. H., & Wientjes, C. J. E. (1994). Emotions and respiratory patterns: Review and critical analysis. *International Journal of Psychophysiology, 17,* 103–128.

Botvinick, M., Braver, T., Barch, D., Carter, C., & Cohen, J. (2001). Conflict monitoring and cognitive control. *Psychological Review, 108,* 624–652.

Brown, K. W., Ryan, R. M., & Creswell, J. D. (2007). Mindfulness: Theoretical foundations and evidence for its salutary effects. *Psychological Inquiry, 18,* 211–237.

Bushman, B. J. (2002). Does venting anger feed or extinguish the flame?: Catharsis, rumination, distraction, anger, and aggressive responding. *Personality and Social Psychology Bulletin, 28,* 724–731.

Cacioppo, J. T., Berntson, G. G., & Klein, D. J. (1992). What is an emotion?: The role of somatovisceral afference, with special emphasis on somatovisceral "illusions." *Review of Personality and Social Psychology, 14,* 63–98.

Cahn, B. R., & Polich, J. (2006). Meditation states and traits: EEG, ERP, and neuroimaging studies. *Psychological Bulletin, 132,* 180–211.

Campbell, W. K., & Sedikides, C. (1999). Self-threat magnifies the self-serving bias: A meta-analytic integration. *Review of General Psychology, 3,* 23–43.

Carstensen, L. L., Fung, H., & Charles, S. (2003). Socioemotional selectivity theory and the regulation of emotion in the second half of life. *Motivation and Emotion, 27,* 103–123.

Carver, C. S., & Scheier, M. F. (1998). *On the self-regulation of behavior.* New York: Cambridge University Press.

Chen, M., & Bargh, J. A. (1999). Nonconscious avoidance and approach behavioral consequences of the automatic evaluation effect. *Personality and Social Psychology Bulletin, 25,* 215–224.

Dandeneau, S. D., Baldwin, M. W., Baccus, J. R., Sakellaropoulo, M., & Pruessner, J. C. (2007). Cutting stress off at the pass: Reducing stress and hypervigilance to social threat by manipulating attention. *Journal of Personality and Social Psychology, 93,* 651–666.

Derakshan, N., Eysenck, M. W., & Myers, L. B. (2007). Emotional information processing in repressors: The vigilance–avoidance theory. *Cognition and Emotion, 21,* 1585–1614.

Derryberry, D. (1993). Attentional consequences of outcome-related motivational states: Congruent, incongruent, and focusing effects. *Motivation and Emotion, 17,* 65–89.

Erber, R. (1996). The self-regulation of moods. In L. L. Martin & A. Tesser (Eds.), *Striving and feeling: Interactions between goals and affect* (pp. 251–275). Hillsdale, NJ: Erlbaum.

Erber, R., & Tesser, A. (1992). Task effort and the regulation of mood: The absorption hypothesis. *Journal of Experimental Social Psychology, 28,* 339–359.

Esch, T., Fricchione, G. L., & Stefano, G. B. (2003). The therapeutic use of the relaxation response in stress-related diseases. *Medical Science Monitor, 9,* 23–34.

Frankl, V. E. (1975). *The unconscious god: Psychotherapy and theology.* New York: Simon & Schuster.

Freud, S. (1961). *Beyond the pleasure principle.* New York: Norton. (Original work published 1920)

Frijda, N. (2006). *The laws of emotion.* New York: Erlbaum.

Greeno, C. G., & Wing, R. R. (1994). Stress-induced eating. *Psychological Bulletin, 115,* 444–464.

Gröpel, P., Kuhl, J., & Kazén, M. (2004). Toward an integrated self: Age differences and the role of action orientation. *Conference Proceedings of the Third International SELF Research Conference* [CD-ROM]. Sydney: SELF Research Centre.

Gross, J. J. (1998). Antecedent- and response-focused emotion regulation: Divergent consequences for experience, expression, and physiology. *Journal of Personality and Social Psychology, 74,* 224–237.

Gross, J. J. (2001). Emotion regulation in adulthood: Timing is everything. *Current Directions in Psychological Science, 10,* 214–219.

Gross, J. J. (Ed.). (2007). *Handbook of emotion regulation.* New York: Guilford Press.

John, O. P., & Gross, J. J. (2004). Healthy and unhealthy emotion regulation: Personality processes, individual differences, and lifespan development. *Journal of Personality, 72,* 1301–1334.

Jostmann, N., Koole, S. L., Van der Wulp, N., & Fockenberg, D. (2005). Subliminal affect regulation: The moderating role of action versus state orientation. *European Psychologist, 10,* 209–217.

Kabat-Zinn, J. (1990). *Full catastrophe living: Using the wisdom of your body and mind to face stress, pain, and illness.* New York: Dell.

Klein, K., & Boals, A. (2001). Expressive writing can increase working memory capacity. *Journal of Experimental Psychology: General, 130,* 520–533.

Koole, S. L. (2009). The psychology of emotion regulation: An integrative review. *Cognition and Emotion, 23,* 4–41.

Koole, S. L., & Coenen, L. H. M. (2007). Implicit self and affect regulation: Effects of action orientation and subliminal self priming in an affective priming task. *Self and Identity, 6,* 118–136.

Koole, S. L. Govorun, O., Cheng, C., & Gallucci, M. (2009). Pulling your self together: Meditation enhances the congruence between implicit and explicit self-esteem. *Journal of Experimental Social Psychology, 45,* 1220–1226.

Koole, S. L., & Jostmann, N. B. (2004). Getting a grip on your feelings: Effects of action orientation and external demands on intuitive affect regulation. *Journal of Personality and Social Psychology, 87,* 974–990.

Koole, S. L., McCullough, M., Kuhl, J., & Roelofsma, P. (2010). Why religion's burdens are light: From religiosity to implicit self-regulation. *Personality and Social Psychology Review, 14,* 95–107.

Kopp, C. B. (1989). Regulation of distress and negative emotions: An integrative review. *Developmental Psychology, 25,* 343–354.

Kuhl, J. (2000). A functional-design approach to motivation and self-regulation: The dynamics of personality systems interactions. In M. Boekaerts, P. R. Pintrich, & M. Zeidner (Eds.), *Handbook of self-regulation* (pp. 111–169). San Diego, CA: Academic Press.

Kunda, Z. (1990). The case for motivated inference. *Psychological Bulletin, 108,* 480–498.

Larsen, R. J. (2000). Toward a science of mood regulation. *Psychological Inquiry, 11,* 129–141.

Lazarus, R. S. (1991). Progress on a cognitive–motivational–relational theory of emotion. *American Psychologist, 46,* 819–834.

LeDoux, J. E. (2002). *Synaptic self: How our brains become who we are.* New York: Viking.

Liberman, A., & Chaiken, S. (1992). Defensive processing of personally relevant health messages. *Personality and Social Psychology Bulletin, 18,* 669–679.

MacLeod, C., Koster, E. H. W., & Fox, E. (2009). Whither cognitive bias modification research? *Journal of Abnormal Psychology, 118,* 89–99.

Maslow, A. H. (1968). *Toward a psychology of being* (2nd ed.). New York: Van Nostrand Reinhold.

Mathews, A., & MacLeod, C. (2005). Cognitive vulnerability to emotional disorders. *Annual Review of Clinical Psychology, 1,* 167–195.

Mauss, I., Levenson, R. W., McCarter, L., Wilhelm, F., & Gross, J. J. (2005). The tie that binds?: Coherence among emotion experience, behavior, and physiology. *Emotion, 5,* 175–190.

Mauss, I. B., Bunge, S. A., & Gross, J. J. (2007). Automatic emotion regulation. *Social and Personality Psychology Compass, 1,* 146–167.

McClure, S. M., Botvinick, M. M., Yeung, N., Greene, J. D., & Cohen, J. D. (2007). Conflict monitoring in cognition–emotion competition. In J. J. Gross (Ed.), *Handbook of emotion regulation* (pp. 204–226). New York: Guilford Press.

McCrae, R. R., Costa, P. T., Jr., Ostendorf, F., Angleitner, A., Hrebrikova, M., Avia, M. D., et al. (2000). Nature over nurture: Temperament, personality, and lifespan development. *Journal of Personality and Social Psychology, 78,* 173–186.

Mikulincer, M., Shaver, P. R., & Pereg, D. (2003). Attachment theory and affect regulation: The dynamics, development, and cognitive consequences of attachment-related strategies. *Motivation and Emotion, 27,* 77–102.

Miller, E. K., & Cohen, J. D. (2001). An integrative theory of prefrontal cortex function. *Annual Review of Neuroscience, 24,* 167–202.

Mohr, C. D., Brannan, D., Mohr, J., Armeli, S., & Tennen, H. (2008). Evidence for positive mood buffering among college student drinkers. *Personality and Social Psychology Bulletin, 34,* 1249–1259.

Neumann, R., Förster, J., & Strack, F. (2003). Motor compatibility: The bidirectional link between behavior and evaluation. In J. Musch & K. C. Klauer (Eds.), *The psychology of evaluation: Affective processes in cognition and emotion* (pp. 371–391). Mahwah, NJ: Erlbaum.

Niedenthal, P. M., Barsalou, L. W., Winkielman, P., Krauth-Gruber, S., & Ric, F. (2005). Embodiment in attitudes, social perception, and emotion. *Personality and Social Psychology Review, 9,* 184–211.

Nolen-Hoeksema, S., Wisco, B. E., & Lyubomirsky, S. (2008). Rethinking rumination. *Perspectives on Psychological Science, 3,* 400–424.

Oaten, M., & Cheng, K. (2006a). Academic study improves regulatory strength. *Basic and Applied Social Psychology, 28,* 1–16.

Oaten, M., & Cheng, K. (2006b). Longitudinal gains in self-control from regular physical exercise. *British Journal of Health Psychology, 11,* 717–733.

Oaten, M., & Cheng, K. (2007). Improvements in self-control from financial monitoring. *Journal of Economic Psychology, 28,* 487–501.

Ochsner, K. N., Bunge, S. A., Gross, J. J., & Gabrieli, J. D. E. (2002). Rethinking feelings: An fMRI study of the cognitive regulation of emotion. *Journal of Cognitive Neuroscience, 14,* 1215–1299.

Ochsner, K. N., & Gross, J. J. (2008). Cognitive emotion regulation: Insights from social cognitive and affective neuroscience. *Currents Directions in Psychological Science, 17,* 153–158.

Parkinson, B., & Totterdell, P. (1999). Classifying affect-regulation strategies. *Cognition and Emotion, 13,* 277–303.

Paulhus, D. L., & Levitt, K. (1987). Desirable responding triggered by affect: Automatic egotism? *Journal of Personality and Social Psychology, 52,* 245–259.

Pawlow, L. A., & Jones, G. E. (2002). The impact of abbreviated progressive muscle relaxation on salivary cortisol. *Biological Psychology, 60,* 1–16.

Pennebaker, J. W., & Chung, C. K. (2007). Expressive writing, emotional upheavals, and health. In H. Friedman & R. Silver (Eds.), *Handbook of health psychology* (pp. 263–284). New York: Oxford University Press.

Philippot, P., Chapelle, C., & Blairy, S. (2002). Respiratory feedback in the generation of emotion. *Cognition and Emotion, 16,* 605–627.

Posner, M. I., & Snyder, C. R. (1975). Attention and cognitive control. In R. L. Solso (Ed.), *Infor-*

mation processing and cognition: The Loyola Symposium (pp. 55–85). Hillsdale, NJ: Erlbaum.

Pyszczynski, T., & Greenberg, J. (1987). Toward an integration of cognitive and motivational perspectives on social inference: A biased hypothesis-testing model. In L. Berkowitz (Ed.), *Advances in experimental social psychology* (Vol. 20, pp. 297–340). Hillsdale, NJ: Erlbaum.

Rafaeli-Mor, E., & Steinberg, J. (2002). Self-complexity and well-being: A review and research synthesis. *Personality and Social Psychology Review, 6,* 31–58.

Ramel, W., Goldin, P. R., Carmona, P. E., & McQuaid, J. R. (2004). The effects of mindfulness meditation on cognitive processes and affect in patients with past depression. *Cognitive Therapy and Research, 28,* 433–455.

Rankin, C. H. (2009). Introduction to a special issue of neurobiology of learning and memory on habituation. *Neurobiology of Learning and Memory, 92,* 125–126.

Rausch, S. M., Gramling, S. E., & Auerbach, S. M. (2006). Effects of a single session of large-group meditation and progressive muscle relaxation training on stress reduction, reactivity, and recovery. *International Journal of Stress Management, 13,* 273–290.

Richards, J. M., & Gross, J. J. (2000). Emotion regulation and memory: The cognitive costs of keeping one's cool. *Journal of Personality and Social Psychology, 79,* 410–424.

Robinson, M. D., Schmeichel, B. J., & Inzlicht, M. (2010). How does the self control itself? Questions and considerations based on a cognitive control perspective. *Social and Personality Psychology Compass, 4,* 189–200.

Roese, N. J., & Olson, J. M. (2007). Better, stronger, faster: Self-serving judgment, affect regulation, and the optimal vigilance hypothesis. *Perspectives on Psychological Science, 2,* 124–141.

Rothbart, M., Ziaie, H., & O'Boyle, C. (1992). Self-regulation and emotion in infancy. In N. Eisenberg & R. Fabes (Eds.), *Emotion and its regulation in early development: New directions for child development* (pp. 7–23). San Francisco: Jossey-Bass/Pfeiffer.

Rothermund, K., Voss, A., & Wentura, D. (2008). Counter-regulation in affective attentional bias: A basic mechanism that warrants flexibility in motivation and emotion. *Emotion, 8,* 34–46.

Sapolsky, R. M. (2007). Stress, stress-related disease, and emotional regulation. In J. J. Gross (Ed.), *Handbook of emotion regulation* (pp. 606–615). New York: Guilford Press.

Schmeichel, B. J. (2007). Attention control, memory updating, and emotion regulation temporarily reduce the capacity for executive control. *Journal of Experimental Psychology: General, 136,* 241–255.

Schmeichel, B. J., Demaree, H. A., Robinson, J. L., & Pu, J. (2006). Ego depletion by response exaggeration. *Journal of Experimental Social Psychology, 42,* 95–102.

Sheppes, G., Catran, E., & Meiran, N. (2009). Reappraisal (but not distraction) is going to make you sweat: Physiological evidence for self control effort. *International Journal of Psychophysiology, 71,* 91–96.

Sheppes, G., & Meiran, N. (2007). Better late than never?: On the dynamics of online regulation of sadness using distraction and cognitive reappraisal. *Personality and Social Psychology Bulletin, 33,* 1518–1532.

Sheppes, G., & Meiran, N. (2008). There is no such thing as a free lunch: Divergent cognitive costs for online reappraisal and distraction. *Emotion, 8,* 870–874.

Southam-Gerow, M. A., & Kendall, P. C. (2002). Emotion regulation and understanding: Implications for child psychopathology and therapy. *Clinical Psychology Review, 22,* 189–222.

Tamir, M., Chiu, C., & Gross, J. J. (2007). Business or pleasure?: Utilitarian versus hedonic considerations in emotion regulation. *Emotion, 7,* 546–554.

Tamir, M., John, O. P., Srivastava, S., & Gross, J. J. (2007). Implicit theories of emotion: Affective and social outcomes across a major life transition. *Journal of Personality and Social Psychology, 92,* 731–744.

Tang, Y., & Posner, M. I. (2009). Attention training and attention state training. *Trends in Cognitive Science, 13*, 222–227.

Tang, Y. Y., Ma, Y., Fan, Y., Feng, H., Wang, J., Feng, S., et al. (2009). Central and autonomic nervous system interaction is altered by short-term meditation. *Proceedings of the National Academy of Sciences USA, 106*, 8865–8870.

Tang, Y. Y., Ma, Y., Wang, J., Fan, Y., Feng, S., Lu, Q., et al. (2007). Short term meditation training improves attention and self regulation. *Proceedings of the National Academy of Sciences USA, 104*(43), 17152–17156.

Taylor, S. E., & Lobel, M. (1989). Social comparison activity under threat: Downward evaluation and upward contacts. *Psychological Review, 96*, 569–575.

Terracciano, A., Costa, P. T., Jr., & McCrae, R. R. (2005). Personality plasticity after age 30. *Personality and Social Psychology Bulletin, 32*, 999–1009.

Tesser, A. (2000). On the confluence of self-esteem maintenance mechanisms. *Personality and Social Psychology Review, 4*, 290–299.

Thayer, R. E., Newman, J. R., & McClain, T. M. (1994). Self-regulation of mood: Strategies for changing a bad mood, raising energy, and reducing tension. *Journal of Personality and Social Psychology, 67*, 910–925.

Tice, D. M., & Bratslavsky, E. (2000). Giving in to feel good: The place of emotion regulation in the context of general self-control. *Psychological Inquiry, 11*, 149–159.

Tice, D. M., Bratslavsky, E., & Baumeister, R. F. (2001). Emotional distress regulation takes precedence over impulse control: If you feel bad, do it! *Journal of Personality and Social Psychology, 80*, 53–67.

Tugade, M. M., & Frederickson, B. L. (2004). Resilient individuals use positive emotions to bounce back from negative emotional experiences. *Journal of Personality and Social Psychology, 86*, 320–333.

van Dillen, L. F., Heslenfeld, D., & Koole, S. L. (2009). Tuning down the emotional brain: An fMRI study of the effects of task load on the processing of negative and neutral images. *NeuroImage, 45*, 1212–1219.

van Dillen, L. F., & Koole, S. L. (2007). Clearing the mind: A working memory model of distraction from negative emotion. *Emotion, 7*, 715–723.

van Dillen, L. F., & Koole, S. L. (2009). How automatic is "automatic vigilance"?: Effects of working memory load on interference of negative emotional information. *Cognition and Emotion, 23*, 1106–1117.

Weinberger, D. A., Schwartz, G. E., & Davidson, R. J. (1979). Low-anxious, high-anxious and repressive coping styles: Psychometric patterns and behavioral and physiological responses to stress. *Journal of Abnormal Psychology, 88*, 369–380.

Westen, D. (1994). Toward an integrative model of affect regulation: Applications to social-psychological research. *Journal of Personality, 62*, 641–647.

Westen, D., Kilts, C., Blagov, P., Harenski, K., & Hamann, S. (2006). The neural basis of motivated reasoning: An fMRI study of emotional constraints on political judgment during the U.S. Presidential election of 2004. *Journal of Cognitive Neuroscience, 18*, 1947–1958.

CHAPTER 3

Giving In to Temptation
The Emerging Cognitive Neuroscience of Self-Regulatory Failure

DYLAN D. WAGNER
TODD F. HEATHERTON

When it comes to exercising self-control, it is often the case that inhibiting a behavior is more difficult than engaging in one. This occurs despite the fact that all one is required to do is, simply put, nothing. The deceptive ease with which people manage to avoid indulging every craving, voicing every thought, or giving in to the vicissitudes of every emotion belies the sheer amount of effort that must be expended to stay in control. Should people's ability to regulate themselves somehow be compromised, the damage to their social lives would be devastating. Even behaviors as trivial as not looking at a mole on an employer's face or not telling one's mother-in-law jokes involving brothels would be nigh impossible to resist. While, at first blush, it might seem unfathomable that people could suddenly be robbed of their self-control, the reality is that with certain brain injuries anyone could suffer from the deficits in self-regulation just described. We are all just one unlucky cerebrovascular stroke away from believing it a good idea to open a eulogy with a dirty limerick.

The neural substrates of self-regulatory ability have hitherto received little attention in self-regulation research. Of the varying disciplines that study self-regulation (e.g., developmental psychology, educational psychology, social psychology), nearly all have remained agnostic regarding the underlying neural mechanisms that allow self-regulation to occur. This is not to say there has not been research on the neuroscience of the elementary processes involved in self-regulation. Neuroscientists of many stripes have long studied the brain mechanisms that underlie elementary forms of motor and cognitive control, generally under the rubric of "executive function." However, this line of research seldom explores how these faculties play out in more complex situations, such as social interactions, controlling prejudices or inhibiting emotions—topics that more traditionally are under the purview of social psychologists. With the emergence of cognitive neuroscience in the 1980s this began to change as first developmental psychologists and, more recently, social psychologists began to look to the brain to further their understanding of the basic mechanisms involved in the phenomena they study (Cacioppo, Berntson, Sheridan, & McClintock, 2000; Johnson, 1997). It is not immediately clear why it took so long for self-regulation researchers to seek out neural mechanisms, as neurologists and neuropsychologists have long recognized the importance of the brain, particularly the frontal lobes, in the organization and regulation of behavior (e.g., Kleist, 1934). Reports of extraordinary cases of dysregulated social behavior following brain injury go back as far as the 19th century (Harlow, 1868; Welt, 1888), and many early neuropsychologists put the prefrontal cortex at the center of their theories of self-control (Fuster, 1980; Jarvie, 1954; Luria, 1960, 1973). Although neuropsychologists have made great strides in understanding the relationship between brain and behavior, it is often the case that these theories are blind to the social contexts in which most of our thoughts and actions are embedded. Only recently have researchers begun to apply modern cognitive neuroscience methods to the problem of how the brain makes self-regulation possible and, just as importantly, what happens in the brain when self-regulation fails.

In this chapter we present an overview of prefrontal brain systems supporting self-regulation in social and affective domains, with an emphasis on recent research demonstrating what happens in these brain regions when self-regulation breaks down. The prefrontal cortex (PFC) covers a large area of the frontal lobe and is involved in many processes, such as working memory, attention control, inhibiting prepotent responses, and planning—all of which fall under the umbrella term *executive function* (Miller & Cohen, 2001; Tranel, Anderson, & Benton, 1994). Although there is significant overlap between self-regulation and executive function, this chapter is principally concerned with the involvement of the PFC in self-regulation; that is, in controlling social behaviors, thoughts, emotions, and appetitive cravings (e.g., food and drugs). We begin by reviewing neuropsychological cases of self-regulation impairments following damage to each of the three principal divisions of the PFC, along with their basic neuroanatomy. Following this, we turn to studies of the neural substrates of self-regulation and self-regulatory failure across three domains: moods and emotions, thoughts and prejudices, and appetitive behaviors (e.g., food and drug cravings). Finally, we end by discussing the implications of this research for limited resource models of self-regulation.

NEUROPSYCHOLOGICAL INSIGHTS INTO THE FUNCTIONAL ORGANIZATION OF SELF-REGULATION

The most widely accepted definition of PFC is that it is the portion of the frontal lobe that lies anterior to primary and secondary motor cortex. The PFC, unlike other regions of the brain, is unique in that it shares connections with a wide range of systems involved in generating and modulating behavior (e.g., motor and sensory systems, subcortical regions involved in emotion and reward, and medial temporal regions involved in learning and memory). More than any other region, the PFC has a history of being associated with many of humankind's highest faculties. Initially it was thought that the PFC was the seat of human intelligence and that its large size relative to that of other species (Rilling, 2006) explained why human intellect far outstrips that of all other animals. This theory has waxed and waned over the last century as neuropsychologist continually fail to find any deficits of general intelligence in patients with frontal lobe lesions (Eslinger & Damasio, 1985; Hebb & Penfield, 1940; Stuss & Benson, 1986). More recently, it has been argued that fluid intelligence, the aspect of intelligence involved in reasoning and problem solving, is reliant upon the PFC. While there is some support for this theory (Duncan, Burgess, & Emslie, 1995), there is also compelling evidence that focal damage to any of the subregions of the frontal lobe has no effect whatsoever on measures of intelligence, fluid or otherwise (Tranel, Manzel, & Anderson, 2008). It seems that whatever it is the frontal lobes are doing, it is unlikely to be general intelligence.

Evidence that the PFC plays a critical role in organizing and controlling behavior stretches back as far as the mid-19th century (although less systematic accounts can be traced back to the 14th century; see Lanfranchi, 1315). Early case reports of patients with damage to the PFC revealed deficits so bizarre that many doubted their veracity. For example, the famous case of Phineas Gage was initially dismissed as a "Yankee invention" by a noted English surgeon of the time. Early case studies focused on the striking personality changes exhibited by these patients, with many examples of formerly pleasant people becoming profane, egoistic, and insensitive to social norms following damage to the PFC. Reflecting the general tone of these patients' behavior, one early observer termed this constellation of symptoms *Witzelsucht*, which roughly means facetiousness and refers to a patient's tendency to make inappropriate jokes (Oppenheim, 1890). Another type of symptom commonly observed after damage to the PFC was that of a dramatic loss of motivational drive. These patients had great difficulty with spontaneously generating behaviors and lacked initiative to such a degree that they often failed to wash or dress themselves. Early theorists of prefrontal function assumed these two distinct types of self-regulation failure were manifestations of the same underlying "prefrontal syndrome," but as diagnostic techniques improved and the number of patient studies increased, it became clear that the different neuropsychological deficits observed in these patients had their origin in damage to distinct regions of the PFC.

While there remains debate concerning the precise anatomical boundaries of the PFC and its subregions, researchers are largely in agreement on three principal subdivision of the PFC: the ventromedial PFC (VMPFC), the lateral PFC (LPFC; dorsal and ventral convexities), and the anterior cingulate cortex (ACC). Knowledge of the underlying pattern of anatomical connectivity between regions of the PFC is essential to understanding how these regions come together to make self-regulation possible. We turn now to an overview of the neuroanatomy and psychological changes wrought by damage to each of these three regions.

Ventromedial Prefrontal Cortex

The VMPFC consists primarily of the inferior aspect of the medial PFC and the orbitofrontal cortex, both of which are cytoarchitecturally similar structures (Ongur & Price, 2000). Patients with damage to the VMPFC have difficulty regulating social, affective, and appetitive behaviors. This is borne out by the connectivity pattern in the VMPFC, which is highly interconnected with subcortical limbic areas, such as the amygdala (Amaral & Price, 1984; Carmichael & Price, 1995). In addition, the VMPFC shares connections with reward-processing regions in the ventral striatum (Haber, Kunishio, Mizobuchi, & Lynd-Balta, 1995), as well as regions involved in appetite and visceral sensation, such as the hypothalamus and the insula (Barbas, Saha, Rempel-Clower, & Ghashghaei, 2003; Gabbott, Warner, Jays, & Bacon, 2003).

Prior to the 20th century there were few systematic studies of the changes in personality and behavior brought about by damage to the PFC. Most early examples are case studies, such as that of Phineas Gage, the American railroad foreman whose tamping iron (an iron bar approximately 3 inches in diameter) was propelled through his cranium when the explosive charge he had been preparing accidentally ignited. The rod's passing damaged the VMPFC and possibly a portion of the ACC (Damasio, Grabowski, Frank, Galaburda, & Damasio, 1994; Harlow, 1848). Remarkably, Gage survived the injury, though not without complications, as he acquired a near fatal infection during his convalescence (Macmillan, 2000). Gage's case is notable for being the earliest case of disinhibited behavior arising from a brain injury. Prior to his injury, Gage was amiable, honest, and reliable; however, following the accident, his personality underwent a radical alteration and was described as "gross, profane, coarse and vulgar, to such a degree that his society was intolerable to decent people" (Anonymous, 1851, p. 89; attributed to Harlow, see Macmillan, 2000). The importance of Gage's case to a theory of frontal lobe function was not immediately recognized and would have languished in obscure American medical journals had not the neurologist David Ferrier (1878) highlighted Gage's case in his prestigious Goulstonian Lecture, delivered to the Royal College of Physicians in London. While unquestionably important, the case of Phineas Gage does suffer from a paucity of evidence; the only known descriptions of his behavior are those written by his doctor, 8 years after Gage's death (Harlow, 1868).

A far more compelling case for social disinhibition following damage the VMPFC was made in 1888 by Leonore Welt, who describes the case of a man who sustained severe head trauma after falling 100 feet from a window. This patient showed personality changes similar to those of Phineas Gage, becoming cantankerous and threatening, and often playing cruel practical jokes on the other patients (Welt, 1888). Shortly after his release from the hospital, the patient succumbed to an unrelated illness and his brain was subject to a postmortem examination. Studying his brain, Welt found evidence of extensive VMPFC damage and posited that this injury was the source of the patient's personality changes. This particular case is important for being the first published report of a brain injury as the basis for a personality change and confirmation by postmortem examination; it inspired others to consider the importance of the precise location of damage to the etiology of personality changes following brain injury.

Since these early case reports, a large number of studies have confirmed the basic finding of social disinhibition following damage to the VMPFC. While initially neurologists had difficulty arriving at a precise description of the symptoms, focusing on certain aspects of the disorder, such as inappropriate humor and use of profanity (Jastrowitz, 1888; Oppenheim, 1890) or the tendency to boast (Brickner, 1934), display aggression (Rylander, 1939), steal and lie (Kleist, 1934), or engage in sexual exhibitionism (Ackerly, 1937), over time neuropsychologists converged on the view that damage to the VMPFC leads to a breakdown in self-control and restraint, with a particular emphasis on failure to obey social norms (Blumer & Benson, 1975; Jarvie, 1954).

In addition to difficulties controlling social behavior, these patients may also fail to regulate their primary physiological drives. For example, patients with damage to the VMPFC may engage in sexual exhibitionism and make inappropriate and occasionally aggressive sexual advances (Grafman et al., 1996; Hécaen, 1964; Jarvie, 1954; Rylander, 1939). There is also evidence of excessive overeating, leading to unhealthy weight gain (Erb, Gwirtsman, Fuster, & Richeimer, 1989; Kirschbaum, 1951; Woolley et al., 2007). Interestingly, these patients do not lack knowledge of common social norms (Saver & Damasio, 1991). Theirs is a problem not of memory but of maintaining control over their behavior in everyday situations.

Lateral Prefrontal Cortex

The LPFC, unlike the VMPFC, has no direct connections to limbic regions involved in emotion; instead the LPFC projects primarily to other regions in the PFC, namely, to secondary motor regions involved in action planning (Barbas & Pandya, 1987; Petrides & Pandya, 1999), as well as the VMPFC and ACC (McDonald, Mascagni, & Guo, 1996). Given this region's known role in elementary executive processes, such as working memory (Smith & Jonides, 1999) and inhibiting responses (Garavan, Ross, & Stein, 1999), it would appear that the LPFC, through its rich connections with ACC, VMPFC, and secondary motor areas, is principally involved in planning and maintaining behaviors. For self-regulation, this means holding regulatory strategies in mind and ensuring that these are not derailed by distractions, such as when a restrained eater suddenly finds him- or herself ambushed by appetizing foods.

Patients suffering from damage to lateral portions of the PFC present a very different symptomatology than do patients with VMPFC damage. These patients display profound difficulties in planning behavior and inhibiting goal-irrelevant distractions. Moreover, they often appear to lack motivation and seem listless and apathetic. One early case illustrating these deficits is described by the noted Canadian neurosurgeon Wilder Penfield and is of a patient who underwent a neurosurgical resection involving lateral portions of the PFC. Following recovery, it was noted that the patient demonstrated much difficulty playing games that involved the maintenance of multiple goals in memory, such as bridge (Penfield & Evans, 1935). Moreover, the patient appeared to lose all initiative, displaying a profound apathy toward seeking employment. This case is remarkably similar to one reported half a century later, in which a college student, having recovered from damage to the right PFC, repeatedly failed classes and eventually dropped out of college. He later reported that despite understanding the material, he simply could not muster the interest it would take to be successful (Stuss & Benson, 1986).

One of the more interesting cases of LPFC damage is that of Penfield's sister, on whom he himself performed the resection of a right prefrontal glioma. Following her recovery, Penfield noted no real change in her personality. Only later did Penfield observe that she displayed a profound difficulty in performing everyday household tasks. This was brought to his attention during a family gathering, in which Penfield's sister found herself confused by the task of preparing a meal (Penfield & Evans, 1935). It appeared that his sister suffered from an inability to plan complex tasks and to maintain the necessary steps in mind, leaving certain dishes unfinished and forgetting to begin others at the appropriate time.

Unlike patients with damage to the VMPFC, LPFC patients have no problem engaging in social interactions or understanding social and emotional cues (Bar-On, Tranel, Denburg, & Bechara, 2003). Their deficits are more in line with the core faculties of what has come to be known as *executive function* (Miller & Cohen, 2001), and their difficulty in organizing and regulating behavior can be traced to deficits in working memory, task switching, and inhibitory control. Accordingly, these patients have difficulty in tasks that have changing demands, and they often perseverate in behaviors that have become irrelevant to the current goals of the task (Barceló & Knight, 2002; Milner, 1963). These patients also perform poorly on tasks relying on inhibitory control. For instance, patients with LPFC damage are impaired on the Stroop task (Perret, 1974; Vendrell et al., 1995), in which they have to read the name of a color word printed in a conflicting ink color (e.g., the word *red* printed in blue ink). These patients also have difficulty generating novel items, such as nonverbalizable designs, and tend to perseverate on the same type of design throughout the task (Jones-Gotman & Milner, 1977).

Perhaps the best overall example of the constellation of deficits exhibited by patients with LPFC damage comes from observing their performance on everyday tasks outside the lab. In a cleverly designed study, Shallice and Burgess (1991) instructed patients to perform an array of real-world errands (e.g., shopping for items on a list, asking for directions, and meeting someone at a specified time) while being unobtrusively tailed by two observers who made note of their performance. The only rule the patients had to follow was that they could only enter shops in which they intended to purchase an item. As might be expected given Penfield's early observations of the deficits exhibited by his sister, these patients showed a remarkable inability to complete even the most rudimentary daily errands. Errors committed by the patients included failing to purchase items on their list, entering the same shop multiple times, and leaving a shop without paying (Shallice & Burgess, 1991). This clever, real-world neuropsychological test serves to illustrate how the many facets of LPFC function must work together to allow us to accomplish even the most mundane of goal-directed behaviors.

Anterior Cingulate Cortex

The ACC is the rostral portion of cingulate cortex resting above the corpus callosum. It is interconnected with a wide range of brain structures involved in cognition, emotion, and motor execution. However, unlike other regions of the PFC, the ACC receives little input from regions involved in sensory processing (Carmichael & Price, 1995). The ACC is intimately connected to the LPFC and VMPFC, and the adjacent motor cortex. In addition, the ACC shares many important connections with limbic regions involved in emotion, and ventral striatal regions implicated in reward processing (Ongur, An, & Price, 1998; Vogt & Pandya, 1987). In many ways the ACC sits at the anatomical crossroads of cognitive control, affective control, motor planning, and arousal, and thus is ideally suited to exert an influence over these regions in response to environmental demands (Paus, 2001).

Knowledge of the cognitive and behavioral effects of ACC damage is constrained by the relative paucity of patients with pure focal damage to the ACC. It is uncommon for this region to be damaged in closed-head injuries, and damage caused by strokes tends to encroach upon surrounding cortex (e.g., the medial PFC and secondary motor cortices). One source of information regarding ACC function comes from patients who have undergone cingulotomies for the treatment of intractable pain or psychiatric disorders (Ballantine, Cassidy, Flanagan, & Marino, 1967; Corkin, 1979; Le Beau & Pecker, 1949; Whitty, Duffield, Tow, & Cairns, 1952).

One of the most catastrophic disorders to arise from damage to the ACC is akinetic mutism, in which patients suffer from a devastating inability to spontaneously generate actions or speech (Barris & Schuman, 1953). Patients with akinetic mutism do not suffer from paralysis; rather, they have a striking inability to generate behaviors. They rarely move, eat only if fed, and speak only when directly asked a question. Moreover, they display little or no emotion and fail to withdraw from painful stimuli. This disorder arises primarily when the ACC and adjacent supplementary motor areas suffer extensive damage. Cases of focal ACC damage are similar in character but far less catastrophic (Laplane, Degos, Baulac, & Gray, 1981). These cases of relatively pure ACC damage are marked by a general apathy, blunted affect, and difficulty in maintaining goal-directed behavior (Cohen, Kaplan, Moser, Jenkins, & Wilkinson, 1999; Cohen, Kaplan, Zuffante, et al., 1999; Cohen, McCrae, & Phillips, 1990; Laplane et al., 1981; Wilson & Chang, 1974). Family members report that these patients appear to have lost their "drive" and frequently note a dramatic loss of interest in activities and hobbies the patient formerly found pleasurable (Cohen, Kaplan, Moser, et al., 1999; Tow & Whitty, 1953). On the surface, many of these symptoms appear similar to those of patients with damage to lateral portions of the PFC. However, patients with damage to the ACC are characterized primarily by their loss of motivational drive, and while similar symptoms occur in patients with LPFC damage, they are not nearly as severe.

Given the paucity of patients with focal ACC damage, much of the theorizing concerning ACC function is built upon recent findings from cognitive neuroscience. One of the most consistent findings from brain activation studies is that the ACC is involved in detecting conflict among competing responses and monitoring for errors in performance (Carter et al., 1998; Gehring & Knight, 2000; MacDonald, Cohen, Stenger, & Carter, 2000; for a review, see Carter & van Veen, 2007). This has led many to theorize that the primary role of the ACC is to detect situations where response conflict is likely and then to signal the need for increased cognitive control, such as when overriding habitual behaviors or overcoming temptations (Botvinick, Braver, Barch, Carter, & Cohen, 2001; Kerns et al., 2004; Paus, 2001; Peterson et al., 1999). Moreover, it is hypothesized that under situations of cognitive conflict, the ACC communicates directly with the LPFC to bring current behavior in line with overarching goals (Ridderinkhof, Ullsperger, Crone, & Nieuwenhuis, 2004).

THE COGNITIVE NEUROSCIENCE
OF SELF-REGULATION AND SELF-REGULATORY FAILURE

In the previous section we reviewed neuropsychological case studies demonstrating the roles of VMPFC, LPFC, and ACC in self-regulation. This research demonstrates that damage to any one of these regions can have catastrophic effects on a person's ability to regulate behaviors across a variety of domains, from following social norms to carrying out mundane, everyday tasks (e.g., cooking a meal or shopping for groceries). The ability to maintain our goals in mind, to correct for errors in performance and, ultimately, to bring our thoughts and behaviors in line with our intentions, relies on the complex interplay between each of the aforementioned PFC regions. Careful study of the deficits exhibited by patients with focal brain damage can give us important insights into the underlying cognitive operations that these damaged regions normally support. However, to understand how the healthy PFC enables self-regulation and what happens in the brain when self-regulation fails, as it so often does, we must turn to the study of healthy populations and the methods of cognitive neuroscience.

Myriad methods have been employed to answer these questions. Commonly used techniques such as functional magnetic resonance imaging (fMRI) and positron emission tomography (PET) allow for the localization of brain activity to specific regions, with a relatively high degree of spatial resolution. Other methods, such as cortical morphometry and diffusion tensor imaging, allow researchers to study the relationship between cognition and structural metrics (e.g., thickness of cortical gray matter). In the following section we examine how these methods have been used to investigate the neural substrates of self-regulation in three separate domains: emotions, thoughts and stereotypes, and appetitive behaviors. In addition, we highlight recent research examining what happens in the brain when self-regulation breaks down.

Neural Bases of Emotion Regulation

Keeping emotions in check is a vital part of maintaining harmonious social relationships. Were our ability to do so suddenly knocked out, our relationships would likely turn very ugly indeed. Research on the neural substrates of this complex ability has honed in on a model of emotion regulation involving top-down regulation by the PFC of limbic regions involved in affect (Davidson, Putnam, & Larson, 2000; Ochsner & Gross, 2005; see McRae, Ochsner & Gross, Chapter 10, this volume). A consistent finding across a wide range of studies is an inverse correlation between the PFC and activity in the amygdala, a limbic region sensitive to emotionally arousing stimuli. The precise region of PFC involved in modulating the amgydala varies across studies but is invariably either the LPFC (Hariri, Mattay, Tessitore, Fera, & Weinberger, 2003; Ochsner, Bunge, Gross, & Gabrieli, 2002; Ochsner et al., 2004) or the VMPFC (Johnstone, van Reekum, Urry, Kalin, & Davidson, 2007; Urry et al., 2006). In light of our earlier discussion of the anatomical connectivity of these two regions, specifically regarding the fact that the LPFC has no direct connections to limbic regions, it would appear that the LPFC exerts its regulatory influence indirectly. Recent evidence for this indirect pathway was reported by Johnstone and colleagues (2007), who found that the relationship between LPFC and the amygdala during emotion regulation is mediated by the VMPFC.

Additional support for a critical role of the VMPFC in regulating limbic regions comes from research examining the relationship between individual differences in emotion regulation and the morphometry (e.g., cortical thickness, gray matter density) of the VMPFC. In one such study, the authors employed a fear extinction paradigm whereby participants were exposed to a cue that was formerly paired with a shock while psychophysiological measures of arousal (e.g., skin conductance) were collected. The magnitude of the arousal response upon being reexposed to the cue (now no longer predictive of shock) was inversely correlated with the thickness of the cortical manifold in VMPFC (Milad et al., 2005). Put another way, increased VMPFC thickness predicted greater extinction of fear-related memories. A similar correlation was found between the ability to regulate negative emotion and cortical gray matter density in the VMPFC (Mak, Wong, Han & Lee, 2009).

Mood disorders, such as major depressive disorder (MDD) and borderline personality disorder (BPD), present interesting cases of impaired emotion regulation. Research on patients with these mood disorders has consistently shown a breakdown in the inverse functional coupling between VMPFC and the amygdala, leading to exaggerated activation of the amygdala in response to negative emotional material (Donegan et al., 2003;

Johnstone et al., 2007; Silbersweig et al., 2007). This finding of a dysfunctional VMPFC–amygdala circuit finds additional support in a recent study of patients with BPD, using FDG-PET, a neuroimaging method that allows for the measurement of resting glucose metabolism. In contrast to healthy controls, patients with BPD showed no coupling of metabolism in the VMPFC and amygdala (New et al., 2007). These findings demonstrate that even when patients with BPD are not actively regulating emotions, the normal functional coupling between the VMPFC and amygdala is impaired.

A final example of the uncoupling of this VMPFC–amygdala circuit comes from a study of the deleterious effects of sleep deprivation on emotion regulation. In this research, sleep-deprived and control participants underwent fMRI scanning while viewing negative emotional material. As in the patients with mood disorders mentioned earlier, sleep-deprived patients demonstrated an exaggerated amygdala response compared to control participants and impaired functional connectivity between the VMPFC and amygdala (Yoo, Gujar, Hu, Jolesz, & Walker, 2007).

Social psychological research on self-regulation has a long history of studying the deleterious effects of emotion regulation (specifically, emotion inhibition) on participants' subsequent ability to perform tasks requiring self-regulation (Vohs, Baumeister, & Ciarocco, 2005; Vohs & Heatherton, 2000). Given these findings, it is reasonable to expect that tasks requiring effortful self-regulation might lead to a subsequent impairment in emotion regulation. A recent brain imaging study from our lab suggests that this is indeed the case. In this study, participants were assigned to one of two groups, one of which was required to engage in a difficult attention control task (modeled after the video in Baumeister, Bratslavsky, Muraven, & Tice, 1998) prior to viewing negative emotional material. The control group performed the same set of tasks and watched the same video, but without being required to control attention. Compared to controls, we found that participants whose self-regulatory resources were depleted by the attention control task showed reduced recruitment of LPFC regions involved in emotion regulation and an exaggerated amygdala response to neutral emotional material (Wagner & Heatherton, 2010). While not strictly in accord with the research on patients with mood disorder, described earlier, these findings do suggest that emotion regulation draws from the same limited resource as other acts of self-regulation, a possibility we discuss at greater length later in the chapter.

Regulation of Thoughts and Prejudices

As reviewed earlier, damage to the VMPFC can lead to disinhibited social behavior, characterized by inappropriate humor (e.g., *Witzelsucht*), verbal threats, and even aggressive sexual advances. It is an unsettling prospect to consider that the only thing keeping us from expressing this form of "acquired sociopathy" (Damasio, Tranel, & Damasio, 1990) is a relatively small patch of cortex in the front of the brain. The paucity of case reports of VMPFC damage leading to "acquired benevolence" or exaggerated prosocial behavior raises the specter that without the ability to regulate our thoughts, we would find that teeming underneath the veneer of civility lies a predominantly selfish and puerile mind. Fortunately, people are generally adept at controlling their thoughts and overriding their prejudices. Nevertheless, many of life's most dreaded moments occur during those lapses in control, when suddenly we realize that telling our mother-in-law what we really think of her favorite political party is probably not such a good idea.

Cognitive neuroscientists have long studied the neural basis of response inhibition, relying primarily on the go/no-go task, in which certain cues indicate a go response (usually a button press), while others require the participant to inhibit responding. Research using this task has consistently found activation in both the ACC and LPFC (Casey et al., 1997; Kiehl, Liddle, & Hopfinger, 2000). The ACC in particular is thought to be involved in response competition between conflicting cues, and in monitoring for errors in performance, while activity in the LPFC reflects the actual inhibition of responses during the no-go trials (Liddle, Kiehl, & Smith, 2001). Surprisingly, few attempts have been made to apply this framework to the problem of thought suppression.

In the first study to examine the neural substrates of actively suppressing thoughts, Wyland, Kelley, Macrae, Gordon, and Heatherton (2003) found increased ACC activity during periods of active thought suppression compared to periods of unrestrained thought. One problem with interpreting these results is that because subjects were not instructed to report thought intrusions during the suppression period, it is unclear whether ACC activity was related to failures of thought suppression or was instead signaling the need for additional cognitive control (see Botvinick et al., 2001). To parse out these two interpretations, Mitchell and colleagues (2007) conducted a similar study. However, this time, participants were instructed to respond whenever they experienced intrusions of a prespecified thought. Results from this study are in agreement with the previously described research on response inhibition, demonstrating increased activity in the LPFC during periods of thought suppression, while the ACC was found to respond only during instances of thought intrusions. These findings provide converging evidence that the ACC monitors for conflict, while the LPFC is involved in actively regulating and suppressing thoughts (Mitchell et al., 2007).

Controlling attitudes and prejudices differs from thought regulation in that stereotypes are often automatically activated upon encountering outgroup members (Devine, 1989; Devine, Plant, Amodio, Harmon-Jones, & Vance, 2002; Fiske, 1998; Greenwald, McGhee, & Schwartz, 1998; Payne, 2001). Moreover, outgroup members, particularly racial outgroup members, are often perceived as threatening (Brewer, 1999; cf. Ackerman et al., 2006). Research examining the neural correlates of prejudice has largely focused on prefrontal top-down regulation of amygdala activity to members of a racial outgroup, although similar findings exist for members of stigmatized groups, such as unattractive people and the obese (Krendl, Macrae, Kelley, Fugelsang, & Heatherton, 2006). An important factor to keep in mind when reviewing this research is that people differ in implicit racial attitudes, and this difference has been shown to moderate amygdala activity in response to racial outgroup members (Cunningham et al., 2004; Phelps et al., 2000). An excellent example of this comes from a study examining the depleting effects of interracial interactions on the propensity to recruit control regions of the PFC when evaluating racial outgroup members. In this study, participants engaged in an interracial interaction with a black confederate, in which they were asked to discuss racially charged topics. Following the interaction, participants completed a Stroop task. Interestingly, participants with more negative implicit attitudes toward blacks showed decreased performance on the Stroop task, indicating that, for them, the interracial interaction was cognitively depleting. Participants also participated in an ostensibly unrelated fMRI study in which they viewed black and white faces. As with other similar studies (e.g., Cunningham et al., 2004), they showed increased recruitment of the LPFC and ACC when viewing black faces. More importantly, activity in these regions was positively correlated with both participants' scores on the Implicit Association Test (IAT) and with their Stroop interference scores (Richeson et al., 2003). These results suggest that for those with fewer implicit attitudes toward blacks, there is less need to recruit PFC regions involved in cognitive control to override stereotypes that they simply do not seem to have.

Social psychological models of person categorization (e.g., Devine, 1989; Fiske, 1998; Lepore & Brown, 1997) posit that upon perceiving an outgroup member, stereotypes and attitudes concerning that group are automatically activated and lead to prejudicial behavior unless inhibitory processes act to override these stereotypes. Interestingly, many of the neuroscience findings on race-related brain activation share striking similarities with this framework. For instance, in a study of race evaluation, Cunningham and colleagues (2004) found evidence for top-down regulation of the amygdala by regions of the PFC during explicit processing of black faces (525-millisecond exposure) but not during implicit processing (30-millisecond exposure). Amygdala activity during the implicit condition was greatest for black faces; however, during explicit presentation, activity in the amygdala failed to differentiate between black and white faces. Instead they found greater recruitment of the LPFC to black faces, and this LPFC activity was inversely correlated with activity in the amygdala (Cunningham et al., 2004). These results are interpreted as indicating that the amygdala response to black faces is largely automatic, but it can be inhibited by the LPFC if participants are aware of the stimulus. This finding maps onto social psychological models of person categorization, whereby amygdala activity reflects automatic activation of racially biased attitudes that must then be actively regulated by the LPFC to override these automatic stereotypes.

Control of Cravings and Appetitive Behaviors

That we are able to take the time to read dry academic chapters when we could be running around in a hedonistic frenzy, smoking, drinking, or gorging ourselves on the chocolate opulence to be found at the nearest supermarket is a testament to our ability to regulate our appetitive desires. Of course, we do not always do this very well, and when our cravings get the better of us, unhealthy addictions may form.

While much attention has been paid to the disinhibited social behavior and poor decision making displayed by patients with VMPFC damage, another equally noteworthy class of symptoms is the difficulty these patients show in inhibiting appetitive behaviors. For instance, patients with VMPFC damage may engage in sexual exhibitionism (Ackerly, 1937), or aggressive sexual advances (Grafman et al., 1996; Hécaen, 1964) and may in some cases also present with excessive overeating (e.g., hyperphagia) (Erb et al., 1989). A similar pattern is found in patients with frontotemporal dementia, an occasional symptom of which is unrestrained eating. Moreover, the magnitude of hyperphagia exhibited by these patients has been linked to the degree of cortical degeneration in the VMPFC (Woolley et al., 2007).

As noted earlier, the VMPFC and ACC share many reciprocal connections with midbrain regions that are important for reward (e.g., nucleus accumbens). The nucleus accumbens, along with the ventral tegmental area (VTA), form part of what is known as the *mesolimbic dopamine system*. Both animal neurophysiology and human neuroimaging work have shown that a universal feature of rewarding stimuli, be they natural rewards or drugs of abuse, is that they activate dopamine release in the nucleus accumbens (Boileau et al., 2003; Carelli, Ijames, & Crumling, 2000; Di Chiara & Imperato, 1988; Imperato &

Di Chiara, 1986; Pfaus et al., 1990; Schilstrom, Svensson, Svensson, & Nomikos, 1998; Solinas et al., 2002) or, in the case of neuroimaging work, lead to increased activation in this same region (Berns, McClure, Pagnoni, & Montague, 2001; Breiter et al., 1997; O'Doherty, Dayan, Friston, Critchley, & Dolan, 2003; Stein et al., 1998; Zubieta et al., 2005). This holds true even when participants are simply viewing photographic "cues" of rewarding stimuli, such as attractive members of the opposite sex (Cloutier, Heatherton, Whalen, & Kelley, 2008), erotic images (Karama et al., 2002) or images of drugs (David et al., 2007; Garavan et al., 2000; Myrick et al., 2008). This paradigm, given the name *cue reactivity*, has become an important tool in research on the neural correlates of craving and control in drug addicts (Childress et al., 1999; Garavan et al., 2000; Maas et al., 1998; Wexler et al., 2001), smokers (David et al., 2007; Due, Huettel, Hall, & Rubin, 2002), and obese persons (Rothemund et al., 2007; Stoeckel et al., 2008). Finally, a number of studies have shown that cue-related brain activity is predictive of self-reported cravings for the desired items (McClernon, Hiott, Huettel, & Rose, 2005; Myrick et al., 2008; Wang et al., 2004). Furthermore, a recent study from our lab has extended these findings to show that cue-related activity in the nucleus accumbens to appetizing food images is predictive of weight gain 6 months later (Demos, Kelley, & Heatherton, in press). However, it is unclear at present whether this represents a failure to recruit top-down control regions in the PFC, or whether the participants who gained weight display an exaggerated sensitivity to the reward value of food items (cf. Beaver et al., 2006).

What happens when participants try to inhibit their response to food or drug cues? As might be expected from results in other domains, self-regulation of appetitive desires recruits PFC control systems regardless of whether the rewarding stimulus is food (Stoeckel et al., 2008), erotic images (Beauregard, Levesque, & Bourgouin, 2001), or drugs (Brody et al., 2007; David et al., 2005; Garavan et al., 2000; Wrase et al., 2002). Moreover, activity in these regions appears to be related to whether people are successful at inhibiting cravings. For example, successful dieters have been shown to spontaneously recruit the LPFC when viewing images of appetizing foods, whereas unsuccessful dieters do not (DelParigi et al., 2007). This finding suggests that what makes these dieters successful is that they appear to spontaneously recruit regulatory regions in response to food cues, and that this automatic regulation strategy helps to control food cravings.

A pervasive finding in research on restrained eating is that forcing chronic dieters to break their diet, usually by having them consume a high-calorie milkshake "preload," can lead to bouts of unrestrained eating (Heatherton, Herman, & Polivy, 1991, 1992; Heatherton, Polivy, Herman, & Baumeister, 1993; Herman & Mack, 1975). This has been shown primarily to be a cognitive effect, as dieters who are told that the preload contains few calories do not subsequently overeat (Polivy, 1976). Theories of drug addiction suggest that the reason why drug addicts fail to control their consumption is that midbrain reward areas become hypersensitized to drug cues (Stoeckel et al., 2008) and are uncoupled from top-down control regions in the PFC (Bechara, 2005; Koob & Le Moal, 1997, 2008). This theory was tested by a recent study from our lab in which we compared cue reactivity to appetizing foods in restrained and unrestrained eaters. Half of the participants in each group drank a high-calorie milkshake preload, effectively breaking the restrained eaters' diets. Interestingly, activity in the nucleus accumbens mirrored the behavioral findings mentioned earlier (e.g., Heatherton et al., 1991, 1992; Herman & Mack, 1975). Restrained eaters whose diets were broken by the milkshake preload demonstrated increased food-cue-related activity in the nucleus accumbens compared to both unrestrained eaters and restrained eaters whose diet had not been broken (Demos et al., in press). Moreover, restrained eaters showed greater activity in LPFC regions involved in top-down control, but this did not differentiate between persons whose diets had been broken and those whose diets were still intact. This last finding suggests that restrained eaters whose diets have been broken are still recruiting top-down control regions, but these regions have become uncoupled from midbrain reward areas and are no longer able to effectively regulate food cue reactivity.

An interesting proposition that has emerged from recent theorizing about the underlying mechanism of self-regulatory strength is whether a person can be buffered from self-regulatory breakdown by an artificial increase in self-regulatory resources. The theory in question posits that effortful self-regulation relies on current levels of circulating blood glucose (Gailliot & Baumeister, 2007). Early findings have shown that administering glucose after an effortful self-regulation task mitigates the depletion effects that this task would otherwise produce (Gailliot et al., 2007). We sought to investigate this proposition by examining food-cue-related brain activity in restrained eaters who underwent self-regulatory depletion. In this study, half of the participants were given a high-glucose lemonade drink and the other half, a similar-tasting artificially sweetened lemonade drink. Participants were unaware of the nature of the drink manipulation and were simply told that we were interested in the effects of hydration on brain activity. Thus, if self-regulation relies on glucose stores, which become depleted by acts of effortful self-regulation, then administering glucose should reduce the impact of self-regulatory depletion on food cue reactivity in restrained eaters. Results from this study replicated our earlier findings, in that participants who drank the artificially sweetened lemonade (i.e., did not received glucose) showed increased food cue reactivity following self-regulatory resource depletion by an effortful emotion inhibition task (Heatherton, Demos, Amble, & Wagner, 2010). The participants in the glucose condition, on the other hand, failed to show this exaggerated nucleus accumbens response and instead demonstrated increased activity in prefrontal control systems (e.g., the VMPFC and the ACC). These findings suggest that, indeed, glucose does buffer against the effects of self-regulatory depletion, allowing people to maintain self-regulatory focus despite continued effort expenditure.

IMPLICATIONS FOR A LIMITED RESOURCE MODEL OF SELF-REGULATION

Successful regulation of thoughts, emotions, and cravings relies on a common system of prefrontal control regions that comprise the ACC, the LPFC, and the VMPFC. Although we addressed each of these domains in isolation, there is ample evidence that self-regulation relies on a domain-general resource that can become depleted by successive attempts at self-regulation (Baumeister & Heatherton, 1996; Muraven & Baumeister, 2000; Vohs & Heatherton, 2000). The new research reviewed in this chapter on the cognitive neuroscience of self-regulatory failure supports this depletion model of self-regulation. For instance, we saw that expending self-regulatory resources on a difficult attention control task leads to reduced recruitment of LPFC and to impaired emotion regulation (Wagner & Heatherton, 2010). Similarly, depleting self-regulatory resources in restrained eaters (this time using an emotion regulation task) leads to reduced recruitment of the PFC (ACC and VMPFC) and exaggerated food-cue-related activity in the nucleus accumbens (Heatherton et al., 2010).

That engaging in self-regulation in one domain can impair self-regulation in a wholly different domain is not in itself a new finding. Behavioral research on self-regulation has shown that engaging in an effortful emotion suppression task can break diets (Vohs & Heatherton, 2000) and lead to poor impression management during interpersonal interactions (Vohs et al., 2005). Similarly, having participants engage in effortful thought suppression impairs impulse control and leads participants to consume more alcohol (Muraven, Collins, & Nienhaus, 2002) while having participants engage in an interracial interaction can impair performance on subsequent tests of executive function (Richeson & Shelton, 2003). Although still in its infancy, what research on the brain basis of self-regulation failure adds to this model is the finding that self-regulatory depletion works by reducing or disrupting PFC regions involved in top-down control. Over a number of studies we have consistently seen that a signature of self-regulatory failure appears to be a failure to appropriately engage control systems in the PFC.

But what exactly is the resource whose depletion leads to reduced PFC recruitment? One suggestion, hinted at earlier, is that successful self-regulation relies on adequate levels of circulating blood glucose (Gailliot & Baumeister, 2007). In a series of behavioral experiments, Gailliot and colleagues (2007) have shown that engaging in effortful self-regulation tasks reduces circulating blood glucose levels, and that artificially raising these levels not only eliminates the effects of self-regulatory depletion on a subsequent cognitive task (Gailliot et al., 2007) but also reduces expressions of prejudice (Gaillot, Peruche, Plant, & Baumeister, 2009). As discussed earlier, recent research from our lab has similarly shown that giving participants a glucose drink prior to a depletion task reduces the impact of depletion on PFC activity. Participants in the glucose condition continued to recruit PFC to regulate food-cue-related responses in midbrain control areas, while participants in the artificial sweetener condition did not (Heatherton et al., 2010).

The application of this theory to self-regulation is recent; however, the impact of glucose on cognitive performance has a long history. For instance, prior research has demonstrated that administering glucose improves performance on memory tasks (Benton & Owens, 1993) and on tasks requiring response inhibition (Benton, Owens, & Parker, 1994). That glucose is consumed during effortful tasks should also come as no surprise because glucose metabolism is the primary contrast in neuroimaging research using PET. Moreover, a common finding in PET research is that of greater glucose metabolism as task difficulty increases (Jonides et al., 1997). Thus, it seems likely that self-regulatory resource depletion occurs because effortful tasks temporarily reduce brain glucose stores. Moreover, since tasks that require self-regulation, by definition, require the range of control functions ascribed to the PFC, depletion effects should be greatest when both the depleting task and the subsequent self-regulation task recruit the same region of the brain. While this has yet to be tested, PET neuroimaging, with its ability to directly measure glucose metabolism, is an ideal method for investigating the link between local glucose depletion and subsequent impairments in self-regulation.

CONCLUSIONS

Failure to maintain control over one's thoughts, emotions, and desires can have disastrous consequences for the individual. Patients with focal damage to the PFC present an extreme case of what life would be like without the ability to regulate our behaviors.

Clinical case studies have provided essential clues to the cognitive operations subserved by the PFC. However, to understand the complex interplay between regions of the PFC involved in initiating, planning, and regulating behavior necessitates a cognitive neuroscience approach. In this chapter we focused on three distinct regions of the PFC and how findings from cognitive neuroscience shed light on their role in self-regulation. First is the VMPFC, which shares important reciprocal connections with subcortical regions involved in emotion and reward, and is critical for regulating behavior in social, affective, and appetitive domains; second is the LPFC, which, with its important role in core aspects of executive function (e.g., working memory), is necessary for planning behavior and maintaining regulatory goals; and finally, the ACC, a region that is richly interconnected with cognitive, affective, and motor regions, monitors our performance and signals the need for recruiting control systems to regulate our behavior.

In this chapter we put special emphasis on recent work investigating what happens in the brain when regulatory systems fail. The general framework that emerges from this research is that lapses in control lead to a breakdown of prefrontal down-regulation of stimulus-driven responses in subcortical regions involved in emotion, threat, and reward. This breakdown of top-down control can lead to a host of undesirable behaviors, such as mood disorders, drug addiction, and racial prejudice.

Perhaps the most successful way to induce self-regulatory failure has been through the depletion of self-regulatory resources. Although still in its infancy, the neuroscience of self-regulatory failure has shown promising results. Moreover, as our understanding of the brain systems involved in self-regulation failure matures, we find ourselves forced to consider the question: Just what exactly is being depleted? One possible theory that might explain these findings is that self-regulation relies on circulating blood glucose. We reviewed behavioral and neuroscientific research on the effects of glucose depletion and of glucose load on self-regulation, and concluded that this theory shows much promise. In summary, we look forward to research on the brain basis of self-regulatory failure, in the hope that it will shed light on why we fail at self-control and what we can do to become better at it.

REFERENCES

Ackerly, S. (1937). Instinctive, emotional and mental changes following prefrontal lobe extirpation. *American Journal of Psychiatry, 92,* 717–729.

Ackerman, J. M., Shapiro, J. R., Neuberg, S. L., Kenrick, D. T., Becker, D. V., Griskevicius, V., et al. (2006). They all look the same to me (unless they're angry): From out-group homogeneity to out-group heterogeneity. *Psychological Science, 17*(10), 836–840.

Amaral, D. G., & Price, J. L. (1984). Amygdalo-cortical projections in the monkey (*Macaca fascicularis*). *Journal of Comparative Neurology, 230*(4), 465–496.

Anonymous. (1851). Remarkable case of injury. *American Phrenological Journal, 13,* 89.

Ballantine, H. T., Jr., Cassidy, W. L., Flanagan, N. B., & Marino, R., Jr. (1967). Stereotaxic anterior cingulotomy for neuropsychiatric illness and intractable pain. *Journal of Neurosurgery, 26*(5), 488–495.

Barbas, H., & Pandya, D. N. (1987). Architecture and frontal cortical connections of the premotor cortex (Area 6) in the rhesus monkey. *Journal of Comparative Neurology, 256*(2), 211–228.

Barbas, H., Saha, S., Rempel-Clower, N., & Ghashghaei, T. (2003). Serial pathways from primate prefrontal cortex to autonomic areas may influence emotional expression. *BMC Neuroscience, 4,* 25.

Barceló, F., & Knight, R. T. (2002). Both random and perseverative errors underlie WCST deficits in prefrontal patients. *Neuropsychologia, 40*(3), 349–356.

Bar-On, R., Tranel, D., Denburg, N. L., & Bechara, A. (2003). Exploring the neurological substrate of emotional and social intelligence. *Brain, 126*(Pt. 8), 1790–1800.

Barris, R. W., & Schuman, H. R. (1953). Bilateral anterior cingulate gyrus lesions: Syndrome of the anterior cingulate gyri. *Neurology, 3*(1), 44–52.

Baumeister, R. F., Bratslavsky, E., Muraven, M., & Tice, D. M. (1998). Ego depletion: Is the active self a limited resource? *Journal of Personality and Social Psychology, 74*, 1252–1265.

Baumeister, R. F., & Heatherton, T. F. (1996). Self-regulation failure: An overview. *Psychological Inquiry, 7*(1), 1–15.

Beauregard, M., Levesque, J., & Bourgouin, P. (2001). Neural correlates of conscious self-regulation of emotion. *Journal of Neuroscience, 21*(18), RC165.

Beaver, J. D., Lawrence, A. D., van Ditzhuijzen, J., Davis, M. H., Woods, A., & Calder, A. J. (2006). Individual differences in reward drive predict neural responses to images of food. *Journal of Neuroscience, 26*(19), 5160–5166.

Bechara, A. (2005). Decision making, impulse control and loss of willpower to resist drugs: A neurocognitive perspective. *Nature Neuroscience, 8*(11), 1458–1463.

Benton, D., & Owens, D. S. (1993). Blood glucose and human memory. *Psychopharmacology, 113*(1), 83–88.

Benton, D., Owens, D. S., & Parker, P. Y. (1994). Blood glucose influences memory and attention in young adults. *Neuropsychologia, 32*(5), 595–608.

Berns, G. S., McClure, S. M., Pagnoni, G., & Montague, P. R. (2001). Predictability modulates human brain response to reward. *Journal of Neuroscience, 21*(8), 2793–2798.

Blumer, D., & Benson, D. (1975). Personality changes with frontal and temporal lesions. In *Psychiatric aspects of neurologic disease* (pp. 151–169). New York: Grune & Stratton.

Boileau, I., Assaad, J. M., Pihl, R. O., Benkelfat, C., Leyton, M., Diksic, M., et al. (2003). Alcohol promotes dopamine release in the human nucleus accumbens. *Synapse, 49*(4), 226–231.

Botvinick, M. M., Braver, T. S., Barch, D. M., Carter, C. S., & Cohen, J. D. (2001). Conflict monitoring and cognitive control. *Psychological Review, 108*(3), 624–652.

Breiter, H. C., Gollub, R. L., Weisskoff, R. M., Kennedy, D. N., Makris, N., Berke, J. D., et al. (1997). Acute effects of cocaine on human brain activity and emotion. *Neuron, 19*(3), 591–611.

Brewer, M. B. (1999). The psychology of prejudice: Ingroup love or outgroup hate? *Journal of Social Issues, 55*, 429–444.

Brody, A. L., Mandelkern, M. A., Olmstead, R. E., Jou, J., Tiongson, E., Allen, V., et al. (2007). Neural substrates of resisting craving during cigarette cue exposure. *Biological Psychiatry, 62*(6), 642–651.

Cacioppo, J. T., Berntson, G. G., Sheridan, J. F., & McClintock, M. K. (2000). Multilevel integrative analyses of human behavior: Social neuroscience and the complementing nature of social and biological approaches. *Psychological Bulletin, 126*(6), 829–843.

Carelli, R. M., Ijames, S. G., & Crumling, A. J. (2000). Evidence that separate neural circuits in the nucleus accumbens encode cocaine versus "natural" (water and food) reward. *Journal of Neuroscience, 20*(11), 4255–4266.

Carmichael, S. T., & Price, J. L. (1995). Limbic connections of the orbital and medial prefrontal cortex in macaque monkeys. *Journal of Comparative Neurology, 363*(4), 615–641.

Carter, C. S., Braver, T. S., Barch, D. M., Botvinick, M. M., Noll, D., & Cohen, J. D. (1998). Anterior cingulate cortex, error detection, and the online monitoring of performance. *Science, 280*, 747–749.

Carter, C. S., & van Veen, V. (2007). Anterior cingulate cortex and conflict detection: An update of theory and data. *Cognitive, Affective, and Behavioral Neuroscience, 7*(4), 367–379.

Casey, B. J., Trainor, R. J., Orendi, J. L., Schubert, A. B., Nystrom, L. E., Giedd, J. N., et al. (1997). A developmental functional MRI study of prefrontal activation during performance of a go/no-go task. *Journal of Cognitive Neuroscience, 9*(6), 835–847.

Childress, A. R., Mozley, P. D., McElgin, W., Fitzgerald, J., Reivich, M., & O'Brien, C. P. (1999). Limbic activation during cue-induced cocaine craving. *America Journal of Psychiatry, 156*(1), 11–18.

Cloutier, J., Heatherton, T. F., Whalen, P. J., & Kelley, W. M. (2008). Are attractive people rewarding?: Sex differences in the neural substrates of facial attractiveness. *Journal of Cognitive Neuroscience, 20*(6), 941–951.

Cohen, R. A., Kaplan, R. F., Moser, D. J., Jenkins, M. A., & Wilkinson, H. (1999). Impairments of attention after cingulotomy. *Neurology, 53*(4), 819–824.

Cohen, R. A., Kaplan, R. F., Zuffante, P., Moser, D. J., Jenkins, M. A., Salloway, S., et al. (1999). Alteration of intention and self-initiated action associated with bilateral anterior cingulotomy. *Journal of Neuropsychiatry and Clinical Neuroscience, 11*(4), 444–453.

Cohen, R. A., McCrae, V., & Phillips, K. (1990). Neurobehavioral consequences of bilateral medial cingulotomy (Abstract). *Neurology, 40*(Suppl. 1), A198.

Corkin, S. (1979). Hidden-figures-test performance: Lasting effects of unilateral penetrating head injury and transient effects of bilateral cingulotomy. *Neuropsychologia, 17*(6), 585–605.

Cunningham, W. A., Johnson, M. K., Raye, C. L., Gatenby, J. C., Gore, J. C., & Banaji, M. R. (2004). Separable neural components in the processing of black and white faces. *Psychological Science, 15*(12), 806–813.

Damasio, A. R., Tranel, D., & Damasio, H. (1990). Individuals with sociopathic behavior caused by frontal damage fail to respond autonomically to social stimuli. *Behavioural Brain Research, 41*(2), 81–94.

Damasio, H., Grabowski, T., Frank, R., Galaburda, A. M., & Damasio, A. R. (1994). The Return of Gage, Phineas: Clues about the brain from the skull of a famous patient. *Science, 264*, 1102–1105.

David, S. P., Munafo, M. R., Johansen-Berg, H., Mackillop, J., Sweet, L. H., Cohen, R. A., et al. (2007). Effects of acute nicotine abstinence on cue-elicited ventral striatum/nucleus accumbens activation in female cigarette smokers: A functional magnetic resonance imaging study. *Brain Imaging and Behavior, 1*(3–4), 43–57.

David, S. P., Munafo, M. R., Johansen-Berg, H., Smith, S. M., Rogers, R. D., Matthews, P. M., et al. (2005). Ventral striatum/nucleus accumbens activation to smoking-related pictorial cues in smokers and nonsmokers: A functional magnetic resonance imaging study. *Biological Psychiatry, 58*(6), 488–494.

Davidson, R. J., Putnam, K. M., & Larson, C. L. (2000). Dysfunction in the neural circuitry of emotion regulation—a possible prelude to violence. *Science, 289*, 591–594.

DelParigi, A., Chen, K., Salbe, A. D., Hill, J. O., Wing, R. R., Reiman, E. M., et al. (2007). Successful dieters have increased neural activity in cortical areas involved in the control of behavior. *International Journal of Obesity (London), 31*(3), 440–448.

Demos, K. E., Kelley, W. M., & Heatherton, T. F. (in press). Dietary restraint violations influence reward responses in nucleus accumbens and amygdala. *Journal of Cognitive Neuroscience.*

Devine, P. G. (1989). Stereotypes and prejudice—their automatic and controlled components. *Journal of Personality and Social Psychology, 56*(1), 5–18.

Devine, P. G., Plant, E. A., Amodio, D. M., Harmon-Jones, E., & Vance, S. L. (2002). The regulation of explicit and implicit race bias: The role of motivations to respond without prejudice. *Journal of Personality and Social Psychology, 82*(5), 835–848.

Di Chiara, G., & Imperato, A. (1988). Drugs abused by humans preferentially increase synaptic dopamine concentrations in the mesolimbic system of freely moving rats. *Proceedings of the National Academy of Sciences USA, 85*(14), 5274–5278.

Donegan, N. H., Sanislow, C. A., Blumberg, H. P., Fulbright, R. K., Lacadie, C., Skudlarski, P., et al. (2003). Amygdala hyperreactivity in borderline personality disorder: Implications for emotional dysregulation. *Biological Psychiatry, 54*(11), 1284–1293.

Due, D. L., Huettel, S. A., Hall, W. G., & Rubin, D. C. (2002). Activation in mesolimbic and visuospatial neural circuits elicited by smoking cues: Evidence from functional magnetic resonance imaging. *American Journal of Psychiatry, 159*(6), 954–960.

Duncan, J., Burgess, P., & Emslie, H. (1995). Fluid intelligence after frontal lobe lesions. *Neuropsychologia, 33*(3), 261–268.

Erb, J. L., Gwirtsman, H. E., Fuster, J. M., & Richeimer, S. H. (1989). Bulimia associated with frontal-lobe lesions. *International Journal of Eating Disorders, 8*(1), 117–121.

Eslinger, P. J., & Damasio, A. R. (1985). Severe disturbance of higher cognition after bilateral frontal lobe ablation: Patient EVR. *Neurology, 35*(12), 1731–1741.

Ferrier, D. (1878). The Goulstonian Lectures on the localisation of cerebral diseases. *British Medical Journal, 1*, 443–447.

Fiske, S. T. (1998). Stereotyping, prejudice, and discrimination. In D. T. Gilbert, S. T. Fiske, & G. Lindzey (Eds.), *Handbook of social psychology* (Vol. 2, pp. 357–411). Boston: McGraw-Hill.

Fuster, J. M. (1980). *The prefrontal cortex.* New York: Raven.

Gabbott, P. L., Warner, T. A., Jays, P. R., & Bacon, S. J. (2003). Areal and synaptic interconnectivity of prelimbic (Area 32), infralimbic (Area 25) and insular cortices in the rat. *Brain Research, 993*(1–2), 59–71.

Gailliot, M. T., & Baumeister, R. F. (2007). The physiology of willpower: Linking blood glucose to self-control. *Personality and Social Psychology Review, 11*(4), 303–327.

Gailliot, M. T., Baumeister, R. F., DeWall, C. N., Maner, J. K., Plant, E. A., Tice, D. M., et al. (2007). Self-control relies on glucose as a limited energy source: Willpower is more than a metaphor. *Journal of Personality and Social Psychology, 92*(2), 325–336.

Gailliot, M. T., Peruche, B. M., Plant, E. A., & Baumeister, R. F. (2009). Stereotypes and prejudice in the blood: Sucrose drinks reduce prejudice and stereotyping. *Journal of Experimental Social Psychology, 45*(1), 288–290.

Garavan, H., Pankiewicz, J., Bloom, A., Cho, J. K., Sperry, L., Ross, T. J., et al. (2000). Cue-induced cocaine craving: Neuroanatomical specificity for drug users and drug stimuli. *American Journal of Psychiatry, 157*(11), 1789–1798.

Garavan, H., Ross, T. J., & Stein, E. A. (1999). Right hemispheric dominance of inhibitory control: An event-related functional MRI study. *Proceedings of the National Academy of Sciences USA, 96*(14), 8301–8306.

Gehring, W. J., & Knight, R. T. (2000). Prefrontal–cingulated interactions in action monitoring. *Nature Neuroscience, 3*(5), 516–520.

Grafman, J., Schwab, K., Warden, D., Pridgen, A., Brown, H. R., & Salazar, A. M. (1996). Frontal lobe injuries, violence, and aggression: A report of the Vietnam Head Injury Study. *Neurology, 46*(5), 1231–1238.

Greenwald, A. G., McGhee, D. E., & Schwartz, J. L. (1998). Measuring individual differences in implicit cognition: The implicit association test. *Journal of Personality and Social Psychology, 74*(6), 1464–1480.

Haber, S. N., Kunishio, K., Mizobuchi, M., & Lynd-Balta, E. (1995). The orbital and medial prefrontal circuit through the primate basal ganglia. *Journal of Neuroscience, 15*(7, Pt. 1), 4851–4867.

Hariri, A. R., Mattay, V. S., Tessitore, A., Fera, F., & Weinberger, D. R. (2003). Neocortical modulation of the amygdala response to fearful stimuli. *Biological Psychiatry, 53*(6), 494–501.

Harlow, J. M. (1848). Passage of an iron rod through the head. *Boston Medical and Surgical Journal, 39*, 389–393.

Harlow, J. M. (1868). Recovery from the passage of an iron bar through the head. *Publications of the Massachusetts Medical Society, 2,* 327–347.

Heatherton, T. F., Demos, K. E., Amble, C., & Wagner, D. D. (2010). *Administering glucose protects against the effects of self-regulatory depletion: An fMRI study.* Unpublished manuscript, Dartmouth College, Hanover, NH.

Heatherton, T. F., Herman, C. P., & Polivy, J. (1991). Effects of physical threat and ego threat on eating behavior. *Journal of Personality and Social Psychology, 60*(1), 138–143.

Heatherton, T. F., Herman, C. P., & Polivy, J. (1992). Effects of distress on eating: The importance of ego-involvement. *Journal of Personality and Social Psychology, 62*(5), 801–803.

Heatherton, T. F., Polivy, J., Herman, C. P., & Baumeister, R. F. (1993). Self-awareness, task failure, and disinhibition: How attentional focus affects eating. *Journal of Personality, 61*(1), 49–61.

Hebb, D. O., & Penfield, W. (1940). Human behavior after extensive bilateral removal from the frontal lobes. *Archives of Neurology and Psychiatry, 44,* 421–438.

Hécaen, H. (1964). Mental symptoms associated with tumors of the frontal lobe. In J. M. Warren & K. Ackert (Eds.), *The frontal granular cortex and behavior* (pp. 335–352). New York: McGraw-Hill.

Herman, C. P., & Mack, D. (1975). Restrained and unrestrained eating. *Journal of Personality, 43*(4), 647–660.

Imperato, A., & Di Chiara, G. (1986). Preferential stimulation of dopamine release in the nucleus accumbens of freely moving rats by ethanol. *Journal of Pharmacology and Experimental Therapeutics, 239*(1), 219–228.

Jarvie, H. F. (1954). Frontal lobe wounds causing disinhibition: A study of six cases. *Journal of Neurology, Neurosurgery and Psychiatry, 17,* 14–32.

Jastrowitz, J. (1888). Beitrage zur Lokalisation im Grosshirn und uber deren praktische Verwerthung [Contributions to localization in the cerebrum and their practical evaluation]. *Deutsche Medizinische Wochenschrift, 24,* 108–112.

Johnson, M. H. (1997). *Developmental cognitive neuroscience: An introduction.* Cambridge, MA: Blackwell.

Johnstone, T., van Reekum, C. M., Urry, H. L., Kalin, N. H., & Davidson, R. J. (2007). Failure to regulate: Counterproductive recruitment of top-down prefrontal–subcortical circuitry in major depression. *Journal of Neuroscience, 27*(33), 8877–8884.

Jones-Gotman, M., & Milner, B. (1977). Design fluency: The invention of nonsense drawings after focal cortical lesions. *Neuropsychologia, 15*(4–5), 653–674.

Jonides, J., Schumacher, E. H., Smith, E. E., Lauber, E. J., Awh, E., Minoshima, S., et al. (1997). Verbal working memory load affects regional brain activation as measured by PET. *Journal of Cognitive Neuroscience, 9*(4), 462–475.

Karama, S., Lecours, A. R., Leroux, J. M., Bourgouin, P., Beaudoin, G., Joubert, S., et al. (2002). Areas of brain activation in males and females during viewing of erotic film excerpts. *Human Brain Mapping, 16*(1), 1–13.

Kerns, J. G., Cohen, J. D., MacDonald, A. W., III, Cho, R. Y., Stenger, V. A., & Carter, C. S. (2004). Anterior cingulate conflict monitoring and adjustments in control. *Science, 303,* 1023–1026.

Kiehl, K. A., Liddle, P. F., & Hopfinger, J. B. (2000). Error processing and the rostral anterior cingulate: An event-related fMRI study. *Psychophysiology, 37*(02), 216–223.

Kirschbaum, W. R. (1951). Excessive hunger as a symptom of cerebral origin. *Journal of Nervous and Mental Disease, 113,* 95–114.

Kleist, K. (1934). *Gehirnpathologie.* Leipzig: Barth.

Koob, G. F., & Le Moal, M. (1997). Drug abuse: Hedonic homeostatic dysregulation. *Science, 278,* 52–58.

Koob, G. F., & Le Moal, M. (2008). Addiction and the brain antireward system. *Annual Review of Psychology, 59*, 29–53.

Krendl, A. C., Macrae, C. N., Kelley, W. M., Fugelsang, J. A., & Heatherton, T. F. (2006). The good, the bad, and the ugly: An fMRI investigation of the functional anatomic correlates of stigma. *Social Neuroscience, 1*(1), 5–15.

Lanfranchi, G. (1315). *Chirurgia magna.* London: Marshe.

Laplane, D., Degos, J. D., Baulac, M., & Gray, F. (1981). Bilateral infarction of the anterior cingulate gyri and of the fornices: Report of a case. *Journal of the Neurological Sciences, 51*(2), 289–300.

Le Beau, J., & Pecker, J. (1949). La topectomie péricalleuse antérieure dans certaines formes d'agitation psychomotrice au cours de l'épilepsie et de l'arriération mentale [Bilateral anterior pericallosal topectomy in the treatment of certain forms of psychomotor seizures in epilepsy]. *Revue Neurologique, 81*, 1039–1041.

Lepore, L., & Brown, R. (1997). Category and stereotype activation: Is prejudice inevitable? *Journal of Personality and Social Psychology, 72*, 275–287.

Liddle, P. F., Kiehl, K. A., & Smith, A. M. (2001). An event-related fMRI study of response inhibition. *Human Brain Mapping, 12*(2), 100–109.

Luria, A. R. (1960). Verbal regulation of behavior. In *The central nervous system and behavior; transactions.* Madison, NJ: Conference on the Central Nervous System and Behavior.

Luria, A. R. (1973). The frontal lobes and the regulation of behavior. In K. H. Pribam & A. R. Luria (Eds.), *Psychophysiology of the frontal lobes* (pp. 3–28). New York: Academic Press.

Maas, L. C., Lukas, S. E., Kaufman, M. J., Weiss, R. D., Daniels, S. L., Rogers, V. W., et al. (1998). Functional magnetic resonance imaging of human brain activation during cue-induced cocaine craving. *American Journal of Psychiatry, 155*(1), 124–126.

Macmillan, M. (2000). *An odd kind of fame: Stories of Phineas Gage.* Cambridge, MA: MIT Press.

Mak, A. K. Y., Wong, M. M. C., Han, S., & Lee, T. M. C. (2009). Gray matter reduction associated with emotion regulation in female outpatients with major depressive disorder: A voxel-based morphometry study. *Progress in Neuropsychopharmacology and Biological Psychiatry, 33*(7), 1184–1190.

McClernon, F. J., Hiott, F. B., Huettel, S. A., & Rose, J. E. (2005). Abstinence-induced changes in self-report craving correlate with event-related FMRI responses to smoking cues. *Neuropsychopharmacology, 30*(10), 1940–1947.

MacDonald, A. W., Cohen, J. D., Stenger, V. A., & Carter, C. S. (2000). Dissociating the role of dorsolateral prefrontal and anterior cingulated cortex in cognitive control. *Science, 288*, 1835–1838.

McDonald, A. J., Mascagni, F., & Guo, L. (1996). Projections of the medial and lateral prefrontal cortices to the amygdala: A *Phaseolus vulgaris* leucoagglutinin study in the rat. *Neuroscience, 71*(1), 55–75.

Milad, M. R., Quinn, B. T., Pitman, R. K., Orr, S. P., Fischl, B., & Rauch, S. L. (2005). Thickness of ventromedial prefrontal cortex in humans is correlated with extinction memory. *Proceedings of the National Academy of Sciences USA, 102*(30), 10706.

Miller, E. K., & Cohen, J. D. (2001). An integrative theory of prefrontal cortex function. *Annual Review of Neuroscience, 24*, 167–202.

Milner, B. (1963). Effects of different brain lesions on card sorting. *Archives of Neurology, 9*, 90–100.

Mitchell, J. P., Heatherton, T. F., Kelley, W. M., Wyland, C. L., Wegner, D. M., & Macrae, C. N. (2007). Separating sustained from transient aspects of cognitive control during thought suppression. *Psychological Science, 18*(4), 292–297.

Muraven, M., & Baumeister, R. F. (2000). Self-regulation and depletion of limited resources: Does self-control resemble a muscle? *Psychological Bulletin, 126*(2), 247–259.

Muraven, M., Collins, R. L., & Nienhaus, K. (2002). Self-control and alcohol restraint: An initial application of the self-control strength model. *Psychology of Addictive Behaviors, 16*(2), 113–120.

Myrick, H., Anton, R. F., Li, X., Henderson, S., Randall, P. K., & Voronin, K. (2008). Effect of naltrexone and ondansetron on alcohol cue-induced activation of the ventral striatum in alcohol-dependent people. *Archives of General Psychiatry, 65*(4), 466–475.

New, A. S., Hazlett, E. A., Buchsbaum, M. S., Goodman, M., Mitelman, S. A., Newmark, R., et al. (2007). Amygdala–prefrontal disconnection in borderline personality disorder. *Neuropsychopharmacology, 32*(7), 1629–1640.

O'Doherty, J. P., Dayan, P., Friston, K., Critchley, H., & Dolan, R. J. (2003). Temporal difference models and reward-related learning in the human brain. *Neuron, 38*(2), 329–337.

Ochsner, K. N., Bunge, S. A., Gross, J. J., & Gabrieli, J. D. (2002). Rethinking feelings: An fMRI study of the cognitive regulation of emotion. *Journal of Cognitive Neuroscience, 14*(8), 1215–1229.

Ochsner, K. N., & Gross, J. J. (2005). The cognitive control of emotion. *Trends in Cognitive Sciences, 9*(5), 242–249.

Ochsner, K. N., Ray, R. D., Cooper, J. C., Robertson, E. R., Chopra, S., Gabrieli, J. D., et al. (2004). For better or for worse: Neural systems supporting the cognitive down- and up-regulation of negative emotion. *NeuroImage, 23*(2), 483–499.

Ongur, D., An, X., & Price, J. L. (1998). Prefrontal cortical projections to the hypothalamus in macaque monkeys. *Journal of Comparative Neurology, 401*(4), 480–505.

Ongur, D., & Price, J. L. (2000). The organization of networks within the orbital and medial prefrontal cortex of rats, monkeys and humans. *Cerebral Cortex, 10*(3), 206–219.

Oppenheim, H. (1890). Zur Pathologie der Grosshirngeschwülste [On the pathology of cerebral tumors]. *Archiv für Psychiatrie und Nervenkrankheiten, 22,* 27–72.

Paus, T. (2001). Primate anterior cingulate cortex: Where motor control, drive and cognition interface. *Nature Reviews Neuroscience, 2*(6), 417–424.

Payne, B. K. (2001). Prejudice and perception: The role of automatic and controlled processes in misperceiving a weapon. *Journal of Personality and Social Psychology, 81*(2), 181–192.

Penfield, W., & Evans, J. (1935). The frontal lobe in man: A clinical study of maximum removals. *Brain, 58,* 115–133.

Perret, E. (1974). The left frontal lobe of man and the suppression of habitual responses in verbal categorical behaviour. *Neuropsychologia, 12*(3), 323–330.

Peterson, B. S., Skudlarski, P., Gatenby, J. C., Zhang, H., Anderson, A. W., & Gore, J. C. (1999). An fMRI study of Stroop word–color interference: Evidence for cingulate subregions subserving multiple distributed attentional systems. *Biological Psychiatry, 45*(10), 1237–1258.

Petrides, M., & Pandya, D. N. (1999). Dorsolateral prefrontal cortex: Comparative cytoarchitectonic analysis in the human and the macaque brain and corticocortical connection patterns. *European Journal of Neuroscience, 11*(3), 1011–1036.

Pfaus, J. G., Damsma, G., Nomikos, G. G., Wenkstern, D. G., Blaha, C. D., Phillips, A. G., et al. (1990). Sexual behavior enhances central dopamine transmission in the male rat. *Brain Research, 530*(2), 345–348.

Phelps, E. A., O'Connor, K. J., Cunningham, W. A., Funayama, E. S., Gatenby, J. C., Gore, J. C., et al. (2000). Performance on indirect measures of race evaluation predicts amygdala activation. *Journal of Cognitive Neuroscience, 12*(5), 729–738.

Polivy, J. (1976). Perception of calories and regulation of intake in restrained and unrestrained subjects. *Addictive Behaviors, 1*(3), 237–243.

Richeson, J. A., Baird, A. A., Gordon, H. L., Heatherton, T. F., Wyland, C. L., Trawalter, S., et al. (2003). An fMRI investigation of the impact of interracial contact on executive function. *Nature Neuroscience, 6*(12), 1323–1328.

Richeson, J. A., & Shelton, J. N. (2003). When prejudice does not pay: Effects of interracial contact on executive function. *Psychological Science, 14*(3), 287–290.

Ridderinkhof, K. R., Ullsperger, M., Crone, E. A., & Nieuwenhuis, S. (2004). The role of the medial frontal cortex in cognitive control. *Science, 306,* 443–447.

Rilling, J. K. (2006). Human and nonhuman primate brains: Are they allometrically scaled versions of the same design? *Evolutionary Anthropology, 15*(2), 65–77.

Rothemund, Y., Preuschhof, C., Bohner, G., Bauknecht, H. C., Klingebiel, R., Flor, H., et al. (2007). Differential activation of the dorsal striatum by high-calorie visual food stimuli in obese individuals. *NeuroImage, 37*(2), 410–421.

Rylander, G. (1939). *Personality changes after operations on the frontal lobes.* Copenhagen: Munksgaard.

Saver, J. L., & Damasio, A. R. (1991). Preserved access and processing of social knowledge in a patient with acquired sociopathy due to ventromedial frontal damage. *Neuropsychologia, 29*(12), 1241–1249.

Schilstrom, B., Svensson, H. M., Svensson, T. H., & Nomikos, G. G. (1998). Nicotine and food induced dopamine release in the nucleus accumbens of the rat: Putative role of alpha7 nicotinic receptors in the ventral tegmental area. *Neuroscience, 85*(4), 1005–1009.

Shallice, T., & Burgess, P. W. (1991). Deficits in strategy application following frontal lobe damage in man. *Brain, 114*(2), 727–741.

Silbersweig, D., Clarkin, J. F., Goldstein, M., Kernberg, O. F., Tuescher, O., Levy, K. N., et al. (2007). Failure of frontolimbic inhibitory function in the context of negative emotion in borderline personality disorder. *American Journal of Psychiatry, 164*(12), 1832–1841.

Smith, E. E., & Jonides, J. (1999). Storage and executive processes in the frontal lobes. *Science, 283,* 1657–1661.

Solinas, M., Ferre, S., You, Z. B., Karcz-Kubicha, M., Popoli, P., & Goldberg, S. R. (2002). Caffeine induces dopamine and glutamate release in the shell of the nucleus accumbens. *Journal of Neuroscience, 22*(15), 6321–6324.

Stein, E. A., Pankiewicz, J., Harsch, H. H., Cho, J. K., Fuller, S. A., Hoffmann, R. G., et al. (1998). Nicotine-induced limbic cortical activation in the human brain: A functional MRI study. *American Journal of Psychiatry, 155*(8), 1009–1015.

Stoeckel, L. E., Weller, R. E., Cook, E. W., III, Twieg, D. B., Knowlton, R. C., & Cox, J. E. (2008). Widespread reward-system activation in obese women in response to pictures of high-calorie foods. *NeuroImage, 41*(2), 636–647.

Stuss, D. T., & Benson, D. F. (1986). *The frontal lobes.* New York: Raven Press.

Tow, P. M., & Whitty, C. W. (1953). Personality changes after operations on the cingulate gyrus in man. *Journal of Neurology, Neurosurgery and Psychiatry, 16*(3), 186–193.

Tranel, D., Anderson, S. W., & Benton, A. (1994). Development of the concept of "executive function" and its relationship to the frontal lobes. In *Handbook of neuropsychology* (pp. 125–148). Amsterdam: Elsevier.

Tranel, D., Manzel, K., & Anderson, S. W. (2008). Is the prefrontal cortex important for fluid intelligence?: A neuropsychological study using matrix reasoning. *Clinical Neuropsychologist, 22*(2), 242–261.

Urry, H. L., van Reekum, C. M., Johnstone, T., Kalin, N. H., Thurow, M. E., Schaefer, H. S., et al. (2006). Amygdala and ventromedial prefrontal cortex are inversely coupled during regulation of negative affect and predict the diurnal pattern of cortisol secretion among older adults. *Journal of Neuroscience, 26*(16), 4415–4425.

Vendrell, P., Junque, C., Pujol, J., Jurado, M. A., Molet, J., & Grafman, J. (1995). The role of prefrontal regions in the Stroop task. *Neuropsychologia, 33*(3), 341–352.

Vogt, B. A., & Pandya, D. N. (1987). Cingulate cortex of the rhesus monkey: II. Cortical afferents. *Journal of Comparative Neurology, 262*(2), 271–289.

Vohs, K. D., Baumeister, R. F., & Ciarocco, N. J. (2005). Self-regulation and self-presentation:

Regulatory resource depletion impairs impression management and effortful self-presentation depletes regulatory resources. *Journal of Personality and Social Psychology, 88*(4), 632–657.

Vohs, K. D., & Heatherton, T. F. (2000). Self-regulatory failure: A resource-depletion approach. *Psychological Science, 11*(3), 249–254.

Wagner, D. D., & Heatherton, T. F. (2010). *Expending cognitive effort leads to emotion dysregulation.* Manuscript submitted for publication.

Wang, G. J., Volkow, N. D., Telang, F., Jayne, M., Ma, J., Rao, M., et al. (2004). Exposure to appetitive food stimuli markedly activates the human brain. *NeuroImage, 21*(4), 1790–1797.

Welt, L. (1888). Uber charakterveranderungen der menschen infolge von lasionen des stirnhirn [On changes in character as a consequence of lesions of the frontal lobe]. *Deutsches Archiv für Klinische Medizin, 42,* 339–390.

Wexler, B. E., Gottschalk, C. H., Fulbright, R. K., Prohovnik, I., Lacadie, C. M., Rounsaville, B. J., et al. (2001). Functional magnetic resonance imaging of cocaine craving. *American Journal of Psychiatry, 158*(1), 86–95.

Whitty, C. W. M., Duffield, J. E., Tow, P. M., & Cairns, H. (1952). Anterior cingulectomy in the treatment of mental disease. *Lancet, 1,* 475–481.

Wilson, D. H., & Chang, A. E. (1974). Bilateral anterior cingulectomy for the relief of intractable pain: Report of 23 patients. *Confinia Neurologica, 36*(1), 61–68.

Woolley, J. D., Gorno-Tempini, M. L., Seeley, W. W., Rankin, K., Lee, S. S., Matthews, B. R., et al. (2007). Binge eating is associated with right orbitofrontal–insular–striatal atrophy in frontotemporal dementia. *Neurology, 69*(14), 1424–1433.

Wrase, J., Grusser, S. M., Klein, S., Diener, C., Hermann, D., Flor, H., et al. (2002). Development of alcohol-associated cues and cue-induced brain activation in alcoholics. *European Psychiatry, 17*(5), 287–291.

Wyland, C. L., Kelley, W. M., Macrae, C. N., Gordon, H. L., & Heatherton, T. F. (2003). Neural correlates of thought suppression. *Neuropsychologia, 41*(14), 1863–1867.

Yoo, S. S., Gujar, N., Hu, P., Jolesz, F. A., & Walker, M. P. (2007). The human emotional brain without sleep—a prefrontal amygdala disconnect. *Current Biology, 17*(20), R877–R878.

Zubieta, J. K., Heitzeg, M. M., Xu, Y., Koeppe, R. A., Ni, L., Guthrie, S., et al. (2005). Regional cerebral blood flow responses to smoking in tobacco smokers after overnight abstinence. *American Journal of Psychiatry, 162*(3), 567–577.

CHAPTER 4

Self-Regulatory Strength

ISABELLE M. BAUER
ROY F. BAUMEISTER

The answer to the perennial question of what facilitates individual and cultural success might be found in the concept of self-regulation. The benefits of successful self-regulation are great and its costs can be dire. Failures of self-regulation are at the root of many personal and societal ills, such as interpersonal violence, self-defeating behaviors, substance abuse, poor health, underachievement, and obesity (e.g., Tangney, Baumeister, & Boone, 2004). The consequences of failed self-control can therefore create enormous social and economic costs, thus placing a heavy burden on society. In contrast, effective self-regulation allows individuals and cultures to thrive by promoting moral, disciplined, and virtuous behaviors. For example, successful self-regulation allows people to subordinate short-term temptations to long-term goals, to trade the pleasure of immediate gratification for delayed rewards, and to tolerate the frustration that can be associated with persisting in the face of challenges or hard work. Effective self-regulation is also necessary to restrain selfish wishes that could threaten group interests, to curb hostile and aggressive impulses that can undermine prosocial goals, and to overcome natural proclivities that are inherently self-interested for a greater collective good. In light of the personal and social benefits of good self-control, it is perplexing why self-regulation fails so often despite many people's valiant efforts and strong motivation to conquer their instincts and temptations for the sake of behaviors associated with long-term rewards that promote success in life.

To account for such failures of self-control, the limited strength model of self-regulation suggests that people are equipped with a limited supply of willpower that is dedicated to acts of self-control and other operations of the executive system (Baumeister & Heatherton, 1996; Baumeister, Heatherton, & Tice, 1994; Baumeister, Muraven, & Tice, 2000; Baumeister, Vohs, & Tice, 2007; Muraven & Baumeister, 2000; Vohs et al., 2008). Each act of self-control draws from this limited supply, leaving less available for subsequent acts that require self-regulation or the self's active intervention. When this resource becomes depleted, people become vulnerable to self-control failures. In light of the potential personal and social consequences of failed self-control, self-regulatory resources might therefore be vital to the successful development of individuals and collectivities.

SELF-REGULATION AND SELF-REGULATORY STRENGTH

Self-control or *self-regulation* (terms that we use interchangeably) is defined as the capacity to override natural and automatic tendencies, desires, or behaviors; to pursue long-term goals, even at the expense of short-term attractions; and to follow socially prescribed norms and rules. In other words, self-regulation is the capacity to alter the self's responses to achieve a desired state or outcome that otherwise would not arise naturally. Thus, the goal of self-control is to interrupt the self's tendency to operate on automatic pilot and to steer behavior consciously in a desired direction.

Self-regulation can be conceptualized from various perspectives. One influential model of self-regulation describes this capacity in terms of *feedback loops* (known as TOTE loops, an acronym for test–operate–test–exit) (Carver & Scheier, 1981, 1998). According to this model, people evaluate (or test) their current state in relation to internal standards. When a discrepancy between the desired and current states is detected, people can initiate actions to eliminate this discrepancy. Once the discrepancy is reduced, the self-regulation process enters the exit phase and is terminated.

The construct of *self-regulatory strength* is relevant at the stage when a person has detected a discrepancy and is ready to initiate actions to reduce it. At this point, the person must have the inner psychological resources (i.e., self-regulatory strength) necessary to alter behavior in a way that will bring him or her closer to internal standards or goals. This form of self-regulation is one important function of the executive system, which also subsumes other forms of volitional and active capabilities of the self, including planning and problem solving, goal-directed behavior, decision making, as well as logical and intelligent thought. According to the strength model, depletion of limited self-regulatory resources should selectively undermine the controlled and deliberate operations of the executive system, while sparing those involving automatic processes. In brief, the depletion of self-regulatory resources is contingent upon the operations of the active but not the passive self.

The colloquial equivalent of self-regulatory strength is *willpower*. Based on the limited strength model, willpower is in limited supply. Thus, faulty self-regulation stems from the depletion of resources following acts of self-regulation or other executive functions that all draw on this common energy supply. In light of this, the concept of self-regulatory strength, or willpower, has been compared to muscle strength. Like a muscle that grows tired and weak after being exercised, the capacity for self-control also weakens with repeated attempts at self-control.

Competing models of self-regulation have been proposed. For example, one model views the capacity for self-regulation as a skill that remains constant and unchanged across consecutive attempts at self-control, and that can be increased gradually over time through practice. An alternative model conceptualizes self-regulation as a knowledge structure or schema that, when activated or primed, should make available other information that supports self-regulatory goals through the process of spreading activation.

The activation of self-regulation schemas should further support subsequent behaviors that require self-control. Based on the skill and cognitive schema models, self-regulation should be unchanged or facilitated (respectively) after an initial act of self-control rather than being hindered, as the strength model would predict.

These three models of self-regulation have been pitted against each other in several empirical investigations. Contrary to the skill and cognitive schema models, findings have confirmed that self-regulation suffers after an initial attempt at self-control, suggesting that an act of self-control consumes some limited resource. The resulting self-regulatory failures support the strength model of self-regulation, and this phenomenon has been dubbed *ego depletion*. In the following sections, we present research guided by the limited strength model that has identified key operations of the executive system that are reliant on limited self-regulatory resources.

SELF-REGULATORY STRENGTH: EMPIRICAL EVIDENCE

Two decades of research have now discredited the popular wisdom that people can freely control their behaviors, suppress their impulses, conquer their temptations, or overcome their vices if only they put their mind to it, try harder, and persist. Research supporting the limited and exhaustible nature of self-regulation resources is based on a standard paradigm involving the assignment of participants to one of two conditions. In the self-control (depletion) condition, participants perform a task that requires the expenditure of self-control resources, while participants in the control (no-depletion) condition perform an equivalent task that does not require self-control. For example, on the Stroop task, participants in the depletion group have to override the natural tendency to read words in order to name the color of the ink in which the words are printed instead (e.g., the word *blue* printed in red), while participants in the control condition read words that match the ink colors. On the attention control task, participants in the depletion condition watch a silent video of a woman being interviewed with instructions to avoid attending to words flashed at the bottom of the screen, while control participants are instructed to watch the video as if they were watching television. Following the initial task, all participants perform another task that requires self-control, and their performance on this task represents the dependent measure of depletion.

The limited strength model of self-control predicts that depleted participants should perform more poorly on the dependent measure of self-control in comparison to participants in the control condition. The depletion effect has been found to be robust, and it has been documented consistently using various independent and dependent measures of self-control, and by independent research teams across the world. This research has also shown that the types of responses and behaviors that draw on and are sensitive to depletion of self-regulatory resources are varied: They include the regulation of emotions, the control of temptations and impulses, the suppression of thoughts, and the inhibition of stereotypes.

Early evidence in support of the idea that willpower is in limited supply came from a study in which participants were tempted by the aroma of freshly baked chocolate cookies (Baumeister, Bratslavsky, Muraven, & Tice, 1998; Muraven, Tice, & Baumeister, 1998). One group of participants was instructed to resist the urge to sample the cookies but could eat radishes instead, a task that required self-regulation. Their performance was contrasted with that of participants in two different control conditions in which self-control was not required. Participants in one control group were allowed to eat the chocolate treats without constraints, while the other control group was not presented with a food temptation. Results indicated that participants who were forbidden to eat the cookies gave up more quickly on a subsequent unsolvable figure-tracing task in comparison to participants in both control groups, thus displaying poorer self-control.

A subsequent study examined the link between self-control and dieting (Vohs & Heatherton, 2000). Presumably, resisting a food temptation should require more self-regulatory resources among dieters than among nondieters, as the temptation to indulge is pitted against the goal of inhibiting caloric intake among dieters. Consistent with that prediction, dieters who were depleted (i.e., by sitting close to a candy bowl) ate more ice cream and demonstrated less persistence on a cognitive task in comparison to nondepleted dieters (i.e., who sat far away from a candy bowl). In contrast, sitting near a bowl of candies did not impair self-control performance among nondieters. This suggests that temptations are depleting only to the extent that people have the goal of resisting them, setting up a situation in which temptations overwhelm restraints that have become weakened by a prior exertion of self-control.

In a similar vein, another study found that participants who were high in trait chocolate craving and abstained from eating chocolate for 24 hours prior to testing evidenced impaired performance on tasks measuring reaction time and working memory capacity completed in the presence of a chocolate temptation (in comparison to control group participants, who did not abstain from eating chocolate, did not complete the tasks in the presence of a chocolate temptation, and were low in trait craving). These findings once again support the performance patterns indicative of self-regulatory depletion and suggest that depletion is most likely to occur when high trait cravers attempt to curb the automatic tendency to consume a highly tempting food. Under these circumstances, cravers direct limited resources toward managing and controlling salient food cravings at the cost of their performance on tasks associated with high cognitive demands (Kemps, Tiggemann, & Grigg, 2008).

The self-regulatory challenges that are implicated in resisting temptations are relevant to the management of behaviors associated with a variety of addictions and can thus have important clinical applications and implications. For example, a study of a sample of smokers found that participants whose self-control resources had become depleted by the task of resisting a highly tempting food were more likely subsequently to smoke a cigarette during a recess in comparison to smokers who resisted a food low in temptation (Shmueli & Prochaska, 2009). One implication of this work is that the competing demands of smoking cessation and dietary restraint on limited resources can inadvertently precipitate a breakdown in self-regulation that could manifest as a lapse or relapse in the very habits or behaviors targeted for change. Thus, it appears that people may benefit more from modest attempts to regulate single behaviors in succession than from ambitious attempts to change the self by regulating it in multiple ways. In this light, the limited strength model can inform health behavior change practices, as well as treatment interventions for comorbid conditions involving addictions, physical health problems, and/or mental health issues.

This line of research has been extended to the study of other temptations and impulses, including spending, sexual behavior, and alcohol consumption. For example, in a series of studies, depleted participants reported a higher urge and willingness to spend, and they actually purchased a greater number of food items and spent more money on these items in comparison to nondepleted participants, suggesting that impulse buying is susceptible to the depletion of self-control resources (Vohs & Faber, 2007).

In another study, participants who reported lower trait self-control, or whose self-control strength had become depleted by a prior act of self-regulation, were more likely to engage in inappropriate or objectionable sexual behaviors. In comparison to non-depleted participants, depleted participants were more likely to generate inappropriate sexual words on a word anagram, to rate themselves as more likely to engage in sexual infidelity in response to hypothetical scenarios, and to engage in higher levels of physical intimacy with their partner in the privacy of a laboratory setting. These effects were strongest among men, sexually unrestricted individuals, and sexually inexperienced couples, suggesting that self-regulation breakdowns are most likely to occur when weakened restraints become inadequate for bringing under control particularly strong sexual impulses (Gailliot & Baumeister, 2007a).

In another study of male social drinkers, participants who were depleted by a self-control task requiring the suppression of forbidden thoughts drank more beer and had higher blood alcohol content than participants who performed simple math problems that did not require self-control (Muraven, Collins, & Nienhaus, 2002). Together, these findings confirm that resisting temptations requires self-control resources, and even when people self-regulate successfully on one task, they are more likely to succumb to self-control failures shortly thereafter.

While resisting temptations represent a classic example of the tug-of-war between an impulse and self-control, self-regulation is required for a variety of behaviors that involve the inhibition of an incipient response for the sake of another highly prized goal or more adaptive behavior. Thus, low self-regulatory strength is likely to affect performance on any task or behavior that competes with a conflicting or prepotent desire, impulse, or goal. In fact, converging evidence suggests that low self-regulatory strength can impair performance on diverse measures of depletion, including physical endurance, persistence, and emotion regulation.

For example, in a study by Muraven and colleagues (1998), participants in the depletion condition were instructed to increase or decrease their emotional reaction to an upsetting movie, while those in the control group were not instructed to alter their emotional response. All participants were then instructed to squeeze a handgrip for as long as they could, a task that required participants to overcome the natural tendency to let go of the handgrip to be relieved of the physical discomfort associated with squeezing the device. It was found that participants in the depletion groups displayed less physical endurance, as evidenced by their tendency to squeeze the handgrip for less time in comparison to participants in the control condition. This study showed that exerting self-control in the domain of emotion regulation could impair performance in an unrelated domain involving physical stamina.

Extending the research on emotion regulation, a recent study found that the depleting effect of emotion regulation was moderated by the capacity for good self-control. Specifically, participants who suppressed their emotions in response to a disgust-eliciting video displayed less persistence on a subsequent anagram task in comparison to participants in the control group, who watched the video without instructions to regulate their emotions. Crucially, high (but not low) levels of good self-control (as assessed by a self-report measure) attenuated the effect of emotion regulation on persistence in the depletion group. Finally, task persistence in the depletion group (but not in the control group) was associated with self-reported risk behaviors such as aggression, as well as the frequency of alcohol and marijuana use. These findings suggest that good self-control may protect against the depleting effects of self-regulation, and that individual differences in depletion can be associated with real-life consequences (Dvorak & Simons, 2009).

Other research examining the link between thought suppression and self-control found that participants who had to suppress specific thoughts evidenced more difficulty inhibiting the expression of amusement in response to a humorous video in comparison to the control group, in which participants performed a moderately challenging task that did not require self-regulation (solving math problems) (Muraven et al., 1998). Thus, the depleting effect of thought suppression undermined participants' capacity to bring emotional responses under control. This study extended earlier findings in several important ways. First, it showed that tasks involving self-regulation specifically, and not those involving other challenging forms of mental exertion (math problems), have the potential to deplete the limited resource. Second, this study eliminated the alternative possibility that depletion merely increased passivity, as depletion resulted in greater behavioral responses involving smiling and laughing. Finally, regarding alternative explanations for the depletion effect, it does not appear that poor performance after an initial self-control task can be attributed to perceptions of failure on the first task because another study showed that receiving positive, negative, or neutral performance feedback on an initial self-control task did not differentially impair performance on a subsequent task (Wallace & Baumeister, 2002).

Research supporting the depleting effects of thought suppression was extended to a unique instance of thought suppression involving thoughts about death (Gailliot, Schmeichel, & Baumeister, 2006). In this study, depleted participants solved more word fragments with death-related words in comparison to nondepleted participants, which suggests that keeping thoughts of death at bay requires self-regulation. In another study (Gailliot et al., 2006), participants who wrote about death performed worse on tasks requiring self-control (e.g., they solved fewer anagrams) in comparison to participants who wrote about a neutral topic. This suggests that people are motivated to suppress thoughts of death once these are activated, and that this process depletes limited self-regulation resources that are necessary to persist at challenging tasks or to perform other behaviors that require self-control.

While inhibition is one process that reflects executive control, research has shown that different operations of the executive system can affect, and be affected by, prior attempts at executive control. Specifically, a series of studies found that exaggerating the expression of emotions, controlling attention, and inhibiting a dominant response impaired subsequent executive control processes associated with working memory span and updating working memory. In addition, updating working memory impaired the capacity to inhibit emotional responses. These effects were specific to executive control processes, and did not disrupt attention and memory more generally, and they were not accounted for by changes in mood and motivation, or by task difficulty (Schmeichel, 2007). Thus, these findings suggest that diverse executive control processes share and deplete a common underlying resource.

While the extensive body of research reviewed thus far has documented depletion effects after a single self-control task, a recent study has shown that performance on a dependent measure of self-regulation actually improved (rather than worsened, as the depletion model would predict) after two consecutive tasks requiring self-control. These findings were interpreted to support an adaptation view of self-regulation, according to which performance of multiple tasks requiring a high expenditure of self-regulation resources could facilitate learning by influencing expectations about the amount of self-control or effort required in subsequent tasks. As a result, people could adjust their behaviors by expending more effort and resources, thereby resulting in improved performance on a subsequent task (Converse & DeShon, 2009).

Taken together, research has offered strong support for the strength model and has suggested that self-control tasks such as resisting temptations, suppressing thoughts, regulating emotions, persisting despite challenges, and sustaining physical stamina can induce, and suffer from, depletion. These findings further imply that behaviors stemming from unrelated self-control domains draw from a common pool of resources. Thus, successful self-control on one occasion can inadvertently precipitate self-regulatory failures in the short term. In light of the possibility that a process of adaptation may also influence self-regulation, future research might explore the possible interplay between depletion and adaptation as self-regulation unfolds over time.

SELF-CONTROL, INTERPERSONAL PROCESSES, AND CULTURAL LIFE

We have reviewed evidence that the depletion of limited resources can have deleterious personal consequences. We now consider how interpersonal processes and behaviors that support social life also require self-regulatory resources and can be affected by depletion. Living in groups requires that people transform selfish impulses into behaviors that support group interests, substitute aggressive tendencies for prosocial behaviors, and adhere to rules and laws governing social life. Cultural life is thus replete with self-regulatory dilemmas that people have to master to live together and reap the benefits of cultural life.

Accumulating research suggests that prosocial behaviors require a great deal of self-control. For example, depleted participants were less willing to help (e.g., to donate food or money), as evidenced by their responses to hypothetical scenarios and their unwillingness to volunteer their time to assist the victim of a tragedy (DeWall, Baumeister, Gailliot, & Maner, 2008). This suggests that choosing prosocial over selfish motivations consumes resources. Moreover, prosocial behaviors, such as helping, may be undermined when resources are depleted, and this may have downstream consequences for the quality of social bonds.

From a different perspective, research from the consumer psychology literature suggests that acts of benevolence can actually increase as a result of depletion. In a series of studies, participants' initial compliance with a charitable request induced a temporary state of depletion (presumably, yielding to a charitable request involves effortful self-presentation and cognitive demands that deplete self-control resources). The self-regulatory depletion in turn mediated compliance with further requests for charitable acts (e.g., donating money or volunteering) due to a greater reliance on heuristic principles, such as likability or reciprocity (Fennis, Janssen, & Vohs, 2009). This suggests that performing charitable actions can depend on the availability of limited self-regulatory resources.

Another study that examined the effect of self-control on the emergence of antisocial behaviors found that depleted participants were more likely to misrepresent their performance by falsely reporting fewer errors on a task and claiming a greater monetary reward for their performance. In another study, depleted participants were more likely than their nondepleted counterparts to mark their responses on an answer sheet on which the correct responses were erased but nevertheless remained visible, instead of a blank answer sheet (Mead, Baumeister, Gino, Schweitzer, & Ariely, 2009). Depleted participants who chose the premarked answer sheets were also more likely to cheat, as evidenced by the fact that they claimed more correct answers in comparison to nondepleted participants who chose the premarked answer sheet. By placing themselves in a compromising position associated with the temptation to cheat, depleted participants set up a self-regulatory dilemma in which selfish goals were pitted against weakened restraints, ultimately leading to self-regulation failure and the emergence of self-interested and dishonest behavior.

Other socially damaging behaviors have also been shown to be affected by the depletion of resources. For example, in comparison with nondepleted participants, depleted participants were more likely to aggress against others (e.g., blast a participant with loud noise), particularly in the wake of provocation that incited a hostile impulse (DeWall, Baumeister, Stillman, & Gailliot, 2007). In another study, depleted romantic partners were more likely to require their partners to maintain physically uncomfortable and painful poses for longer periods of time than were nondepleted partners, particularly if they were led to believe that their partner negatively evaluated their performance on a task. This suggests that self-regulation resources are needed to prevent people from perpetrating interpersonal violence against romantic partners when hostile impulses arise, at least in the context of a laboratory measure of intimate partner violence (Finkel, DeWall, Slotter, Oaten, & Foshee, 2009).

Other self-regulatory challenges inherent in social and cultural life stem from pitting the tendency to favor ingroup over outgroup members against the need to tolerate interindividual and intergroup diversity. In this respect, in order for people and groups to coexist peacefully, people must inhibit biases and stereotypes (e.g., those related to ethnicity, race, religion, or sexual orientation) that could otherwise threaten harmony and result in subtle or explicit forms of discrimination or hostility. To the extent that these processes require overriding natural tendencies and behaving in ways that are inconsistent with personal values or beliefs, it is likely that these and other processes serving interpersonal functions could deplete self-regulation resources.

Consistent with the idea that processes that can facilitate effective interpersonal exchanges require self-control, research has shown that attempts to manage impressions or to present oneself in a manner that runs counter to one's natural tendencies is effortful and depletes limited self-regulation resources, thereby resulting in deficits of self-regulation (Vohs, Baumeister, & Ciarocco, 2005). Research has also shown that social interactions between people who share different features can entail self-regulatory costs. For example, one study found that white participants who interacted with someone of a different race performed more poorly on a subsequent measure of executive attentional capacity in comparison to participants who engaged in a same-race interaction, suggesting that attempts to negotiate interracial exchanges effectively depletes self-regulation resources (Richeson & Shelton, 2003).

Subsequent work showed that different approaches to interracial interactions can mitigate or augment these self-regulatory costs. For example, one study found that participants who were instructed to avoid expressing prejudice during an interracial exchange, and those who engaged in an interracial interaction without specific instructions performed worse on the Stroop color-naming task than did participants instructed to focus on having a positive interracial exchange (promotion focus) (Trawalter & Richeson, 2006). These findings suggest that resource depletion is not an inevitable consequence of interracial interactions, but that the goal to inhibit or suppress prejudices rather than to enhance the quality of the interaction can have self-regulatory costs. Given the importance of self-regulatory resources for positive social interactions, depletion of these resources could inadvertently undermine rather than promote the quality of the interpersonal bond.

Another line of work has shown that suppressing stereotypes draws on limited self-regulation resources and can thus be undermined by depletion (Govorun & Payne, 2006), as well as interfere with subsequent attempts at self-control (Gordijn, Hindriks, Koomen, Dijksterhuis, & Van Knippenberg, 2004). The suppression of stereotypes has been shown to undermine self-control particularly among people with a low motivation to suppress stereotypes. In one study, participants who expressed high versus low motivation to suppress homosexual stereotypes wrote about the daily activities of a homosexual man without making any reference to stereotypes. The results showed that low-motivation participants solved fewer anagrams than did high-motivation participants after suppressing stereotypes, suggesting that suppressing stereotypes was particularly depleting among participants for whom this task was inconsistent with natural inclinations (Gailliot, Plant, Butz, & Baumeister, 2007).

While the suppression of stereotypes can promote social harmony, effective interpersonal interactions also rely on subtler forms of social coordination that involve synchronizing or tailoring one's behaviors or relational style with the behaviors or style of the interaction partner. Interpersonal interactions can require high or low social coordination, depending on whether the interaction is characterized by high or low maintenance, respectively. In contrast to low-maintenance interactions, high-maintenance interactions require considerable effort to achieve social coordination. Given the effortful and challenging nature of high-maintenance interactions, people may therefore be tempted to withdraw from such interactions or to express their impatience or frustration. Thus, resisting these temptations for the sake of relationship-enhancing behaviors may tax limited self-regulation resources. This was confirmed in several studies showing that the performance of participants who engaged in a high-maintenance social interaction was undermined across several tasks requiring self-regulation in comparison to that of participants who engaged in a low-maintenance social exchange (Finkel et al., 2006). In brief, high-maintenance interpersonal encounters depleted self-regulation resources.

Together, these findings suggest that prosocial or relationship-enhancing behaviors vitally rely on a limited resource, and that a depleted state can interfere with the capacity to override selfish and antisocial responses in favor of socially desirable responses. In brief, self-regulatory strength is necessary if people are to use their inner restraints in the service of elevating prosocial goals over selfish impulses and desires, a challenge that is essential for sustaining cultural life.

DECISION MAKING, REASONING, AND INTELLIGENT THOUGHT

While self-control is a psychological process that draws heavily on limited self-regulation resources, this resource is by no means dedicated exclusively to acts of self-control. We now present evidence of self-regulatory depletion stemming from other processes of the executive system that also rely on the self as an active agent. These functions include decision making, reasoning, and intelligent thought.

While research suggests that the task of making choices is overseen by the self's executive system, it is unlikely that all the choices people make, from the time they awake to the time they fall asleep, necessitate the active involvement of the self, and by extension, the same amount of self-regulation resources. For example, people make choices that are the same every day in a relatively quick and effortless manner (e.g., having toast for breakfast). These types of choices may become automatic over time and may not require the same amount of deliberation and psychological resources they necessitated the first time. In light of this, we suggest that only effortful, involving choices would deplete the stock of limited resources.

In a series of studies testing the hypothesis that active choosing depletes self-regulatory resources (Vohs et al., 2008), one group of participants was asked to make choices among pairs of consumer products, while another group was simply instructed to rate each of the same products. Participants then performed a task that required self-regulation as a measure of ego depletion. For example, participants were instructed to drink as much of a bad-tasting beverage as they could or to submerge an arm in cold water for as long as possible. Both challenges constituted acts of self-control because participants had to overcome their distaste for the beverage or the physical discomfort of holding an arm in icy water to perform well on the tasks. Results showed that participants in the choice condition drank fewer ounces of the bad-tasting beverage and withdrew their arms from the icy water more quickly than did participants in the no-choice condition. Making choices among products therefore depleted the limited resource dedicated to acts of self-regulation and impaired further attempts at self-control.

These findings have been replicated in other domains of choice that could have greater relevance to participants' daily lives. In one study, participants in the choice condition were instructed to choose among descriptions of potential courses they could take to complete the requirements of their program. The control group simply read the course descriptions, without choosing between them. Subsequently, participants were given 15 minutes to study for an upcoming math test. They were simultaneously presented with competing temptations, such as reading magazines and playing video games. They were free to divide the allotted 15 minutes as they desired between studying and engaging in these activities. The results showed that participants in the choice condition spent considerably less time studying for the exam and more time engaged in distracting activities. Another study confirmed that the act of personally selecting one alternative and foregoing another (above and beyond deliberating about different choice options or implementing a predetermined choice) appears to be the key ingredient that hastens the depletion of self-regulation resources. It is possible that deliberation and implementation also deplete resources, but even if they do, the specific act of choosing depletes more, above and beyond those.

Decision making is highly reliant on the capacity to reason logically and to make sophisticated judgments based on multiple pieces of information. Masicampo and Baumeister (2008) capitalized on the well-established attraction effect (Huber, Payne, & Puto, 1982) to demonstrate that when people are depleted, their capacity to reason logically and to make judgments suffers. As a result, they are more likely to succumb to such an irrational decision bias (i.e., the attraction effect). In this study, participants had to decide between two options in the presence of a third "decoy" option, which was similar but objectively inferior to one of the two options. It was found that, in comparison to nondepleted participants, those who were depleted were more likely to be swayed in their choice by the decoy. These participants were thus more likely to rely on a simpler yet misleading heuristic that resulted in selecting an inferior option. In a similar vein, another study showed that depleted participants were more likely to rely on simpler and intuitive decision strategies that circumvent effortful and deliberate processing, as evidenced by their tendency to be swayed and to favor extremes instead of options that reflect a more complex compromise (Pocheptsova, Amir, Dhar, & Baumeister, 2009).

Presumably, intelligent thought is another capacity that requires the self's active involvement and likely underlies many operations of the executive system, such as decision making and reasoning. However, research suggests that not all forms of intelligent thought are equally demanding when it comes to the depletion of resources. Some information processing is relatively automatic and effortless, such as storing and retrieving information from memory, rote memory, and general knowledge. In contrast, higher-order levels of information processing involving fluid intelligence, problem solving, and logical reasoning require controlled processing, and therefore necessitate the active involvement of the self. In light of this distinction, only high-level, controlled forms of information processing should be affected by the depletion of self-regulatory resources, whereas basic forms of information processing should remain intact.

This prediction was tested in a series of studies by Schmeichel, Vohs, and Baumeister (2003). The first study, which broadly examined the effect of self-control on higher-order cognitive capacity, found that depleted participants showed impaired cognitive performance on a logical reasoning task, as measured by items from the Graduate Record Examination (GRE) Analytical test. Follow-up studies specifically examined the differential impact of depletion on simple (requiring the retrieval of information from memory and applying simple rules) versus more elaborate forms of information processing (requiring extrapolating from existing knowledge and reasoning about it). In one study, ego depletion induced by the regulation of emotions to an upsetting video specifically impaired participants' performance on tasks of higher-order but not more basic information processing in comparison to that of nondepleted participants. These results thus confirmed that self-regulatory resources are needed exclusively for the effective operation of cognitive processes that rely on the self's executive function.

These findings support the conclusion that self-regulatory resources are needed for higher-order operations of the executive system. In line with the strength model, depleted participants lacked the resources necessary to perform mental operations involving controlled cognitive processing. Given that complex forms of reasoning, decision making, and intelligent thought are necessary to manage successfully the intricacies of daily and social life, this argues for the importance of self-regulatory resources for promoting adaptive behaviors that could benefit individuals and cultures.

PREVENTING OR OFFSETTING THE EFFECTS OF DEPLETION

We have shown that a variety of adaptive behaviors rely on self-control resources. In addition, the limited nature of this resource has been shown to place constraints on behaviors that support personal and social goals. Given the implications of having insufficient self-control resources, it is important to determine whether this resource can be replenished, and whether people can still regulate themselves when the resource is in short supply. Alternatively, once they are depleted, are people doomed to self-regulation failures that breed antisocial and self-defeating behaviors?

Research argues against such a defeatist view of willpower and suggests instead that people may never become completely depleted to the point that self-regulation failures are inevitable. Evidence in support of this assertion was provided in a study by Muraven, Shmueli, and Burkley (2006), in which participants were initially depleted by a self-control task. Participants in one group were then told they would have to perform two additional tasks, and that the last of these would require considerable self-control. Participants in the other group were also told that they would perform two additional tasks, but without any reference to the amount of self-control required for each task. Participants' performance on the intermediate task was measured. It was found that depleted participants who anticipated having to exert self-control on the last task performed worse on the intermediate task than the other group. Of note, participants who were not depleted by a previous self-control task did not show any differences in their performance on the intermediate task. Depleted participants' worse performance was interpreted to reflect a conservation of resources to ensure adequate performance on the final task. Thus, it appears that people are sensitive to reductions in limited self-control resources and are motivated to conserve the leftover resource should a situation arise in the future in which self-control would be required for an important goal.

While conservation is an adaptive strategy, the high demands placed on this limited resource by the multiple operations of the central executive system could nevertheless hasten self-regulation failures, unless the stock of resources could be periodically replenished. Thus, how do people recover from depletion and restore their capacity for effective self-regulation? In a series of studies, Tice, Baumeister, Shmueli, and Muraven (2007) explored the role of positive affect in improving self-regulation following depletion. They found that depleted participants who underwent a positive mood induction by either watching a comedy video or receiving a surprise gift performed as well on a subsequent self-control task as nondepleted participants, suggesting that positive emotions can restore self-control performance following depletion.

More recently, evidence was furnished by Schmeichel and Vohs (2009) that self-affirmation can also counter depletion effects. In a series of studies, half of depleted and nondepleted participants were asked to write about their most important value (self-affirmation condition). The other half of the participants were asked to write about how and why a value they ranked lower in importance might be important to the average student (no-affirmation condition). As expected, depleted participants who affirmed their core value performed better on a subsequent self-control task in comparison to depleted participants who did not engage in the self-affirmation exercise. There was no difference in the performance of nondepleted participants on the self-control task regardless of whether they affirmed their core value. The researchers further confirmed that self-affirmation facilitated self-control by promoting an abstract level of mental construal that has been linked to good self-control. This suggests that self-affirmation can promote effective self-control by broadening one's perspective in a way that encompasses long-term goals and higher-order values. In this broader light, people's behaviors are more likely to be steered by higher-order goals and values rather than to reflect the press of the immediate situation.

Researchers from other laboratories have also begun to investigate factors that can buffer the effects of ego depletion. For example, Tyler and Burns (2008) found that a 10-minute interval or a 3-minute period of relaxation between self-control tasks could prevent depletion, and that performance decrements could also be overcome by distracting participants' attention during the second self-control task (Alberts, Martijn, Nievelstein, Jansen, & De Vries, 2008). Another line of research guided by self-determination theory showed that inducing an intrinsic, as opposed to an extrinsic, motivation to exert self-control on an initial task was associated with better performance on a second self-control task (Muraven, Gagné, & Rosman, 2008).

Yet another potential way to offset the cost of resource-intensive mental operations is to relegate self-control tasks to the domain of automatic processes. Consistent with this argument, participants who formed automatic associations in the form of an implementation intention (about overriding automatic responses on an initial self-control task) persisted more on an unsolvable tracing puzzle in comparison to the control group, which did not form an implementation intention. Implementation intentions also prevented a subsequent decrement in self-control performance among participants who were already depleted (Webb & Sheeran, 2003). In a similar vein, priming depleted participants with the concept of persistence prevented the standard decrease in self-control performance reflective of ego depletion (Alberts, Martijn, Greb, Merckelbach, & De Vries, 2007). Taken together, these findings suggest the potential for counteracting the effects of depletion, therefore averting imminent failures of self-regulation.

BOOSTING SELF-REGULATORY STRENGTH

While the studies described in the previous section suggest that temporary states of depletion can be managed and to some extent overcome, is it possible to enlarge the overall pool of self-regulatory resources? If, as we suggested, self-control resembles a muscle, then self-regulatory strength should increase with practice over time, just like a muscle gains strength and stamina as a result of exercise.

The first evidence suggesting the potential for increasing self-regulatory strength through practice was furnished in a study by Muraven, Baumeister, and Tice (1999). Participants provided a baseline measure of depletion during an initial assessment. During the next 2 weeks, participants in the experimental groups engaged in one of three self-regulatory exercises (tracking food eaten, improving mood, or improving posture), while the control group did not engage in self-regulatory exercises. Depletion was reassessed after the 2-week period. As expected, participants who engaged in self-regulation exercises showed greater self-regulatory strength (less depletion) at follow-up in comparison to the control group (Muraven et al., 1999).

In another study (Oaten & Cheng, 2006a), participants entered a 2-month self-regulation program consisting of regular physical exercise (e.g., aerobic activity, free weights, and resistance training). In two laboratory sessions (one before and the other following the program), all participants performed an initial self-control task, and their performance on a subsequent self-control task served as the dependent measure of depletion. While results revealed a standard depletion effect at the first session, the depletion effect was attenuated at follow-up among participants who underwent the 2-month physical program. Notably, the gains in self-control transferred to unrelated domains, including emotional well-being, adaptive health behaviors (e.g., smoking, alcohol and caffeine consumption, and healthy eating), and study habits.

Similar findings were reported in response to a study intervention program designed to assist students with implementing a regular study schedule during a period leading up to exams (Oaten & Cheng, 2006b). While depletion was observed at exam time among participants who did not partake in the intervention, students enrolled in the program showed an improvement in self-control. Another study found that a 4-month financial monitoring program could also buffer depletion effects over time. In an effort to facilitate progress toward personalized money management goals, this program required participants to track their monthly income and expenses to calculate their monthly savings, a task that constitutes an important self-regulatory challenge. In comparison to the control group that showed depletion, participants who adhered to this program demonstrated improved self-control at follow-up (Oaten & Cheng, 2007).

In a somewhat different approach, interventions designed to increase self-regulatory strength have been applied in an attempt to offset the burden of resource-costly behaviors that involve the suppression of stereotypes (Gailliot, Plant, et al., 2007). This study was based on the rationale that people with a high motivation to suppress prejudicial thoughts would have accumulated extensive practice with regulating these stereotypes, therefore making this tendency more habitual, and drawing on fewer self-control resources. In contrast, for those with a low motivation, regulating stereotypes would require conscious control, thereby draining limited self-regulation resources.

The study tested the effect of exercising self-control during a 2-week period on depletion that was the result of stereotype suppression among participants with high versus low motivation to suppress stereotypes. During an initial session, participants were instructed to write about a homosexual man without using any related stereotypes. Following this exercise, participants solved letter anagrams, and this served as the dependent measure of depletion. For the next 2 weeks, half of the participants engaged in specific self-regulatory exercises, such as using their nondominant hand or modifying their manner of speaking, while the other half was not given any instructions. The depleting effect of suppressing stereotypes observed at baseline among participants with low motivation was eliminated at follow-up if they had engaged in self-regulation exercises in the intervening 2 weeks. These findings suggest that practice at self-control can make the suppression of stereotypes less effortful among those who are least likely to keep those behaviors in check.

These findings suggest that while self-control may become compromised shortly after the expenditure of this limited resource, consistently practicing self-control may build up the pool of self-regulatory resources. This could increase the amount of resources available in the long run and make people increasingly resistant to self-regulation failures. Thus, the cost of expending resources in the short term could be offset by the long-term gains associated with building up the resource.

TOWARD A PHYSIOLOGICAL ACCOUNT OF EGO DEPLETION

In support of the strength model, we have shown that self-control relies on a limited energy supply that becomes depleted by subsequent attempts at self-regulation. Does this metaphorical energy have a physiological basis that can be detected and measured? Indeed, research has determined that self-control depletes blood glucose levels. Glucose is the fuel consumed by the brain to perform mental activities and functions throughout the body. Findings now suggest that people who have low glucose levels, and those who are unable to metabolize glucose efficiently, show deficits indicative of low self-control (for a review, see Gailliot & Baumeister, 2007b).

In a series of experimental studies, Gailliot, Baumeister, and colleagues (2007) established the link between glucose and self-control. In this research, a baseline measure of blood glucose was collected with blood-sampling lancets and analyzed with a glucose meter. Next, one group of participants engaged in a self-control task, while another group performed an equivalent task that did not require self-control. The nature of this task varied across studies and included laboratory tests (e.g., Stroop task, attention control video, and thought suppression), as well as social behaviors that involved a self-regulation dilemma (e.g., suppressing stereotypes during an interracial interaction). Blood glucose levels were measured once more after the initial task. Across studies, it was found that blood glucose levels dropped significantly among participants depleted by the initial self-control task in comparison to those who were not depleted. Several follow-up studies found that lower glucose levels after depletion predicted worse performance on a subsequent self-control measure, suggesting that low glucose levels precipitated the observed decrements in self-control performance.

In a test of causality, the researchers experimentally manipulated blood glucose levels. After performing an initial task that required self-control (depletion group) or not (control group), half of the participants in each group received lemonade sweetened with either sugar (glucose condition) or Splenda (a sugar substitute that does not contain glucose; placebo condition). It was found that depleted participants who drank the placebo beverage made more errors on the Stroop task compared to their nondepleted counterparts. In contrast, participants who received the glucose drink, and who exerted self-control on the initial task, did not show any impairment in their performance on the Stroop task, suggesting that the glucose drink replenished the depleted resource and thereby counteracted the depletion effect.

Other studies examined the effect of manipulating glucose on behaviors previously shown to rely on limited self-control resources, namely, coping with death-related thoughts and suppressing stereotypes. In one study, participants who initially consumed a placebo drink and were subsequently induced to think about their death left more word fragments unsolved in contrast to participants who were instructed to think about dental pain. In contrast, among participants who consumed the glucose drink, there was no difference in the number of word fragments solved between participants in the mortality salience and those in the dental pain conditions. These findings suggest that an increase in glucose eliminated the self-control impairment that resulted from coping with death-related thoughts. Replicating these findings in a different self-control domain, another study found that participants who drank a glucose drink used fewer stereotypes in describing the activities of a homosexual man in comparison to participants who consumed a placebo drink (Gailliot, Peruche, Plant, & Baumeister, 2008).

Consistent with the idea that other tasks of the executive system draw on limited self-regulatory resources, glucose has also been implicated in decision making. A study found that the tendency to rely on simple yet misleading decision-making heuristics following depletion was attenuated among participants who consumed a drink sweetened with sugar (containing glucose) in comparison to depleted participants who received an artificially sweetened beverage (without glucose) (Masicampo & Baumeister, 2008). This finding confirms that rational choice relies on the same resource (glucose) dedicated to acts of self-control, and that restoring this resource can help to preserve the capacity for rational choice in spite of depletion.

Together, these findings suggest that acts of self-control and other executive functions depend on, and deplete, blood glucose levels. In addition, experimentally manipulating glucose levels affected behaviors and psychological processes known to rely on limited self-regulatory resources. In light of these findings, the focus on biological processes involved in depletion could be a promising avenue for understanding whether factors that counteract the effects of depletion (e.g., positive affect and self-affirmation) exert their positive influence by replenishing the psychological (and physiological) resource, or simply by motivating people to use more of it to ensure good performance. This approach could help to clarify the nature of the resource that is depleted and provide insights into the mechanisms by which this limited resource is restored.

CONCLUSION

Self-regulation is a key ingredient that can facilitate individual and cultural success. The capacity for self-regulation is not unlimited. In support of the strength model, self-regulation and other executive functions that require the self's active intervention rely on the same limited energy supply. Blood glucose has been shown to constitute the physiological equivalent of this psychological resource. When this resource is depleted, there is less of it available for other volitional acts, and people become vulnerable to self-regulation failures. In line with this rationale, self-regulation and other executive functions that support adaptive personal and interpersonal behaviors have been shown to induce, and to suffer from, a state of depletion. Despite the finite nature of self-regulatory resources, research has not only begun to identify specific variables that can offset the effects of depletion, but it has also shown that self-regulatory strength can be increased by practicing self-regulation. We thus conclude that honing people's skills in the art of selectively allocating or conserving this limited resource, being sensitive to its reductions, and taking corrective actions to restore it could go a long way in alleviating the personal and societal ills associated with faulty self-regulation. In this light, the key to personal and cultural advancement may lie in how efficiently people hone these skills, and how well society structures itself to create opportunities for its members to develop the capacity for self-control.

ACKNOWLEDGMENT

The preparation of this chapter was supported by a postdoctoral fellowship awarded to Isabelle M. Bauer from the Social Sciences and Humanities Research Council of Canada (No. 756-2008-0245).

REFERENCES

Alberts, H. J. E. M., Martijn, C., Greb, J., Merckelbach, H., & De Vries, N. K. (2007). Carrying on or giving in: The role of automatic processes in overcoming ego depletion. *British Journal of Social Psychology, 46*, 383–399.

Alberts, H. J. E. M., Martijn, C., Nievelstein, F., Jansen, A., & De Vries, N. K. (2008). Distracting the self: Shifting attention prevents ego depletion. *Self and Identity, 7*, 322–334.

Baumeister, R. F., Bratslavsky, E., Muraven, M., & Tice, D. M. (1998). Ego depletion: Is the active self a limited resource? *Journal of Personality and Social Psychology, 74*, 1252–1265.

Baumeister, R. F., & Heatherton, T. F. (1996). Self-regulation failure: An overview. *Psychological Inquiry, 7*, 1–15.

Baumeister, R. F., Heatherton, T. F., & Tice, D. M. (1994). *Losing control: How and why people fail at self-regulation.* San Diego, CA: Academic Press.

Baumeister, R. F., Muraven, M., & Tice, D. M. (2000). Ego depletion: A resource model of volition, self-regulation, and controlled processing. *Social Cognition, 18*, 130–150.

Baumeister, R. F., Vohs, K. D., & Tice, D. M. (2007). The strength model of self-control. *Current Directions in Psychological Science, 16*, 351–355.

Carver, C. S., & Scheier, M. F. (1981). *Attention and self-regulation: A control theory approach to human behavior.* New York: Springer-Verlag.

Carver, C. S., & Scheier, M. F. (1998). *On the self-regulation of behavior.* New York: Cambridge University Press.

Converse, P. D., & DeShon, R. P. (2009). A tale of two tasks: Reversing the self-regulatory resource depletion effect. *Journal of Applied Psychology, 94*, 1318–1324.

DeWall, C. N., Baumeister, R. F., Gailliot, M. T., & Maner, J. K. (2008). Depletion makes the heart grow less helpful: Helping as a function of self-regulatory energy and genetic relatedness. *Personality and Social Psychology Bulletin, 34*, 1653–1662.

DeWall, C. N., Baumeister, R. F., Stillman, T. F., & Gailliot, M. T. (2007). Violence restrained: Effects of self-regulatory capacity and its depletion on aggressive behavior. *Journal of Experimental Social Psychology, 43*, 62–76.

Dvorak, R. D., & Simons, J. S. (2009). Moderation of resource depletion in the self-control strength model: Differing effects of two modes of self-control. *Personality and Social Psychology Bulletin, 35*, 572–583.

Fennis, B. M., Janssen, L., & Vohs, K. D. (2009). Acts of benevolence: A limited-resource account of compliance with charitable requests. *Journal of Consumer Research, 35*, 906–924.

Finkel, E. J., Campbell, W. K., Brunell, A. B., Dalton, A. N., Scarbeck, S. J., & Chartrand, T. L. (2006). High-maintenance interaction: Inefficient social coordination impairs self-regulation. *Journal of Personality and Social Psychology, 91*, 456–475.

Finkel, E. J., DeWall, C. N., Slotter, E. B., Oaten, M., & Foshee, V. A. (2009). Self-regulatory failure and intimate partner violence perpetration. *Journal of Personality and Social Psychology, 97*, 483–499.

Gailliot, M. T., & Baumeister, R. F. (2007a). The physiology of willpower: Linking blood glucose to self-control. *Personality and Social Psychology Review, 11*, 303–327.

Gailliot, M. T., & Baumeister, R. F. (2007b). Self-regulation and sexual restraint: Dispositionally and temporarily poor self-regulatory abilities contribute to failures at restraining sexual behavior. *Personality and Social Psychology Review, 33*, 173–186.

Gailliot, M. T., Baumeister, R. F., DeWall, C. N., Maner, J. K., Plant, E. A., Tice, D. M., et al. (2007). Self-control relies on glucose as a limited energy source: Willpower is more than a metaphor. *Journal of Personality and Social Psychology, 92*, 325–336.

Gailliot, M. T., Peruche, B. M., Plant, E. A., & Baumeister, R. F. (2008). Stereotypes and prejudice in the blood: Sucrose drinks reduce prejudice and stereotyping. *Journal of Experimental Social Psychology, 45*, 288–290.

Gailliot, M. T., Plant, E. A., Butz, D. A., & Baumeister, R. F. (2007). Increasing self-regulatory strength can reduce the depleting effect of suppressing stereotypes. *Personality and Social Psychology Bulletin, 33*, 281–294.

Gailliot, M. T., Schmeichel, B. J., & Baumeister, R. F. (2006). Self-regulatory processes defend against the threat of death: Effects of mortality salience, self-control depletion, and trait self-control on thoughts and fears of dying. *Journal of Personality and Social Psychology, 91*, 49–62.

Gordijn, E. H., Hindriks, I., Koomen, W., Dijksterhuis, A., & Van Knippenberg, A. (2004). Consequences of stereotype suppression and internal suppression motivation: A self-regulation approach. *Personality and Social Psychology Bulletin, 30*, 212–224.

Govorun, O., & Payne, K. B. (2006). Ego-depletion and prejudice: Separating automatic and controlled components. *Social Cognition, 24*, 111–136.

Huber, J., Payne, J. W., & Puto, C. (1982). Adding asymmetrically dominated alternatives: Violations of regularity and the similarity hypothesis. *Journal of Consumer Research, 9*, 90–98.

Kemps, E., Tiggemann, M., & Grigg, M. (2008). Food cravings consume limited cognitive resources. *Journal of Experimental Psychology: Applied, 14*, 247–254.

Masicampo, E. J., & Baumeister, R. F. (2008). Toward a physiology of dual-process reasoning and judgment: Lemonade, willpower, and expensive rule-based analysis. *Psychological Science, 19*, 255–260.

Mead, N. L., Baumeister, R. F., Gino, F., Schweitzer, M. E., & Ariely, D. (2009). Too tired to tell the truth: Self-control resource depletion and dishonesty. *Journal of Experimental Social Psychology, 45*, 594–597.

Muraven, M., Baumeister, R. F., & Tice, D. M. (1999). Longitudinal improvement of self-regulation through practice: Building self-control through repeated exercise. *Journal of Social Psychology, 139*, 446–457.

Muraven, M., Collins, R. L., & Nienhaus, K. (2002). Self-control and alcohol restraint: An initial application of the self-control strength model. *Psychology of Addictive Behaviors, 16*, 113–120.

Muraven, M., Gagné, M., & Rosman, H. (2008). Helpful self-control: Autonomy support, vitality, and depletion. *Journal of Experimental Social Psychology, 44*, 573–585.

Muraven, M., Shmueli, D., & Burkley, E. (2006). Conserving self-control strength. *Journal of Personality and Social Psychology, 91*, 524–537.

Muraven, M., Tice, D. M., & Baumeister, R. F. (1998). Self-control as limited resource: Regulatory depletion patterns. *Journal of Personality and Social Psychology, 74*, 774–789.

Muraven, M. R., & Baumeister, R. F. (2000). Self-regulation and depletion of limited resources: Does self-control resemble a muscle? *Psychological Bulletin, 126*, 247–259.

Oaten, M., & Cheng, K. (2006a). Improved self-control: The benefits of a regular program of academic study. *Basic and Applied Social Psychology, 28*, 1–16.

Oaten, M., & Cheng, K. (2006b). Longitudinal gains in self-regulation from regular physical exercise. *British Journal of Health Psychology, 11*, 717–733.

Oaten, M., & Cheng, K. (2007). Improvements in self-control from financial monitoring. *Journal of Economic Psychology, 28*, 487–501.

Pocheptsova, A., Amir, O., Dhar, R., & Baumeister, R. F. (2009). Deciding without resources: Resource depletion and choice in context. *Journal of Marketing Research, 46*, 344–355.

Richeson, J. A., & Shelton, J. N. (2003). When prejudice does not pay: Effects of interracial contact on executive function. *Psychological Science, 14*, 287–290.

Schmeichel, B. J. (2007). Attention control, memory updating, and emotion regulation temporarily reduce the capacity for executive control. *Journal of Personality and Social Psychology, 136*, 241–255.

Schmeichel, B. J., & Vohs, K. (2009). Self-affirmation and self-control: Affirming core values counteracts ego depletion. *Journal of Personality and Social Psychology, 96*, 770–782.

Schmeichel, B. J., Vohs, K. D., & Baumeister, R. F. (2003). Intellectual performance and ego depletion: Role of the self in logical reasoning and other information processing. *Journal of Personality and Social Psychology, 85*, 33–46.

Shmueli, D., & Prochaska, J. J. (2009). Resisting tempting foods and smoking behavior: Implications from a self-control theory perspective. *Health Psychology, 28*, 300–306.

Tangney, J. P., Baumeister, R. F., & Boone, A. L. (2004). High self-control predicts good adjustment, less pathology, better grades, and interpersonal success. *Journal of Personality, 72*, 271–322.

Tice, D. M., Baumeister, R. F., Shmueli, D., & Muraven, M. (2007). Restoring the self: Positive affect helps improve self-regulation following ego depletion. *Journal of Experimental Social Psychology, 43*, 379–384.

Trawalter, S., & Richeson, J. A. (2006). Regulatory focus and executive function after interracial interactions. *Journal of Experimental Social Psychology, 42*, 406–412.

Tyler, J. M., & Burns, K. C. (2008). After depletion: The replenishment of the self's regulatory resources. *Self and Identity, 7*, 305–321.

Vohs, K. D., Baumeister, R. F., & Ciarocco, N. (2005). Self-regulation and self-presentation: Regulatory resource depletion impairs impression management and effortful self-presentation depletes regulatory resources. *Journal of Personality and Social Psychology, 88*, 632–657.

Vohs, K. D., Baumeister, R. F., Schmeichel, B. J., Twenge, J. M., Nelson, N. M., & Tice, D. M. (2008). Making choices impairs subsequent self-control: A limited resource account of decision making, self-regulation, and active initiative. *Journal of Personality and Social Psychology, 94*, 883–898.

Vohs, K. D., & Faber, R. J. (2007). Spent resources: Self-regulatory resource availability affects impulse buying. *Journal of Consumer Research, 33*, 537–547.

Vohs, K. D., & Heatherton, T. F. (2000). Self-regulatory failure: A resource-depletion approach. *Psychological Science, 11*, 249–254.

Wallace, H. M., & Baumeister, R. F. (2002). The effects of success versus failure feedback on further self-control. *Self and Identity, 1*, 35–41.

Webb, T. L., & Sheeran, P. (2003). Can implementation intentions help to overcome ego-depletion? *Journal of Experimental Social Psychology, 39*, 279–286.

CHAPTER 5

Willpower in a Cognitive Affective Processing System

The Dynamics of Delay of Gratification

WALTER MISCHEL

OZLEM AYDUK

In this chapter, we examine the processes and conditions in which individuals may overcome stimulus control and the pressures and temptations of the moment for the sake of more valued but delayed, or blocked, goals and outcomes. What makes it possible for some people to give up their addictions, to resist the temptations that threaten their cherished values and goals, to persist in the effort, to maintain their relationship, to overcome the more selfish motivation and take account of other people—in short, to exert "willpower"? And why do others seem to remain the victims of their own vulnerabilities and biographies?

We address these questions guided by the cognitive affective processing model of self-regulation, abbreviated as CAPS (e.g., Mischel, in press; Mischel & Ayduk, 2004; Mischel & Shoda, 1995). In this analysis effective pursuit of delayed rewards and difficult to attain long-term goals depends on the availability and accessibility of certain types of cognitive-attention strategies that are essential for overcoming stimulus control. Here we ask: What strategies and processes make that possible? How do they work and how can they be harnessed in the service of more constructive and effective self-regulation? Absent the availability and accessibility of such strategies, efforts to sustain delay of gratification and self-control are likely to be short-lived and the power of the immediate situation is likely to prevail and elicit the prepotent response—eat the cake, smoke the cigarette, grab the money, succumb to the temptation. In contrast, in effective goal pursuit, these strategies become activated and utilized when the person tries to forego impulsive, automatic reactions in response to immediate situational pressures and temptations for the sake of more valued but temporally delayed goals.

The Delay of Gratification Paradigm

Insights into the conditions and processes that enable effortful control have come from research in the preschool delay paradigm (Mischel, 1974a; Mischel & Baker, 1975; Mischel & Ebbesen, 1970; Mischel, Ebbesen, & Zeiss, 1972; Mischel & Moore, 1973). In this procedure, young children wait for two cookies (or other little treats) that they want and have chosen to get, and which they prefer to a smaller treat, such as one cookie. They then are faced with a dilemma: They are told that the experimenter needs to leave for a while and that they can continue to wait for the larger reward until the experimenter comes back on his or her own, or they are free to ring a little bell to summon the adult at any time and immediately get the smaller treat at the expense of getting the larger preferred reward.

In short, the situation creates a strong conflict between the temptation to stop the delay and take the immediately available smaller reward or to continue waiting for their original, larger, more preferred choice, albeit not knowing how long the wait will be. After children understand the situation, they are left alone in the room until they signal the experimenter. The child, of course, has a continuous free choice, and can resolve the conflict about whether or not to stop waiting at any time by ringing the bell, which immediately brings back the adult. If the child continues to wait, the adult returns spontaneously (15–25 minutes depending on child's age).

This simple and seemingly trivial situation has turned out to be not only compelling for the young child but also surprisingly diagnostic, making it possible to significantly predict conceptually relevant and consequential long-term outcomes from the number of seconds children wait at age 4 years to diverse indices of self-regulation in goal pursuit and social–emotional cognitive competencies decades later in adulthood (e.g., Ayduk et al., 2000; Mischel, Shoda, & Rodriguez, 1989). To illustrate, the number of seconds children can wait in certain diagnostic situations (i.e., when no regulatory strategies are provided by the experimenter and children have to access their own competencies) is significantly predictive of higher Scholastic Aptitude Test (SAT) scores and better social cognitive, personal, and interpersonal competencies years later (Mischel, Shoda, & Peake, 1988; Shoda, Mischel, & Peake, 1990). These links between seconds of preschool delay time and adaptive life outcomes in diverse social and cognitive domains remain stable, persisting into adulthood, as discussed in later sections.

Given the existence and psychological importance of the individual differences tapped in this situation it becomes important to understand what is happening psychologically that makes some children ring soon and others wait for what seems an eternity. What determines who will be under the stimulus control elicited by immediate temptations and who will be able to resist those pressures and sustain the choice to persist for the delayed rewards? We next consider the cognitive-attention control strategies that help and hurt such efforts and examine how they may play out in the proposed self-regulatory system.

Temporal Discounting

The delay of gratification paradigm for the analysis of willpower taps a phenomenon that makes effortful control especially difficult in situations when it is often most needed. It is a factor that undermines the person's motivation to keep important long-term goals in mind when faced with short-term gratifications that are immediately present. This pervasive phenomenon, found in animal species from rats to humans, is *temporal discounting* (Ainslie, 2001; Loewenstein, Read, & Baumeister, 2003; Rachlin, 2000; Trope & Liberman, 2003). Well-known to economists and philosophers as well as to psychologists, this tendency refers to the systematic discounting of the subjective value of a reward, outcome, or goal as the anticipated time delay before its expected occurrence increases.

Temporal discounting is seen clearly in delay of gratification studies in the finding that the perceived subjective value of the delayed reward(s) in young children, and hence their motivation to choose to delay, decreases systematically as the length of the expected delay interval increases (Mischel, 1966, 1974b; Mischel & Metzner, 1962). Similar findings with respect to the effect of time delays on the discounting of subjective value have long been widely documented and recognized as of central importance for understanding problems that range from the psychiatric and medical to the areas of behavioral medicine and behavioral economics (Ainslie, 2001; Loewenstein et al., 2003; Morf & Mischel, 2002; Petry, 2002; Rachlin, 2000; Wulfert, Block, Ana, Rodriguez, & Colsman, 2002). The hot/cool analysis of willpower, described next, was developed in large part to try to understand the basic mechanisms that may underlie the phenomena tapped by the delay paradigm.

Hot/Cool Systems within CAPS

Following the connectionist and parallel distributed processing neural network metaphor, two closely interacting systems—a cognitive "cool" system and an emotional "hot" system—have been proposed as components of the broader CAPS system. The interactions between these two systems are basic in the dynamics of self-regulation in general and of delay of gratification in particular, and underlie the person's ability—or inability—to sustain effortful control in pursuit of delayed goals (Metcalfe & Mischel, 1999).

Briefly, the cool system is an emotionally neutral, "know" system: It is cognitive, complex, slow, and contemplative. Attuned to the informational, cognitive, and spatial aspects of stimuli, the cool system consists of a network of informational, *cool nodes* that are elaborately interconnected to each other, and generate rational, reflective, and strategic behavior. Although the specific biological roots of this system are still being explored, the cool system seems to be associated with hippocampal and frontal lobe processing (Lieberman, Gaunt, Gilbert, & Trope, 2002; Metcalfe & Mischel, 1999).

In contrast, the hot system is a "go" system. It enables quick, emotional processing: simple and fast, and thus useful for survival from an evolutionary perspective by allowing rapid flight or fight reactions, as well as necessary appetitive approach responses. The hot system consists of relatively few representations, or *hot spots* (e.g., unconditioned stimuli), which elicit virtually reflexive avoidance and approach reactions when activated by trigger stimuli. This hot system develops early in life and is the most dominant in the young infant. It is an essentially automatic system, governed by virtually reflexive stimulus–response reactions, which, unless interrupted, preclude effortful control.

Although other theorists (e.g., Epstein, 1994; Lieberman, 2003) have employed somewhat different terms to describe similar sets of opponent self-regulatory processes, there is reasonable consensus that what Metcalfe and Mischel (1999) call the hot system is more affect-based relative to the cool system and generates simple, impulsive, and quick approach–avoidance responses in the presence of eliciting stimuli. The impulsive behavioral products of this system provide ample documentation for the power of stimulus control, and the formidable constraints that many hot (*affect-arousing*) situations place on a person's ability to exert willpower or volitional control. Currently, neural models of information processing suggest that the amygdala—a small, almond-shaped region in the forebrain thought to enable fight-or-flight responses—may be the seat of hot system processing (Gray, 1987; LeDoux, 1996; Metcalfe & Jacobs, 1996), but again the exact loci and circuitry remain to be mapped with increasing precision.

Consistent with a parallel-processing neural network metaphor, the hot/cool analysis assumes that cognition and affect operate in continuous interaction with one another, and emphasizes the close connections of the two subsystems in generating phenomenological experiences as well as behavioral responses. Specifically, in the model, hot spots and cool nodes that have the same external referents are directly connected to one another, and thus link the two systems (Metcalfe & Jacobs, 1996; Metcalfe & Mischel, 1999). Hot spots can be evoked by activation of corresponding cool nodes; alternatively, hot representations can be cooled through intersystem connections to the corresponding cool nodes. Effortful control and willpower become possible to the extent that the cooling strategies generated by the cognitive cool system circumvent hot system activation through such intersystem connections that link hot spots to cool nodes. Thus, consequential for self-control are the conditions under which hot spots do not have access to corresponding cool representations because these conditions are the ones that undermine or prevent cool system regulation of hot impulses.

Effects of System Maturation

Two assumptions are made about the determinants of the balance between hot and cool systems. First, this balance depends critically on the person's developmental phase. The hot system is well developed at birth, whereas the cool system develops with age. Consequently, early in development the baby is primarily responsive to the pushes and pulls of hot stimuli in the external world, as many of the hot spots do not have corresponding cool nodes that can regulate and inhibit hot system processing. This assumption is in line with developmental differences in the maturation rates of the biological centers for these two systems.

With age and maturity, however, the cool system becomes elaborated as many more cool nodes develop and become connected to one another, thereby greatly increasing the network of cool system associations and thus the number of cool nodes corresponding to the hot spots (e.g., Altman & Bayer, 1990; Gaffan, 1992). Empirical evidence from the delay of gratification studies supports these expectations. Whereas delay of gratification in the paradigm described seems almost impossible—and even incomprehensible—for most children younger than 4 years of age (Mischel, 1974b; Mischel & Mischel, 1983), by age 12 almost 60% of children in some studies were able to wait to criterion (25 minutes maximum; Ayduk et al., 2000, Study 2). Furthermore, the child's spontaneous use of cooling strategies such as purposeful self-distraction is positively related to both age and verbal intelligence (Rodriguez, Mischel, & Shoda, 1989). By the time most children reach the age of 6 years, they are less susceptible to stimulus control from mere exposure to the desired objects facing them. As the cool system develops it becomes increasingly possible for the child to generate spontaneously diverse cognitive and attention deployment cooling strategies (e.g., self-distraction, inventing mental games to make the delay less aversive), and thus to be less controlled by whatever is salient in the immediate field of attention (Rodriguez, Mischel, & Shoda, 1989).

Effects of Stress Level

Second, the hot/cool balance depends on the stress level, which in turn depends both on the stress induced by the appraisal of the specific situation and the chronic level characteristic for the person. The theory assumes that whereas at low to moderate levels of stress cool system activation may be enhanced, at high levels it becomes attenuated and even shuts off. In contrast, the hot system becomes activated to the degree that stress is increased (Metcalfe & Jacobs, 1996; Metcalfe & Mischel, 1999). The stress level of the system reflects both individual differences in the person's chronic level of stress and the stress induced within the particular situation.

Consistent with the view that high stress levels tend to attenuate the activation of the cool system, delay of gratification becomes more difficult when children experience additional psychological stress (e.g., by thinking about unhappy things that happened to them), but it becomes easier when stress is decreased, for example, by priming them to "think fun" (Mischel et al., 1972). It is an ironic aspect of willpower and human nature that the cool system is most difficult to access when it is most needed.

The reader who remembers Freud's conception of the id as characterized by irrational, impulsive urges for immediate wish-fulfillment, and its battles with the rational, logical executive ego, will not fail to note their similarity to the hot and cool systems as conceptualized in contemporary thinking (e.g., Epstein, 1994; Metcalfe & Mischel, 1999). The key difference is that what has been learned from research on this topic over the course of the past century now allows us to specify more clearly the cognitive and emotional processes that underlie these two systems and their interactions to enable effective self-regulation. We consider these specific processes next, drawing on experiments using the delay of gratification paradigm.

The hot/cool analysis of the dynamics of willpower summarized earlier was based in part on empirical evidence from the long-term research program on delay of gratification by Mischel and colleagues (e.g., for reviews, see Mischel, 1974b; Mischel & Ayduk, 2002; Mischel, Shoda, & Rodriguez, 1989). This research provides a framework for systematically conceptualizing the processes that undermine or support the successful exertion of willpower in diverse contexts, and provides an account that seems to fit the available data reasonably well. We next consider those data and examine how they speak to the predictions and postdictions suggested by the hot/cool analysis.

PROCESSING DYNAMICS IN DELAY OF GRATIFICATION

Mental Representation of Goals/Rewards

The experiments on mechanisms enabling delay of gratification were motivated originally by the following question, posed more than 30 years ago: How does the mental representation of deferred rewards or goals influence the person's ability to continue to wait or to work for them? The question needed to be asked at that time, when behaviorism was still at its height; although rewards had been assigned huge power as the determinants of behavior, virtually nothing was known about how people's mental representations of them operated and influenced goal-directed behavior. Few theories or even hypotheses were available to guide the search for answers.

A notable exception was Freud (1911/1959), whose writing about the transition from primary (id-based) to secondary (ego-based) processes famously theorized that the ability to endure delay of gratification begins to develop when the young child can construct a "hallucinatory wish-fulfilling image" of the wished-for but delayed object. In Freud's view, this mental image or representation of the object of desire (e.g., the maternal breast) makes it possible for the child to "bind time" and come to sustain delay of gratification volitionally. If so, Mischel and Ebbeson (1970) reasoned, sustained delay behavior in goal pursuit ought to be facilitated by cues that make the delayed rewards more salient and thus more available for mental representation.

Similar expectations came from a second, unexpected source in the research on learning with animals. Struggling with the question of how a rat manages to keep running to get its rewards later, at the end of all those complicated mazes, learning psychologists theorized that behavior toward a goal may be maintained by "fractional anticipatory goal responses" (Hull, 1931). While eschewing the language of cognition, the concept implied some kind of partial representation of the goal as a necessary condition for maintaining the animal's goal pursuit, for example, as the animal in a learning task tries to find its way back to the food at the end of a maze. In this sense, extrapolating to the young child, anticipation and self-instructions through which the delayed rewards are made salient should sustain delay behavior in pursuit of those rewards because it makes them easier to keep in mind and anticipate the gratification of having them. In short, collectively, these views from utterly different literatures suggested that focusing attention on the delayed rewards should facilitate delay of gratification.

To explore this hypothesis and to approximate the presence versus absence of mental representations of the delayed rewards, a series of experiments varied whether or not the reward objects in the choice were available for attention while the children tried to keep waiting for them (Mischel & Ebbesen, 1970). For example, in one condition, both the delayed and immediately available rewards were exposed, whereas in another condition both the delayed and immediate rewards were concealed from children's attention. In the remaining two groups, either the delayed or the immediate rewards were exposed while the other rewards were concealed. Rather than enhancing children's delay time, as was initially hypothesized by both psychodynamic and learning theories, having rewards available for attention in any combination (i.e., whether both were available or just one) dramatically reduced children's wait time.

When first obtained, these results were the opposite of what was predicted, but in retrospect, when viewed from a hot/cool systems framework, they are exactly as should be expected. Presumably availability of the rewards for attention increases their salience, making their consummatory, "hot" representations more accessible. This in turn intensifies the conflict between the stimulus pull of the immediate situation (i.e., to ring the bell and get the small reward) and the desirability of the future goal (i.e., getting the larger, preferred reward), thereby increasing the child's level of frustration or stress. Under such hot system activation, it is harder to resist stimulus control, and most children reverse their initial preference, ring the bell, and settle for the less desired outcome. When the rewards are obscured from sight, however, the conflict and the frustration inherent in the delay situation are diminished, making "willpower" much less difficult, and enabling children to wait longer (Mischel, 1974b). Theoretically, when attention is not focused on the tempting reward stimuli, corresponding hot nodes are less likely to become activated, making sustained delay of gratification less effortful.

By the same rationale, moving attention away from the rewards altogether as in the use of distraction strategies even when the rewards are physically present in the environment should also prevent hot system activation and make the delay situation less difficult to endure for the child. In testing this idea, Mischel and colleagues (1972) provided children experimentally with external or internal distracters. In some conditions preschoolers were given a little toy to play with; in others they were primed with self-distracting pleasant thoughts (e.g., thinking about Mommy pushing them on a swing), or they were not given any distracters while they faced the rewards. Such self-distraction made it much easier for the children to wait (regardless of whether the distracters were external or internal), and they did so readily even though the rewards were available for attention and staring them in the face. The successful dieter who resists the desserts on the tray will not be surprised by these results.

But whereas these results showed the effects of attention to the exposed actual rewards, they still left open the more basic question: What is the effect of their internal *mental* representation? Might it be possible to represent the same stimulus in alternate ways? Foreshadowing the hot/cool formal theory by more than 30 years, a distinction had been made in the research literature between the motivational (the consummatory, arousing, action-oriented, or motivating "go" features) and the informational (cognitive cue) functions of a stimulus (Berlyne, 1960; Estes, 1972).

Drawing on this distinction, Mischel and Moore (1973) reasoned that the actual rewards, or their mental representations by the child as real, puts the child's attention on the hot, arousing, consummatory features of the rewards (whether the immediately available or the delayed ones), and hence elicits the motivational effects (the "go" response: ring the bell, get the treat now). In contrast, a focus on the more cool, abstract, cue features of the rewards might have the effect of reminding the child of the delayed consequences without activating the consummatory trigger reaction, typically elicited by a focus on the motivating hot features. For example, the mental representation of the rewards as pictures emphasizes their cognitive, informational features rather than their consummatory features. Therefore, Mischel and Moore speculated that this kind of cool focus may reduce the conflict between wanting to wait and wanting to ring the bell by shifting attention away from arousing features of the stimulus and on to their informative meaning.

Hot/Cool Representations

Methodologically, the challenge was how to find operations for activating a mental representation at a time when the cognitive revolution was still in its infancy and even the concept of mental representations was still regarded suspiciously. To move beyond the effects of the actual stimulus and try to approximate their mental representations, a first step was to present the rewards in the form of *images*—literally, life-size pictures (formally, "iconic representations") of the immediate and delayed rewards presented from a slide projector on a screen facing the child. These pictorial representations were pitted against the presence of the real rewards themselves during the delay period. As predicted, the results were the opposite of those found when the real rewards were exposed: Exposure to the pictures of the images of the rewards significantly increased children's waiting time, whereas exposure to the actual rewards decreased delay (Mischel & Moore, 1973).

Again in retrospect, these findings are consistent with those expected from the hot/cool system analysis. The slide-presented images of the desired objects (in contrast to the actual objects) are more likely to activate cool nodes that correspond to inherently hot stimuli and attenuate the hot system. Recall that the cool nodes are conceptualized as representing informational, cognitive, and spatial aspects of stimuli. A pictorial depiction of the rewards, of a little stick of pretzel of the sort used in the studies, for example, is likely to activate a cool representation, in sharp contrast to the effects of facing the actual temptations.

Mischel and colleagues speculated that what is true for pictorial representations also should apply to diverse other forms of cognitive, cool appraisals of the "objects of desire" that might activate corresponding cool nodes for the rewards in the delay of gratification paradigm (Moore, Mischel, & Zeiss, 1976). Consequently, if the actual rewards could be construed in such a way that they psychologically become cool, for example, by thinking of them as pictures rather than real, it should help the child to reduce the frustration of the delay situation cognitively rather than being at the mercy of external situational cues.

To examine this prediction, children were faced with actual rewards but this time were cued in advance by the experimenters to pretend that they were pictures by essentially "putting a frame around them in your head" (Moore et al., 1976). In a second condition, the children were shown pictures of the rewards but this time were asked to imagine them as though they were real. Children were able to delay almost 18 minutes when they pretended that the rewards facing them were not real, but pictures. In contrast, they were able to wait for less than 6 minutes if they pretended that the real rewards, rather than the pictures, were in front of them. Theoretically, in the former group, the children were able to exert willpower by mentally activating cool nodes that corresponded to the hot stimulus in front of them (i.e., by cognitively transforming a real treat into "just a picture"). In posttests that asked about why they waited so long, as one child put it "you can't eat a picture."

The transformations of hot, motivating representations into cool, informative ones to facilitate willpower in the delay situation also were demonstrated by Mischel and Baker (1975). In this study, children in one condition were cued with cool, informational or hot, consummatory representations of the rewards during the delay task. For example, children who were waiting for marshmallows were cued to think of them as "white, puffy clouds." Those waiting for pretzels were told to think of them as "little, brown logs." In a second hot ideation condition, the instructions cued children to think about the marshmallows as "yummy, and chewy" and the pretzels as "salty and crunchy." As expected, when children thought about the rewards in hot terms, they were able to wait only for 5 minutes, whereas when they thought about them in cool terms, delay time increased to 13 minutes.

Summary: Attention Control in the Delay Process

Taking these findings collectively, it became clear that delay of gratification depends not on whether or not attention is focused on the objects of desire, but rather on just how they are mentally represented. A focus on their hot features may momentarily increase motivation, but unless it is rapidly cooled by a focus on their cool, informative features (e.g., as reminders of what will be obtained later if the contingency is fulfilled) it is likely to become excessively arousing and trigger the "go" response.

While most of the delay of gratification experiments have involved passive waiting in order to obtain the preferred outcomes, the same mechanisms of attention deployment seem to apply when goal attainment is contingent on the person's work and performance. This was demonstrated recently in experiments in which children were required to complete a work task instead of passively waiting for the experimenter to return in order to get the larger but delayed rewards. Attention focused on the rewards undermined delay of gratification in both working and waiting situations, thus extending the generalizability of the attention control mechanisms that enable such effortful control (Peake, Hebl, & Mischel, 2002).

Flexible Attention Deployment and Discriminative Facility

Studies conducting fine-grain analyses of second-by-second attention deployment during efforts at sustained delay of gratification suggest that self-regulation depends not just on cooling strategies but on *flexible attention deployment* in the process (Peake et al., 2002). For example, Peake and colleagues' (2002) study on delay in working situations showed that when children had to complete a boring, frustrating task, delay ability was facilitated most when attention intermittently shifted to the rewards, as if the children tried to enhance their motivation to remain by reminding themselves about the rewards, but then quickly shifted away to prevent arousal from becoming excessive. Such flexibility in attention deployment is consistent with the view that it is the balanced interactions between the hot and cool systems that sustain delay of gratification and effortful control, as they exert their motivating and cooling effects in tandem (see also Rodriguez, Mischel, & Shoda, 1989).

Evidence that flexible attention deployment is important for effective self-regulation also is consistent with findings showing the role of *discriminative facility* in self-regulation. Discriminative facility refers to the individual's ability to perceive the subtly different demands and opportunities of different kinds of situations, and flexibly adjust coping strategies accordingly. A good deal of research now documents that discriminative facility is basic for adaptive social and emotional coping in diverse contexts (Cantor & Kihlstrom, 1987; Cheng, Chiu, Hong, & Cheung, 2001; Chiu, Hong, Mischel, & Shoda, 1995; Mendoza-Denton, Ayduk, Mischel, Shoda, & Testa, 2001; Shoda, Mischel, & Wright, 1993).

The types of cooling strategies in these studies with preschoolers are, of course, only illustrative of the many adaptive ways to maintain long-term goal pursuit and to overcome stimulus control with agentic self-control. The important point is that diverse, creative cooling strategies can be constructed by the cool system, if it can be accessed before automatic impulsive action is triggered by the hot system that preempts the person from thinking rationally and creatively. In formal terms, goal pursuit in delay of gratification depends both on the activation of motivational processes, as discussed earlier in this chapter, and on the accessibility and activation of the necessary cooling strategies. It depends on the network of organization connecting the motivational processes that lead to choice and goal commitment, to the activation and generation of cooling strategies. When these strategies are accessed they serve to reduce the hot stimulus pull and the frustration aroused in the situation, so that hopeful wishing can be transformed into effective willing.

Automaticity: Taking the Effort out of Effortful Control

In order for these adaptive control efforts in the hot system/cool system interactions to be maintained over time and accessed rapidly when they are urgently needed, they have to be converted from conscious, slow, and effortful to automatic activation, in this sense taking the effort out of "effortful self-control." The conversion process that enables the person to go from good intentions to effective action and goal attainment has been most extensively addressed by Gollwitzer and colleagues in their research on *implementation plans* (see Gollwitzer, 1999; Patterson & Mischel, 1975). Individuals can avoid succumbing to stimulus control by planning out and rehearsing their "implementation intentions" for difficult goal pursuit. These plans specify in detail the various steps needed to protect the person from the obstacles, frustrations, and temptations likely to be encountered, keeping in mind and in awareness the demands of the current goal that is being pursued (Gollwitzer, 1999).

When planned and rehearsed, implementation intentions help self-control because goal-directed action is initiated relatively automatically when the relevant trigger cues become situationally salient. Implementation intentions help self-regulation across a wide range of regulatory tasks such as action initiation (e.g., "I will start writing the paper the day after Thanksgiving"), inhibition of unwanted habitual responses (e.g., "When the dessert menu is served, I will not order the chocolate cake"), and resistance to temptation (e.g., "Whenever the distraction arises, I will ignore it"). In short, Gollwitzer's work indicates that some effortful, deliberative process of linking action plans to specific situational triggers (the "ifs") is needed in the initial phases of automatization. But after this link has been established and rehearsed, effective self-regulatory behavior and cool system strategies can be activated and generated much more readily, even under stressful or cognitively busy situations, without conscious effort. That is, if the specified situational cue remains highly activated, the planned behavior will run off automatically when the actual cue is encountered (Gollwitzer, 1999).

Stability and Meaningfulness of Individual Differences in Self-Regulatory Competencies

There is increasing evidence for the long-term stability and predictive value of individual differences in the self-regulatory competencies assessed in the delay of gratification paradigm early in life. As noted earlier, the number of seconds that preschoolers at age 4 years delayed gratification in the diagnostic condition of the delay paradigm described earlier significantly predicted such outcomes as their SAT scores and ratings of their social–emotional and cognitive competencies in adolescence (Mischel et al., 1988; Shoda et al., 1990). Likewise, in further follow-up studies preschool delay times predicted such outcomes as the attained educational level and use of cocaine-crack when the participants are about 27 years old (Ayduk et al., 2000).

The early antecedents of the ability to delay gratification in preschool, which are visible already in the toddler's behavior, also have been explored. They are meaningfully expressed in the ways in which the toddler deals with the delay of gratification demands produced by brief maternal separation in attachment studies using the Strange Situation (Sethi, Mischel, Aber, Shoda, & Rodriguez, 2000). Thus the same cooling attention control mechanisms demonstrated to be effective in preschool children appear to be visible in the toddler at 18 months and have been linked to delay behavior at age 4 years (Sethi et al., 2000). Furthermore, these mechanisms also have been shown to apply in diverse populations in middle school years, and to have meaningful correlates supporting their validity as predictors of diverse adaptive social, cognitive, and emotional outcomes (Ayduk et al., 2000, 2008; Rodriguez, Mischel, & Shoda, 1989).

Individual differences in the types of self-regulatory behavior tapped in the delay paradigm may be related to distinct patterns of neural and biological reactivity, as well as to aspects of temperament visible in early childhood (e.g., Derryberry, 2002; Derryberry & Rothbart, 1997; Rothbart, Derryberry, & Posner, 1994). For example, a number of studies have shown that the reactivity of the neural circuitry embedded in the limbic system, which underlies people's appetitive and defensive motivational systems, can be modulated by an executive attention control system that is sensitive to effortful intentions (Derryberry & Reed, 2002; Eisenberg, Fabes, Guthrie, & Reiser, 2000). This executive system, believed to be located in the anterior cingulate, appears to be related to the regulation of motivational impulses through "attention flexibility" and is assumed to contribute to the development of the ability to delay gratification, among a variety of other important developmental processes (Derryberry & Rothbart, 1997). It is tempting to speculate that the effective, flexible attention control that seems basic for the ability to delay gratification in goal pursuit also should be related to the neural circuitry that underlies the anterior attention system. To our knowledge, however, no empirical study to date has directly tested this assumptions and it seems important to explore those potential connections.

COOLING STRATEGIES IN EMOTION REGULATION: DEALING WITH DIVERSE AVERSIVE HOT SITUATIONS

The strategies that help people deal with the control of appetitive impulses as in the delay situation also apply to emotional self-regulation for dealing with aversive hot situations and dilemmas, including those produced by one's own vulnerabilities and negative emotions (e.g., fears of abandonment and rejection) in diverse interpersonal contexts. Experimental research reported years ago that an attitude of detachment helps people react more calmly when exposed to gory scenes portraying bloody accidents and death (Koriat, Melkman, Averill, & Lazarus, 1972) or when expecting electric shock (Holmes & Houston, 1974). Since then, experiments have helped to specify further the processes that allow people to regulate their negative emotions. In a typical study to probe the underlying processes in emotion regulation, Gross (1998) brings participants into the laboratory and informs them that they will be watching a movie. The film they will see shows detailed close-up views of severe burn victims or of an arm amputation.

Participants then are divided into different groups and given different instructions prior to viewing the film. For example, in one condition (called "cognitive reappraisal"), they are asked to use a cooling strategy, and to try to think about the movie in a detached unemotional way, objectively, focusing attention on the technical details of the event, not feeling anything personally (e.g., "Pretend that you're a teacher in medical school").

From the perspective of the present model, this is a cognitive cooling strategy, similar to the preschoolers' trying to think about the real treats facing them as if they were "just pictures," or focusing on their cool rather than hot qualities. As predicted, Gross's results supported the value of the cooling strategy. Cooling enabled adaptive regulation of negative emotions better than either a control condition (in which participants were simply asked to watch the movie), or a suppression condition (in which they were asked to try to hide their emotional reactions to the film as they watched it so that anyone seeing them would not know that they were feeling anything at all). The cooling strategy by means of cognitive reappraisal was a much more adaptive way to regulate negative emotions, as seen in measures of the intensity of people's negative experiences as well as in their levels of physiological autonomic nervous system arousal and distress. Thus, individuals who were cued to think about the movie in a way that cools the emotional content experienced fewer feelings of disgust and less physiological activation (evidenced by less blood vessel constriction) when compared to those who attempted to hide completely and suppress their emotional responses to the film faces (Gross, 1998; see also John & Gross, 2004, and Ochsner & Gross, 2008, for reviews).

Along similar lines, recent research on self-distancing also illustrates the adaptive function of cooling strategies in emotion regulation (Ayduk & Kross, 2008; Kross & Ayduk, 2008; Kross, Ayduk, & Mischel, 2005). More specifically, this work shows that focusing on negative past experiences from a self-distanced, third-person perspective as opposed to a self-immersed, first-person perspective serves as a buffer against a variety of negative outcomes, such as heightened negative affect, physiological reactivity, and rumination over time, by facilitating reconstrual of the experience and inhibiting people's tendency to recount the emotionally evocative details of their experience.

A good deal of related research further supports the conclusion that self-distraction, when possible, can be an excellent way to reduce unavoidable stresses like unpleasant medical examinations (Miller, 1987) and coping with severe life crises (Bonanno, 2001; Bonanno, Keltner, Holen, & Horowitz, 1995; Taylor & Brown, 1988). Self-distraction (e.g., watching travel slides or recalling pleasant memories) increases tolerance of experimentally induced physical pain (e.g., Berntzen, 1987; Chaves & Barber, 1974). Similarly, distracting and relaxation-inducing activities, such as listening to music reduce anxiety in the face of uncontrollable shocks (Miller, 1979), help people cope with the daily pain of rheumatoid arthritis (Affleck, Urrows, Tennen, & Higgins, 1992) and even with severe life crises (e.g., Taylor & Brown, 1988). Minimization of negative affect and instead being engaged in everyday tasks following the death of a spouse predicted minimal grief symptoms more than a year after the loss (Bonanno et al., 1995).

Cooling strategies, as illustrated by re-construal mechanisms, can also help one to transform potentially stressful situations to make them less aversive. For example, if surgical patients are encouraged to re-construe their hospital stay as a vacation to relax a while from the stresses of daily life, they show better postoperative adjustment (Langer, Janis, & Wolfer, 1975), just as chronically ill patients who reinterpret their conditions more positively also show better adjustment (Carver, Pozo, Harris, & Noriega, 1993). In sum, when stress and pain are inevitable, the adage to look for the silver lining and to "accentuate the positive" seems wise.

A word of clarification is needed, however, about the distinction between our conceptualization self-distraction as an effective self-regulatory strategy and emotional suppression as viewed by Gross (1998), and thought suppression as discussed by Wegner (1994). Self-distraction of the kind we discuss involves strategically moving attention away from hot information while actively attending to cool aspects of the situation in a way that creates "psychological distance." In this sense, it is different from thought suppression where one simply tries to avoid thinking about an unwanted thought. It is likewise different from emotional suppression where the individual is merely asked to not reveal his or her affective reactions without an alternative stimulus on which attention can be purposefully focused. Indeed, research on thought suppression indicates that when people are provided with focused distraction strategies (i.e., are given an alternative thought to focus on every time the to-be-suppressed idea comes to mind) they are buffered against the typical rebound effect (Wegner, Schneider, Carter, & White, 1987).

IMPLICATIONS OF EFFORTFUL CONTROL FOR COPING WITH PERSONAL VULNERABILITIES AND INTERPERSONAL DIFFICULTIES

Most of the delay of gratification studies have focused on conflicts between immediately available smaller rewards and delayed larger outcomes in essentially simple "less now" versus "more later" dilemmas. Similar psychological processes, however, underlie the subtler interpersonal conflicts that threaten to undermine many human relationships both in the workplace and in intimate relations. Good intentions to maintain harmony and to work cooperatively toward common goals all too often are sabotaged by the explosion of anger, hostility, and jealousy within the daily tensions of life. It is in the heat of the moment that the need to inhibit hot, automatic—potentially destructive—reactions becomes most difficult in interpersonal relationships, particularly when those relationships are of high importance to the self.

These situations often create conflicts between the tendency to make immediate, self-centered responses, as opposed to focusing on the long-term consequences and implications for the partner and the preservation of the relationship itself (e.g., Arriaga & Rusbult, 1998). In the present model of self-regulation, a constructive approach to such conflicts requires cooling hot system activation by accessing cooling strategies that allow the long-term goals to be pursued, so that " . . . immediate, self-interested preferences are replaced by preferences that take into account broader concerns, including considerations to some degree that transcend the immediate situation" (Arriaga & Rusbult, 1998, p. 928). Basically, to attain interpersonal accommodation requires delay of gratification—making and sustaining a choice between immediate but smaller self-interest and a delayed but larger interest (larger in the sense that it is good both for the self and for the relationship).

Supporting this analysis, evidence suggests that cooling attention control processes that underlie delay ability also help in the regulation of defensive reactions in interpersonal contexts. To illustrate, we explored the hypothesis that delay ability serves as a protective buffer against the interpersonal vulnerability of *rejection sensitivity*, or RS. Viewed from a CAPS perspective, RS is a chronic processing disposition characterized by anxious expectations of rejection (Downey & Feldman, 1996) and a readiness to encode even ambiguous events in interpersonal situations (e.g., partner momentarily seems inattentive) as indicators of rejection that rapidly trigger automatic hot reactions (e.g., hostility–anger, withdrawal–depression, self-silencing (Ayduk, Downey, Testa, Yen, & Shoda, 1999; Ayduk, May, Downey, & Higgins, 2003; Ayduk, Mischel, & Downey, 2002).

Probably rooted in prior rejection experiences, these dynamics are readily activated when high-RS people encounter interpersonal situations in which rejection is a possibility, triggering in them a sense of threat and foreboding. In such a state, the person's defensive, fight-or-flight system is activated (Downey, Mougios, Ayduk, London, & Shoda, 2004), and attention narrows on detection of threat-related cues. This in turn makes the high-RS person ready to perceive the threatening outcome—and to engage in behaviors (e.g., anger, hostility, exit threats) likely ultimately to confirm their worst fears by wrecking the relationship (Downey, Freitas, Michealis, & Khouri, 1998). Repeated rejection and disillusionment with relationships tend to lead to identity problems and erode self-worth, and both self-concept confusion and low self-esteem are common characteristics of people high in RS (e.g., Ayduk, Gyurak, & Luerssen, 2009; Ayduk et al., 2000).

In short, RS may predispose vulnerable individuals to react in automatic and reflexively impulsive hot ways rather than engage in reflective, goal-oriented, or instrumental responses in interpersonal interactions. According to our self-regulatory processing model, however, whether this characteristic pattern unfolds or not should depend on the availability of self-regulatory competencies (see Ayduk & Gyurak, 2008, for further discussion). To the extent that high RS individuals are capable of accessing the strategies that enable them to attenuate negative arousal, they may be able to inhibit some of their destructive behavioral patterns.

These theoretically expected processing dynamics are depicted in Figure 5.1. Panel A shows a high-RS network in which potential trigger features (e.g., partner seems bored and distracted) activate anxious rejection expectations and are encoded as rejection that quickly activates hot thoughts ("She doesn't love me anymore") and negative affect. Attention control and cooling strategies are relatively inaccessible and/or have weak inhibitory links to the RS dynamics, allowing this vulnerability to have an unmediated effect on eliciting destructive behavior. In contrast, Panel B depicts a high-RS network where attention control and cooling strategies are highly accessible and deactivate the RS dynamics via strong inhibitory links so that the event is not encoded as rejection, and hot thoughts and feelings are inhibited. Consequently the individual's dispositional vulnerability—the tendency to behave in a destructive manner—is attenuated and the negative consequences of this disposition are circumvented.

To explore these expectations empirically, in one set of studies self-regulatory ability was assessed by measuring the child's waiting time in the delay of gratification situation at age 4 years (Ayduk et al., 2000, Study 1; Ayduk et al., 2008, Study 2). This longitudinal study showed that among vulnerable (high-RS) individuals, the number of seconds participants were able to wait as preschoolers in the delay situation predicted their adult resiliency against the potentially destructive effects of RS. That is, high-RS adults who had high delay ability in preschool had more positive functioning (high self-esteem, self-worth, and coping ability, and lower vulnerability to borderline personality features) compared with similarly high-RS adults who were not able to delay in preschool. Furthermore, high-RS participants showed higher levels of cocaine-crack use and lower levels of education than those low in RS, only if they were unable to delay gratification in preschool. That is, high-RS people who had high preschool delay ability had relatively lower levels of drug use and higher education levels, and in these respects were similar to low-RS participants.

A similar pattern of results was found in a second study with middle school children from a different cohort and from a very different socioeconomic and ethnic population (Ayduk et al., 2000, Study 2). Namely, whereas high-RS children with low delay ability were more aggressive toward their peers and thus had less positive peer relationships than children low in RS, high-RS children who were able to delay longer were even less aggressive and more liked by their peers than low-RS children. Consistent with the moderating role of delay ability in the RS dynamics, a cross-sectional study of preadolescents boys with behavioral problems characterized by heightened hostile reactivity to potential interpersonal threats also showed that the spontaneous use of cooling strategies in the delay task (i.e., looking away from the rewards and self-distraction) predicted reduced verbal and physical aggression (Rodriguez, Mischel, Shoda, & Wright, 1989).

In a more direct experimental test of the effect of hot and cool systems on hostile reactivity to rejection, college students imagined an autobiographical rejection experience focusing on either their physiological and emotional reactions during the experience (hot ideation) or contextual features of the physical setting where this experience happened (cool ideation). In a subsequent lexical decision task, hostility and anger words were less accessible to those individuals primed with cool ideation than to those primed with hot ideation. More important, this was true for both high-RS and low-RS participants. The same pattern of anger reduction in the cool condition was found in people's self-report measures of angry mood and in the level of angry affect expressed in their descriptions of the rejection experience (Ayduk, Mischel, & Downey, 2002).

In sum, these correlational and experimental findings, taken collectively, suggest that how high RS translates into behavior over the course of development depends on the accessibility of self-regulatory competencies like those tapped by the delay of gratification paradigm. In the present model the extent to which an individual is likely to engage in the destructive interpersonal behavior, to which the RS vulnerability readily leads, depends on the connection—or lack of connection—between the activation of the RS dynamic and the activation of the relevant attention control strategies. If these two subsystems are interconnected within the network's organization, the cooling strategies can modulate the hot reactivity of the RS dynamic, as illustrated by Figure 5.1, and the individual may be protected against the maladaptive behavioral consequences of this vulnerability.

What is true for the RS vulnerability also may apply to diverse other dispositional vulnerabilities. A growing body of research is examining similar interaction patterns between self-regulation competencies and other personality variables for diverse set of behavioral outcomes. To illustrate, Derryberry and Reed (2002) report that attention control (measured by a self-report measure of flexible shifting and focusing of attention) helps regulate attention biases of high-anxious individuals in processing threat-related information. Whereas anxious individuals with poor attention control show a bias to focus on threat-related cues, anxious participants with good attention control are better able to shift their attention away from threat information, showing the buffering effects of attention control on trait anxiety. Consistently, Eisenberg and colleagues find that dispositional negative emotionality and attention control predict children's social functioning both additively and multiplicatively (see Eisenberg, Fabes, Guthrie, & Reiser, 2002, for review). More specifically, children high in negative emotionality and low in attention control seem to be at greatest risk for difficulties with peers, and externalizing as well as internalizing problems, while high regulation seems to buffer against the effect of negative emotionality on problem behaviors.

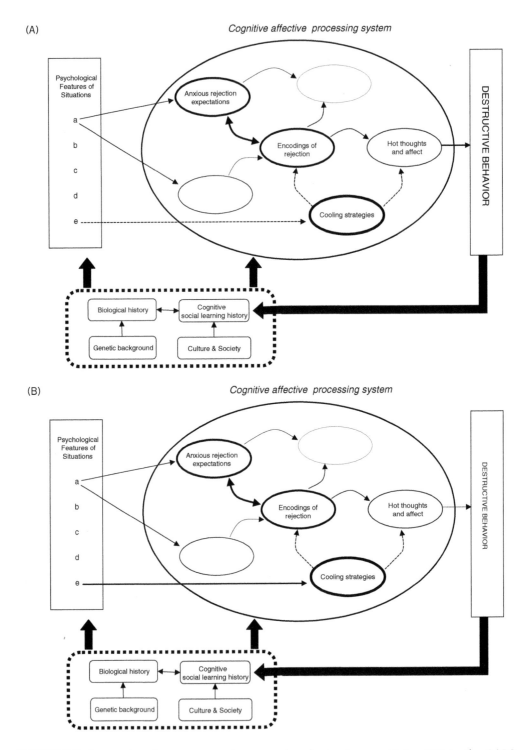

(A)

Cognitive affective processing system

(B)

Cognitive affective processing system

FIGURE 5.1. Interactions between attention control and rejection sensitivity (RS) in the CAPS network. (A) A high-RS network where attention control and cooling strategies are relatively inaccessible and/or weakly connected, through inhibitory links, to the RS dynamics, allowing them to have an unmediated effect on eliciting destructive behavior. (B) A high-RS network where attention control and cooling strategies are highly accessible and connect to the RS dynamics via strong inhibitory links, attenuating the individual's tendency to behave in a destructive manner.

CONCLUDING REMARKS

In the CAPS model of self-regulation, willpower requires the joint operation of regulatory motivation and competencies. Whereas strength of desire, and goal commitment, are necessary first steps in order to be able to sustain those intentions to completion, often under hot, frustrating, temptation-filled conditions, the individual has to access rapidly and flexibly utilize certain cognitive-attention deployment strategies whose key ingredients we have attempted to articulate. Furthermore, the interaction between motivation and competencies is not a one-time serial process, nor is there only one choice to be made (e.g., when the individual decides whether or not to delay gratification in the first place). Rather the process of sustaining effortful control plays out over time, as choices shift when the experience proves to be more difficult than initially anticipated, and as the power of the situation exerts its effect. In a connectionist, dynamic view of self-regulation, motivational and cognitive-attention control processes operate simultaneously and in a mutually recursive manner: The strength and commitment to one's long-term goals, and their importance within the goal hierarchies of the total system, affect how much effort may be expended in utilizing available self-regulatory skills. At the same time, utilization of attention control mechanisms and the subsequent inhibition of hot system processing helps one to stay committed to the initial goal by making all the relevant cognitive affective units (CAUs)—self-efficacy beliefs, control expectancies, value of the goal, and so on—highly salient and accessible.

To reiterate, for the effortful control processes necessary to maintain willpower to be accessed rapidly when they are urgently needed, and maintained over time, they have to be converted from conscious, slow, and effortful to automatic activation, in this sense taking the effort out of "effortful self-control." Fortunately, as reviewed earlier in this chapter, the processes that enable this conversion (e.g., through planning and rehearsal) have become increasingly clear (see Gollwitzer, 1999; Patterson & Mischel, 1975). We also want to reemphasize that effective self-regulation and adaptive coping depend on the particulars of the continuous interactions between the motivating effects of the emotional, hot system and the strategic competencies enabled by the cognitive, cool system, not on the predominance of either system with the shut down of the other. It is true that in many situations in which the person wants to exercise self-control and finds it most difficult to do so, the hot system is activated by the situational pressures of the moment (the tempting pastry tray is in one's face) and cooling strategies may be urgently needed—at least some of the time. But it would be a misreading to think that adaptive goal pursuit is served by shutting down the hot system altogether and having the cool system prevail.

At the level of brain research, the work of Damasio and colleagues documents in detail the importance of both systems and their continuous interactions (e.g., Bechara, Damasio, Damasio, & Lee, 1999). For example, their somatic marker hypothesis suggests that both the ventromedial prefrontal cortex (VMF; a "cool system" structure in our conceptualization) and the amygdala (locus of the "hot" system) are essential parts of a neural circuitry that is necessary for advantageous decision making. In the "gambling tasks" in these studies, subjects choose between decks of cards that yield either immediate or delayed gratification (i.e., high immediate gain but larger future loss vs. lower immediate gain but a smaller future loss). Although we cannot elaborate the details here, briefly these studies show how both the patients with damage to the VMF and those with damage to the amygdala make disadvantageous decisions in the gambling game (i.e., choose immediate gratification), but this is the consequence of different kinds of impairments.

Patients with amygdala damage cannot effectively experience somatic (emotional states) either after winning or losing money, and never develop conditioned affective reactions (i.e., increased skin conductance reflecting high arousal); subsequently, the potential impact of this kind of somatic information on decision making is precluded. Patients with VMF damage, on the other hand, show somatic states in response to reward and punishment but they cannot integrate all of this information in an effective and coherent manner; thus, the somatic states (although experienced) cannot be used as feedback in subsequent decision making. These studies make it clear that patients who have impairment in what we call the hot system, and those with damage in the cool system, both encounter serious problems with delay behavior: Clearly we need both systems and their interactions to make the choice to delay gratification for a larger yet distal good and to sustain effort toward its attainment.

Long ago, a distinguished humanist, Lionel Trilling (1943), also addressed both the gains and losses that either the absence or the excess of willpower can yield. After noting the place of passion in life and "the strange paradoxes of being human," he emphasized that "the will is not everything," and spoke of the "panic and emptiness which make their onset when the will is tired from its own excess" (p. 139). And as research in recent years suggests, using willpower may indeed have fatiguing consequences (e.g., Baumeister, Gailliot, & Tice, 2009). Excessively postponing gratification can become a stifling, joyless choice, but an absence of will leaves people the victims of their biographies. Often the choice to delay or not is difficult and effortful, yet in the absence of the competencies needed to sustain delay and to exercise the will when there is a wish to do so, the choice itself is lost.

In this chapter we have tried to show that while many of the ingredients of willpower, and particularly the processing dynamics that enable regulatory competence and delay of gratification, have long been mysterious, some of the essentials now are becoming clear. Self-regulatory ability assessed in the delay of gratification paradigm reflects stable individual differences in regulatory strength that are visible early in life and cut across different domains of behavior (e.g., eating, attachment, aggression). Much is also known about the basic attention control mechanisms that underlie and govern this self-regulatory competence. These control rules help to demystify willpower and point to the processes that enable it. Furthermore, the implications of regulatory ability—or its lack—for the self are straightforward, influencing self-concepts and self-esteem, interpersonal strategies (e.g., aggression), coping, and the ability to buffer or protect the self against the maladaptive consequences of chronic personal vulnerabilities such as rejection sensitivity.

An urgent question remains unanswered: Can self-regulation and the ability to delay gratification be taught? We already know that attention control strategies are experimentally modifiable (Ayduk et al., 2002; Mischel et al., 1989). Also, modeling effective control strategies can have positive consequences, generalizing to behavior outside of the lab in the short run for at least a period of a month or so (Bandura & Mischel, 1965). What we do not know yet is whether—and how—socialization, education, and therapy can effectively be utilized to help individuals gain the necessary attention control competencies to make willpower more accessible when they need and want it. For both theoretical and practical reasons it is time to pursue this question. We hope the answers will turn out to be affirmative—and not too long delayed.

ACKNOWLEDGMENTS

The preparation of this chapter was supported by Grant No. MH39349 from the National Institute of Mental Health. We would like to thank Ethan Kross for his constructive comments on several drafts of this chapter.

REFERENCES

Affleck, G., Urrows, S., Tennen, H., & Higgins, P. (1992). Daily coping with pain from rheumatoid arthritis: Patterns and correlates. *Pain, 51,* 221–229.

Ainslie, G. (2001). *Breakdown of will.* Cambridge, UK: Cambridge University Press.

Altman, J., & Bayer, S. A. (1990). Migration and distribution of two populations of hippocampal granule cell precursors during the perinatal and postnatal periods. *Journal of Comparative Neurology, 301,* 365–381.

Arriaga, X. B., & Rusbult, C. E. (1998). Standing in my partner's shoes: Partner perspective taking and reactions to accommodative dilemmas. *Personality and Social Psychology Bulletin, 24,* 927–948.

Ayduk, O., Downey, G., Testa, A., Yen, Y., & Shoda, Y. (1999). Does rejection sensitivity elicit hostility in rejection sensitive women? *Social Cognition, 17,* 245–271.

Ayduk, O., & Gyurak, A. (2008). Applying the cognitive-affective systems (CAPS) approach to conceptualizing rejection sensitivity. *Social and Personality Psychology Compass, 2/5,* 2016–2033.

Ayduk, O., Gyurak, A., & Luerssen, A. (2009). Rejection sensitivity moderates the impact of rejection on self-concept clarity. *Personality and Social Psychology Bulletin, 35*(11), 1467–1478.

Ayduk, O., & Kross, E. (2008). Enhancing the pace of recovery: Self-distanced analysis of negative experiences reduces blood pressure reactivity. *Psychological Science, 19,* 229–231.

Ayduk, O., May, D., Downey, G., & Higgins, T. (2003). Tactical differences in coping with rejection sensitivity: The role of prevention pride. *Personality and Social Psychology Bulletin, 29,* 435–448.

Ayduk, O., Mendoza-Denton, R., Mischel, W., Downey, G., Peake, P., & Rodriguez, M. L. (2000). Regulating the interpersonal self: Strategic self-regulation for coping with rejection sensitivity. *Journal of Personality and Social Psychology, 79,* 776–792.

Ayduk, O., Mischel, W., & Downey, G. (2002). Attentional mechanisms lining rejection to hostile reactivity: The role of the "hot" vs. "cool" focus. *Psychological Science, 13,* 443–448.

Ayduk, O., Zayas, V., Downey, G., Cole, A. B., Shoda, Y., & Mischel, W. (2008). Rejection sensitivity and executive control: Joint predictors of borderline personality features. *Journal of Research in Personality, 42,* 151–168.

Bandura, A., & Mischel, W. (1965). Modification of self-imposed delay of reward through exposure to live and symbolic models. *Journal of Personality and Social Psychology, 2,* 698–705.

Baumeister, R. F., Gailliot, M. T., & Tice, D. M. (2009). Free willpower: A limited resource theory of volition, choice, and self-regulation. In E. Morsella, J. Bargh, & P. Gollwitzer (Eds.), *Oxford handbook of human action* (pp. 487–508). New York: Oxford University Press.

Bechara, A., Damasio, H., Damasio, A. R., & Lee, G. (1999). Different contributions of the human amygdala and ventromedial prefrontal cortex to decision-making. *Journal of Neuroscience, 19,* 5473–5481.

Berlyne, D. (1960). *Conflict, arousal, and curiosity.* New York: McGraw-Hill.

Berntzen, D. (1987). Effects of multiple cognitive coping strategies on laboratory pain. *Cognitive Therapy and Research, 11,* 613–623.

Bonanno, G. A. (2001). Grief and emotion: A social–functional perspective. In M. S. Stroebe &

R. O. Hansson (Eds.), *Handbook of bereavement research: Consequences, coping, and care* (pp. 493–515). Washington, DC: American Psychological Association.

Bonanno, G. A., Keltner, D., Holen, A., & Horowitz, M. J. (1995). When avoiding unpleasant emotions might not be such a bad thing: Verbal–autonomic response dissociation and midlife conjugal bereavement. *Journal of Personality and Social Psychology, 69,* 975–989.

Cantor, N., & Kihlstrom, J. F. (1987). *Personality and social intelligence.* Englewood Cliffs, NJ: Prentice-Hall.

Carver, C. S., Pozo, C., Harris, S. D., & Noriega, V. (1993). How coping mediates the effect of optimism on distress: A study of women with early stage breast cancer. *Journal of Personality and Social Psychology, 65,* 375–390.

Chaves, J. F., & Barber, T. X. (1974). Cognitive strategies, experimenter modeling, and expectation in the attenuation of pain. *Journal of Abnormal Psychology, 83,* 356–363.

Cheng, C., Chiu, C. Y., Hong, Y. Y., & Cheung, J. S. (2001). Discriminative facility and its role in the perceived quality of interactional experiences. *Journal of Personality, 69,* 765–786.

Chiu, C., Hong, Y., Mischel, W., & Shoda, Y. (1995). Discriminative facility in social competence: Conditional versus dispositional encoding and monitoring-blunting of information. *Social Cognition, 13,* 49–70.

Derryberry, D. (2002). Attention and voluntary self-control. *Self and Identity, 1,* 105–111.

Derryberry, D., & Reed, M. A. (2002). Anxiety-related attentional biases and their regulation by attention control. *Journal of Abnormal Psychology, 111,* 225–236.

Derryberry, D., & Rothbart, M. (1997). Reactive and effortful processes in the organization of temperament. *Development and Psychopathology, 9,* 633–652.

Downey, G., & Feldman, S. (1996). Implications of rejection sensitivity for intimate relationships. *Journal of Personality and Social Psychology, 70,* 1327–1343.

Downey, G., Freitas, A., Michealis, B., & Khouri, H. (1998). The self-fulfilling prophecy in close relationships: Do rejection sensitive women get rejected by romantic partners? *Journal of Personality and Social Psychology, 75,* 545–560.

Downey, G., Mougios, V., Ayduk, O., London, B., & Shoda, Y. (2004). Rejection sensitivity and the defensive motivational system: Insights from the startle response to rejection cues. *Psychological Science, 15,* 668–673.

Eisenberg, N., Fabes, R. A., Guthrie, I. K., & Reiser, M. (2000). Dispositional emotionality and regulation: Their role in predicting quality of social functioning. *Journal of Personality and Social Psychology, 78,* 136–157.

Eisenberg, N., Fabes, R. A., Guthrie, I. K., & Reiser, M. (2002). The role of emotionality and regulation in children's social competence and adjustment. In A. Caspi (Ed.), *Paths to successful development: Personality in the life course* (pp. 46–70). New York: Cambridge University Press.

Epstein, S. (1994). Integration of the cognitive and psychodynamic unconscious. *American Psychologist, 49,* 709–724.

Estes, W. K. (1972). Reinforcement in human behavior. *American Scientist, 60,* 723–729.

Freud, S. (1911). Formulations regarding the two principles of mental functioning. In *Collected papers* (Vol. IV, pp. 13–21). New York: Basic Books. (Original work published 1959)

Gaffan, D. (1992). Amygdala and the memory of reward. In J. P. Aggleton (Ed.), *The amygdala: Neurobiological aspects of emotion, memory, and mental dysfunction* (pp. 471–483). New York: Wiley-Liss.

Gollwitzer, P. M. (1999). Implementation intentions: Strong effects of simple plans. *American Psychologist, 54,* 493–503.

Gray, J. A. (1987). *The psychology of fear and stress* (2nd ed.). New York: McGraw-Hill.

Gross, J. J. (1998). Antecedent- and response-focused emotion regulation: Divergent consequences for experience, expression, and physiology. *Journal of Personality and Social Psychology, 74,* 224–237.

Holmes, D. S., & Houston, B. K. (1974). Effectiveness of situation redefinition and affective isolation in coping with stress. *Journal of Personality and Social Psychology, 29,* 212–218.

Hull, C. L. (1931). Goal attraction and directing ideas conceived as habit phenomena. *Psychological Review, 38,* 487–506.

John, O. P., & Gross, J. J. (2004). Healthy and unhealthy emotion regulation: Personality processes, individual differences, and life span development [Special issue]. *Journal of Personality, 72*(6), 1301–1333.

Koriat, A., Melkman, R., Averill, J. R., & Lazarus, R. S. (1972). The self-control of emotional reactions to a stressful film. *Journal of Personality, 40,* 601–619.

Kross, E., & Ayduk, O. (2008). Facilitating adaptive emotional analysis: Distinguishing distanced-analysis of depressive experiences from immersed-analysis and distraction. *Personality and Social Psychology Bulletin, 34,* 924–938.

Kross, E., Ayduk, O., & Mischel, W. (2005). When asking "why" doesn't hurt: Distinguishing rumination from reflective processing of negative emotions. *Psychological Science, 16,* 709–715.

Langer, E. J., Janis, I. L., & Wolfer, J. A. (1975). Reduction of psychological stress in surgical patients. *Journal of Experimental Social Psychology, 11,* 155–165.

LeDoux, J. (1996). *The emotional brain.* New York: Touchstone.

Lieberman, M. D. (2003). Reflective and reflexive judgment processes: A social cognitive neuroscience approach. In J. P. Forgas, K. Williams, & W. von Hippel (Eds.), *Social judgments: Implicit and explicit processes* (pp. 44–67). Philadelphia: Psychology Press.

Lieberman, M. D., Gaunt, R., Gilbert, D. T., & Trope, Y. (2002). Reflection and reflexion: A social cognitive neuroscience approach to attributional inference. In M. Zanna (Ed.), *Advances in experimental social psychology* (Vol. 34, pp. 199–249). New York: Academic Press.

Loewenstein, G., Read, D., & Baumeister, R. (Eds.). (2003). *Time and decision: Economic and psychological perspectives on intertemporal choice.* New York: Russell Sage Foundation.

Mendoza-Denton, R., Ayduk, O., Mischel, W., Shoda, Y., & Testa, A. (2001). Person × situation interactionism in self-encoding (I am . . . when . . .): Implications for affect regulation and social information processing. *Journal of Personality and Social Psychology, 80,* 533–544.

Metcalfe, J., & Jacobs, J. W. (1996). A "hot/cool-system" view of memory under stress. *PTSD Research Quarterly, 7,* 1–6.

Metcalfe, J., & Mischel, W. (1999). A hot/cool system analysis of delay of gratification: Dynamics of willpower. *Psychological Review, 106,* 3–19.

Miller, S. M. (1979). Coping with impending stress: Physiological and cognitive correlates of choice. *Psychophysiology, 16,* 572–581.

Miller, S. M. (1987). Monitoring and blunting: Validation of a questionnaire to assess styles of information seeking under threat. *Journal of Personality and Social Psychology, 52,* 344–353.

Mischel, W. (1966). Theory and research on the antecedents of self-imposed delay of reward. In B. A. Maher (Ed.), *Progress in experimental personality research* (Vol. 3, pp. 85–131). New York: Academic Press.

Mischel, W. (1974a). Cognitive appraisals and transformations in self-control. In B. Weiner (Ed.), *Cognitive views of human motivation* (pp. 33–49). New York: Academic Press.

Mischel, W. (1974b). Processes in delay of gratification. In L. Berkowitz (Ed.), *Advances in experimental social psychology* (Vol. 7, pp. 249–292). New York: Academic Press.

Mischel, W. (in press). Self-control. In P. A. M. Van Lange, A. W. Kruglanski, & E. T. Higgins (Eds.), *Theories of social psychology.* Thousand Oaks, CA: Sage.

Mischel, W., & Ayduk, O. (2002). Self-regulation in a cognitive-affective personality system: Attentional control in the service of the self. *Self and Identity, 1,* 113–120.

Mischel, W., & Ayduk, O. (2004). Willpower in a cognitive-affective processing system: The dynamics of delay of gratification. In R. F. Baumeister & K. D. Vohs (Eds.), *Handbook of self-regulation: Research, theory, and applications* (pp. 99–129). New York: Guilford Press.

Mischel, W., & Baker, N. (1975). Cognitive appraisals and transformations in delay behavior. *Journal of Personality and Social Psychology, 31,* 254–261.

Mischel, W., & Ebbesen, E. B. (1970). Attention in delay of gratification. *Journal of Personality and Social Psychology, 16,* 239–337.

Mischel, W., Ebbesen, E. B., & Zeiss, A. R. (1972). Cognitive and attentional mechanisms in delay of gratification. *Journal of Personality and Social Psychology, 21,* 204–218.

Mischel, W., & Metzner, R. (1962). Preference for delayed reward as a function of age, intelligence, and length of delay interval. *Journal of Abnormal and Social Psychology, 64,* 425–431.

Mischel, H. N., & Mischel, W. (1983). The development of children's knowledge of self-control strategies. *Child Development, 54,* 603–619.

Mischel, W., & Moore, B. (1973). Effects of attention to symbolically-presented rewards on self-control. *Journal of Personality and Social Psychology, 28,* 172–179.

Mischel, W., & Shoda, Y. (1995). A cognitive-affective system theory of personality: Reconceptualizing situations, dispositions, dynamics, and invariance in personality structure. *Psychological Review, 102,* 246–268.

Mischel, W., Shoda, Y., & Peake, P. (1988). The nature of adolescent competencies predicted by preschool delay of gratification. *Journal of Personality and Social Psychology, 54,* 687–696.

Mischel, W., Shoda, Y., & Rodriguez, M. L. (1989). Delay of gratification in children. *Science, 244,* 933–938.

Moore, B., Mischel, W., & Zeiss, A. (1976). Comparative effects of the reward stimulus and its cognitive representation in voluntary delay. *Journal of Personality and Social Psychology, 34,* 419–424.

Morf, C. C., & Mischel, W. (2002). Special issue: Self-concept, self-regulation, and psychological vulnerability. *Self and Identity, 1,* 103–199.

Ochsner, K. N., & Gross, J. J. (2008). Cognitive emotion regulation: Insights from social cognitive and affective neuroscience. *Current Directions in Psychological Science, 17*(2), 153–158.

Patterson, C. J., & Mischel, W. (1975). Plans to resist distraction. *Developmental Psychology, 11,* 369–378.

Peake, P., Hebl, M., & Mischel, W. (2002). Strategic attention deployment in waiting and working situations. *Developmental Psychology, 38,* 313–326.

Petry, N. M. (2002). Discounting of delayed rewards in substance abusers: Relationship to antisocial personality disorder. *Psychopharmacology, 162,* 425–432.

Rachlin, H. (2000). *The science of self-control.* Cambridge, MA: Harvard University Press.

Rodriguez, M. L., Mischel, W., & Shoda, Y. (1989). Cognitive person variables in the delay of gratification of older children at-risk. *Journal of Personality and Social Psychology, 57,* 358–367.

Rodriguez, M. L., Mischel, W., Shoda, Y., & Wright, J. (1989, April). *Delay of gratification and children's social behavior in natural settings.* Paper presented at the annual meeting of the Eastern Psychological Association, Boston.

Rothbart, M. K., Derryberry, D., & Posner, M. (1994). A psychobiological approach to the development of temperament. In T. D. Wachs (Ed.), *Temperament: Individual differences at the interface of biology and behavior* (pp. 83–116). Washington, DC: American Psychological Association.

Sethi, A., Mischel, W., Aber, J. L., Shoda, Y., & Rodriguez, M. L. (2000). The role of strategic attention deployment in development of self-regulation: Predicting preschoolers delay of gratification from mother–toddler interactions. *Developmental Psychology, 36,* 767–777.

Shoda, Y., Mischel, W., & Peake, P. (1990). Predicting adolescent cognitive and self-regulatory competencies from preschool delay of gratification: Identifying diagnostic conditions. *Developmental Psychology, 26,* 978–986.

Shoda, Y., Mischel, W., & Wright, J. (1993). The role of situational demands and cognitive competencies in behavior organization and personality coherence. *Journal of Personality and Social Psychology, 65*, 1023–1035.

Taylor, S. E., & Brown, J. D. (1988). Illusion and well-being: A social psychological perspective on mental health. *Psychological Bulletin, 103*, 193–210.

Trilling, L. (1943). *E. M. Forster*. New York: New Directions.

Trope, Y., & Liberman, N. (2003). Temporal construal. *Psychological Review, 110*, 403–421.

Wegner, D. M. (1994). Ironic processes of mental control. *Psychological Review, 101*, 34–52.

Wegner, D. M., Schneider, D. J., Carter, S., III, & White, T. L. (1987). Paradoxical effects of thought suppression. *Journal of Personality and Social Psychology, 53*, 5–13.

Wulfert, E., Block, J. A., Ana, E. S., Rodriguez, M. L., & Colsman, M. (2002). Delay of gratification: Impulsive choices and problem behaviors in early and late adolescence. *Journal of Personality, 70*, 533–552.

CHAPTER 6

Self-Regulation and Behavior Change
Disentangling Behavioral Initiation and Behavioral Maintenance

ALEXANDER J. ROTHMAN
AUSTIN S. BALDWIN
ANDREW W. HERTEL
PAUL T. FUGLESTAD

On a day-to-day basis, people face myriad behavioral challenges. Some challenges require people to form and execute a novel response, whereas others require them to continue an ongoing pattern of behavior. At first glance, one might surmise that it is easier to maintain a response to a familiar challenge than to respond to a new challenge. Given their familiarity with the situation, people should have a better sense of what to do and what they are capable of doing. Moreover, the strength of the contingency between the response and the eliciting situation should only increase as the behavior is repeated over time. From this perspective, successfully enacting a behavior should afford future success; over time, a self-sustaining pattern of behavior (i.e., a *habit*) will form. Accordingly, the notion of *habit* has been invoked as the logical consequence of a series of successfully enacted behaviors (Ajzen, 2002; Wood & Neal, 2007). But does this account adequately capture the processes that underlie the transition from behavioral initiation to behavioral maintenance and, ultimately, to habit formation? Is it correct to assume that the decision criteria that guide behavioral decision making are invariant over time?

The premise that a successfully initiated behavior will be maintained over time can be found either implicitly or explicitly in most, if not all, models of behavioral decision making (Rothman, 2000). Yet this premise is at variance with behavioral data obtained across a range of domains. Specifically, people who have successfully initiated a new pattern of behavior more often than not fail to sustain that behavior over time (e.g., Jeffery et al., 2000; Ockene et al., 2000; Marlatt & Donovan, 2005). Furthermore, intervention strategies that have been shown to help people initiate changes in their behavior have not had a similar impact on rates of behavioral maintenance (e.g., McCaul, Glasgow, & O'Neill, 1992; Perri, Nezu, Patti, & McCann, 1989).

The observation that initial behavioral success does not ensure continued success suggests that greater attention must be given to the manner in which newly enacted behaviors evolve into a habit. Although *behavioral maintenance* can be operationally defined as a series of similar decisions to take action, the processes that guide people's behavioral decisions need not be invariant over time. In this chapter, we first review how investigators have traditionally conceptualized the processes that underlie the ongoing self-regulation of behavior. To date, if anything, different phases in the behavior change process have been described. Although there is value in specifying the behavioral markers that characterize people at each point in the behavior change process, these descriptions must be complemented by an understanding of the factors that regulate transitions through each phase. We propose that once people have chosen to initiate a new pattern of behavior, four distinct phases in the behavior change process can be identified. Furthermore, the primary determinants of the behavior shift as people transition from one phase to the next. To this end, we examine a series of hypotheses regarding the differential influence of specific factors throughout the behavior change process. We hope that this framework will motivate a new generation of theorizing and empirical investigations that will afford a better specification of the factors that facilitate or inhibit behavioral maintenance.

CURRENT THEORETICAL APPROACHES TO BEHAVIORAL MAINTENANCE

Most models of health behavior, for example, social cognitive theory (SCT; Bandura, 1986), the theory of planned behavior (TPB; Ajzen, 1991), the theory of reasoned action (TRA; Ajzen & Fishbein, 1980), and the transtheoretical model of behavior change (TTM; Prochaska, DiClemente, & Norcross, 1992), have focused on elucidating how people determine whether to adopt a given behavior.[1] The decision to adopt a new behavior is predicated on an analysis of the relative costs and benefits associated with different courses of action. Consistent with their conceptual framework, these theoretical perspectives have primarily been used to explain why people engage in a particular unhealthy or healthy behavioral practice—for example, why people choose to enroll in a smoking cessation program (Norman, Conner, & Bell, 1999). Very limited consideration has been given to modeling an ongoing sequence of behaviors, such as the pattern of behavioral decisions that underlie efforts to quit smoking. For instance, TRA (Ajzen & Fishbein, 1980) and TPB (Ajzen, 1991) make no formal distinction between decisions regarding the initiation of a behavior and those regarding the maintenance of that behavior over time. Although investigators have used these approaches to examine long-term behavioral outcomes, these investigations have focused on whether people's behavioral practices become sufficiently stable, such that behavior is a function of itself and no longer contingent on a set of mediating thoughts or feelings (Ajzen, 2002; Wood, Quinn, & Kashy, 2002).

According to SCT (Bandura, 1986), self-efficacy beliefs are a crucial determinant of both the initiation and the maintenance of a change in behavior. Confidence in one's ability to take action serves to sustain effort in the face of obstacles. The successful implementation of changes in behavior bolsters people's confidence, which in turn facilitates further action, whereas failure experiences serve to undermine personal feelings of efficacy. Although the reciprocal relation between perceived self-efficacy and behavior is well documented, this relation needs to be reconciled with the observation that successfully enacted changes in behavior are not always maintained.

Although stage models have identified maintenance as a distinct stage in the behavior change process, the primary focus of these models has been to recognize that people differ in their readiness to take action (Prochaska et al., 1992; Weinstein, 1988). In the TTM (Prochaska et al., 1992), a distinction is made between people in the action and in the maintenance stages, yet this distinction rests solely on the length of time a behavior has been adopted. Accordingly, the set of cognitive and behavioral strategies predicted to facilitate initial action is similarly predicted to help sustain that action over time (Prochaska & Velicer, 1997).

Taken together, the dominant theoretical approaches to the study of health behavior offer little guidance as to how the processes that govern the initiation and the maintenance of behavior change might differ. Because maintenance has been operationalized as action sustained over time, it is predicted to rely on the same set of behavioral skills and motivational concerns that facilitate the initial change in behavior.

Rothman (2000) has argued that there may be important differences in the decision criteria that guide the initiation and maintenance of behavior change, and that these differences may explain why people who successfully adopt a new pattern of behavior frequently fail to maintain that pattern of behavior over time. Behavioral decisions, by definition, involve a choice between different behavioral alternatives. What differentiates decisions concerning initiation from those concerning maintenance are the criteria on which the decision is based. Decisions regarding behavioral initiation involve a consideration of whether the potential benefits afforded by a new pattern of behavior compare favorably to one's current situation; thus, the decision to initiate a new behavior depends on a person's holding *favorable expectations* regarding future outcomes. This premise is well-grounded in a broad tradition of research endeavors indicating that the more optimistic people are about the value of the potential outcomes afforded by the new pattern of behavior and their ability to obtain those outcomes, the more likely they are to initiate changes (Rothman & Salovey, 2007). Because the decision to initiate a new behavior is predicated on obtaining future outcomes, it can be conceptualized as an approach-based self-regulatory process in which progress toward one's goal is indicated by a reduction in the discrepancy between one's current state and a desired reference state.

Whereas decisions regarding behavioral initiation are based on expected outcomes, decisions regarding behavioral maintenance involve a consideration of people's experiences engaging in the new pattern of behavior and a determination of whether those experiences are sufficiently desirable to warrant continued action. Consistent with Leventhal's self-regulatory model of illness behavior (Leventhal & Cameron, 1987), the decision to continue a pattern of behavior reflects an ongoing assessment of the behavioral, psychological, and physiological experiences afforded by the behavior change process. People's assessment of these experiences is ultimately indexed by their satisfaction with the experiences afforded by the new pattern of behavior, and they will maintain a change in behavior only if they are satisfied with what they have accomplished. The feeling of satisfaction indicates that the initial decision to change the behavior was correct; furthermore, it provides justification for the continued effort people must put forth to monitor their behavior and minimize vulnerability to relapse. To the extent that people choose to maintain a behavior to preserve a favorable situation, the decision processes that underlie behavioral maintenance may be conceptualized as an avoidance-based self-regulatory process in which people strive to maintain a discrepancy between their current state and an undesired reference state.

Because different decision criteria are proposed to guide behavioral initiation and behavioral maintenance, factors that may facilitate one behavioral outcome may not have a similar effect on the other. In particular, people's outcome expectancies may have a pernicious effect on decisions regarding behavioral maintenance. Optimistic outcome expectations are likely to motivate people to make changes in their behavior and, in fact, intervention strategies often work to heighten these expectancies. However, these expectations may also serve as the standard against which people evaluate the outcomes afforded by the new pattern of behavior. To the extent that people's satisfaction with the behavior depends on their experiences meeting or exceeding their expectations, the unrealistically optimistic expectations that initially inspired people to make a change in their behavior may ultimately elicit feelings of dissatisfaction and disappointment, thus undermining behavioral maintenance.

Although Rothman (2000) discussed the potential value of distinguishing between predictors of behavioral initiation and behavioral maintenance, the manner in which people transition from one phase to the next was not well delineated. The absence of a complete description of the behavior change process hinders both theoretical and empirical efforts to specify the factors that guide people's behavioral decisions. To be effective, a conceptual framework must provide investigators with both a set of features that can be used to identify what phase a person is in and a set of determinants that uniquely predict transition between each phase (Weinstein, Rothman, & Sutton, 1998). To this end, we propose unpacking the behavior change process into a series of four phases: initial response, continued response, maintenance, and habit. These phases capture the behavioral processes that begin once someone has embarked on a course of action, transitioning out of what Prochaska and colleagues (1992) have characterized as the preparation stage. In some cases this point of transition is marked by an explicit action, such as enrolling in a formal program (e.g., an exercise program) or purchasing a piece of equipment (e.g., a treadmill), whereas in other cases, it is marked solely by a public or private affirmation to engage in a particular pattern of behavior (e.g., committing to exercise 3 days a week).

The structure of the four phases identified was informed, in part, by a consensus description of the phases that individuals pass through during treatment for major depressive disorder (Frank et al., 1991). At a general level, the four proposed phases reflect our belief that distinctions needed to be made within prior conceptualizations of both behavioral initiation and behavioral maintenance. Regarding behavioral initiation, we have distinguished between the decisions that underlie a person's efforts to initiate successfully a new pattern of behavior (i.e., the initial response phase) and the efforts involved with managing the new behavior and confronting the challenges associated with developing a sense of control over one's actions (i.e., the continued response phase). Regarding behavioral maintenance, we have distinguished between a phase in which people choose to maintain a pattern of behavior based on a repeated assessment of the behavior's value (i.e., the maintenance phase) and a phase in which people continue to maintain the behavior, but without any consideration of a behavioral alternative (i.e., the habit phase). Table 6.1 provides a description of the defining features of each phase, as well as a general outline of the factors believed to regulate people's ability to transition successfully to the next phase.

TABLE 6.1. The Four Phases of the Behavior Change Process

Phase	Initial response	Continued response	Maintenance	Habit
Defining feature of phase	Initial effort to change behavior (e.g., enrolling in a program)	Continued effort to establish new behavior	Sustained effort to continue newly established behavior	Self-perpetuating pattern of behavior
Primary determinants of transition to next phase[a]	Efficacy beliefs (++) Outcome expectations (+) Personality/ situation (+/–)	Initial rewards (+) Sustained self-efficacy beliefs (+) Sustained outcome expectations (+) Demands of the behavior change process (– –) Personality/situation (+/– –)	Satisfaction with new behavior (++) Personality/ situation (+/–)	Prior behavior (++)
Marker of end of phase/ beginning of next phase[a]	First reliable performance of the desired behavior	Consistent performance of the desired behavior and complete confidence in one's ability to perform the behavior	Consistent behavior without consideration of the value of the behavior	

Note. "++" and "– –" indicate factors that have strong facilitating and inhibiting effects on behavior change, respectively. "+" and "–" indicate factors that have moderate facilitating and inhibiting effects on behavior change, respectively.
[a]Habit, the last phase of the sequence, is expected to persist as long as the behavior is sustained.

UNPACKING THE BEHAVIOR CHANGE PROCESS

The first phase of the behavior change process, *initial response*, begins as soon as people embark on an effort to change their behavior and continues until they first manifest a significant change. For example, a person might enroll in a smoking cessation program and subsequently report having been smoke-free for 7 consecutive days. The successful performance of the desired behavior (e.g., not smoking) serves as an indication that the participant has responded favorably to the treatment or intervention. Although how the behavioral outcome is operationally defined will vary across domains, the measure should indicate that a person has reliably performed the desired behavior and the behavioral response therefore is not due to chance. People who fail to emit the desired behavioral response (e.g., someone who is unable to remain smoke-free for 7 consecutive days) are considered nonresponsive to the treatment or intervention and fail to transition to the next phase. It is assumed that these people revert back to a consideration of whether they want to begin a new attempt to modify their behavior.

Because researchers have primarily focused their efforts on identifying predictors of initial behavior change, the factors that predict successfully completing the initial response phase are relatively well understood. Specifically, the likelihood that people will initiate a change in their behavior has been shown to be a function of both confidence in their ability to execute the behavior and their belief that engaging in the new pattern of behavior will meaningfully improve their lives (Rothman & Salovey, 2007). This thesis has also been supported by a pair of interventions demonstrating that experimentally heightening people's expectations elicits stronger rates of behavioral initiation (Finch et al., 2005; Hertel et al., 2008).

In many ways, the onset of this phase of the behavior change process is characterized by a sense of optimism and hope. Because the ability to adopt an optimistic mindset is an important determinant of initial success (Taylor & Gollwitzer, 1995), any factor that undermines a person's ability to generate and sustain this perspective, such as a facet of one's personality (e.g., pessimism) or of one's life situation (e.g., an unsupportive partner), should in turn make it more difficult for the person to pass through this phase.

Once a person has reliably performed the desired behavior, the second phase of the behavioral process, *continued response*, begins. This phase is characterized by a tension between a person's ability and motivation to enact the new pattern of behavior consistently, and the challenges and unpleasant experiences that leave him or her vulnerable to lapses and relapses. It is during this period of time that people strive to gain a sense of mastery over their new behavior. The length of time people remain in this phase is likely to differ across both domains and persons. Some people may find it easy to master the new pattern of behavior, whereas others may find it a continual struggle. Similarly, some behavioral domains involve a complex series of behavioral modifications, which should lengthen this phase, whereas other domains involve a very limited set of challenges, which should shorten this phase. The point at which people transition out of this phase occurs when they not only perform the new pattern of behavior consistently but also do so with complete confidence in their ability to manage their behavior.

A key aspect of the continued response phase is that people have to face the reality of engaging in the new pattern of behavior, including the possibility or actuality of slips and lapses. People begin to shift their attention from their expectations regarding the behavior to their experiences with it. Although people's desire to change their behavior and confidence in their ability to implement that change continue to influence behavior, it is critical that people sustain these beliefs in the face of their experience performing the new pattern of behavior. To the extent that people find the new behavior to be unpleasant or feel that it requires a considerable amount of mental and/or physical energy, their commitment to and confidence in their behavior may weaken, thus, making it difficult for them to complete this phase of the behavior change process.

Because people's experiences with the behavior begin to affect behavioral decision making, careful consideration must be given to the nature and the timing of the consequences afforded by a new pattern of behavior. Any favorable outcomes elicited by the behavior (e.g., compliments from others) should help sustain people's motivation to change their behavior. However, in many cases, the primary benefits afforded by the new pattern of behavior arise only after extended action. Because the costs associated with a behavior are often closely tied to the process of enacting the behavior (e.g., having to get up early to exercise), they tend to appear with the onset of the behavior. The heightened salience of these costs can make this phase of the behavior change process particularly difficult and unpleasant, and may elicit a set of experiences that are in sharp contrast to the optimism and hope that characterized people's initial willingness to commit to the behavior change process. Given the greater prevalence of negative information about the new behavior, any aspect of a person's personality or life situation that makes it difficult for him or her to remain optimistic about the behavior change process is likely to have the most debilitating impact during this phase. For example, people may find they can initiate a behavior in the absence of social support, or even in the presence of unsupportive others, but that these conditions greatly hinder their ability to sustain these efforts over time (see Rothman, Hertel, Baldwin, & Bartels, 2008, for further discussion of this issue).

People who are unable to complete the continued response phase are thought to have relapsed and returned to their prior behavioral practices. However, successfully completing this phase of the behavior change process can be taken as a sign of recovery. People have put their prior, unwanted habits behind them and are engaging in a new, healthy pattern of behavior. Moreover, they are doing so with a sense that they are in control of their actions. Up until now, engaging in the new pattern of behavior reflected a struggle against pressures to relapse, but with the onset of a new phase in the behavior change process, the decision to engage in the unwanted behavior becomes more volitional.

The *maintenance* phase is characterized by the desire to sustain this new, successful pattern of behavior. Because people who have reached this phase are not struggling to perform the behavior, there is an important shift in the determinants of their behavior. Having demonstrated that they can successfully perform the behavior over an extended period of time, people feel less need to verify their ability to engage in the behavior. Hence, the decision to continue the behavior becomes less a function of a person's ability to perform the behavior and more a function of the behavior's perceived value (see Baldwin et al., 2006). It is at this phase in the behavior change process that people complete the shift from focusing on what they expect the behavior to afford to what outcomes the behavior has in fact afforded (Rothman, 2000). Enough time has passed since the onset of the behavior, so the consequences of the new behavior are now informative. Thus, people begin to form an integrated assessment of the relative costs and benefits afforded by the behavior to determine whether the behavior is worth continuing. To the extent that people conclude they are satisfied with the new behavior, they will choose to sustain the behavior and preserve the gains that have accrued (Finch et al., 2005; Hertel et al., 2008).

During the maintenance phase, people continue to monitor the consequences of their behavior and should be sensitive to changes in the perceived benefits and costs associated with the behavior (Baldwin, Rothman, Hertel, Keenan, & Jeffery, 2009). For example, starting to receive fewer and fewer compliments as friends and family begin to take the new behavior for granted may undermine people's feelings of satisfaction. Similarly, how people think about the behavior may shift as they habituate to the pleasure associated with their new experiences. Unlike the prior two phases of the behavior change process, people can remain in the maintenance phase indefinitely. As long as people feel the need to evaluate continually their perception of the relative costs and benefits of the behavior, they will remain in this phase. Because the value of continuing the pattern of behavior is continually reassessed, it is always possible that a person will choose to end the behavior after concluding that it is no longer worthwhile. At this phase, the return of the prior, unhealthy behavior is considered a recurrence rather than a relapse; that is, it represents a new episode, or instance, of the behavior as opposed to a continuation of a prior pattern of behavior.

The transition to *habit*, the final phase in the behavior change process, occurs when people are no longer actively concerned about their ability to engage in the behavior or their evaluation of the outcomes afforded by the behavior. At this point in time, people engage in the behavior in the absence of any regular analysis of whether they should or should not continue to take action (Wood et al., 2002). In other words, the behavior sustains itself. This is not to say that people in this phase do not value the behavior; rather, they no longer need to verify its value. Consistently wearing seat belts when riding in a car, which is considered a prototypical habit, fits nicely within this framework because it is relatively easy for people to reach the point that they question neither their ability to use a seat belt nor its value as a safety device.

Because people in this phase assume that their behavior is worthwhile, they should be less sensitive to fluctuations in the outcomes afforded by the behavior than are those who remain in the maintenance phase of the behavior change process. Consistent with this perspective, Ferguson and Bibby (2002) observed that the subsequent behavior of occasional but not habitual blood donors was affected by having seen people faint during blood donation. It is assumed that once people have reached the habit phase, they will continue in this phase until an event of sufficient magnitude causes them to reconsider the value of their behavior. Should this occur, people shift back into the maintenance phase and reconsider whether the behavior in question is of sufficient value to sustain (Wood, Tam, & Guerrero Witt, 2005).

DISENTANGLING BEHAVIORAL INITIATION
AND BEHAVIORAL MAINTENANCE: A METHODOLOGICAL NOTE

The premise that the primary determinants of people's behavior may shift over time has important methodological implications. First and foremost, given the principle of parsimony, the burden of proof rests with investigators who assert that the determinants of behavior vary across phases of the behavior change process. Cross-sectional comparisons of individuals at different phases can be informative, but systematic longitudinal and experimental work is needed to test predictions regarding the determinants of each transition (Weinstein, Lyon, Sandman, & Cuite, 1998). Second, any systematic analysis of the behavior change process, by definition, requires a methodology that provides a rich description of the ongoing relation between people's thoughts and feelings, and their behavior. Psychologists have relied on methods that enable them to delineate the manner in which people's behavior is regulated by their psychological state, but the context for these accounts is almost always a single, often brief interval of time. Insufficient attention has been paid to how the process unfolds over several time intervals. More frequent assessment of psychological constructs would enable investigators to examine the conditions under which people are and are not able to sustain their favorable views of the behavior (a crucial determinant of successful behavior change). In contrast, behavioral epidemiologists often track individuals' behavior over extended periods of time. Yet the predominant methods and research designs involve infrequent assessments, thus providing minimal information regarding people's ongoing experiences as they manage their behavior (but see Shiffman & Stone, 1998). For example, despite the extensive volume of research on weight control behavior, remarkably little is known about people's experiences as they make ongoing changes in their dietary and exercise practices (Jeffery, Kelly, Rothman, Sherwood, & Boutelle, 2004). Given the complementary nature of the approaches associated with these two disciplines, the development of interdisciplinary initiatives led jointly by psychologists and epidemiologists may provide excellent opportunities to examine these issues (e.g., Finch et al., 2005; Hertel et al., 2008).

Testing predictions regarding the differential determinants of initial and long-term behavior change also necessitates that investigators capture the unique effect that a particular psychological state (e.g., self-efficacy) has on each phase of the behavior change process. To date, claims regarding the determinants of behavioral maintenance are typically based on tests of whether a psychological state (e.g., self-efficacy at baseline) can predict a distal behavioral outcome (e.g., smoking status 18 months later). Yet this analytic approach is inconclusive regarding the factors that underlie behavioral maintenance because it cannot determine whether, in the current example, people's initial feelings of self-efficacy contribute to their willingness to maintain their behavior over and above its effect on their initial behavioral efforts. With the development of theoretical models that specify differential predictors of behavior over time, the need arises to disentangle the direct relation between a psychological state and a distal outcome from the indirect relation between these two constructs that is mediated by people's initial behavioral efforts (e.g., see Baldwin et al., 2006; Hertel et al., 2008).

THE IMPLICATIONS OF A FOUR-PHASE BEHAVIORAL FRAMEWORK FOR FOUR SUBSTANTIVE RESEARCH PROGRAMS ON BEHAVIORAL SELF-REGULATION

Although research on behavioral decision making has only begun to examine how people move from initiating to maintaining a pattern of behavior, several substantive areas of research address issues germane to the ongoing self-regulation of behavior. Here, we consider four areas of research that have examined the relation between a psychological state and people's ability to regulate their behavior: (1) self-efficacy, (2) regulatory focus, (3) self-regulatory strength, and (4) intrinsic–extrinsic motivation. In reviewing these areas, we examine the degree to which investigators have theoretically and empirically examined distinctions between behavioral initiation and behavioral maintenance, and generate predictions concerning the role that each of these constructs might play within our four-phase model of the behavior change process.

Self-Efficacy and Behavior Change

The premise that people's behavior is contingent on their perceived ability to execute actions in support of the behavior (i.e., *self-efficacy*) has had a fundamental impact on both research and theory regarding behavior change (Bandura, 1997). In fact, self-efficacy, or variables that appear to operate as proxies for the construct, can be found in many, if not all, theories of behavior change (Rothman & Salovey, 2007). As discussed earlier in the chapter, there is strong empirical support for the thesis that people's confidence in their ability to engage in a behavior positively predicts subsequent behavior, and that successfully enacting a behavior heightens people's confidence to perform the behavior (Bandura, 1997). However, is it appropriate to conclude that self-efficacy is an equally valuable predictor of behavior at all points in the behavior change process?

Investigators have consistently demonstrated that self-efficacy is a robust predictor of behavioral initiation, but most empirical investigations have failed to consider whether it has an effect at specific points in the behavior change process. The precaution adoption process model (PAPM) is one of the few conceptual frameworks that explicitly predicts when self-efficacy will be a valuable predictor of behavior (Weinstein, 1988). In an empirical test of the PAPM, self-efficacy to test for radon gas was a critical determinant of behavioral initiation (i.e., ordering a test), but only once people had committed to performing the behavior. People who were not yet committed to testing for radon did not benefit from an intervention aimed at self-efficacy (Weinstein et al., 1998). In the context of our four-phase model of behavior change, the findings obtained by Weinstein and colleagues (1998) are consistent with the prediction that a heightened sense of self-efficacy is necessary if people are to complete the initial response phase of the behavior change process.

According to our model, confidence in one's ability to perform a behavior is also a critical determinant of success during the continued response phase. In particular, it is essential that people maintain their sense of self-efficacy as they grapple with the challenges posed by the new pattern of behavior. Consistent with this premise, self-efficacy beliefs are thought to be closely linked to people's ability to manage lapses and the threat of relapse during the initial days of the behavior change (e.g., relapse prevention; Marlatt & Donovan, 2005), and empirical evidence in the domain of smoking cessation suggests that daily changes in self-efficacy are critical in dealing with lapses during this important phase of the behavior change process (Shiffman et al., 2000).

According to the proposed four-phase model of behavior change, the predictive value of self-efficacy shifts as people move from initiating to maintaining a behavior. Once people have shown that they can successfully manage their behavior, the decision to maintain it is thought to have less to do with variability in people's perceptions of their ability to perform the behavior, and more to do with their willingness or desire to sustain it. Recent empirical evidence supports this prediction. The clearest evidence comes from an empirical test of the prediction among people enrolled in a smoking cessation trial (Baldwin et al., 2006). Measures of self-efficacy and satisfaction with cessation were assessed concurrently at various time points during the trial and used to predict people's cessation status. A critical aspect of these predictions is that they were tested separately in two groups of people: those who were actively trying to quit smoking (i.e., people in the initial and continuing response phases) and those who had already successfully quit (i.e., people in the maintenance phase). Among people in the initial and continuing response phases, self-efficacy was a significant predictor of future cessation success as expected. But among people in the maintenance phase, self-efficacy was no longer a significant predictor of maintained cessation. Instead, satisfaction predicted maintenance of cessation.

Although we are not aware of other data that provide as clear a test of the shifting influence of self-efficacy, additional data suggest that the influence of self-efficacy becomes less important once people have attained some success with the behavior. For example, Linde, Rothman, Baldwin, and Jeffery (2006) reported that diet- and exercise-related self-efficacy predicted diet and exercise behavior, respectively, during the active treatment portion of a weight loss trial. But during the treatment follow-up period, self-efficacy was no longer predictive of the weight-related behaviors. Similarly, Baer, Holt, and Lichtenstein (1986) reported that smoking cessation self-efficacy predicted future cessation status in a sample of people trying to quit smoking but did not predict whether people who were able to quit smoking subsequently maintained cessation (see Rothman, Baldwin, & Hertel, 2004, for further discussion of the effect of self-efficacy on behavioral maintenance).

Regulatory Focus and Behavior Change

Regulatory focus theory (Higgins, 1997) proposes that goal-directed behavior is regulated through two *distinct* motivational systems, promotion and prevention. *Promotion focus* involves concerns for advancement, growth, and accomplishment. Individuals who are high in promotion focus eagerly pursue desired outcomes, performing well on tasks that involve seeking gains. Complementing promotion focus, *prevention focus* involves concerns for security, duty, and meeting obligations. Individuals who are high in prevention focus are vigilant in avoiding undesired outcomes, performing well on tasks that involve monitoring for losses to preserve desired outcomes (Brodscholl, Kober, & Higgins, 2007; Shah, Higgins, & Friedman, 1998).

When examined within the context of our four-phase model of behavior change, promotion focus should facilitate initiating behavioral change, whereas prevention focus should facilitate maintaining behavioral change. People higher in promotion focus, but not prevention focus, should find it easier to initiate changes that focus on the achievement of benefits and gains, whereas people higher in prevention focus, but not promotion focus, should find it easier to maintain changes that guard against potential losses and preserve desired outcomes.

Grounded in this theoretical approach, Fuglestad, Rothman, and Jeffery (2008b) examined whether promotion and prevention foci would predict rates of initiation and maintenance in longitudinal studies of smoking cessation and weight loss. In the domain of smoking cessation, people higher in promotion focus, but not prevention focus, had better quit rates across the first 6 months of follow-up. Results were similar for weight loss: People higher in promotion focus, but not prevention focus, were better able to initiate successful weight loss across the active intervention and first 6 months of follow-up. Providing further support for the role of promotion focus in initiation, for people who had lost weight but were still far from their weight loss goal, promotion focus predicted continued weight loss over the next year. In response to slips (i.e., smoking again after initial cessation, gaining weight after initial weight loss), people higher in promotion focus were more successful in quitting smoking again and losing weight again (Fuglestad, Rothman, & Jeffery, 2008a, 2009). In terms of the continued response phase, these findings suggest that people higher in promotion focus are better able than people lower in promotion focus to remain motivated and optimistic as they strive to master new behaviors to attain desired outcomes.

Complementing the role of promotion focus in the initiation of behavioral change, prevention focus, but not promotion focus, predicted greater success at maintaining a change in behavior. Of smokers who had been able to quit for at least 2 months, those higher in prevention focus were more likely to remain smoke-free over the following year. In weight loss, when participants had lost weight and were close to their weight loss goal, prevention focus predicted keeping lost weight off over the next year. Furthermore, in both interventions, people high in prevention focus were more likely never to slip over the course of follow-up if they had been successful for a few months (Fuglestad et al., 2008a, 2009). Together, these findings suggest that once a person has successfully initiated behavioral change and attained a desired outcome (e.g., a goal weight), higher prevention focus is beneficial for maintaining behavioral change and preserving desired outcomes.

These findings speak to the issue of how quickly initiation transitions to maintenance across various behavioral domains. As observed by Fuglestad and colleagues (2008b), promotion focus continued to predict weight loss as long as one was far from attaining a desired weight, suggesting that behavioral initiation can last a relatively long time as one strives to master effortful behaviors and attain desired outcomes. On the other hand, smoking cessation and behaviors such as condom use, cancer screening, and sunscreen use may have relatively shorter initiation phases and relatively longer maintenance phases because these behaviors are relatively easy to perform but are not immediately reward-ing (the perceived costs may outweigh the perceived benefits). As such, prevention focus should play a more prominent role in the performance of these behaviors.

Self-Regulatory Strength and Behavior Change

Behavior change involves not only adopting a new pattern of behavior but also curbing a prior pattern of behavior. Baumeister and his colleagues (Baumeister, Heatherton, & Tice, 1994; Muraven & Baumeister, 2000) have argued that to override, inhibit, or alter a dominant response tendency, people must possess a sufficient degree of self-regulatory strength, which is conceptualized as a limited, but renewable, cognitive resource that is drained whenever someone attempts to regulate his or her emotions, thoughts, or behav-ior. Because deficits in self-regulatory strength are thought to be a primary determinant of self-regulatory failure, relapses are predicted to be more likely when people are faced with repeated demands to manage their thoughts, feelings, or behavior. Support for this premise has been obtained from a series of empirical investigations across a range of behavioral domains (e.g., Baumeister, Bratslavsky, Muraven, & Tice, 1998; Muraven, Tice, & Baumeister, 1998).

When considered in the context of the four-phase model we have specified in the behavior change process, self-regulatory strength would seem to be more important in the initial response and continued response phases compared to the maintenance and habit phases. During the initial response phase, people are likely to have difficulty initiat-ing a new pattern of behavior successfully, if they are in a situation that involves other sig-nificant self-regulatory demands. In fact, from a self-regulatory strength perspective, one would predict that to the extent that people overlay additional self-regulatory demands on the behavior change process (e.g., attempting to hide the new behavior from friends or family), they will have less success completing this phase. Given that the threat posed by lapses and relapses is predicted to occur during the continued response phase, self-regulatory strength should be an important determinant of whether people are able to complete this phase of the behavior change process. In fact, most of the empirical work concerning self-regulatory strength has involved tasks analogous to the demands of this phase. To the extent to which people feel that the new behavior requires continued effort and considerable self-regulatory resources, they may find it difficult to sustain their confi-dence and commitment to the behavior. Moreover, even if people have allocated sufficient resources to continue their new behavior, they may find that this results in a resource deficit and undermines their ability to respond to the simultaneous and ongoing needs of their family, friends, or employers. The dissatisfaction that subsequently emanates from these domains may not only heighten people's need for self-regulatory strength but also lower their evaluation of the new behavior.

Because people's behavioral practices during the maintenance and habit phases reflect more their evaluation of the behavior than their ability to perform it, the cognitive resources that were necessary to perform the new behavior consistently in the first two phases are no longer needed. This does not mean that the behavior does not continue to require effort and commitment; rather, there is a steep drop in people's needs to override or inhibit an underlying behavior. The new pattern of behavior transforms into the dominant response. In fact, the onset of the maintenance phase would appear to be the time at which people can begin to take on additional self-regulatory demands, without critically undermining the new behavior.

Motivation and Behavior Change

People's motivation for engaging in a pattern of behavior has traditionally been considered an important determinant of their ability to initiate and maintain a pattern of behavior. Specifically, investigators have distinguished between two classes of motivation: external and internal. *External motivation* refers to either extrinsic motivation that arises from the desire to gain (avoid) an externally imposed reward (punishment), or controlled motivation that arises from the desire to please others. *Internal motivation* refers to either the desire to obtain internally imposed rewards (intrinsic motivation) or the motivation to engage in a behavior to satisfy one's own needs (autonomous motivation; Deci & Ryan, 1985). Investigators have traditionally asserted that people are more likely to sustain a pattern of behavior over time if it is based on intrinsic or autonomous motivation compared to extrinsic or controlled motivation. The benefit associated with an internal motivation is that a person's assessment of the behavior is more under his or her control and less contingent on outside reinforcement.

When examined within the context of our four-phase model of the behavior change process, it would appear that internal motivation may exert a more positive influence than external motivation on behavior during the maintenance phase. However, it is less clear whether behavior during the first two phases of the behavior change process is differentially affected by these two classes of motivations. During the initial response phase, participants focus on the outcomes they expect to experience. Given the focus on future outcomes, the perceived desirability of the outcome is likely to be more important than whether the rewards reflect internal or external contingencies. With the onset of the continued response phase, people whose behavior reflects intrinsic or autonomous motivational needs may find it easier to sustain their confidence in and feelings about the behavior. This should be particularly true when the costs associated with engaging in the new behavior are more salient than the associated benefits. Under these conditions, people may find it easier to sustain themselves through this unpleasant period if their actions are motivated by their own needs and desires as opposed to the needs and desires of others. However, the differential impact of these two classes of motivational concerns may be attenuated to the extent that people enjoy engaging in the new behavior. In fact, to the extent that people derive a sense of satisfaction from engaging in the new pattern of behavior, they may choose to take a greater sense of personal ownership of the task and, over time, develop a stronger sense of intrinsic motivation.

The empirical literature concerning the impact of internal and external motivation on behavior change provides some insight into the relation between these constructs and behavior change. Across several studies, the degree to which people are motivated by internal concerns has been shown to predict the successful initiation and maintenance of behavior change (e.g., Williams, Freedman, & Deci, 1998; Williams, Niemiec, Patrick, Ryan, & Deci, 2009; Williams, Rodin, Ryan, Grolnick, & Deci, 1998). Evidence regarding the effect of external motivation on behavior change is inconsistent at best (Curry, Grothaus, & McBride, 1997; Williams, Freedman, et al., 1998; Williams, Rodin, et al., 1998). However, the structure of the research designs and/or analytic strategies employed in these studies precludes drawing any specific conclusions regarding the effect that internal and external motivation has on each unique phase of the behavior change process. In addition, a more detailed assessment of people's experience with the behavior change process would offer an opportunity to determine how behavioral experiences influence motivation, and whether particular classes of behavioral experiences enable people to shift from an external to an internal motivation for behavior change.

LOOKING TOWARD THE FUTURE

Even a cursory review of the goals outlined in *Healthy People 2010* (U.S. Department of Health and Human Services, 2001) reveals the practical benefits that would arise, for both individuals and society, if people would not only initiate but also maintain changes in their behavioral practices. Even modest, sustained changes in people's lifestyles would afford substantial reductions in disease morbidity and mortality, as well as reduced health care costs. Yet efforts to promote long-term behavior change effectively are constrained by our theoretical understanding of the factors that regulate people's behavioral practices over time. Investigators need to specify more thoroughly and test the implications drawn from their theoretical models regarding ongoing behavioral practices. In order to encourage this line of work, we have delineated a series of testable predictions regarding the factors that may regulate people's ability to go from successfully initiating a new behavior to making it a habit. We hope this framework inspires investigators to undertake theoretical and empirical investigations that will ultimately enable us to specify more clearly the factors that inhibit and facilitate long-term behavior change, which, in turn, can inform the design and implementation of intervention approaches that reliably elicit healthy changes in behavioral practices.

ACKNOWLEDGMENT

The initial preparation of this chapter was supported in part by Grant No. NS38441 from the National Institute of Neurological Disorders and Stroke.

NOTE

1. Because health behavior is the primary domain in which conceptual and empirical attention has been given to behavioral maintenance, we have chosen to ground our discussion in this area. However, the issues addressed in this chapter should generalize to other behavioral domains.

REFERENCES

Ajzen, I. (1991). The theory of planned behavior. *Organizational Behavior and Human Decision Processes, 50*, 179–211.

Ajzen, I. (2002). Residual effects of past on later behavior: Habituation and reasoned action perspectives. *Personality and Social Psychology Review, 6*, 107–122.

Ajzen, I., & Fishbein, M. (1980). *Understanding attitudes and predicting social behavior.* Englewood Cliffs, NJ: Prentice-Hall.

Baer, J. S., Holt, C. S., & Lichtenstein, E. (1986). Self-efficacy and smoking reexamined: Construct validity and clinical utility. *Journal of Consulting and Clinical Psychology, 54*, 846–852.

Baldwin, A. S., Rothman, A. J., Hertel, A. W., Keenan, N. K., & Jeffery, R. W. (2009). Longitudinal associations between people's cessation-related experiences and their satisfaction with cessation. *Psychology and Health, 24*, 187–201.

Baldwin, A. S., Rothman, A. J., Hertel, A. W., Linde, J. A., Jeffery, R. W., Finch, E., et al. (2006). Specifying the determinants of the initiation and maintenance of behavior change: An examination of self-efficacy, satisfaction, and smoking cessation. *Health Psychology, 25*, 626–634.

Bandura, A. (1986). *Social foundations of thought and action: A social cognitive theory.* Englewood Cliffs, NJ: Prentice-Hall.

Bandura, A. (1997). *Self-efficacy: The exercise of control.* New York: Freeman.

Baumeister, R. F., Bratslavsky, E., Muraven, M., & Tice, D. M. (1998). Ego depletion: Is the active self a limited resource? *Journal of Personality and Social Psychology, 74*, 1252–1265.

Baumeister, R. F., Heatherton, T. F., & Tice, D. M. (1994). *Losing control: How and why people fail at self-regulation.* San Diego, CA: Academic Press.

Brodscholl, J. C., Kober, H., & Higgins, E. T. (2007). Strategies of self-regulation in goal attainment versus goal maintenance. *European Journal of Social Psychology, 37*, 628–648.

Curry, S. J., Grothaus, L. C., & McBride, C. M. (1997). Reasons for quitting: Intrinsic and extrinsic motivation for smoking cessation in a population-based sample of smokers. *Addictive Behaviors, 22*, 727–739.

Deci, E. L., & Ryan, R. M. (1985). *Intrinsic motivation and self-determination in human behavior.* New York: Plenum Press.

Ferguson, E., & Bibby, P. A. (2002). Predicting future blood donor returns: Past behavior, intentions, and observer effects. *Health Psychology, 21*, 513–518.

Finch, E. A., Linde, J. A., Jeffery, R. W., Rothman, A. J., King, C. M., & Levy, R. L. (2005). The effects of outcome expectations and satisfaction on weight loss and maintenance: Correlational and experimental analyses. *Health Psychology, 24*, 608–616.

Frank, E., Prien, R. F., Jarrett, R. B., Keller, M. B., Kupfer, D. J., Lavori, P. W., et al. (1991). Conceptualization and rationale for consensus definitions of terms in major depressive disorder: Remission, recovery, relapse, and recurrence. *Archives of General Psychiatry, 48*, 851–855.

Fuglestad, P. T., Rothman, A. J., & Jeffery, R. W. (2008a, February). *The effect of regulatory focus on responding to and avoiding slips in a longitudinal study of smoking cessation.* Paper presented at the annual meeting of the Society for Personality and Social Psychology, Albuquerque, NM.

Fuglestad, P. T., Rothman, A. J., & Jeffery, R. W. (2008b). Getting there and hanging on: The effect of regulatory focus on performance in smoking and weight loss interventions. *Health Psychology, 27*, S260–S270.

Fuglestad, P. T., Rothman, A. J., & Jeffery, R. W. (2009, February). *The effect of regulatory focus on responding to weight gain and remaining persistent in a longitudinal study of weight loss.* Presented at the annual meeting of the Society for Personality and Social Psychology, Tampa, FL.

Hertel, A. W., Finch, E., Kelly, K., King, C., Lando, H., Linde, J., et al. (2008). The impact of outcome expectations and satisfaction on the initiation and maintenance of smoking cessation: An experimental test. *Health Psychology, 27*, S197–S206.

Higgins, E. T. (1997). Beyond pleasure and pain. *American Psychologist, 52*, 1280–1300.

Jeffery, R. W., Drewnowski, A., Epstein, L. H., Stunkard, A. J., Wilson, G. T., Wing, R. R., et al. (2000), Long-term maintenance of weight loss: Current status. *Health Psychology, 19*, 5–16.

Jeffery, R. W., Kelly, K. M., Rothman, A. J., Sherwood, N. E., & Boutelle, N. (2004). The weight loss experience: A descriptive analysis. *Annals of Behavioral Medicine, 27*, 100–106.

Leventhal, H., & Cameron, L. (1987). Behavioral theories and the problem of compliance. *Patient Education and Counseling, 10*, 117–138.

Linde, J. A., Rothman, A. J., Baldwin, A. S., & Jeffery, R. W. (2006). The impact of self-efficacy on behavior change and weight change among overweight participants in a weight loss trial. *Health Psychology, 25*, 282–291.

Marlatt, G. A., & Donovan, D. M. (Eds.). (2005). *Relapse prevention: Maintenance strategies in the treatment of addictive behaviors* (2nd ed.). New York: Guilford Press.

McCaul, K. D., Glasgow, R. E., & O'Neill, H. K. (1992). The problem of creating habits: Establishing health protective dental behaviors. *Health Psychology, 11*, 101–110.

Muraven, M., & Baumeister, R. F. (2000). Self-regulation and depletion of limited resources: Does self-control resemble a muscle? *Psychological Bulletin, 126*, 247–259.

Muraven, M., Tice, D. M., & Baumeister, R. F. (1998). Self-control as limited resource: Regulatory depletion patterns. *Journal of Personality and Social Psychology, 74*, 774–789.

Norman, P., Conner, M., & Bell, R. (1999). The theory of planned behavior and smoking cessation. *Health Psychology, 18*, 89–94.

Ockene, J. K., Emmons, K. M., Mermelstein, R. J., Perkins, K. A., Bonollo, D. S., Vorhees, C. C., et al. (2000). Relapse and maintenance issues for smoking cessation. *Health Psychology, 19*, 17–31.

Perri, M. G., Nezu, A. M., Patti, E. T., & McCann, K. L. (1989). Effect of length of treatment on weight loss. *Journal of Consulting and Clinical Psychology, 57*, 450–452.

Prochaska, J. O., DiClemente, C. C., & Norcross, J. C. (1992). In search of how people change: Applications to addictive behaviors. *American Psychologist, 47*, 1102–1114.

Prochaska, J. O., & Velicer, W. F. (1997). The transtheoretical model of health behavior change. *American Journal of Health Promotion, 12*, 38–48.

Rothman, A. J. (2000). Toward a theory-based analysis of behavioral maintenance. *Health Psychology, 19*, 1–6.

Rothman, A. J., Baldwin, A. S., & Hertel, A. W. (2004). Self-regulation and behavior change: Disentangling behavioral initiation and behavioral maintenance. In R. F. Baumeister & K. D. Vohs (Eds.), *Handbook of self-regulation: Research, theory, and applications* (pp. 130–148). New York: Guilford Press.

Rothman, A. J., Hertel, A. W., Baldwin, A. S., & Bartels, R. D. (2008). Understanding the determinants of health behavior change: Integrating theory and practice. In J. Y. Shah & W. L. Gardner (Eds.), *Handbook of motivation science* (pp. 494–507). New York: Guilford Press.

Rothman, A. J., & Salovey, P. (2007). The reciprocal relation between principles and practice: Social psychology and health behavior. In A. W. Kruglanski & E. T. Higgins (Eds.), *Social psychology: Handbook of basic principles* (2nd ed., pp. 826–849). New York: Guilford Press.

Shah, J., Higgins, E. T., & Friedman, R. S. (1998). Performance incentives and means: How regulatory focus influences goal attainment. *Journal of Personality and Social Psychology, 74*, 285–293.

Shiffman, S., Balabanis, M. H., Paty, J. A., Engberg, J., Gwaltney, C. J., Liu, K. S., et al. (2000). Dynamic effects of self-efficacy on smoking lapse and relapse. *Health Psychology, 19*, 315–323.

Shiffman, S., & Stone, A. A. (1998). Introduction to special section: Ecological momentary assessment in health psychology. *Health Psychology, 17*, 3–5.

Taylor, S. E., & Gollwitzer, P. M. (1995). Effects of mindset on positive illusions. *Journal of Personality and Social Psychology, 69*, 213–226.

U.S. Department of Health and Human Services. (2001). *Healthy people 2010: National health promotion and disease prevention objectives.* Washington, DC: U.S. Government Printing Office.

Weinstein, N. D. (1988). The precaution adoption process. *Health Psychology, 7*, 355–386.

Weinstein, N. D., Lyon, J. E., Sandman, P. M., & Cuite, C. L. (1998). Experimental evidence for stages of health behavior change: The precaution adoption process model applied to home radon testing. *Health Psychology, 17*, 445–453.

Weinstein, N. D., Rothman, A. J., & Sutton, S. R. (1998). Stage theories of health behavior: Conceptual and methodological issues. *Health Psychology, 17*, 290–299.

Williams, G. C., Freedman, Z. R., & Deci, E. L. (1998). Supporting autonomy to motivate patients with diabetes glucose control. *Diabetes Care, 21*, 1644–1651.

Williams, G. C., Niemiec, C. P., Patrick, H., Ryan, R. M., & Deci, E. L. (2009). The importance of supporting autonomy and perceived competence in facilitating long-term tobacco abstinence. *Annals of Behavioral Medicine, 37*, 315–324.

Williams, G. C., Rodin, G. C., Ryan, R. M., Grolnick, W. S., & Deci, E. L. (1998). Autonomous regulation and long-term medication adherence in adult outpatients. *Health Psychology, 17*, 269–276.

Wood, W., & Neal, D. T. (2007). A new look at habits and the habit–goal interface. *Psychological Review, 114*, 843–863.

Wood, W., Quinn, J. M., & Kashy, D. A. (2002). Habits in everyday life: Thought, emotion, and action. *Journal of Personality and Social Psychology, 83*, 1281–1297.

Wood, W., Tam, L., & Guerrero Witt, M. (2005). Changing circumstances, disrupting habits. *Journal of Personality and Social Psychology, 88*, 918–933.

PART II

COGNITIVE, PHYSIOLOGICAL, AND NEUROLOGICAL DIMENSIONS OF SELF-REGULATION

CHAPTER 7

Nonconscious Self-Regulation, or the Automatic Pilot of Human Behavior

ESTHER K. PAPIES
HENK AARTS

Writing a chapter on nonconscious processes of self-regulation means addressing some of the most central issues in current theory and research in psychology in general, and social psychology in particular. The term *regulation* refers to the notion that some process or procedure controls something in a given direction. This direction is often conceptualized in terms of a standard or goal to which the current state can be compared to adjust one's behavior (Carver & Scheier, 1981). The "self" as an entity in psychological processes has long interested psychologists and philosophers alike (James, 1890) and is still an important topic in several strands of psychology (see Baumeister, 1998). Recent research on the "self," inspired especially by developments in the area of social and cognitive neuroscience, has been used to explore areas in the brain involved in self-related processing and in distinguishing the "self" from others (e.g., Decety & Sommerville, 2003; see Legrand & Ruby, 2009, for an overview). The idea of the "self" has also gained a prominent role in research on the regulation of behavior, where studies on "self-regulation" abound.

The term *self-regulation* often refers to "the exertion of control over the self by the self," which involves altering the way an individual feels, thinks, or behaves in order to pursue short- or long-term interests. In this view of self-regulation, the "self" is seen as an active agent and controller (i.e., the "pilot" of one's behavior) (Baumeister, 1998; James, 1890). Traditionally, the regulation of one's behavior in the pursuit of personal goals has been assumed to happen in a consciously controlled fashion, including the willpower needed to overcome one's initial impulsive reactions to stimuli (Mischel, Cantor, & Feldman, 1996; Muraven & Baumeister, 2000), and these goal-directed processes of regulation have been contrasted with automatic processes that follow an individual's impulses (e.g., Metcalfe & Mischel, 1999; Muraven & Baumeister, 2000; Strack & Deutsch, 2004).

Over the course of about the last three decades, however, evidence has indicated that much of the regulation of our cognition and behavior can also occur in a nonconscious fashion (i.e., without conscious awareness of the triggers and of the processes guiding our behavior). Initially, it was assumed that only rather simple or well-practiced skills could be executed by this "automatic pilot" of human behavior, such as brushing one's teeth or driving a car (see Bargh, 1996). Recently, however, it has become evident that more complex behaviors, such as thought and action in social situations, and the regulation of behavior in pursuit of a wide range of personal goals, can also be performed effectively without the need for conscious awareness (Aarts, 2007; Bargh, 1990). The overwhelming evidence for such processes in human behavior, and the efficiency with which these processes seem to navigate us through our daily lives, has even led many researchers to subscribe to the original notion of William James (1890) that the largest part of our behavior is guided by such an automatic pilot, saving the resources of our limited consciousness for intervention in urgent and exceptional matters.

In this chapter, we systematically discuss some of the intriguing research in the area of nonconscious self-regulation and examine the nature, as well as the working mechanisms, of the "automatic pilot" that seems to be guiding it. This way, we use the latest advances in this field to elucidate to some degree how it is possible that our motivated behavior can direct us toward our goals so effectively, yet do so without our conscious awareness. To be sure, there can be no doubt that conscious awareness can sometimes be useful for attaining one's goals. For example, conscious awareness of one's goals and of the obstacles that keep one from attaining them, allows one to mobilize and integrate one's resources in a novel way, or to set out a completely new course of action (Dijksterhuis & Aarts, 2010). In support of this point, conscious planning has been shown to be useful for goal attainment, even when this requires a course of action that implies a diversion from one's habitual behavior (Gollwitzer & Sheeran, 2006; Papies, Aarts, & de Vries, 2009). However, recent developments cited in the literature suggest that in most situations, such conscious control is neither necessarily present, nor indeed required to regulate one's behavior successfully in accordance with one's goals.

Approaching self-regulation from this perspective touches upon intriguing questions regarding the origin of control over such processes and the role of the "self" as the active agent of regulation (see, e.g., Bargh & Ferguson, 2000; Baumeister, 1998; Baumeister, Schmeichel, & Vohs, 2007). Specifically, whereas people often derive the sense of self-regulation ("It's me who is doing the control") from their conscious experiences of self-agency, recent research suggests that such self-agency experiences originate in the unconscious and are the result of an inference that occurs fluently and perfunctorily after action performance, and they are thus not per se accurate in terms of the actual cause of the behavior (Wegner, 2002). Thus, how do our conscious experiences of agency relate to the fact that much of the regulation of our behavior unfolds outside conscious awareness? We briefly address this issue in the last part of this chapter. In the meantime, however, we treat self-regulation as the regulation of cognition and behavior that occurs within a given individual in the service of goal pursuit.

In this chapter, then, we systematically discuss mechanisms of nonconscious self-regulation, from the initial perception of goal-relevant cues in the environment to the execution of goal-directed behavior in dynamic circumstances. Rather than merely describe nonconscious goal pursuit as a phenomenon, we present a process framework to explain how goal pursuit can function in a nonconscious fashion, integrating perceptual, cognitive, motivational, and motor processes. In addition, we present empirical evidence that supports the framework presented here and can help us to understand the complex and fascinating phenomenon of nonconscious, goal-directed behavior and its behavioral manifestations. We start out by examining how goals are represented in order to determine which features of goal representations actually motivate human behavior nonconsciously. Here, we show that both the accessibility of the specific content of the goal and an affective cue signaling its desirability are crucial for triggering nonconscious motivation to pursue the goal. Next, we turn toward the execution of nonconscious goal pursuit and show that goals can be pursued by habitual behaviors that nonetheless are flexible and can be adjusted in an ongoing manner. Moreover, we discuss how goal pursuit in dynamic circumstances is facilitated by cognitive mechanisms of working memory and executive control, which allow for active maintenance, shielding, and monitoring of one's goals and goal-relevant information. Finally, we turn toward the experiences of self-agency that accompany much of our behavior and discuss how research on nonconscious goal pursuit can inform our insight on processes of agency and willful action.

THE REPRESENTATION OF GOALS

Goals can be conceptualized as mental representations of certain behaviors or outcomes that are desirable to pursue or to attain (Bargh, 1997; Custers & Aarts, 2005; Fishbach & Ferguson, 2007). The representations of these desirable end states can differ in their level of abstractness: while socializing or having a slim figure is a representation of a goal that usually require a series of behaviors to be achieved, getting hold of a bottle of water or producing matching symbols on a slot machine are results that can be attained by a simple hand movement or a button press. Research in several domains of psychology has confirmed the original ideomotor notion of William James and shown that human actions are represented in the brain in terms of their observable effects, associated with the motor program needed to produce the effect (Hommel, Musseler, Aschersleben, & Prinz, 2001; Jeannerod, 2001; Prinz, 1997; Vallacher & Wegner, 1987). As a consequence, merely thinking about a certain outcome can activate the behavioral program needed to achieve that outcome. In addition, representing actions in terms of their potentially desirable results allows us to direct our behavior by anticipating its effect, so that goals can serve as the standard and reference point for behavior to make sure that the ongoing actions actually produce the desired results.

However, not every behavior or outcome that is represented in terms of a result of concrete actions operates as a goal for an individual. An outcome has to be rewarding to actually motivate behavior, or at least perceived that way by the individual. An important question that arises, then, is how the rewarding value of an outcome is actually determined, and how this is done in the absence of conscious deliberation. In more traditional approaches to this issue, such as the expectancy value principle (Fishbein & Ajzen, 1975), a person is assumed to weigh consciously the pros and cons of a certain outcome and thus arrive at a deliberate judgment regarding its desirability. However, how does this work with regard to nonconscious goals? In the absence of conscious awareness, how does an individual know what state to pursue or what outcomes to strive for?

In order to answer this question, researchers have introduced a variety of concepts, such as the *active self-account* (Wheeler, DeMarree, & Petty, 2007), which argues that a prime will affect behavior if it is integrated in the active, currently accessible self-concept of a person. Other researchers have introduced terms like *implicit volition* (Moskowitz, Li, & Kirk, 2004), *implicit intentions* (Wood, Quinn, & Kashy, 2002), or the *automated will* (Bargh, Gollwitzer, Lee Chai, Barndollar, & Troetschel, 2001) to describe the nonconscious origins of motivation. Essentially, these approaches suggest that the process of forming the intention to pursue a goal can occur outside of conscious awareness, thus extending the capacities of nonconscious processes to include functions that previously were exclusive to the realm of consciousness. As such, these terms remain rather descriptive and do not inform us about the potential mechanisms that enable full-blown motivated behavior to occur without conscious awareness.

Approaching this issue from a different angle and following the conceptualization of a goal as a desired outcome or behavior, recent research into the underlying mechanisms of nonconscious goal pursuit has focused on the role of positive affective signals as indicators that a given state is worth pursuing (e.g., Custers & Aarts, 2005; Ferguson, 2007; see also Foerster, Liberman, & Friedman, 2007). Affective signals play a fundamental role in directing human behavior and are processed quickly and without the need for conscious awareness upon perception of a stimulus (Chen & Bargh, 1999; Damasio, 1994; Fazio, Sanbonmatsu, Powell, & Kardes, 1986; Zajonc, 1980). Positive affect has been shown to play a central role in incentive learning and the neurological mechanisms involved in reward processing and motivation (see Berridge, 2007), suggesting that positive affective signals may be crucial for conveying information about the desirability and thus the motivational value of a potential goal state. We conceptualize a goal, therefore, as consisting of the cognitive representation of an outcome or behavior that can serve as a reference point for one's actions, coupled with a signal of positive affect that indicates this reference point is desirable to attain.

In addition to being represented as outcomes or behaviors associated with positive affect, goals are embedded in knowledge structures containing goal-relevant information. Indeed, when activating a goal in social psychological studies, we most likely do not prime a single concept, but rather a rich conceptual structure containing behavioral, motor, affective, interactional, and other information (Bargh, 2006). These knowledge structures also include situational and contextual cues indicating opportunities for goal pursuit (Aarts & Dijksterhuis, 2000; Austin & Vancouver, 1996; Bargh, 1990; Bargh & Gollwitzer, 1994; Kruglanski et al., 2002). For example, the goal of socializing can be mentally associated with contextual cues, such as bars or birthday parties; the goal of high academic performance can be associated with the thought of one's seminar room at the university; and a delicious chocolate cake can evoke the goal of hedonic enjoyment or, conversely, of following a diet (e.g., Bargh et al., 2001; Fishbach, Friedman, & Kruglanski, 2003; Papies, Stroebe, & Aarts, 2007, 2008b). Such cognitive links between certain environmental cues and the mental representation of goals develop when goals are repeatedly and consistently pursued in certain situations. As a result of frequent coactivation, features of critical situations then become associated with the goal representations, so that these goals can be activated automatically when the relevant situation is encountered (Bargh, 1990; Hebb, 1949).

An abundance of empirical evidence shows that activating a goal construct can indeed lead to motivated behavior. In one of the first series of studies on this topic, Bargh and colleagues (2001) subtly activated the goal of achievement and observed participants' subsequent behavior on an intellectual task. More specifically, participants were asked to solve word puzzles in which words related to achievement (e.g., *strive, succeed*) were presented or not, thereby subtly activating the concept of achievement without drawing participants' attention to it. The researchers found that in a later task, achievement-primed participants displayed more motivated behavior to perform well than did control participants. Importantly, debriefing showed that participants were not aware of the achievement primes or of the way that the word puzzles could have influenced their later behavior. Fitzsimons and Bargh (2003) and Shah (2003) later showed that the motivation to achieve could also be triggered when participants were primed with the name of a significant other who was strongly associated with the goal of doing well in college, such as one's mother or father (see also Kraus & Chen, 2009). Other studies have confirmed that a variety of social cues, such as names of attachment figures, goal-directed behavior of other people, the experience of social exclusion, or names and exemplars of social categories, can function as primes to trigger motivated behavior in participants (Aarts, Chartrand, et al., 2005; Aarts, Gollwitzer, & Hassin, 2004; Custers, Maas, Wildenbeest, & Aarts, 2008; Gillath et al., 2006; Lakin, Chartrand, & Arkin, 2008; Moskowitz, Gollwitzer, Wasel, & Schaal, 1999; Moskowitz & Ignarri, 2009; Papies & Hamstra, in press).

Concepts such as academic achievement or helping another person, which were primed in the studies mentioned earlier, are most likely inherently positive to the study participants, so that activating them can lead directly to motivated behavior. Thus, to assess the unique contribution of positive affective signals toward motivated behavior, other studies examined whether this is more likely to occur when a goal state is more positive. In one set of studies, Ferguson (2007) measured participants' implicit affective responses toward potential goals, for example, the goal of being thin, then examined their motivation toward pursuing this end state. Results showed that participants who valued this goal more positively displayed more goal-directed behavior toward it, such as resistance to high-fat food in daily life, stronger intentions to diet, and consumption of less fattening food in a taste test in the laboratory. Likewise, participants who had a more positive response toward being egalitarian were found to display less prejudice toward older adults. In a similar vein, Custers and Aarts (2005) showed that priming a behavioral state that is initially neutral can trigger motivated behavior, but only when it is unobtrusively coupled with positive affect, for example, through an evaluative conditioning procedure (Custers & Aarts, 2005). Thus, the degree to which a goal is associated with positive affect translates the mere accessibility of the goal into actual motivation, so that only when a behavioral state is represented as actually being a desired state does priming trigger the motivation to pursue it as a goal.

These findings point toward two possible routes for priming effects on behavior. While activating the cognitive representation of a behavioral state might trigger the associated behavior by means of the common code for the results of one's action and motor programs (Hommel et al., 2001; Jeannerod, 2001), actual goal-directed behavior requires additionally the motivating power of positive affective signals. A recent study directly disentangled this effect of the ideomotor principle from actual motivated behavior (Aarts, Custers, & Marien, 2008). Here, words related to the concept of exertion (e.g., *exert, vigor*) were primed subliminally and paired with positive or with neutral words. Subsequently, participants were given a handgrip and instructed to squeeze it in response to a cue on the computer screen. The study revealed that participants who had been primed with the concept of exertion started squeezing the handgrip faster than participants who had not been primed, suggesting that the prime triggered the behavior by relying on the close association of the end state with the associated motor program. However, participants for whom the concept of exertion had also been paired with positive affect displayed actual motivated behavior: They exerted more force than the other participants when squeezing the handgrip. This additional effect of positive affective signals shows that outside participants' awareness, positive affect served to motivate participants directly, so that they put additional effort into their behavior, going beyond the mere priming of a neutral end state.

In conclusion, the broad array of studies on goal priming shows that goal-directed behavior emerges when a prime activates the mental representation of a behavior associated with positive affect, confirming that these are the two crucial components of goal representations to initiate and regulate behavior outside of conscious awareness.

THE EXECUTION OF GOAL-DIRECTED BEHAVIOR

So far, we have seen how the activation of a goal representation can lead to motivated behavior in pursuit of that goal. However, once a goal is activated, how is its pursuit accomplished? How is subsequent behavior directed and organized to enable actual goal attainment? In the knowledge structures in which goals are embedded, goal representations are cognitively associated with not only situational cues that can trigger them but also actions, procedures, objects, and opportunities that can facilitate their actual pursuit and attainment (Aarts & Dijksterhuis, 2000; Bargh, 1997; Cooper & Shallice, 2006; Kruglanski et al., 2002). For example, the goal of socializing can be associated with going out, being cheerful, and ordering beer in bar, and the goal of earning money can be associated with actions such as getting a job, getting up early to go to work, or playing a slot machine. These knowledge structures are built by repeatedly attaining a goal by means of certain action chains, leading to enduring associations between goal representations and skillful goal-directed behaviors. Such associations enable us to pursue goals nonconsciously and without the need for deliberation because the activation of a goal can directly trigger the activation of associated behaviors and thus, effective pursuit of a goal.

The nonconscious execution of goal-directed behavior has been commonly understood and appreciated in terms of habits; that is, goals prime behavior as a result of practice and the routinization of skills. At the lowest level of analysis, *habits* can be regarded as stimulus–response links established and reinforced by rewards that follow certain responses to a stimulus. If, for example, one feels nicely refreshed after drinking a glass of water on a hot day, the sight of a glass of water may later evoke the action of grabbing it in order to drink. Eventually, when a behavior has repeatedly and successfully been executed in response to a certain stimulus and the stimulus–response association has become well-ingrained in procedural memory, the perception of the stimulus may automatically trigger the execution of the associated behavior. In other words, once the habit is sufficiently strong, it can operate independently of the reward that initially served to reinforce the link between the stimulus and the response (Dickinson, Balleine, Watt, Gonzales, & Boakes, 1995). This enables the efficient performance of instrumental actions in a similar context later on, without the need for conscious awareness.

However, not all behaviors can be executed successfully by such single responses to certain stimuli. If a behavior is more complex, then it may require skills that comprise several sequential responses, with one response triggering the next in an effortless fashion (Aarts & Custers, 2009; Cooper & Shallice, 2006). When one prepares coffee in the morning, for example, pouring the water may trigger getting a filter from the cupboard; putting the filter in the machine triggers getting the coffee powder, and so forth. Such action chains can be conceptualized as open-loop mechanisms that enable the efficient execution of behavior when the exact sequence of actions is required every time the behavior is performed. In these types of habits, once initiated, the behavior runs to completion in a rather ballistic fashion and does not allow for adjustments of the ongoing process.

However, although such response chains may be sufficient for the execution of some routine behavioral patterns, they fail as soon as a small change in the environment requires only the slightest adjustment of one's behavior. Because the execution of goal-directed behavior more often than not happens under such dynamic conditions, researchers have suggested that another type of habitual behavior operates via a feedback control system, in which one's actions can be adjusted in an ongoing manner. More specifically, in such closed-loop processes, the result of one action forms the input for the next one, thereby allowing for constant adjustments and efficient regulation of skillful actions in changing circumstances (e.g., Fourneret & Jeannerod, 1998; Frith, Blakemore, & Wolpert, 2000; Powers, 1973). When driving one's car, for example, the required behavior is largely the same every time one takes the usual route to work. Still, slightly different actions are needed on different occasions, such as when the traffic light is red instead of green, there is a slow car in front, or a steady side wind requires adjusting one's steering wheel. Such adjustments of one's habitual behavior can be made in a nonconscious manner by monitoring the results of one's actions and using perceptual feedback to fine-tune the execution of the necessary skills and responses (Aarts & Custers, 2009; Bargh & Ferguson, 2000). Thus, once a course of action is triggered to reach a certain goal, the execution of goal-directed behavior is monitored and adjusted by such a perceptual feedback control system, thus ensuring that the same goals can be attained under different circumstances.

When pursuing a goal, however, how is the selection of a course of action made in the first place? Out of a variety of behaviors that could potentially lead to the attainment of a goal, how does the mental system supporting nonconscious goal pursuit decide which path to follow? All else being equal, we are likely to do things as we did them before, and this is certainly true for nonconscious goal-directed behavior. Repeatedly pursuing a goal via a certain course of behavior forges a strong cognitive link between the goal representation and the representation of this behavior, so that activation of a goal can automatically lead to the activation of the habitual means for goal pursuit. This way, for example, we do not have to think deliberately how to get to work in the morning because the goal of going to work automatically activates the idea of using a bike or car; we do not have to consider all available supermarkets when having to do the groceries, since the goal of grocery shopping automatically activates the representation of the store we usually go to. Thus, habitual behavior involves not only the skilled execution (driven by either open- or closed-loop processes) but also the initial selection of a means for goal pursuit, which can be automatized based on earlier behavior and later executed in an efficient, nonconscious fashion.

The idea that habitual behavior also comprises the automatic selection of a course of action has received empirical support in a number studies and was first tested in the domain of travel behavior (e.g., Aarts & Dijksterhuis, 2000). Here, participants who had been primed with certain travel goals (e.g., going to attend a lecture) showed increased activation of certain means for traveling (e.g., biking). However, this effect occurred only among those students who habitually used the bicycle to reach their travel goals. These findings were replicated and extended in the domain of the habitual drinking of alcohol among students in the United Kingdom (Sheeran et al., 2005), where activating the goal of socializing increased the accessibility of the concept of drinking, but only among those student participants who were regular drinkers of alcohol in social situations. In addition, after a socializing prime, these students were more likely to choose a voucher for alcohol rather than for coffee or tea as a reward for their participation in the experiment. These results indicate that the activation of a goal automatically activates its associated habitual means, making the repeated selection of this means for goal pursuit more likely.

The processes discussed so far have indicated how goal-directed habits diminish the role of conscious processes in the regulation of behavior. Indeed, research that examines the performance of repetitive behaviors, such as purchasing fast food, physical exercise, or condom use, has shown that this is to a large degree predicted by the strength of one's habits toward these behaviors At the same time, conscious intentions have been found to be predictive of such behaviors as well, which suggests that while habits are important in the regulation of behavior, some part of our behavior is still under conscious control (e.g., Danner, Aarts, & de Vries, 2008; Norman, Armitage, & Quigley, 2007; Ouellette & Wood, 1998). Therefore, when examining the extent to which human behavior is under intentional or habitual control, it may be much more informative to consider not only the independent contributions but especially the interaction between habits and intentions in the prediction of behavior, and to examine the role of intentions when people also have strong habits for a certain behavior. A small number of studies now report on this and have confirmed that while intentions are indeed predictive of behavior when habits are weak, they do not predict behavior when habits are strong (Danner et al., 2008; Norman & Conner, 2006; Verplanken, Aarts, van Knippenberg, & Moonen, 1998; Wood, Tam, & Guerrero Witt, 2005). Thus, as a goal-directed behavior is executed more frequently in a stable context and increases in habit strength, conscious intentions and attention become less influential in guiding it, and the instigation and execution of goal-directed habitual behavior can be guided nonconsciously.

WHEN HABITS FAIL: ADAPTIVE FLEXIBILITY IN NONCONSCIOUS GOAL PURSUIT

Thus far, nonconscious goal pursuit has mainly been analyzed and studied as habits: routines and skills, once the goal is activated by the situation, follow a well-practiced path to completion that allows for adjustment to changing environments by a perceptual–motor feedback process. Sometimes, however, the situation does not allow direct execution of habitual means, or it imposes a different approach to attain our goals. In that case, we may need to postpone our nonconsciously activated goals, shield them from distracting cues or overcome tempting alternatives and keep an eye on the progress of our goals. Given that habits may fail, how do we still manage to strive for our desired outcomes? Do such situations automatically require the intervention of consciousness? Actually, this seems rather unlikely given the dynamic environments that we can steer through so effectively despite the limitations of our capacity for conscious processes (Bargh & Morsella, 2008; Kahneman, 1973). Recent developments indicate that nonconscious goals may operate via cognitive processes that allow for the efficient maintenance and use of goal-relevant information, specifically by following the principles of executive control (Aarts & Hassin, 2005; Bargh, 2005; Hassin, Aarts, Eitam, Custers, & Kleiman, 2009; Miller & Cohen, 2001). This suggests that although such mechanisms need attention, they do not rely on conscious awareness, as earlier approaches assumed (Bargh, 2006; Dijksterhuis & Aarts, 2010; Hassin, Bargh, Engell, & McCulloch, 2009), so that they can also support the regulation of nonconscious processes.

Research on working memory processes has revealed that adaptive cognition and behavior benefit from three essential functions of the so-called "workspace of the mind": the active maintenance of relevant information, the allocation of attention to task-relevant information and inhibition of task-irrelevant information, and processes of monitoring and feedback processing (Hassin et al., 2009; Miller & Cohen, 2001; Miyake & Shah, 1999). In support of the argument that such processes play a role in the efficient regulation of nonconscious goal pursuit, it has been shown that the activation of a goal leads to the active maintenance of this goal in mind, to shielding it against potentially interfering information, and to the nonconscious monitoring of relevant processes in the service of goal pursuit.

Aarts, Custers, and Holland (2007), for example, primed participants with the goal of socializing or not, and probed the accessibility of the mental representation of this goal 2.5 minutes later. Participants who had been primed with this goal displayed a higher accessibility of the goal construct, suggesting that an active maintenance mechanism had kept the goal alive in mind. Interestingly, participants for whom the goal of socializing had been made less desirable did not show this effect of sustained activation. Earlier studies have shown that nonconsciously activated goals also affect behavior after a delay of several minutes (Aarts et al., 2004; Bargh et al., 2001). Crucially, such sustained activation distinguishes the processing of goals from mere semantic knowledge, which remains active for only a short period, then shows a rapid decay in level of activation (Atkinson & Birch, 1970; Higgins, Bargh, & Lombardi, 1985; Srull & Wyer, 1979). However, one can easily see why it would be functional to keep the representation of a goal that has motivational, rewarding significance mentally active over an extended period of time: Even when goal pursuit is not immediately possible, this allows one to monitor one's environment for new opportunities and grab them once they arise, thus increasing the chances for goal attainment.

Indeed, activating a goal has been shown to lead to preferential processing of goal-relevant stimuli, as attentional processing of such stimuli is enhanced (Moskowitz, 2002; Papies, Stroebe, & Aarts, 2008a; Raymond & O'Brien, 2009), and goal-instrumental objects are perceived as bigger in size and also evaluated more positively when one's motivation to attain the primed goal is high (Ferguson & Bargh, 2004; Fishbach, Shah, & Kruglanski, 2004; Veltkamp, Aarts, & Custers, 2008). Without the need for conscious awareness, such effects on attentional, perceptual, and evaluative processes make it more likely that an individual will detect and use goal-relevant means and opportunities in the environment, thus facilitating goal attainment when the goal is actively maintained over a critical period of time.

Effective goal pursuit can also benefit from mechanisms that shield one's focal goal from distractions, such as attractive opportunities for pursuing alternative goals. In order to examine how nonconscious goals are protected from such temptations, Shah, Friedman, and Kruglanski (2002) showed that priming participants with a personal goal (e.g., studying) led to the inhibition of an alternative goal that could not be pursued at the same time (e.g., socializing; for similar findings, see Fishbach et al., 2003; Papies et al., 2008b). Similarly, once a goal has been attained, goal-related information is no longer relevant and is inhibited to prevent interference with other processes (see Foerster et al., 2007). Finally, in support of nonconscious monitoring processes during goal pursuit, it has been shown that participants who are chronically working on a certain goal (e.g., the goal of looking neat) spontaneously activate actions to reach this goal (e.g., ironing) when it appears necessary (i.e., when confronted with a situation that is discrepant with that goal: wearing a wrinkled shirt; Custers & Aarts, 2007a; see also Fourneret & Jeannerod, 1998; Hassin, Bargh, et al., 2009).

More indirect evidence that nonconscious goal pursuit relies on mechanisms of working memory comes from research showing that goal priming may not only enhance performance on a related working memory task (Eitam, Hassin, & Schul, 2008) but also impair performance on an unrelated task that relies on the working memory capacity to rehearse relevant information actively and inhibit interfering information (Hassin, Bargh, et al., 2009; see Smith & Jonides, 1999). The results of this study demonstrated that performance on the working memory task was impaired when participants had been subliminally primed with a goal they were highly motivated to attain. Thus, participants seemed to allocate attentional resources to the processes instigated by the activation of the goal and, as a result, these resources were no longer available to support performance on the working memory task introduced later.

The observation that nonconscious goal pursuit is supported by executive processes suggests that the operation of higher cognitive processes does not rely much on the conscious state of the individual. However, this raises the intriguing and fundamental question of whether these processes are effortful and demand mental resources. Contemporary social cognition research often assumes that nonconscious processes are efficient and do not claim mental resources. This view may hold when we merely consider nonconscious goal pursuit as automatic behavior that results from habitual, reflexive processes. However, this "automaticity" argument may be too simplistic; that is, all else being equal, engaging in nonconscious goal pursuit can have costs: The execution of the processes alluded to earlier renders them less available for other tasks. Nonconscious goal pursuit may thus rely on mental resources, and as such represents a class of mental processes in which lack of awareness and effort do not go hand in hand. In other words, goals modulate attention processes, irrespective of the (conscious or unconscious) source of the activation of the goal (Aarts, 2007; Badagaiyan, 2000; Hassin, Aarts, et al., 2009; Lau, Rogers, Haggard, & Passingham, 2004). This concurs with recent views suggesting that consciousness and attention are distinct faculties (Dijksterhuis & Aarts, 2010; Koch & Tsuchiya, 2007; Lamme, 2003).

THE SENSE OF AGENCY IN SELF-REGULATION

Up to now we have discussed how people can pursue their goals outside of conscious awareness. However, the idea that our goal pursuits materialize unconsciously is not without problems and may sound rather counterintuitive. After all, our actions and the outcomes they produce are often accompanied by conscious experiences of self-agency. The experience of *self-agency*—that is, the feeling that one causes one's own actions and their outcomes—has an intimate relationship with self-awareness and constitutes an important building block for our concept of free choice and our belief that our behavior is governed by "consciousness" or some other type of inner agent, such as "the will" or "the self." How, then, can much of our behavior unfold outside conscious awareness if we have those pervasive agency experiences?

One way to address this issue is by arguing that nonconscious goals do not reach self-agency experiences; hence, self-agency only emerges from intentional action: We consciously intend to produce a specific action or outcome, and when the perception of the action or outcome corresponds with this intention, we feel self-agency (e.g., Bandura, 1986; Carver & Scheier, 1998; Deci & Ryan, 1985). In this view, experiences of self-agency are the obvious result of consciously forming and pursuing one's goals. Although the establishment of self-agency resulting from intentional action requires specific mechanisms that have been elucidated only recently, research adopting this perspective has shown that the processing of self-agency draws on a variety of authorship indicators (Wegner & Sparrow, 2004), such as direct bodily feedback (e.g., Gandevia & Burke, 1992; Georgieff & Jeannerod, 1998), direct bodily feedforward (e.g., Blakemore & Frith, 2003; Blakemore, Wolpert, & Frith, 2002), and visual and other indirect feedback (e.g., Daprati et al., 1997). In essence, these signals all provide us with information about the intended outcome of our actions.

However, while dismissing the possibility that self-agency does not involve and ensue from nonconscious, goal-directed processes may be one strategy to solve the fundamental issue of how we establish a sense of personal authorship, recent research offers a somewhat different perspective. This research argues that our conscious experience of self-agency is an inference that occurs fluently and perfunctorily after action performance and is not accurate per se (Prinz, 2003; Wegner, 2002). This inferential character of experiences of self-agency has become apparent in a number of recent studies (Aarts, Custers, & Marien, 2009; Aarts, Custers, & Wegner, 2005; Aarts, Oikawa, & Oikawa, 2010; Custers, Aarts, Oikawa, & Elliot, 2009; Dijksterhuis, Preston, Wegner, & Aarts, 2008; Jones, de Wit, Fernyhough, & Meins, 2008; Sato & Yasuda, 2005; Wegner & Wheatley, 1999), demonstrating that these experiences are the result of a match between the outcome (or goal) of an action, and knowledge about the outcome that was active just prior to its occurrence, even though the outcome is primed subliminally, outside of conscious awareness.

In one study (Aarts, Custers, et al., 2005) showing this effect, participants and the computer each moved a single gray square in opposite directions on a rectangular path consisting of eight white tiles. Participants could press a key to stop the rapid movement of the squares, which would turn one of the eight tiles black. From a participant's perspective, this black tile could represent the location of either his or her square or the computer's square at the time the participant pressed the stop key. Thus, the participant or the computer could have caused the square to stop on the position (outcome), rendering the exclusivity of causes of outcomes ambiguous (Wegner & Wheatley, 1999). In actuality, however, the computer always determined the stops, so actual participant control was absent. In this task, participants either consciously set the intention to stop on a position, or they were subliminally primed with that position just before they saw the presented stop on the corresponding location. To measure experiences of self-agency, participants then rated the extent to which they felt that they have caused the square to stop. Results showed that both intention and priming led to an increased sense of self-agency, suggesting that online self-agency experiences were primarily based on a match between preactivated and actual outcomes, irrespective of whether the source of this activation was conscious or unconscious. This, together with other findings, indicates that agency experiences not only arise from conscious goals but also accompany the unconscious activation of goal representations, leading us to believe that the outcomes of our behaviors are consciously intended, whereas, in fact, they are influenced by cues in our environment outside of our conscious awareness.

It is important to emphasize that considering ourselves as the cause of our own actions and the resulting outcomes is not necessarily illusory because desired outcome representations (i.e., goals) activated outside awareness are also more likely to guide the actions that produce that outcome than when these representations are not activated (Aarts et al., 2004; Bargh et al., 2001; Custers & Aarts, 2007b). If, for instance, we want another person to like us, this changes our behavior toward that person in the service of the given goal, even though we may not be aware of the goal and the effects of pursuing it. Hence, self-agency and nonconscious goal pursuit may go hand in hand as nonconscious activation of goals promotes both goal attainment and agency experiences. As a result, agency experiences in such situations may not be deceptive, but rather are an accurate assessment of the source that produced the outcome. Thus, whereas the experience of self-agency can be a guess, sometimes this guess is right. In that case, experiences of self-agency may serve us well because they can help us to identify the results of our actions in social situations when we lack conscious knowledge of producing them. More importantly, the experience of agency, deriving from either conscious intentions or nonconscious goals, is a crucial source of our general belief that we can and do influence our own behavior, which has been shown to be associated with well-being and health (Taylor & Brown, 1988).

In addition, the belief that we have control over our behavior and its outcomes can also motivate us to look ahead and to plan our actions consciously, which can be beneficial for self-regulation in some circumstances, for example, when a situation demands a completely new course of action, or when previous goal-directed actions are obstructed. Action planning can then facilitate goal achievement by creating new action representations that include both sensorimotor information regarding one's future behavior and information regarding situational cues that can serve to initiate and guide behavior without much conscious thought (e.g., Gollwitzer & Sheeran, 2006; Papies et al., 2009). Indeed, without repeatedly experiencing a sense of control over important outcomes, we may be much less likely to see the point of reverting to such an effortful means of directing our behavior, which can clearly help successful goal pursuit. Future research may increase our understanding of how conscious planning can interact with nonconscious processes of self-regulation, and provide demonstrations of how such knowledge can be applied to enhancing self-regulation in important domains such as health behavior (see also Papies et al., 2008b).

CONCLUSIONS

Human goal-directed behavior originates to a large degree outside of conscious awareness. We have seen in this chapter how the pursuit of nonconscious goals can be initiated and regulated in a highly efficient fashion, without the recruitment of conscious awareness, by the interplay of situational cues, mental representations of desired states, and routinized behaviors that can be executed in an efficient yet flexible fashion. In addition, nonconscious self-regulation is supported by processes of executive control that ensure attainment of our goals also in situations where relying on well-practiced habits does not suffice. Although we often experience a sense of self-agency concerning our own behavior, these experiences seem to be a by-product rather than a necessarily accurate assessment of the mechanisms driving our goal-directed actions. While this emerging insight fits well with the recent advances in the research on goal-directed behavior (e.g., Aarts et al., 2009), it does pose a significant challenge for our understanding of the nature or even the actual existence of the "automatic pilot" of human behavior. Over the past years, the advance in social cognitive research methods has greatly contributed to our understanding of the processes underlying nonconscious self-regulation. In a similar way, future research efforts may benefit increasingly from research into the neural processes underlying consciousness and our experiences of "self" to help us extend our understanding of the "pilot" of this regulation.

ACKNOWLEDGMENT

The preparation of this chapter was supported by VICI Grant No. 453-06-002 from the Netherlands Organization for Scientific Research.

REFERENCES

Aarts, H. (2007). On the emergence of human goal pursuit: The nonconscious regulation and motivation of goals. *Social and Personality Psychology Compass, 1*, 183–201.

Aarts, H., Chartrand, T. L., Custers, R., Danner, U., Dik, G., Jefferis, V. E., et al. (2005). Social stereotypes and automatic goal pursuit. *Social Cognition, 23*, 465–490.

Aarts, H., & Custers, R. (2009). Habit, action, and consciousness. In W. P. Banks (Ed.), *Encyclopedia of consciousness* (pp. 315–328). Oxford, UK: Elsevier.

Aarts, H., Custers, R., & Holland, R. W. (2007). The nonconscious cessation of goal pursuit: When goals and negative affect are coactivated. *Journal of Personality and Social Psychology, 92*, 165–178.

Aarts, H., Custers, R., & Marien, H. (2008). Preparing and motivating behavior outside of awareness. *Science, 319*, 1639.

Aarts, H., Custers, R., & Marien, H. (2009). Priming and authorship ascription: When nonconscious goals turn into conscious experiences of self-agency. *Journal of Personality and Social Psychology, 96*, 967–979.

Aarts, H., Custers, R., & Wegner, D. M. (2005). On the inference of personal authorship: Enhancing experienced agency by priming effect information. *Consciousness and Cognition, 14*, 439–458.

Aarts, H., & Dijksterhuis, A. (2000). Habits as knowledge structures: Automaticity in goal-directed behavior. *Journal of Personality and Social Psychology, 78*, 53–63.

Aarts, H., Gollwitzer, P. M., & Hassin, R. R. (2004). Goal contagion: Perceiving is for pursuing. *Journal of Personality and Social Psychology, 87*, 23–37.

Aarts, H., & Hassin, R. R. (2005). Automatic goal inference and contagion: On pursuing goals one perceives in other people's behavior. In J. P. Forgas, K. D. Williams, & S. M. Laham (Eds.), *Social motivation: Conscious and unconscious processes* (pp. 153–167). New York: Cambridge University Press.

Aarts, H., Oikawa, M., & Oikawa, H. (2010). Cultural and universal routes to authorship ascription: Effects of outcome priming on experienced self-agency in the Netherlands and Japan. *Journal of Cross-Cultural Psychology, 41,* 87–98.

Atkinson, J. W., & Birch, D. (1970). *The dynamics of action.* New York: Wiley.

Austin, J. T., & Vancouver, J. B. (1996). Goal constructs in psychology: Structure, process, and content. *Psychological Bulletin, 120,* 338–375.

Badagaiyan, R. D. (2000). Executive control, willed actions, and nonconscious processing. *Human Brain Mapping, 9,* 38–41.

Bandura, A. (1986). *Social foundations of thought and action: A social cognitive theory.* Englewood Cliffs, NJ: Prentice Hall.

Bargh, J. A. (1990). Auto-motives: Preconscious determinants of social interaction. In E. T. Higgins & R. M. Sorrentino (Eds.), *Handbook of motivation and cognition: Vol. 2. Foundations of social behavior* (pp. 93–130). New York: Guilford Press.

Bargh, J. A. (1996). Automaticity in social psychology. In E. T. Higgins & A. W. Kruglanski (Eds.), *Social psychology: Handbook of basic principles* (pp. 169–183). New York: Guilford Press.

Bargh, J. A. (1997). The automaticity of everyday life. In R. S. Wyer, Jr. (Ed.), *Advances in social cognition* (Vol. 10, pp. 1–61). Mahwah, NJ: Erlbaum.

Bargh, J. A. (2005). Bypassing the will: Towards demystifying the nonconscious control of social behavior. In R. R. Hassin, J. Uleman, & J. A. Bargh (Eds.), *The new unconscious* (pp. 37–58). New York: Oxford University Press.

Bargh, J. A. (2006). What have we been priming all these years?: On the development, mechanisms, and ecology of nonconscious social behavior. *European Journal of Social Psychology, 36,* 147–168.

Bargh, J. A., & Ferguson, M. J. (2000). Beyond behaviorism: On the automaticity of higher mental processes. *Psychological Bulletin, 126,* 925–945.

Bargh, J. A., & Gollwitzer, P. M. (1994). Environmental control of goal-directed action: Automatic and strategic contingencies between situations and behavior. In W. D. Spaulding (Ed.), *Integrative views of motivation, cognition, and emotion: Nebraska Symposium on Motivation* (Vol. 41, pp. 71–124). Lincoln: University of Nebraska Press.

Bargh, J. A., Gollwitzer, P. M., Lee Chai, A., Barndollar, K., & Troetschel, R. (2001). The automated will: Nonconscious activation and pursuit of behavioral goals. *Journal of Personality and Social Psychology, 81,* 1014–1027.

Bargh, J. A., & Morsella, E. (2008). The unconscious mind. *Perspectives on Psychological Science, 3,* 73–79.

Baumeister, R. F. (1998). The self. In D. T. Gilbert, S. T. Fiske, & G. Lindzey (Eds.), *The handbook of social psychology* (4th ed., Vol. 1, pp. 680–740). New York: McGraw-Hill.

Baumeister, R. F., Schmeichel, B. J., & Vohs, K. D. (2007). Self-regulation and the executive function. In A. W. Kruglanski & E. T. Higgins (Eds.), *Social psychology: Handbook of basic principles* (2nd ed., pp. 516–539). New York: Guilford Press.

Berridge, K. C. (2007). The debate over dopamine's role in reward: The case for incentive salience. *Psychopharmacology, 191,* 391–431.

Blakemore, S.-J., & Frith, C. D. (2003). Self-awareness and action. *Current Opinion in Neurobiology, 13,* 219–224.

Blakemore, S.-J., Wolpert, D. M., & Frith, C. D. (2002). Abnormalities in the awareness of action. *Trends in Cognitive Sciences, 6,* 237–242.

Carver, C. S., & Scheier, M. F. (1981). *Attention and self-regulation: A control theory approach to human behavior.* New York: Springer-Verlag.

Carver, C. S., & Scheier, M. F. (1998). *On the self-regulation of behavior.* New York: Cambridge University Press.

Chen, M., & Bargh, J. A. (1999). Consequences of automatic evaluation: Immediate behavioral predispositions to approach or avoid the stimulus. *Personality and Social Psychology Bulletin, 25,* 215–224.

Cooper, R. P., & Shallice, T. (2006). Hierarchical schemas and goals in the control of sequential behavior. *Psychological Review, 113,* 887–916.

Custers, R., & Aarts, H. (2005). Positive affect as implicit motivator: On the nonconscious operation of behavioral goals. *Journal of Personality and Social Psychology, 89,* 129–142.

Custers, R., & Aarts, H. (2007a). Goal-discrepant situations prime goal-directed actions if goals are temporarily or chronically accessible. *Personality and Social Psychology Bulletin, 33,* 623–633.

Custers, R., & Aarts, H. (2007b). In search of the nonconscious sources of goal pursuit: Accessibility and positive affective valence of the goal state. *Journal of Experimental Social Psychology, 43,* 312–318.

Custers, R., Aarts, H., Oikawa, M., & Elliot, A. (2009). The nonconscious road to perceptions of performance: Achievement priming augments outcome expectancies and experienced self-agency. *Journal of Experimental Social Psychology, 45,* 1200–1208.

Custers, R., Maas, M., Wildenbeest, M., & Aarts, H. (2008). Nonconscious goal pursuit and the surmounting of physical and social obstacles. *European Journal of Social Psychology, 38,* 1013–1022.

Damasio, A. R. (1994). *Descartes' error: Emotion, reason, and the human brain.* New York: Putnam.

Danner, U. N., Aarts, H., & de Vries, N. K. (2008). Habit vs. intention in the prediction of future behaviour: The role of frequency, context stability and mental accessibility of past behaviour. *British Journal of Social Psychology, 47,* 245–265.

Daprati, E., Franck, N., Georgieff, N., Proust, J., Pacherie, E., & Dalery, J. (1997). Looking for the agent: An investigation into consciousness of action and self-consciousness in schizophrenic patients. *Cognition, 65,* 71–86.

Decety, J., & Sommerville, J. A. (2003). Shared representations between self and other: A social cognitive neuroscience view. *Trends in Cognitive Sciences, 7,* 527–533.

Deci, E. L., & Ryan, R. M. (1985). *Intrinsic motivation and self-determination in human behavior.* New York: Plenum Press.

Dickinson, A., Balleine, B., Watt, A., Gonzales, F., & Boakes, R. A. (1995). Motivational control after extended instrumental training. *Animal Learning and Behavior, 23,* 197–206.

Dijksterhuis, A., & Aarts, H. (2010). Goals, attention, and (un)consciousness. *Annual Review of Psychology, 16,* 467–490.

Dijksterhuis, A., Preston, J., Wegner, D. M., & Aarts, H. (2008). Effects of subliminal priming of self and God on self-attribution of authorship for events. *Journal of Experimental Social Psychology, 44,* 2–9.

Eitam, B., Hassin, R. R., & Schul, Y. (2008). Nonconscious goal pursuit in novel environments: The case of implicit learning. *Psychological Science, 19,* 261–267.

Fazio, R. H., Sanbonmatsu, D. M., Powell, M. C., & Kardes, F. R. (1986). On the automatic activation of attitudes. *Journal of Personality and Social Psychology, 50,* 229–238.

Ferguson, M. J. (2007). On the automatic evaluation of end-states. *Journal of Personality and Social Psychology, 92,* 596–611.

Ferguson, M. J., & Bargh, J. A. (2004). Liking is for doing: The effects of goal pursuit on automatic evaluation. *Journal of Personality and Social Psychology, 87,* 557–572.

Fishbach, A., & Ferguson, M. J. (2007). The goal construct in social psychology. In A. W. Kruglanski & E. T. Higgins (Eds.), *Social psychology: Handbook of basic principles* (2nd ed., pp. 490–515). New York: Guilford Press.

Fishbach, A., Friedman, R. S., & Kruglanski, A. W. (2003). Leading us not unto temptation: Momentary allurements elicit overriding goal activation. *Journal of Personality and Social Psychology, 84,* 296–309.

Fishbach, A., Shah, J. Y., & Kruglanski, A. W. (2004). Emotional transfer in goal systems. *Journal of Experimental Social Psychology, 40,* 723–738.

Fishbein, M., & Ajzen, I. (1975). *Belief, attitude, intention and behavior: An introduction to theory and research.* Reading, MA: Addison-Wesley.

Fitzsimons, G. M., & Bargh, J. A. (2003). Thinking of you: Nonconscious pursuit of interpersonal goals associated with relationship partners. *Journal of Personality and Social Psychology, 84,* 148–164.

Foerster, J., Liberman, N., & Friedman, R. S. (2007). Seven principles of goal activation: A systematic approach to distinguishing goal priming from priming of non-goal constructs. *Personality and Social Psychology Review, 11,* 211–233.

Fourneret, P., & Jeannerod, M. (1998). Limited conscious monitoring of motor performance in normal subjects. *Neuropsychologia, 36,* 1133–1140.

Frith, C. D., Blakemore, S.-J., & Wolpert, D. M. (2000). Abnormalities in the awareness and control of action. *Philosophical Transactions of the Royal Society of London, 355,* 1771–1788.

Gandevia, S., & Burke, D. (1992). Does the nervous system depend on kinesthetic information to control natural limb movements. *Behavioral and Brain Sciences, 15,* 614–632.

Georgieff, N., & Jeannerod, M. (1998). Beyond consciousness of external reality: A "who" system for consciousness of action and selfconsciousness. *Consciousness and Cognition, 7,* 465–477.

Gillath, O., Mikulincer, M., Fitzsimons, G. M., Shaver, P. R., Schachner, D. A., & Bargh, J. A. (2006). Automatic activation of attachment-related goals. *Personality and Social Psychology Bulletin, 32,* 1375–1388.

Gollwitzer, P. M., & Sheeran, P. (2006). Implementation intentions and goal achievement: A meta-analysis of effects and processes. In M. P. Zanna (Ed.), *Advances in experimental social psychology* (Vol. 38, pp. 69–119). San Diego, CA: Elsevier Academic Press.

Hassin, R. R., Aarts, H., Eitam, B., Custers, R., & Kleiman, T. (2009). Non-conscious goal pursuit, working memory, and the effortful control of behavior. In J. A. Bargh, E. Morsella, & P. M. Gollwitzer (Eds.), *Oxford handbook of human action: Mechanisms of human action* (Vol. 2, pp. 549–568). New York: Oxford University Press.

Hassin, R. R., Bargh, J. A., Engell, A. D., & McCulloch, K. C. (2009). Implicit working memory. *Consciousness and Cognition, 18,* 665–678.

Hebb, D. O. (1949). *Organization of behavior.* New York: Wiley.

Higgins, E. T., Bargh, J. A., & Lombardi, W. J. (1985). Nature of priming effects on categorization. *Journal of Experimental Psychology: Learning, Memory, and Cognition, 11,* 59–69.

Hommel, B., Musseler, J., Aschersleben, G., & Prinz, W. (2001). The Theory of Event Coding (TEC): A framework for perception and action planning. *Behavioral and Brain Sciences, 24,* 849–878.

James, W. (1890). *The principles of psychology.* New York: Dover.

Jeannerod, M. (2001). Neural simulation of action: A unifying mechanism for motor cognition. *NeuroImage, 14,* S103–S109.

Jones, S. R., de Wit, L., Fernyhough, C., & Meins, E. (2008). A new spin on the Wheel of Fortune: Priming of action–authorship judgements and relation to psychosis-like experiences. *Consciousness and Cognition, 17,* 576–586.

Kahneman, D. (1973). *Attention and effort.* Englewood Cliffs, NJ: Prentice-Hall.

Koch, C., & Tsuchiya, N. (2007). Attention and consciousness: Two distinct brain processes. *Trends in Cognitive Sciences, 11,* 16–22.

Kraus, M. W., & Chen, S. (2009). Striving to be known by significant others: Automatic activation of self-verification goals in relationship contexts. *Journal of Personality and Social Psychology, 97,* 58–73.

Kruglanski, A. W., Shah, J. Y., Fishbach, A., Friedman, R., Chun, W. Y., & Sleeth Keppler, D. (2002). A theory of goal systems. In M. P. Zanna (Ed.), *Advances in experimental social psychology* (Vol. 34, pp. 331–378). San Diego, CA: Academic Press.

Lakin, J. L., Chartrand, T. L., & Arkin, R. M. (2008). I am too just like you: Nonconscious mimicry as an automatic behavioral response to social exclusion. *Psychological Science, 19,* 816–822.

Lamme, V. A. F. (2003). Why visual attention and awareness are different. *Trends in Cognitive Sciences, 7,* 12–18.

Lau, H. C., Rogers, R. D., Haggard, P., & Passingham, R. E. (2004). Attention to intention. *Science, 303,* 1208–1210.

Legrand, D., & Ruby, P. (2009). What is self-specific?: Theoretical investigation and critical review of neuroimaging results. *Psychological Review, 116,* 252–282.

Metcalfe, J., & Mischel, W. (1999). A hot/cool-system analysis of delay of gratification: Dynamics of willpower. *Psychological Review, 106,* 3–19.

Miller, E. K., & Cohen, J. D. (2001). An integrative theory of prefrontal cortex function. *Annual Review of Neuroscience, 24,* 167–202.

Mischel, W., Cantor, N., & Feldman, S. (1996). Principles of self-regulation: The nature of willpower and self-control. In E. T. Higgins & A. W. Kruglanski (Eds.), *Social psychology: Handbook of basic principles* (pp. 329–360). New York: Guilford Press.

Miyake, A., & Shah, P. (1999). *Models of working memory: Mechanisms of active maintenance and executive control.* New York: Cambridge University Press.

Moskowitz, G. B. (2002). Preconscious effects of temporary goals on attention. *Journal of Experimental Social Psychology, 38,* 397–404.

Moskowitz, G. B., Gollwitzer, P. M., Wasel, W., & Schaal, B. (1999). Preconscious control of stereotype activation through chronic egalitarian goals. *Journal of Personality and Social Psychology, 77,* 167–184.

Moskowitz, G. B., & Ignarri, C. (2009). Implicit volition and stereotype control. *European Review of Social Psychology, 20,* 97–145.

Moskowitz, G. B., Li, P., & Kirk, E. R. (2004). The implicit volition model: On the preconscious regulation of temporarily adopted goals. In M. P. Zanna (Ed.), *Advances in experimental social psychology* (Vol. 36, pp. 317–413). San Diego, CA: Elsevier Academic Press.

Muraven, M., & Baumeister, R. F. (2000). Self-regulation and depletion of limited resources: Does self-control resemble a muscle? *Psychological Bulletin, 126,* 247–259.

Norman, P., Armitage, C. J., & Quigley, C. (2007). The theory of planned behavior and binge drinking: Assessing the impact of binge drinker prototypes. *Addictive Behaviors, 32,* 1753–1768.

Norman, P., & Conner, M. (2006). The theory of planned behaviour and binge drinking: Assessing the moderating role of past behaviour within the theory of planned behaviour. *British Journal of Health Psychology, 11,* 55–70.

Ouellette, J. A., & Wood, W. (1998). Habit and intention in everyday life: The multiple processes by which past behavior predicts future behavior. *Psychological Bulletin, 124,* 54–74.

Papies, E. K., Aarts, H., & de Vries, N. K. (2009). Planning is for doing: Implementation intentions go beyond the mere creation of goal-directed associations. *Journal of Experimental Social Psychology, 45,* 1148–1151.

Papies, E. K., & Hamstra, P. (in press). Goal priming and eating behavior: Enhancing self-regulation by environmental cues. *Health Psychology.*

Papies, E. K., Stroebe, W., & Aarts, H. (2007). Pleasure in the mind: Restrained eating and spontaneous hedonic thoughts about food. *Journal of Experimental Social Psychology, 43,* 810–817.

Papies, E. K., Stroebe, W., & Aarts, H. (2008a). The allure of forbidden food: On the role of attention in self-regulation. *Journal of Experimental Social Psychology, 44,* 1283–1292.

Papies, E. K., Stroebe, W., & Aarts, H. (2008b). Healthy cognition: Processes of self-regulatory success in restrained eating. *Personality and Social Psychology Bulletin, 34,* 1290–1300.

Powers, W. T. (1973). *Behavior: The control of perception.* Chicago: Aldine.

Prinz, W. (1997). Perception and action planning. *European Journal of Cognitive Psychology, 9,* 129–154.

Prinz, W. (2003). How do we know about our own actions? In S. Maasen, W. Prinz, & G. Roth (Eds.), *Voluntary action: Brains, minds, and sociality* (pp. 21–33). New York: Oxford University Press.

Raymond, J. E., & O'Brien, J. L. (2009). Selective visual attention and motivation: The consequences of value learning in an attentional blink task. *Psychological Science, 20*, 981–988.

Sato, A., & Yasuda, A. (2005). Illusion of sense of self-agency: Discrepancy between the predicted and actual sensory consequences of actions modulates the sense of self-agency, but not the sense of self-ownership. *Cognition, 94*, 241–255.

Shah, J. Y. (2003). Automatic for the people: How representations of significant others implicitly affect goal pursuit. *Journal of Personality and Social Psychology, 84*, 661–681.

Shah, J. Y., Friedman, R., & Kruglanski, A. W. (2002). Forgetting all else: On the antecedents and consequences of goal shielding. *Journal of Personality and Social Psychology, 83*, 1261–1280.

Sheeran, P., Aarts, H., Custers, R., Rivis, A., Webb, T. L., & Cooke, R. (2005). The goal-dependent automaticity of drinking habits. *British Journal of Social Psychology, 44*, 47–63.

Smith, E. E., & Jonides, J. (1999). Storage and executive processes in the frontal lobes. *Science, 283*, 1657–1661.

Srull, T. K., & Wyer, R. S., Jr. (1979). The role of category accessibility in the interpretation of information about persons: Some determinants and implications. *Journal of Personality and Social Psychology, 37*, 1660–1672.

Strack, F., & Deutsch, R. (2004). Reflective and impulsive determinants of social behavior. *Personality and Social Psychology Review, 8*, 220–247.

Taylor, S. E., & Brown, J. D. (1988). Illusion and well-being: A social psychological perspective on mental health. *Psychological Bulletin, 103*, 193–210.

Vallacher, R. R., & Wegner, D. M. (1987). What do people think they're doing?: Action identification and human behavior. *Psychological Review, 94*, 3–15.

Veltkamp, M., Aarts, H., & Custers, R. (2008). Perception in the service of goal pursuit: Motivation to attain goals enhances the perceived size of goal-instrumental objects. *Social Cognition, 26*, 720–736.

Verplanken, B., Aarts, H., van Knippenberg, A., & Moonen, A. (1998). Habit versus planned behavior: A field experiment. *British Journal of Social Psychology, 37*, 111–128.

Wegner, D. M. (2002). *The illusion of conscious will*. Cambridge, MA: MIT Press.

Wegner, D. M., & Sparrow, B. (2004). Authorship processing. In M. Gazzaniga (Ed.), *The cognitive neurosciences* (pp. 1201–1209). Cambridge, MA: MIT Press.

Wegner, D. M., & Wheatley, T. (1999). Apparent mental causation: Sources of the experience of will. *American Psychologist, 54*, 480–492.

Wheeler, S. C., DeMarree, K. G., & Petty, R. E. (2007). Understanding the role of the self in prime-to-behavior effects: The active-self account. *Personality and Social Psychology Review, 11*, 234–261.

Wood, W., Quinn, J. M., & Kashy, D. A. (2002). Habits in everyday life: Thought, emotion, and action. *Journal of Personality and Social Psychology, 83*, 1281–1297.

Wood, W., Tam, L., & Guerrero Witt, M. (2005). Changing circumstances, disrupting habits. *Journal of Personality and Social Psychology, 88*, 918–933.

Zajonc, R. B. (1980). Feeling and thinking: Preferences need no inferences. *American Psychologist, 35*, 151–175.

CHAPTER 8

Promotion and Prevention Systems
Regulatory Focus Dynamics within Self-Regulatory Hierarchies

ABIGAIL A. SCHOLER
E. TORY HIGGINS

Donald has a problem. His wife is nagging him about the home improvement projects he had promised to have completed last month; over and over his New Year's resolutions have remained just that—resolutions; he has important deadlines coming up at work; and the exercise bike is gathering more dust than sweat. Alas, Donald is not unusual in all that he has to juggle. Life presents a seemingly endless series of challenges and opportunities for us to manage. While our ability to be effective in the face of such demands can astound us, so too can all of the ways in which we often fall short dumbfound us.

In this chapter, we explore how thinking about hierarchies of self-regulation can help elucidate both what astounds and dumbfounds us about how we succeed or fail at getting along in the world. In particular, we garner insights from research on regulatory focus theory (Higgins, 1997) to highlight factors that both sustain and disrupt effective self-regulation. While it is tempting to try to identify some single factor that underlies self-regulatory effectiveness, we hope in this chapter to provide a perspective that highlights the complex *dynamics* within regulatory systems that contribute to effective self-regulation. We begin by reviewing the basic tenets of regulatory focus theory as an example of a hierarchical model of self-regulation. We then explore how both horizontal and vertical dynamics within regulatory focus play a role in a number of significant self-regulatory challenges: initiating and maintaining change, confronting temptation, and dealing with failure. We conclude by discussing the implications of this research for interventions and future research.

REGULATORY FOCUS THEORY

Building on earlier distinctions (e.g., Bowlby, 1969, 1973; Higgins, 1987; Mowrer, 1960), regulatory focus theory distinguishes between two coexisting regulatory systems (promotion, prevention) that serve critically important but different survival needs (Higgins, 1997). As we discuss in more detail below, the systems differ in what fundamentally motivates (nurturance vs. security) and in what regulatory strategies are preferred (eagerness vs. vigilance). These key differences have a number of consequences for self-regulatory processes.

The *promotion* orientation regulates nurturance needs and is concerned with growth, advancement, and accomplishment. Individuals in a promotion focus are striving toward ideals, wishes, and aspirations. They are concerned with the presence and absence of positive outcomes (gain/nongain) and are more sensitive to positive deviations from the status quo or neutral state (the difference between "0" and "+1") than to negative deviations from that state (the difference between "0" and "−1") (Higgins, 1997).

In contrast, the *prevention* orientation regulates security needs. Individuals in a prevention focus are concerned with safety and responsibility, and with attending to their oughts, duties, and responsibilities. They are concerned with the absence and presence of negative outcomes (nonloss/loss) and are more sensitive to the difference between "0" and "−1" than to the difference between "0" and "+1" (cf. Brendl & Higgins, 1996; Higgins, 1997).

Importantly, although the two systems are concerned with the regulation of different needs, promotion and prevention orientations each involve *both* approaching desired end states (e.g., approaching accomplishment or safety, respectively) and avoiding undesired end states (e.g., avoiding nonfulfillment or danger, respectively). This has two significant implications. First, the value or personal relevance of some desired end states may be greater in one system than in the other (see Higgins, 2002). For instance, promotion-focused individuals may value the desired end state of having all the latest and greatest technology more than do prevention-focused individuals (cf. Herzenstein, Posavac, & Brakus, 2007). Second, the *same* desired end state can be represented in different ways by prevention- versus promotion-focused individuals. For example, the same desired end state (e.g., being physically fit) may be represented as a duty or responsibility for prevention-focused individuals, but as an ideal or aspiration for promotion-focused individuals.

Promotion and prevention orientations can arise either from *chronic* accessibility (individual differences) or from *temporary* accessibility (situational factors). Consequently, regulatory focus is studied both as a personality variable (chronic strength or predominance of prevention and promotion orientations) and as a situational variable. In keeping with a general principles approach to personality and social psychology (Higgins, 1990, 1999), we believe that what ultimately matters in terms of predicting behavior is the regulatory *state* that one is in, whether that arises from chronic or temporary accessibility.

Individual differences in the chronic strength of the promotion and prevention systems arise in part from different styles of caretaker–child interactions (see Calkins & Leerkes, Chapter 19, this volume; Higgins, 1987, 1997; Keller, 2008; Manian, Papadakis, Strauman, & Essex, 2006; Manian, Strauman, & Denney, 1998). Caretaker–child interactions that involve a promotion focus emphasize desired end states as ideals (hopes, wishes, and aspirations). Caretakers communicate, explicitly and implicitly, that what matters is making good things happen—the presence versus absence of positive outcomes. In contrast, caretaker–child interactions that involve a prevention focus emphasize desired end states as oughts (duties, responsibilities, and obligations). Caretakers communicate that what matters is keeping bad things from happening—the absence versus presence of negative outcomes. Indeed, in both prospective and retrospective studies of caretaker–child interactions and regulatory focus, nurturing and bolstering parenting styles are associated with stronger ideal self-beliefs in children (Manian et al., 2006) and stronger promotion focus in adults (Keller, 2008). In contrast, critical and punitive parenting styles are associated with stronger ought self-beliefs in children (Manian et al., 2006) and stronger prevention focus in adults (Keller, 2008).

A number of measures have now been developed to assess chronic differences in regulatory focus. Two commonly employed measures—the Regulatory Focus Strength Measure (Higgins, Shah, & Friedman, 1997) and the Regulatory Focus Questionnaire (RFQ; Higgins et al., 2001)—assess different aspects of individuals' chronic tendencies. The RFQ captures differences in individual histories of success in the promotion versus prevention systems. Thus, a higher score on the Promotion scale reflects promotion pride, a subjective history of success with promotion-related eagerness, "promotion working," so to speak, whereas a higher score on the Prevention Pride scale reflects "prevention working," or a subjective history of success with prevention-related vigilance.

In contrast, the Regulatory Focus Strength Measure assesses differences in the chronic accessibility of ideals (promotion system) or oughts (prevention system). Scores on strength provide information about the accessibility of these systems, but do not reveal an individual's history of success or failure within the system. Thus, it is possible that someone could be low in promotion pride but show high ideal strength on the strength measure. Presumably, this would be an individual whose promotion ideals are chronically accessible, but who has not experienced (subjective) success using promotion-related eager means.

Other measures to assess chronic differences in regulatory focus have also been developed (e.g., Cunningham, Raye, & Johnson, 2005; Lockwood, Jordan, & Kunda, 2002; Ouschan, Boldero, Kashima, Wakimoto, & Kashima, 2007). These measures differ in the extent to which they emphasize particular facets of the regulatory focus systems. As recently highlighted by Summerville and Roese (2008), some regulatory focus measures place greater emphasis on the extent to which individuals are motivated by or are sensitive to ideals versus oughts (e.g., Higgins et al., 2001), whereas other measures place greater emphasis on the extent to which individuals are sensitive to the gain/nongain versus nonloss/loss distinction (e.g., Lockwood et al., 2002). Exploring when and why these measures converge and diverge in terms of predicting behavior is an important question for future research.

Promotion and prevention regulatory states can also be temporarily induced. As with chronic measures of regulatory focus, a number of different approaches for manipulating regulatory focus have been employed. Promotion and prevention orientations can be induced by framing an identical set of task payoffs for success or failure as involving "gain/nongain" (promotion) or "nonloss/loss" (prevention) (e.g., Shah & Higgins, 1997; Shah, Higgins, & Friedman, 1998). Promotion and prevention states can also be induced by priming ideals or oughts (Higgins, Roney, Crowe, & Hymes, 1994; Liberman, Molden, Idson, & Higgins, 2001), or even implicitly by having participants complete a maze that highlights nurturance versus security concerns (Friedman & Förster, 2001). Having individuals remember episodes in their past when they have been successful within either the promotion system or the prevention system (using items from the RFQ) can also induce temporary promotion or prevention states, respectively (Higgins et al., 2001).

LEVELS OF SELF-REGULATION: THE REGULATORY FOCUS HIERARCHY

Regulatory focus theory joins other self-regulatory models that have emphasized in different ways the importance of differentiating among levels of self-regulation (e.g., Cantor & Kihlstrom, 1987; Carver & Scheier, 1998, and Chapter 1, this volume; Elliot, 2006; Elliot & Church, 1997; Kruglanski et al., 2002; Miller, Galanter, & Pribram, 1960; Pervin, 1989; Vallacher & Wegner, 1985). Although these approaches differ in their preferred terminology and in the number of distinctions they wish to make, all emphasize the importance of recognizing that the levels of self-regulation are defined by different concerns (e.g., goals, strategies, behavioral enactment) and are independent (there are multiple options at a lower level for serving a higher level). In this section, we review levels of self-regulation as defined by regulatory focus theory (see also Higgins, 1997; Scholer & Higgins, 2008), emphasizing distinctions among system, strategic, and tactical levels of self-regulation.

The *system level* defines an individual's overarching motivational concern or goal. Goals serve as the end states, standards, or references points that guide behavior (see Kruglanski, 1996). Perhaps the most ubiquitous distinction made at the system level is whether individuals are regulating in relation to a desired end state (e.g., a goal to be in good physical shape) or an undesired end state (e.g., a goal to avoid being fat). However, the system level also defines the domain of regulation ("physical fitness") and the underlying motivational concerns of the individual (e.g., accomplishment, safety).

As noted earlier, at the system level, regulatory focus theory is orthogonal to the distinction between approaching desired end states and avoiding undesired end states. Promotion and prevention orientations each involve *both* approaching desired end states (e.g., approaching accomplishment or safety, respectively) and avoiding undesired end states (e.g., avoiding nonfulfillment or danger, respectively). However, promotion and prevention do differ at the system level in terms of whether desired end states involve nurturance concerns (aspirations, accomplishments) versus security concerns (responsibilities, safety).

THE "HOW" OF GOAL PURSUIT: STRATEGIES AND TACTICS

The goals that individuals hold are enacted in the means or plans used for goal pursuit (i.e., the "how" of goal pursuit). Within regulatory focus theory, we have distinguished between different levels of "how"—strategies and tactics (Higgins, 1997; Scholer & Higgins, 2008; Scholer, Stroessner, & Higgins, 2008). *Strategies* are the links between goals at a higher level and tactics, or behavior, at a lower level. Strategies reflect the general plans or means for goal pursuit. *Tactics* are the instantiation of a strategy in a given context, capturing the means or process at a more concrete, in-context level (Cantor & Kihlstrom, 1987; Higgins, 1997). Because the levels in the hierarchy are independent, the same strategy can be served by multiple tactics. Similarly, the same tactic can serve multiple strategies. Distinguishing between these two different levels of "how" within goal pursuit highlights some of the significant dynamics of these regulatory systems.

At the strategic level, differences between promotion and prevention focus relate to different preferences for using, respectively, *eager approach* strategies (approaching matches to desired end states, approaching mismatches to undesired end states) or *vigilant avoidance* strategies (avoiding mismatches to desired end states, avoiding matches to undesired end states) (Crowe & Higgins, 1997; Ledgerwood & Trope, Chapter 12, this volume; Liberman et al., 2001; Molden & Higgins, 2005). The *eager strategic means* preferred by individuals in a promotion focus reflect their concerns with advancement and accomplishment, their pursuit of ideals and growth, and their relative sensitivity to the difference between "0" and "+1." The *vigilant strategic means* preferred by individuals in a prevention focus reflect their concerns with safety and responsibility, their need to guard against mistakes, and their relative sensitivity to the difference between "0" and "−1."

Consequently, even if promotion-focused and prevention-focused individuals are pursuing the same desired end state (e.g., good health), they have different preferred strategies for doing so. Promotion-focused Peter will prefer to seize eagerly all possible opportunities for advancing his health, whereas prevention-focused Paula will prefer to avoid vigilantly all possible pitfalls that threaten her health. Knowing whether someone is using an eager or a vigilant strategy, however, does not tell one how that strategy is enacted at the tactical level.

Eagerness and vigilance are enacted in specific situations by the tactics that individuals adopt. One can protect and maintain a vigilant strategy by imagining the possibility of failure or by carefully considering what is necessary. One can boost eagerness by imagining success or by bolstering positive self-evaluations. Individuals may adopt different supporting tactics because of differing situational opportunities or constraints, or because a particular tactic better supports strategic and motivational concerns. For instance, depending on the nature of the situation, either risky tactics or conservative tactics may better support an underlying vigilant strategy (Scholer et al., 2008; Scholer, Zou, Fujita, Stroessner, & Higgins, in press). For example, when all is well, playing it safe tactically by adopting a conservative bias best serves a vigilant strategy because it minimizes the possibility of mistakes. However, when the context is negative or threatening, making a mistake (i.e., missing a negative signal) undermines strategic vigilance. In this context, strategic vigilance is served by doing anything necessary, including being tactically risky, to get back to safety.

It is important to note that, consistent with most hierarchical models of self-regulation, the tactical level is not the lowest level of self-regulation and is not necessarily synonymous with behavior. A risky tactic, for example, may result in different kinds of behaviors depending on what is being demanded or afforded in a given context. A risky tactic may be reflected in not only the behavior of adopting a liberal threshold for acceptance when a recognition judgment is demanded but also in the behavioral preference for a risky choice over a sure thing when a gambling decision is demanded (e.g., Kahneman & Tversky, 1979). Thus, although the tactical level reflects a more concrete instantiation of the strategic level, even the tactical level can be reflected more concretely in different specific behaviors.

In sum, when conceiving the "how" of self-regulation, it is possible to distinguish between different levels of regulation. Strategies differ from tactics or behavior because they are about the broad-level descriptions of the means ("Be eager!") rather than the more specific tactical instantiations (e.g., "Be risky—be willing to make a mistake to seize an opportunity for advancement") and the even more precise behavioral instantiations of those tactics (e.g., "Say yes when Tina asks you if you want to try salsa dancing"). In this chapter, we focus our discussion on distinctions and relations among the system, strategic, and tactical levels within regulatory focus.

HORIZONTAL AND VERTICAL DYNAMICS WITHIN REGULATORY FOCUS

A hierarchical model of self-regulation illuminates distinct types of self-regulatory dynamics that can occur both within and between levels of the regulatory focus hierarchy. For instance, conflicts can exist *within* levels in a self-regulatory hierarchy, which we refer to as *horizontal conflicts*. Conflicts can also exist *between* levels in the hierarchy, which we refer to as *vertical conflicts*. Effective resolution of both horizontal and vertical conflicts is critical for optimal self-regulatory functioning.

A horizontal conflict is any conflict that exists within a level in a self-regulatory hierarchy—between goals, between strategies, and between tactics. At the system level, horizontal conflicts can occur between reference points (e.g., between aiming for an A vs. avoiding an F), between life domains (e.g., performing well in *school* vs. getting along with siblings at *home*), or between differing regulatory focus motivational concerns (e.g., between pursuing one's *aspiration* to be a rock star vs. upholding one's *duty* to provide for a new spouse). At the level of strategies and tactics, horizontal conflicts can occur because of the trade-offs associated with different strategies or tactics. Resolution of such conflicts can have important implications for goal pursuit and performance. For instance, Wallace, Little, and Shull (2008) found that, under normal conditions, prevention focus is related to good safety performance and promotion focus is related to good production performance in a simulation game. Under high task complexity, the trade-offs between these concerns are difficult to avoid, such that prevention also is related to decreased production and promotion also is related to decreased safety.

Vertical conflicts are conflicts that occur *between* levels in a hierarchy, such as between goals and strategies, or between strategies and tactics. Vertical conflicts occur when there is incompatibility or nonfit between levels. For instance, a vertical conflict is present when an individual pursues a promotion system goal with a nonfitting vigilant strategy (Higgins, 2000). Although promotion-focused individuals prefer eager strategies and prevention-focused individuals prefer vigilant strategies, vertical conflicts are possible because of the independence between levels in the hierarchy (Scholer & Higgins, 2008). When such conflicts are successfully resolved and individuals use means that fit their underlying motivational orientation, they experience *regulatory fit* (Higgins, 2000), which strengthens their engagement in goal pursuit and makes them "feel right" about what they are doing (Higgins, 2000, 2006). Regulatory fit affects the value of the goal pursuit activity, subsequent object appraisals, and task performance (Freitas & Higgins, 2002; Higgins, Idson, Freitas, Spiegel, & Molden, 2003; Shah et al., 1998).

In the remainder of the chapter, we discuss how horizontal and vertical dynamics within regulatory focus play out in a variety of significant self-regulatory challenges. Successful resolution of regulatory focus conflicts (both horizontal and vertical) can impact how individuals initiate and maintain change, confront temptation, and cope with failure.

INITIATING AND MAINTAINING CHANGE

Being open to change, initiating change, and maintaining change are core issues in self-regulation (cf. Rothman, 2000; Rothman, Baldwin, & Hertel, 2004). Individuals often struggle to stop behaviors (e.g., smoking) and start new ones (e.g., exercising). Dynamics within regulatory focus influence a number of core change issues: openness to change in general, the effectiveness of different change strategies, the weighting of relevant factors in one's decision to change, and the influence of persuasion attempts.

Change Is Not Only for the Promotion-Hearted

At first glance, it makes intuitive sense that promotion would align more naturally with openness to change than would prevention. Promotion-focused individuals care about advancement, going for hits, and are more likely to dive into pursuits with eager abandon. Consistent with this intuition, significant empirical evidence supports this "natural" marriage between promotion and change. Promotion-focused individuals are more open to new products than are prevention-focused individuals (Herzenstein et al., 2007) and are more successful at initiating weight loss and smoking cessation (Fuglestad, Rothman, & Jeffery, 2008). Promotion-focused individuals are more willing to give up an activity on which they are working or a prize they currently possess for a new activity or prize; in contrast, prevention-focused individuals are more committed to maintaining and preserving the status quo (Chernev, 2004; Crowe & Higgins, 1997; Liberman, Idson, Camacho, & Higgins, 1999). Indeed, Vaughn, Baumann, and Klemann (2008) found that openness to experience (cf. John & Srivastava, 1999) was positively correlated with pursuit of promotion goals and negatively correlated with pursuit of prevention goals, which has also been found cross-culturally (see Higgins, 2008).

The story is not so straightforward, however. The prevention system has also been implicated in the successful regulation of change (Freitas, Liberman, Salovey, & Higgins, 2002; Fuglestad et al., 2008; Poels & Dewitte, 2008). Prevention-focused individuals have even been shown to initiate goal pursuit *more* quickly than do promotion-focused individuals (Freitas, Liberman, Salovey, et al., 2002; Poels & Dewitte, 2008). Fuglestad and colleagues (2008) also found that prevention-focused individuals are more successful than promotion-focused individuals at *maintaining* changes after successful initiation (weight loss and smoking cessation).

How can we reconcile these apparently conflicting findings? All else being equal, at the system level, promotion concerns probably do align more naturally with change than do prevention concerns. Thus, it makes sense that a general openness to change tends to be in concordance with the promotion system (Herzenstein et al., 2007; Higgins, 2008; Vaughn et al., 2008). Change as shiny newness (cf. Herzenstein et al., 2007) and advancement (Liberman et al., 1999) is a fit for promotion. However, change can also serve as a tactic *in the service of* either promotion or prevention concerns. Consequently, there are contexts in which initiating or maintaining change may sometimes better serve prevention than promotion systems. For example, because prevention-focused individuals are more likely to see goals as necessary duties and obligations, they should generally feel more pressure to initiate goal pursuit (Freitas, Liberman, Salovey, et al., 2002; Poels & Dewitte, 2008). Duties and necessities cannot (should not) be as easily postponed as hopes and dreams.

However, recent work by Fuglestad and colleagues (2008) suggests that this prevention advantage in initiating goal pursuit may itself be affected by the nature of the change decision. In two interventions for intractably difficult-to-change health behaviors (weight loss, smoking cessation), promotion focus, but not prevention focus, was associated with successful initiation of change (as defined by more weight loss and higher quit rates in the first 6 months). Fuglestad and colleagues suggest that because successful initiation of such behaviors is often motivated by the perception of substantial gains (Foster, Wadden, Vogt, & Brewer, 1997), promotion-focused individuals may rise to the initiation challenge more eagerly than do prevention-focused individuals under these circumstances. In contrast, prevention focus was related to the successful *maintenance* of these change behaviors. Because successful behavior maintenance for changes such as weight loss and smoking cessation requires preventing backslides (Rothman, 2000), prevention-focused individuals may be more equipped for the challenges of this phase of change.

More generally, both the way in which the change is construed (a necessary change vs. an ideal change) and the perception of one's current state (as negative, neutral, or positive) are important determinants of whether promotion versus prevention concerns will be more likely to motivate behavior. When individuals find themselves in a state of loss or negativity (below the status quo), prevention-focused individuals should be willing to do *whatever is necessary* to get back to the status quo. For prevention-focused individuals, the measure of acceptable change is whether it returns them to the status quo. In contrast, promotion-focused individuals are motivated to make progress away from the current state, but the status quo holds no special meaning as the state they want to reach. Rather, a measure of acceptable change is whether there is advancement away from the current state.

Given these regulatory focus differences in concerns, when individuals have fallen below the status quo, as in a stock investment paradigm, prevention-focus strength, but not promotion-focus strength, predicts a willingness to take risks that may possibly return participants to the status quo (Scholer et al., in press). In sum, when change allows an individual to avoid losses, prevention-focused individuals should be more motivated than promotion-focused individuals. However, when change allows an individual to attain something more positive, promotion-focused individuals should be more motivated (cf. Tseng & Kang, 2008).

Change That Fits and Using Fit to Change

It is not only the horizontal dynamics between promotion and prevention that determine whether change will occur. Vertical fit and nonfit between the system, strategic, and tactical levels also plays a significant role in the effective regulation of change. Regulatory fit creates a number of conditions that can support change. Because change is often difficult, anything that increases the likelihood that people *like* what they are doing may help in the maintenance of change. Freitas and Higgins (2002) found that when people used strategies that fit their motivational orientation (e.g., vigilant strategies in prevention), they not only experienced greater enjoyment in goal action but were also more willing to continue with that action. Furthermore, regulatory fit can both increase perceived success in goal pursuit (Freitas & Higgins, 2002) and actual success, such as soccer players performing better on a penalty shooting task when they are in a state of fit versus nonfit (Plessner, Unkelbach, Memmert, Baltes, & Kolb, 2009).

Regulatory fit also yields greater cognitive flexibility and exploration of alternative strategies in goal pursuit (Maddox, Baldwin, & Markman, 2006; Markman, Baldwin, & Maddox, 2005; Markman, Maddox, Worthy, & Baldwin, 2007; Worthy, Maddox, & Markman, 2007). Individuals in a state of fit exhibited more cognitive flexibility in both classification learning tasks and an adaptation of the Iowa Gambling Task (Bechara, Damasio, Damasio, & Anderson, 1994). This greater flexibility supports the possibility of change (e.g., openness to switching tactics). However, when increased flexibility harms performance, then regulatory fit can lead to worse performance than nonfit (Maddox et al., 2006).

The feelings of rightness and wrongness created by regulatory fit and nonfit, respectively, also influence the stop rules that individuals employ when deciding whether to continue exerting effort in goal pursuit (Vaughn, Malik, Schwartz, Petkova, & Trudeau, 2006). For an enjoyment stop rule (an intrinsic decision rule such as "Am I enjoying this task?"), regulatory fit generally results in greater effort due to the participant feeling right about his or her evaluation of the task (e.g., "I'm doing this task because I enjoy it and I'm feeling right, so I'll keep on doing it!"). For a sufficiency-based stop rule (a decision rule such as "Have I met my goal?"), however, regulatory *nonfit* generally results in greater effort due to the participant feeling wrong ("I'm doing this task to get it done and I'm feeling wrong, so I haven't done enough yet and need to keep working!"). Thus, regulatory fit can produce more or less effort depending on how the stop rules are construed. Thus, when considering regulatory fit effects on change, the demands of the task must be taken into account.

Regulatory fit can also be used to make messages advocating for change more effective. Individuals are often persuaded by others to make changes in their lives. Consequently, finding ways to make persuasion attempts more effective is critical for those who design and implement interventions. Several studies have demonstrated that when messages or interventions take advantage of regulatory fit principles, individuals are more likely to increase their consumption of fruits and vegetables (Cesario, Grant, & Higgins, 2004; Latimer, Rivers, et al., 2008; Spiegel, Grant-Pillow, & Higgins, 2004), increase physical activity (Latimer, Williams-Piehota, et al., 2008), reduce intentions to smoke (Kim, 2006; Zhao & Pechmann, 2007), floss their teeth (Uskul, Sherman, & Fitzgibbon, 2009), increase motivation to engage in healthy behaviors generally (Lockwood, Chasteen, & Wong, 2005), comply with tax laws (Holler, Hoelzl, Kirchler, Leder, & Mannetti, 2008), positively evaluate and purchase target products (Chang & Chou, 2008; Jain, Lindsey, Agrawal, & Maheswaran, 2007; Lee & Aaker, 2004; Yi & Baumgartner, 2008), increase academic motivation (Lockwood et al., 2002), and even evaluate biblical passages as more meaningful (Reber, Lima, & Fosse, 2007).

Messages that "fit"—either because the message fits the receiver's chronic orientation (e.g., Latimer, Williams-Piehota, et al., 2008) or because a message primes both a regulatory system (e.g., promotion) and the related strategy (e.g., eagerness) (Spiegel et al., 2004)—appear to increase the effectiveness of self-regulation through several channels. Individuals who receive a message under conditions of regulatory fit have been shown to "feel right" about their experience of the message (Cesario et al., 2004; Cesario & Higgins, 2008), to experience greater processing fluency (Labroo & Lee, 2006; Lee & Aaker, 2004), to have more positive feelings towards the focal activity (Latimer, Rivers, et al., 2008), to show greater accessibility for the message (Lee & Aaker, 2004), and to feel that it is more diagnostic (e.g., useful) for making behavioral choices (Zhao & Pechmann,

2007). Conditions that use regulatory nonfit to make people "feel wrong" while reading a message make the message more effective by causing the recipients to read the message arguments more thoroughly (e.g., Koenig, Cesario, Molden, Kosloff, & Higgins, 2009). Although there is much yet to be understood about how regulatory fit can be applied most effectively in persuasive contexts (see Aaker & Lee, 2006; Cesario, Higgins, & Scholer, 2007; Lee & Higgins, 2009), there is little doubt that vertical dynamics within the self-regulatory hierarchy affect the self-regulation of change.

Choices, Choices: Regulatory Focus and Decision Factors

Historical perspectives on what factors matter for goal commitment have emphasized a value × expectancy framework in which the value of a goal affects commitment more when there is a high, rather than low, expectancy of goal attainment (e.g., Azjen, 1991; Ajzen & Fishbein, 1980; Gollwitzer, Heckhausen, & Ratajczak, 1990; Janis & Mann, 1977; Locke & Latham, 1990). Shah and Higgins (1997), however, demonstrated that the traditional expectancy × value interaction varies as a function of regulatory focus. Because promotion-focused individuals are focused on maximizing outcomes, they are especially motivated by high expectancy of goal attainment when attainment is highly valued, thus demonstrating the classic expectancy × value effect on goal commitment. However, prevention-focused individuals view their goals as necessities when the outcome is highly valued. It does not matter whether the goals are high or low expectancy—duty simply calls. Thus, prevention-focused individuals actually show a negative expectancy × value multiplicative effect on goal commitment, such that the effect of high (vs. low) expectancy on commitment becomes *smaller* as the value of goal attainment increases. For example, when the goal is a child's safety, the parent must take action regardless of the likelihood of success—change needs to be instituted regardless of how difficult it might be.

Promotion- and prevention-focused individuals also vary in the type of information they desire when making decisions or choosing to change. Whereas prevention-focused individuals find substantive information (i.e., reasons) more convincing (e.g., information about core product features), promotion-focused individuals are more likely to be swayed by their affective responses to the target (Pham & Avnet, 2004, 2009). Whereas promotion-focused individuals prefer enriched options that offer the possibility of really strong attributes (even at the expense of some negative ones), prevention-focused individuals prefer impoverished options that are relatively neutral (Zhang & Mittal, 2007). This suggests that whether people are open to change is also a function of how information about change options is presented.

CONFRONTING TEMPTATION

When temptation rears its delightful but dangerous head, promotion- and prevention-focused individuals have different preferred strategies for attempting to exert self-control. For example, when confronted with a classic self-control dilemma (e.g., being tempted by pizza while on a diet), promotion-focused individuals are more likely to endorse tactics that advance the diet goal (eagerly approaching a match to the goal), whereas prevention-focused individuals are more likely to avoid tactics vigilantly that could impede the goal

(Higgins et al., 2001). Whether or not these tactics are effective is partly due to the nature of the temptation.

In some situations, prevention-focused individuals may be better able to resist temptations because avoiding obstacles to goal attainment is a preferred means of prevention-focused self-regulation. For instance, inducing a prevention focus reduces the likelihood that impulsive eaters exposed to chocolate cake will exhibit intentions to indulge (Sengupta & Zhou, 2007). Furthermore, prevention-focused individuals even enjoy a task that requires resisting tempting diversions more than do promotion-focused individuals (Freitas, Liberman, & Higgins, 2002). However, Dholakia, Gopinath, Bagozzi, and Nataraajan (2006) have shown that for some temptations, promotion-focused individuals may be better able to engage in self-control because, while reporting a greater desire for the tempting object, their use of long-term approach strategies were more effective than prevention-related avoidance strategies.

The effectiveness of strategies is determined by not only their fit with the situation but also their vertical fit within the system. When individuals regulate in a state of regulatory fit, they are better able to manage subsequent challenges (Hong & Lee, 2008). Hong and Lee (2008) found that participants in a state of regulatory fit exhibited greater subsequent self-regulatory strength than did participants in a state of nonfit (as assessed by how long they could squeeze a handgrip; see Muraven, Tice, & Baumeister, 1998).

COPING WITH FAILURE

Failures are experienced and represented differently in prevention and promotion (e.g., Higgins, 1997; Strauman & Higgins, 1987). In prevention, it is a failure to attain or maintain a satisfactory "0" state: the presence of a negative. In promotion, it is a failure to make progress in advancing to a better "+1" state: the absence of a positive. Consequently, failure results in distinct emotional and motivational responses for prevention-focused and promotion-focused individuals (Brockner & Higgins, 2001; Higgins, 1987, 1997, 2001; Shah & Higgins, 2001).

Distinct Emotional Effects of Failure

Promotion and prevention failures have distinct emotional signatures. Because failure in a promotion focus reflects the absence of a positive outcome (nongain), it results in dejection-related emotions such as sadness and disappointment. Because failure in a prevention focus reflects the presence of a negative outcome (loss), it results in agitation-related emotions such as anxiety and worry. Several studies have found that priming ideal (promotion) discrepancies leads to increases in dejection, whereas priming ought (prevention) discrepancies leads to increases in agitation (Higgins, Bond, Klein, & Strauman; 1986; Strauman & Higgins, 1987). Being socially rejected (a loss) leads to increased anxiety and withdrawal, but being socially ignored (a nongain) leads to sadness and attempts to reengage (Molden, Lucas, Gardner, Dean, & Knowles, 2009). Simply encountering an individual who resembles a parent can activate self-discrepancies associated with that parent's ideals or oughts for the individual, producing dejected affect for parent-related ideal self-discrepancies and agitated affect for parent-related ought self-discrepancies (see Reznik & Andersen, 2007; Shah, 2003).

Although nongains and losses are both painful, losses are more intense than nongains (Idson, Liberman, & Higgins, 2004). This greater intensity of prevention failure impacts how individuals anticipate and respond to failure. For example, prevention-focused individuals appear to be more susceptible to self-handicapping than are promotion-focused individuals (Hendrix & Hirt, 2009). In addition, after experiencing an unfavorable outcome that is represented as a loss, individuals are more upset if the process yielding that outcome was fair rather than unfair (Cropanzano, Paddock, Rupp, Bagger, & Baldwin, 2008). Cropanzano and colleagues (2008) propose that the fair process does not allow one to attribute failure easily to external causes. Consequently, it is particularly threatening for prevention-focused individuals. Molden and Higgins (2008) have also shown that prevention-focused individuals are more likely to engage in self-serving attributions after failure, not only because failure itself is threatening but also because their vigilance reduces the number of possible causes they consider.

Distinct Effects of Failure at the Strategic Level

For promotion-focused individuals, not only is failure negative affectively but it also reduces the strategic eagerness that sustains or fits the promotion system. This produces attempts to bolster eagerness, such as by being optimistic (Grant & Higgins, 2003). When failures accumulate, the chronic nonfit from reduced eagerness weakens engagement and deintensifies the value of goals and activities, which produces the "the loss of interest" or anhedonia of depression (Higgins, 2006; Strauman, 2002; Strauman et al., 2006). In contrast, prevention failure, although very affectively negative, increases the strategic vigilance that fits prevention (Idson, Liberman, & Higgins, 2000), which, under chronic conditions, strengthens engagement and intensifies negative events, even to the extent of producing generalized anxiety disorder (Higgins, 2006).

These different responses to failure should also affect performance because promotion failure is a nonfit that weakens engagement, and prevention failure is a fit that strengthens engagement. Indeed, Idson and Higgins (2000) found that promotion-focused individuals showed a decline in performance after failure feedback relative to success feedback. In contrast, prevention-focused individuals showed the opposite pattern— better performance after failure feedback than after success feedback (see also Van-Dijk & Kluger, 2004).

Notably, promotion-focused individuals do not simply give up after failure; instead, they use tactics to regain their eagerness. For example, after failure feedback in an ongoing performance situation, promotion-focused individuals use tactics to maintain high self-esteem (Scholer, Ozaki, & Higgins, 2010) and show only slight decreases in performance expectancies (Förster, Grant, Idson, & Higgins, 2001). In contrast, in order to maintain vigilance, prevention-focused individuals respond to failure by lowering expectancies *even more* (Förster et al., 2001) and by maintaining relatively lower self-esteem in ongoing performance situations (after success or failure feedback) (Scholer, Ozaki, et al., 2010).

Regrets and Forgiveness: Moving Past Failure

One of the intriguing differences between promotion and prevention-focused individuals is the kind of failure that haunts them. We can think back to what we did not do (e.g.,

"If only I *had* done X, then Y), or think back to what we wish we had not done (e.g., "If only I *hadn't* done X, then Y) (Roese, 1997). Counterfactuals that reverse a previous inaction that missed an opportunity for a gain, known as *additive counterfactuals*, involve imagining a move from what was a "0" to a "+1" instead. In contrast, counterfactuals that reverse a previous action that produced a loss, known as *subtractive counterfactuals*, involve imagining a move from what was a "–1" to a "0" instead. Roese, Hur, and Pennington (1999) found that participants who considered promotion-related setbacks (their own or fictional examples) generated more additive (eager) counterfactuals, whereas participants who considered prevention-related setbacks generated more subtractive (vigilant) counterfactuals. Similarly, being socially rejected (a loss) leads to subtractive counterfactuals, whereas being socially ignored (a nongain) leads to additive counterfactuals (Molden et al., 2009).

These differential responses to failure also impact the likelihood that individuals will forgive the transgressions of others. When people ask for forgiveness, they can either emphasize the absence of gains (e.g., "I don't feel good about what I did to you") or the presence of losses (e.g., "I feel terrible about what I did to you"). Santelli, Struthers, and Eaton (2009) found that when the nature of the repentance is a fit with an individual's regulatory focus orientation, he or she is more likely to forgive a transgressor. In other words, the vertical fit between an individual's orientation and the apology offered by someone else matters for relational well-being (see also Houston, 1990).

CONCLUDING THOUGHTS

The importance of both horizontal and vertical dynamics within the regulatory focus hierarchy suggests two critical factors to consider when designing interventions that can improve self-regulation. First, interventions can target multiple levels within the hierarchy. In other words, if an individual is struggling to lose weight, the goal, strategies, or tactics could be targeted for change. It might help the individual to think about losing weight as a duty versus an aspiration. It could be that vigilant rather than eager strategies would be more effective in managing the daily donut offerings of the break room. It might be that the particular tactics used in service of that vigilance need to be reconsidered.

While all of these approaches may be effective, it is also likely that change is more easily introduced at some levels than others. This possibility needs to be examined in future research. Another possibility that needs examination is that interventions might be more effective if they target more than one level simultaneously. Indeed, this could be necessary to ensure regulatory fit. For instance, a promotion-focused individual who has trouble meeting the safety standards at work might be aided by the inducement of a prevention focus. However, if that person continued to use eager strategies, there would be vertical nonfit. By inducing both a prevention focus and strategic vigilance, the resulting regulatory fit could optimize effectiveness.

Perhaps the most effective approach would be to take advantage of the hierarchical systems as a whole by "working backwards from what you want" (Higgins, 2009). For example, if one wants individuals to emphasize innovation in their performance, then one wants them, tactically, to be open to new alternatives. Working backwards, an eager strategic inclination would support the tactic of being open to new alternatives. Working backwards again, if the individuals had a promotion orientation, then they would naturally prefer an eager strategy that would fit their promotion focus. Now, if the performance were framed as an accomplishment in which advancements could be made, then the induced promotion orientation would prefer an eager strategy that would support the tactic of being open to new alternatives. All of the different levels would work together as an organization of motives for the desired purpose. This approach might be more effective than the standard approach of using incentives to motivate because the hierarchical system *itself* would provide the motivation. This needs to be tested in future research.

REFERENCES

Aaker, J. L., & Lee, A. Y. (2006). Understanding regulatory fit. *Journal of Marketing Research, 43*, 15–19.

Ajzen, I. (1991). The theory of planned behavior. *Organizational Behavior and Human Decision Processes, 50*, 179–211.

Ajzen, I., & Fishbein, M. (1980). *Understanding attitudes and predicting social behavior.* Englewood Cliffs, NJ: Prentice-Hall.

Bechara, A., Damasio, A. R., Damasio, H., & Anderson, S. W. (1994). Insensitivity to future consequences following damage to human prefrontal cortex. *Cognition, 50*, 7–15.

Bowlby, J. (1969). *Attachment and loss: Vol. 1. Attachment.* New York: Basic Books.

Bowlby, J. (1973). *Attachment and loss: Vol. 2. Separation: Anxiety and anger.* New York: Basic Books.

Brendl, C. M., & Higgins, E. T. (1996). Principles of judging valence: What makes events positive or negative? In M. P. Zanna (Ed.), *Advances in experimental social psychology* (Vol. 28, pp. 95–160). San Diego, CA: Academic Press.

Brockner, J., & Higgins, E. T. (2001). Emotions and management: A regulatory focus perspective. *Organizational Behavior and Human Decision Processes, 86*, 35–66.

Cantor, N., & Kihlstrom, J. F. (1987). *Personality and social intelligence.* Englewood Cliffs, NJ: Prentice-Hall.

Carver, C. S., & Scheier, M. F. (1998). *On the self-regulation of behavior.* Cambridge, UK: Cambridge University Press.

Cesario, J., Grant, H., & Higgins, E. T. (2004). Regulatory fit and persuasion: Transfer from "feeling right." *Journal of Personality and Social Psychology, 86*, 388–404.

Cesario, J., & Higgins, E. T. (2008). Making message recipients feel right: How nonverbal cues can increase persuasion. *Psychological Science, 19*, 415–420.

Cesario, J., Higgins, E. T., & Scholer, A. A. (2007). Regulatory fit and persuasion: Basic principles and remaining questions. *Social and Personality Psychology Compass, 2*, 444–463.

Chang, C.-C., & Chou, Y.-J. (2008). Goal orientation and comparative valence in persuasion. *Journal of Advertising, 37*, 73–87.

Chernev, A. (2004). Goal orientation and consumer preference for the status quo. *Journal of Consumer Research, 31*, 557–565.

Cropanzano, R., Paddock, L., Rupp, D. E., Bagger, J., & Baldwin, A. (2008). How regulatory focus impacts the process-by-outcome interaction for perceived fairness and emotions. *Organizational Behavior and Human Decision Processes, 105*, 36–51.

Crowe, E., & Higgins, E. T. (1997). Regulatory focus and strategic inclinations: Promotion and prevention in decision-making. *Organizational Behavior and Human Decision Processes, 69*, 117–132.

Cunningham, W. A., Raye, C. L., & Johnson, M. K. (2005). Neural correlates of evaluation associated with promotion and prevention regulatory focus. *Cognitive, Affective, and Behavioral Neuroscience, 5*, 202–211.

Dholakia, U. M., Gopinath, M., Bagozzi, R. P., & Nataraajan, R. (2006). The role of regulatory focus in the experience and self-control of desire for temptations. *Journal of Consumer Psychology, 16*, 163–175.

Elliot, A. J. (2006). The hierarchical model of approach-avoidance motivation. *Motivation and Emotion, 30*, 111–116.

Elliot, A. J., & Church, M. A. (1997). A hierarchical model of approach and avoidance achievement motivation. *Journal of Personality and Social Psychology, 72*, 218–232.

Förster, J., Grant, H., Idson, L. C., & Higgins, E. (2001). Success/failure feedback, expectancies, and approach/avoidance motivation: How regulatory focus moderates classic relations. *Journal of Experimental Social Psychology, 37*, 253–260.

Foster, G. D., Wadden, T. A., Vogt, R. A., & Brewer, G. (1997). What is a reasonable weight loss?: Patients expectations and evaluations of obesity treatment outcomes. *Journal of Consulting and Clinical Psychology, 65*, 79–85.

Freitas, A. L., & Higgins, E. T. (2002). Enjoying goal-directed action: The role of regulatory fit. *Psychological Science, 13*, 1–6.

Freitas, A. L., Liberman, N., & Higgins, E. (2002). Regulatory fit and resisting temptation during goal pursuit. *Journal of Experimental Social Psychology, 38*, 291–298.

Freitas, A. L., Liberman, N., Salovey, P., & Higgins, E. (2002). When to begin?: Regulatory focus and initiating goal pursuit. *Personality and Social Psychology Bulletin, 28*, 121–130.

Friedman, R. S., & Förster, J. (2001). The effects of promotion and prevention cues on creativity. *Journal of Personality and Social Psychology, 81*, 1001–1013.

Fuglestad, P. T., Rothman, A. J., & Jeffery, R. W. (2008). Getting there and hanging on: The effect of regulatory focus on performance in smoking and weight loss interventions. *Health Psychology, 27*, S260–S270.

Gollwitzer, P. M., Heckhausen, H., & Ratajczak, H. (1990). From weighing to willing: Approaching a change decision through pre- or postdecisional mentation. *Organizational Behavior and Human Decision Processes, 45*, 41–65.

Hendrix, K. S., & Hirt, E. R. (2009). Stressed out over possible failure: The role of regulatory fit on claimed self-handicapping. *Journal of Experimental Social Psychology, 45*, 51–59.

Herzenstein, M., Posavac, S. S., & Brakus, J. (2007). Adoption of new and really new products: The effects of self-regulation systems and risk salience. *Journal of Marketing Research, 44*, 251–260.

Higgins, E. T. (1987). Self-discrepancy: A theory relating self and affect. *Psychological Review, 94*, 319–340.

Higgins, E. T. (1990). Personality, social psychology, and person–situation relations: Standards and knowledge activation as a common language. In L. A. Pervin (Ed.), *Handbook of personality: Theory and research* (pp. 301–338). New York: Guilford Press.

Higgins, E. T. (1997). Beyond pleasure and pain. *American Psychologist, 52*, 1280–1300.

Higgins, E. T. (1999). Persons or situations: Unique explanatory principles or variability in general principles? In D. Cervone & Y. Shoda (Eds.), *The coherence of personality: Social-cognitive bases of consistency, variability, and organization* (pp. 61–93). New York: Guilford Press.

Higgins, E. T. (2000). Making a good decision: Value from fit. *American Psychologist, 55*, 1217–1230.

Higgins, E. T. (2001). Promotion and prevention experiences: Relating emotions to nonemotional motivational states. In J. P. Forgas (Ed.), *Handbook of affect and social cognition* (pp. 186–211). Mahwah, NJ: Erlbaum.

Higgins, E. T. (2002). How self-regulation creates distinct values: The case of promotion and prevention decision making. *Journal of Consumer Psychology, 12*, 177–191.

Higgins, E. T. (2006). Value from hedonic experience and engagement. *Psychological Review, 113*, 439–460.

Higgins, E. T. (2008). Culture and personality: Variability across universal motives as the missing link. *Social and Personality Psychology Compass, 2*, 608–634.

Higgins, E. T. (2009). *Beyond pleasure and pain: The new science of motivation.* Unpublished manuscript, Columbia University, New York, NY.

Higgins, E. T., Bond, R. N., Klein, R., & Strauman, T. (1986). Self-discrepancies and emotional vulnerability: How magnitude, accessibility, and type of discrepancy influence affect. *Journal of Personality and Social Psychology, 51*, 5–15.

Higgins, E. T., Friedman, R. S., Harlow, R. E., Idson, L. C., Ayduk, O. N., & Taylor, A. (2001). Achievement orientations from subjective histories of success: Promotion pride versus prevention pride. *European Journal of Social Psychology, 31*, 3–23.

Higgins, E. T., Idson, L. C., Freitas, A. L., Spiegel, S., & Molden, D. C. (2003). Transfer of value from fit. *Journal of Personality and Social Psychology, 84*, 1140–1153.

Higgins, E. T., Roney, C. J. R., Crowe, E., & Hymes, C. (1994). Ideal versus ought predilections for approach and avoidance distinct self-regulatory systems. *Journal of Personality and Social Psychology, 66*, 276–286.

Higgins, E. T., Shah, J., & Friedman, R. (1997). Emotional responses to goal attainment: Strength of regulatory focus as moderator. *Journal of Personality and Social Psychology, 72*, 515–525.

Holler, M., Hoelzl, E., Kirchler, E., Leder, S., & Mannetti, L. (2008). Framing of information on the use of public finances, regulatory fit of recipients and tax compliance. *Journal of Economic Psychology, 29*, 597–611.

Hong, J., & Lee, A. Y. (2008). Be fit and be strong: Mastering self-regulation through regulatory fit. *Journal of Consumer Research, 34*, 682–695.

Houston, D. A. (1990). Empathy and the self: Cognitive and emotional influences on the evaluation of negative affect in others. *Journal of Personality and Social Psychology, 59*, 859–868.

Idson, L. C., & Higgins, E. T. (2000). How current feedback and chronic effectiveness influence motivation: Everything to gain versus everything to lose. *European Journal of Social Psychology, 30*, 583–592.

Idson, L. C., Liberman, N., & Higgins, E. T. (2004). Imagining how you'd feel: The role of motivational experiences from regulatory fit. *Personality and Social Psychology Bulletin, 30*, 926–937.

Jain, S. P., Lindsey, C., Agrawal, N., & Maheswaran, D. (2007). For better of for worse?: Valenced comparative frames and regulatory focus. *Journal of Consumer Research, 34*, 57–65.

Janis, I. L., & Mann, L. (1977). *Decision making: A psychological analysis of conflict, choice, and commitment.* New York: Free Press.

John, O. P., & Srivastava, S. (1999). The Big Five trait taxonomy: History, measurement, and historical perspectives. In L. A. Pervin & O. P. John (Eds.), *Handbook of personality psychology: Theory and research* (2nd ed., pp. 102–138). New York: Guilford Press.

Kahneman, D., & Tversky, A. (1979). Prospect theory: An analysis of decision under risk. *Econometrica, 47*, 263–292.

Keller, J. (2008). On the development of regulatory focus: The role of parenting styles. *European Journal of Social Psychology, 38*, 354–364.

Kim, Y.-J. (2006). The role of regulatory focus in message framing in antismoking advertisements for adolescents. *Journal of Advertising, 35*, 143–151.

Koenig, A. M., Cesario, J., Molden, D. C., Kosloff, S., & Higgins, E. T. (2009). Incidental experiences of regulatory fit and the processing of persuasive appeals. *Personality and Social Psychology Bulletin, 35*, 1342–1355.

Kruglanski, A. W. (1996). Goals as knowledge structures. In P. M. Gollwitzer & J. A. Bargh (Eds.), *The psychology of action: Linking cognition and motivation to behavior* (pp. 599–619). New York: Guilford Press.

Kruglanski, A. W., Shah, J. Y., Fishbach, A., Friedman, R., Chun, W. Y., & Sleeth-Keppler, D.

(2002). A theory of goal systems. In M. P. Zanna (Ed.), *Advances in experimental social psychology* (Vol. 34, pp. 331–378). San Diego, CA: Academic Press.

Labroo, A., & Lee, A. (2006). Between two brands: A goal fluency account of brand evaluation. *Journal of Marketing Research, 43*, 374–385.

Latimer, A. E., Rivers, S. E., Rench, T. A., Katulak, N. A., Hicks, A., Hodorowski, J. K., et al. (2008). A field experiment testing the utility of regulatory fit messages for promoting physical activity. *Journal of Experimental Social Psychology, 44*, 826–832.

Latimer, A. E., Williams-Piehota, P., Katulak, N. A., Cox, A., Mowad, L. Z., Higgins, E. T., et al. (2008). Promoting fruit and vegetable intake through messages tailored to individual differences in regulatory focus. *Annals of Behavioral Medicine, 35*, 363–369.

Lee, A. Y., & Aaker, J. L. (2004). Bringing the frame into focus: The influence of regulatory fit on processing fluency and persuasion. *Journal of Personality and Social Psychology, 86*, 205–218.

Lee, A. Y., & Higgins, E. T. (2009). The persuasive power of regulatory fit. In M. Wänke (Ed.), *Social psychology of consumer behavior* (pp. 319–333). New York: Psychology Press.

Liberman, N., Idson, L. C., Camacho, C. J., & Higgins, E. T. (1999). Promotion and prevention choices between stability and change. *Journal of Personality and Social Psychology, 77*, 1135–1145.

Liberman, N., Molden, D. C., Idson, L. C., & Higgins, E. (2001). Promotion and prevention focus on alternative hypotheses: Implications for attributional functions. *Journal of Personality and Social Psychology, 80*, 5–18.

Locke, E. A., & Latham, G. P. (1990). *A theory of goal setting and task performance.* Englewood Cliffs, NJ: Prentice-Hall.

Lockwood, P., Chasteen, A. L., & Wong, C. (2005). Age and regulatory focus determine preferences for health-related role models. *Psychology and Aging, 20*, 376–389.

Lockwood, P., Jordan, C. H., & Kunda, Z. (2002). Motivation by positive or negative role models: Regulatory focus determines who will best inspire us. *Journal of Personality and Social Psychology, 83*, 854–864.

Maddox, W., Baldwin, G. C., & Markman, A. B. (2006). A test of the regulatory fit hypothesis in perceptual classification learning. *Memory and Cognition, 34*, 1377–1397.

Manian, N., Papadakis, A. A., Strauman, T. J., & Essex, M. J. (2006). The development of children's ideal and ought self-guides: Parenting, temperament, and individual differences in guide strength. *Journal of Personality, 74*, 1619–1645.

Manian, N., Strauman, T. J., & Denney, N. (1998). Temperament, recalled parenting styles and self-regulation: Testing the developmental postulates of self-discrepancy theory. *Journal of Personality and Social Psychology, 75*, 1321–1332.

Markman, A. B., Baldwin, G. C., & Maddox, W. (2005). The interaction of payoff structure and regulatory focus in classification. *Psychological Science, 16*, 852–855.

Markman, A. B., Maddox, W., Worthy, D. A., & Baldwin, G. C. (2007). Using regulatory focus to explore implicit and explicit processing in concept learning. *Journal of Consciousness Studies, 14*, 132–155.

Miller, G. A., Galanter, E., & Pribram, K. H. (1960). *Plans and the structure of behavior.* New York: Holt.

Molden, D. C., & Higgins, E. T. (2005). Motivated thinking. In K. Holyoak & Morrison (Eds.), *Handbook of thinking and reasoning* (pp. 295–326). New York: Cambridge University Press.

Molden, D. C., & Higgins, E. T. (2008). How preferences for eager versus vigilant judgment strategies affect self-serving conclusions. *Journal of Experimental Social Psychology, 44*, 1219–1228.

Molden, D. C., Lucas, G. M., Gardner, W. L., Dean, K., & Knowles, M. L. (2009). Motivations for prevention or promotion following social exclusion: Being rejected versus being ignored. *Journal of Personality and Social Psychology, 96*, 415–431.

Mowrer, O. H. (1960). *Learning theory and behavior.* New York: Wiley.

Muraven, M., Tice, D. M., & Baumeister, R. F. (1998). Self-control as limited resource: Regulatory depletion patterns. *Journal of Personality and Social Psychology, 74,* 774–789.

Ouschan, L., Boldero, J. M., Kashima, Y., Wakimoto, R., & Kashima, E. S. (2007). Regulatory Focus Strategies Scale: A measure of individual differences in the endorsement of regulatory strategies. *Asian Journal of Social Psychology, 10,* 243–257.

Pervin, L. A. (1989). Goal concepts in personality and social psychology: A historical introduction: In L. A. Pervin (Ed.), *Goal concepts in personality and social psychology* (pp. 1–17). Hillsdale, NJ: Erlbaum.

Pham, M. T., & Avnet, T. (2004). Ideals and oughts and the weighting of affect versus substance in persuasion, *Journal of Consumer Research, 30,* 503–518.

Pham, M. T., & Avnet, T. (2009). Contingent reliance on the affect heuristic as a function of regulatory focus. *Organizational Behavior and Human Decision Processes, 108,* 267–278.

Plessner, H., Unkelbach, C., Memmert, D., Baltes, A., & Kolb, A. (2009). Regulatory fit as a determinant of sport performance: How to succeed in a soccer penalty-shooting. *Psychology of Sport and Exercise, 10,* 108–115.

Poels, K., & Dewitte, S. (2008). Hope and self-regulatory goals applied to an advertising context: Promoting prevention stimulates goal-directed behavior. *Journal of Business Research, 61,* 1030–1040.

Reber, R., Lima, A., & Fosse, B. H. (2007). Effects of regulatory focus on endorsement of religious beliefs. *Scandinavian Journal of Psychology, 48,* 539–545.

Reznik, I., & Andersen, S. M. (2007). Agitation and despair in relation to parents: Activating emotional suffering in transference. *European Journal of Personality, 21,* 281–301.

Roese, N. J. (1997). Counterfactual thinking. *Psychological Bulletin, 121,* 133–148.

Roese, N. J., Hur, T., & Pennington, G. L. (1999). Counterfactual thinking and regulatory focus: Implications for action versus inaction and sufficiency versus necessity. *Journal of Personality and Social Psychology, 77,* 1109–1120.

Rothman, A. J. (2000). Toward a theory-based analysis of behavioral maintenance. *Health Psychology, 19,* 64–69.

Rothman, A. J., Baldwin, A. S., & Hertel, A. W. (2004). Self-regulation and behavior change: Disentangling behavioral initiation and behavioral maintenance. In R. F. Baumeister & K. D. Vohs (Eds.), *Handbook of self-regulation: Research, theory, and applications* (pp. 130–148). New York: Guilford Press.

Santelli, A. G., Struthers, C., & Eaton, J. (2009). Fit to forgive: Exploring the interaction between regulatory focus, repentance, and forgiveness. *Journal of Personality and Social Psychology, 96,* 381–394.

Scholer, A. A., & Higgins, E. T. (2008). Distinguishing levels of approach and avoidance: An analysis using regulatory focus theory. In A. J. Elliot (Ed.), *Handbook of approach and avoidance motivation* (pp. 489–503). New York: Psychology Press.

Scholer, A. A., Ozaki, Y., & Higgins, E. T. (2010). *Inflating and deflating the self: Strategic expression and defense of self-esteem.* Manuscript submitted for publication.

Scholer, A. A., Stroessner, S. J., & Higgins, E. (2008). Responding to negativity: How a risky tactic can serve a vigilant strategy. *Journal of Experimental Social Psychology, 44,* 767–774.

Scholer, A. A., Zou, X., Fujita, K., Stroessner, S. J., & Higgins, E. T. (in press). When risk-seeking becomes a motivational necessity. *Journal of Personality and Social Psychology.*

Sengupta, J., & Zhou, R. (2007). Understanding impulsive eaters' choice behaviors: The motivational influences of regulatory focus. *Journal of Marketing Research, 44,* 297–308.

Shah, J. (2003). The motivational looking glass: How significant others implicitly affect goal appraisals. *Journal of Personality and Social Psychology, 85,* 424–439.

Shah, J., & Higgins, E. (1997). Expectancy × value effects: Regulatory focus as determinant of magnitude and direction. *Journal of Personality and Social Psychology, 73,* 447–458.

Shah, J., & Higgins, E. T. (2001). Regulatory concerns and appraisal efficiency: The general impact of promotion and prevention. *Journal of Personality and Social Psychology, 80*, 693–705.

Shah, J., Higgins, T., & Friedman, R. S. (1998). Performance incentives and means: How regulatory focus influences goal attainment. *Journal of Personality and Social Psychology, 74*, 285–293.

Spiegel, S., Grant-Pillow, H., & Higgins, E. (2004). How regulatory fit enhances motivational strength during goal pursuit. *European Journal of Social Psychology, 34*, 39–54.

Strauman, T. J. (2002). Self-regulation and depression. *Self and Identity, 1*, 151–157.

Strauman, T. J., & Higgins, E. (1987). Automatic activation of self-discrepancies and emotional syndromes: When cognitive structures influence affect. *Journal of Personality and Social Psychology, 53*, 1004–1014.

Strauman, T. J., Vieth, A. Z., Merrill, K. A., Kolden, G. G., Woods, T. E., Klein, M. H., et al. (2006). Self-system therapy as an intervention for self-regulatory dysfunction in depression: A randomized comparison with cognitive therapy. *Journal of Consulting and Clinical Psychology, 74*, 367–376.

Summerville, A., & Roese, N. J. (2008). Self-report measures of individual differences in regulatory focus: A cautionary note. *Journal of Research in Personality, 42*, 247–254.

Tseng, H.-C., & Kang, L.-M. (2008). How does regulatory focus affect uncertainty towards organizational change? *Leadership and Organization Development Journal, 29*, 714–738.

Uskul, A. K., Sherman, D., & Fitzgibbon, J. (2009). The cultural congruency effect: Culture, regulatory focus, and the effectiveness of gain- vs. loss-framed health messages. *Journal of Experimental Social Psychology, 45*, 535–541.

Vallacher, R. R., & Wegner, D. M. (1985). *A theory of action identification*. Hillsdale, NJ: Erlbaum.

Van-Dijk, D., & Kluger, A. N. (2004). Feedback sign effect on motivation: Is it moderated by regulatory focus? *Applied Psychology: An International Review, 53*, 113–135.

Vaughn, L. A., Baumann, J., & Klemann, C. (2008). Openness to experience and regulatory focus: Evidence of motivation from fit. *Journal of Research in Personality, 42*, 886–894.

Vaughn, L. A., Malik, J., Schwartz, S., Petkova, Z., & Trudeau, L. (2006). Regulatory fit as input for stop rules. *Journal of Personality and Social Psychology, 91*, 601–611.

Wallace, J., Little, L. M., & Shull, A. (2008). The moderating effects of task complexity on the relationship between regulatory foci and safety and production performance. *Journal of Occupational Health Psychology, 13*, 95–104.

Worthy, D. A., Maddox, W., & Markman, A. B. (2007). Regulatory fit effects in a choice task. *Psychonomic Bulletin and Review, 14*, 1125–1132.

Yi, S., & Baumgartner, H. (2008). Motivational compatibility and the role of anticipated feelings in positively valenced persuasive message framing. *Psychology and Marketing, 25*, 1007–1026.

Zhang, Y., & Mittal, V. (2007). The attractiveness of enriched and impoverished options: Culture, self-construal, and regulatory focus. *Personality and Social Psychology Bulletin, 33*, 588–598.

Zhao, G., & Pechmann, C. (2007). The impact of regulatory focus on adolescents' response to antismoking advertising campaigns. *Journal of Marketing Research, 44*, 671–687.

CHAPTER 9

Planning Promotes Goal Striving

PETER M. GOLLWITZER
GABRIELE OETTINGEN

Determining the factors that promote successful goal striving is one of the fundamental questions studied by self-regulation and motivation researchers (Bargh, Gollwitzer, & Oettingen, 2010; Gollwitzer & Moskowitz, 1996; Oettingen & Gollwitzer, 2001). A number of theories, and supporting empirical data, suggest that the type of goal chosen and the commitment to that goal are important determinants in whether an individual carries out the behaviors necessary for goal attainment (e.g., Ajzen, 1985; Bandura, 1997; Carver & Scheier, 1998; Elliot, 2008; Locke & Latham, 2006; Molden & Dweck, 2006; Oettingen, Pak, & Schnetter, 2001). Within these models, choosing or accepting a goal or standard is the central act of will in the pursuit of goals. We agree with this contention but argue in this chapter that further acts of will should facilitate goal attainment, in particular, when goal striving is confronted with implemental problems (e.g., difficulties getting started because of failure to use opportunities to do so; sticking to ongoing goal striving in the face of distractions, temptations, and competing goals). Such acts of will can take the form of making plans that specify when, where, and how an instrumental goal-directed response is to be enacted. More specifically, the person may take control over (i.e., self-regulate) goal striving by making if–then plans (i.e., form implementation intentions) that specify an anticipated critical situation and link it to an instrumental goal-directed response.

IMPLEMENTATION INTENTIONS: STRATEGIC AUTOMATICITY IN GOAL STRIVING

Gollwitzer (1993, 1999) has proposed a distinction between goal intentions and implementation intentions. *Goal intentions* (goals) have the structure of "I intend to reach Z!" whereby Z may relate to a certain outcome or behavior to which the individual feels committed. *Implementation intentions* (plans) have the structure of "If situation X is encountered, then I will perform the goal-directed response Y!" Both goal and implementation intentions are set in an act of will: The former specifies the intention to meet a goal or standard; the latter refers to the intention to perform a plan. Commonly, implementation intentions are formed in the service of goal intentions because they specify the where, when, and how of a respective goal-directed response. For instance, a possible implementation intention in the service of the goal intention to eat healthy food could link a suitable situational context (e.g., one's order is taken at a restaurant) to an appropriate behavior (e.g., asking for a low-fat meal). As a consequence, a strong mental link is established between the critical cue of the waiter taking the order and the goal-directed response of asking for a low-fat meal.

Accordingly, to form an implementation intention, one needs to identify a future goal-relevant situational cue (e.g., a good opportunity to act, an obstacle to goal pursuit) and link a related goal-directed response to that cue (e.g., how to respond to the opportunity, how to overcome the obstacle). Whereas goal intentions merely specify desired end states ("I want to achieve goal X!"), the if-component of an implementation intention specifies when and where one wants to act on this goal, and the then-component of the plan specifies how this will be done. Implementation intentions thus delegate control over the initiation of the intended goal-directed behavior to a specified opportunity by creating a strong link between a situational cue and a goal-directed response.

Implementation intentions have been found to help people close the gap between setting goals and actually realizing these goals. Evidence that forming if–then plans enhances rates of goal attainment and behavioral performance has now been obtained in several studies. A recent meta-analysis (Gollwitzer & Sheeran, 2006) involving over 8,000 participants in 94 independent studies revealed a medium-to-large effect size ($d = 0.65$) of implementation intentions on goal achievement in a variety of domains (e.g., interpersonal, environmental, health) on top of the effects of mere goal intentions. The size of the implementation intention effect is noteworthy given that goal intentions by themselves already have a facilitating effect on behavior enactment (Webb & Sheeran, 2006).

Mechanisms of Implementation Intention Effects

Research on the underlying mechanisms of implementation intention effects has discovered that implementation intentions facilitate goal attainment on the basis of psychological mechanisms that relate to the anticipated situation (specified in the if-part of the plan), the intended behavior (specified in the then-part of the plan), and the mental link forged between the if-part and the then-part of the plan. Because forming an implementation intention implies the selection of a critical future situation, the mental representation of this situation becomes highly activated and hence more accessible (Gollwitzer, 1999). This heightened accessibility of the if-part of the plan has been observed in several studies testing this hypothesis by using different experimental paradigms. For instance, Webb and Sheeran (2004, Studies 2 and 3) observed that implementation intentions improve cue detection (fewer misses and more hits), without stimulating erroneous responses to similar cues (false alarms and correct rejections). Using a dichotic listening paradigm, Achtziger, Bayer, and Gollwitzer (2010) found that words describing the anticipated critical situation were highly disruptive to focused attention in implementation-intention participants compared to mere goal-intention participants (i.e., the shadowing performance of the attended materials decreased in implementation-intention participants). Moreover, in a cued recall experiment they observed that participants more effectively recalled the available situational opportunities to attain a set goal given that these opportunities had been specified in if–then links (i.e., in implementation intentions).

In a study by Parks-Stamm, Gollwitzer, and Oettingen (2007), participants had to identify five-letter words in a recorded story that was quickly read aloud. Before listening to the story, all participants familiarized themselves with the two most common five-letter words *Laura* and *mouse*. In the implementation-intention condition, they additionally included these words in if–then plans ("If I hear the word *Laura*, then I will immediately press the *L*; if I hear the word *mouse*, then I will immediately press the *M*"). It was predicted and found that implementation intentions would not only increase performance in response to the two critical five-letter words but also inhibit responses to the remaining five-letter words. Finally, Wieber and Sassenberg (2006) wondered whether critical cues would attract attention when they occurred during the pursuit of an unrelated goal (similar to the dichotic listening study by Achtziger et al. [2010] reported earlier). In two studies, the disruption of attention through implementation intentions was investigated by presenting critical situations (stimuli that were part of an implementation intention for an unrelated task) as task-irrelevant distractors along with task-relevant stimuli in a so-called flanker paradigm (Eriksen & Eriksen, 1974). In the first study, participants had to perform a categorization task (flowers vs. insects). Half of the participants formed implementation intentions ("If I see the word *flower*, then I will press the left control key!" and "If I see *insect*, then I will press the right control key!"). The other half of the participants formed control intentions (mere goal intentions; e.g., "I will respond to *flower* as quickly and accurately as possible!" and "I will respond to *insect* as quickly and accurately as possible!" and "I will press the left control key as quickly and accurately as possible!" and "I will press the right control key as quickly and accurately as possible!"). Next, participants worked on the ostensibly unrelated flanker task, in which they had to make word versus nonword decisions while both neutral and critical stimuli were presented as task-irrelevant distractors. The results indicated that the presence of a critical stimulus slowed down participants' responses; however, this effect only occurred when they had formed implementation intentions, not when they had formed mere goal intentions. In the second study, these findings were replicated using a flanker task with vowel versus consonant classifications.

There are even some studies testing whether the heightened accessibility of the mental representation of critical cues as specified in an implementation intention mediates the attainment of the respective goal intention. For instance, Aarts, Dijksterhuis, and Midden (1999), using a lexical decision task, found that the formation of implementation intentions led to faster lexical decision times for those words that described the specified critical situation. Furthermore, the heightened accessibility of the critical situation (as measured by faster lexical decision responses) mediated the beneficial effects of implementation intentions on goal attainment. More recent studies indicate that forming implementation intentions not only heightens the activation (and thus the accessibility) of the mental presentation of the situational cues specified in the if-component but it also forges a strong associative link between the mental representation of the specified opportunity and the mental representation of the specified response (Webb & Sheeran, 2007, 2008). These associative links seem to be quite stable over time (Papies, Aarts, & de Vries, 2009), and they allow for priming the mental representation of the specified response (the plan's then-component) by subliminal presentation of the specified critical situational cue (if-component) (Webb & Sheeran, 2007). Moreover, mediation analyses suggest that cue accessibility and the strength of the cue–response link together mediate the impact of implementation intention formation on goal attainment (Webb & Sheeran, 2007, 2008).

Gollwitzer (1999) suggested that the upshot of the strong associative (critical situation goal-directed response) links created by forming implementation intentions is that—once the critical cue is encountered—the initiation of the goal-directed response specified in then-component of the implementation intention exhibits features of automaticity, including immediacy, efficiency, and redundancy of conscious intent. When people have formed an implementation intention, they can act *in situ*, without having to deliberate on when and how they should act. Evidence that if–then planners act quickly (Gollwitzer & Brandstätter, 1997, Experiment 3), deal effectively with cognitive demands (i.e., speed-up effects are still evidenced under high cognitive load; Brandstätter, Lengfelder, & Gollwitzer, 2001), and do not need consciously to intend to act in the critical moment is consistent with this idea (i.e., implementation intention effects are observed even when the critical cue is presented subliminally [Bayer, Achtziger, Gollwitzer, & Moskowitz, 2009] or when the respective goal is activated outside of awareness [Sheeran, Webb, & Gollwitzer, 2005, Study 2]).

With respect to *immediacy* of action initiation, for instance, Gollwitzer and Brandstätter (1997, Study 3) observed that participants who had been induced to form implementation intentions that specified viable opportunities for presenting counterarguments to a series of racist remarks made by a confederate did initiate counterarguments sooner than participants who had formed the mere goal intention to counterargue. To test the postulated *efficiency* of action initiation, Brandtstätter and colleagues (2001, Studies 3 and 4) used a go/no-go task embedded as a secondary task in a dual-task paradigm. Participants formed the goal intention to press a button as fast as possible if numbers appeared on the computer screen, but not if letters were presented. Participants in the implementation-intention condition additionally made the plan to press the response button particularly fast if the number 3 was presented. Implementation-intention participants showed a substantial increase in speed of responding to the number 3 compared to the control group, regardless of whether the simultaneously demanded primary task (a memorization task in Study 3 and a tracking task in Study 4) was either easy or difficult to perform. Apparently, the immediacy of responding induced by implementation intentions is also efficient in the sense that it does not require much in the way of cognitive resources (i.e., can be performed even when demanding dual tasks have to be performed at the same time). Finally, with respect to the postulated *redundancy of conscious intent*, Bayer and colleagues (2009) conducted experiments in which the critical situation specified in the if-component was presented subliminally. Results indicated that subliminal presentation of the critical situation led to a speed-up in responding in implementation-intention but not in mere goal-intention participants. These effects suggest that when planned via implementation intentions, the initiation of goal-directed responses becomes triggered by the presence of the critical situational cue, without the need for further conscious intent.

The postulated and observed component processes underlying implementation intention effects (enhanced cue accessibility, strong cue–response links, automation of responding) mean that if–then planning allows people to see and to seize good opportunities to move toward their goals. Fashioning an if–then plan thus *strategically automates* goal striving; people intentionally make if–then plans that delegate control of goal-directed behavior to preselected situational cues, with the explicit purpose of reaching their goals. This delegation hypothesis has recently been tested by studies that collected brain data (electroencephalography [EEG], functional magnetic resonance imaging [fMRI]).

Schweiger Gallo, Keil, McCulloch, Rockstroh, and Gollwitzer (2009, Study 3) used dense-array EEG. Behavioral data indicated that implementation intentions specifying an ignore response in the then-component helped control fear in response to pictures of spiders in participants with spider phobia; importantly, the obtained electrocortical correlates revealed that those participants who bolstered their goal intention to stay calm with an ignore-implementation intention showed significantly reduced early activity in the visual cortex in response to spider pictures, as reflected in a smaller P1 (assessed at 120 milliseconds [msec] after a spider picture was presented). This suggests that implementation intentions indeed lead to strategic automation of the specified goal-directed response (in the present case, an ignore response) when the critical cue (in the present case, a spider picture) is encountered, as conscious effortful action initiation is known to take longer than 120 msec (i.e., at least 300 msec; see Bargh & Chartrand, 2000).

Further support for the delegation hypothesis was obtained in an fMRI study reported by Gilbert, Gollwitzer, Cohen, Oettingen, and Burgess (2009), in which participants had to perform a prospective memory task on the basis of either goal or implementation intention instructions. Acting on the basis of goal intentions was associated with brain activity in the lateral rostral prefrontal cortex, whereas acting on the basis of implementation intentions was associated with brain activity in the medial rostral prefrontal cortex. Brain activity in the latter area is known to be associated with bottom-up (stimulus) control of action, whereas brain activity in the former area is known to be related to top-down (goal) control of action (Burgess, Dumontheil, & Gilbert, 2007).

Finally, the delegation hypothesis concerning the operation of implementation intentions has also been supported by studies using critical samples—that is, individuals with poor self-regulatory abilities, such as people with schizophrenia or substance abuse disorders (Brandstätter et al., 2001, Studies 1 and 2), people with frontal lobe damage (Lengfelder & Gollwitzer, 2001), and children with attention-deficit/hyperactivity disorder (ADHD) (Gawrilow & Gollwitzer, 2008; Paul et al., 2007). For instance, Brandstätter and colleagues (2001, Study 1) asked hospitalized opiate addicts under withdrawal to write a short curriculum vitae (CV) before the end of the day; whereas half of the participants formed relevant implementation intentions (they specified when and where they would start to write what), the other half (control group) formed irrelevant implementation intentions (when and where they would eat what for lunch). Eighty percent of the relevant implementation-intention participants had written a short CV at the end of the day, whereas none of the participants with the irrelevant implementation intention succeeded in doing so.

Implementation intentions have also been found to benefit children with ADHD, who are known to have difficulties with tasks that require response inhibition (e.g., go/no-go tasks). For example, it was observed that the response inhibition performance in the presence of stop signals can be improved in children with ADHD by forming implementation intentions (Gawrilow & Gollwitzer, 2008, Studies 1 and 2). This improved response inhibition is reflected in electrocortical data as well (Paul et al., 2007). Typically, the P300 component evoked by no-go stimuli has greater amplitude than the P300 evoked by go stimuli. This difference is less pronounced in children with ADHD. Paul and colleagues

(2007) found that if–then plans improved response inhibition and increased the P300 difference (no-go/go) in children with ADHD.

Potential Alternative Mechanisms

Additional process mechanisms to the stimulus perception and response initiation processes documented in the findings described earlier have been explored. For instance, furnishing goals with implementation intentions might produce an increase in goal commitment or self-efficacy, which in turn causes heightened goal attainment. However, this hypothesis has not received any empirical support. For instance, when Brandstätter and colleagues (2001, Study 1) analyzed whether heroin addicts suffering from withdrawal benefit from forming implementation intentions to submit a newly composed CV before the end of the day, they also measured participants' commitment to do so. Whereas the majority of the implementation-intention participants succeeded in handing in the CV in time, none of the goal-intention participants succeeded in this task. These two groups, however, did not differ in terms of their goal commitment ("I feel committed to compose a CV" and "I have to complete this task"), measured after the goal- and implementation-intention instructions had been administered. This finding was replicated with young adults who participated in a professional development workshop (Oettingen, Hönig, & Gollwitzer, 2000, Study 2), and analogous results were reported in research on the effects of implementation intentions on meeting health promotion and disease prevention goals (e.g., Orbell, Hodgkins, & Sheeran, 1997). Indeed, a recent meta-analysis of 66 implementation intention studies that assessed goal commitment or self-efficacy after the formation of if–then plans revealed negligible effects on both of these variables (Webb & Sheeran, 2008); accordingly, neither an increase in goal commitment nor self-efficacy qualify as potential mediators of implementation intention effects.

IMPLEMENTATION INTENTIONS AND OVERCOMING THE TYPICAL PROBLEMS OF GOAL STRIVING

Successful goal striving is not secured solely by strongly committing oneself to appropriate goals (i.e., goals that are desirable and also feasible). There is always the second issue of implementing a chosen goal (i.e., goal striving), and one wonders what people can do to enhance their chances of being successful at this phase of goal pursuit. The answer we suggest in this chapter is the following: People need to prepare themselves in advance, so that their chances to overcome arising difficulties of goal implementation are kept high. But what are these difficulties or problems? At least four problems stand out. These problems include getting started with goal striving, staying on track, calling a halt, and not overextending oneself. For all of these problems, the self-regulation strategy of forming implementation intentions has been shown to be beneficial (see meta-analysis by Gollwitzer & Sheeran, 2006).

Given that forming implementation intentions automates goal striving, people who form implementation intentions should actually have it easier when they are confronted with these four central problems of goal implementation. Indeed, numerous studies suggest that problems of *getting started* on one's goals can be solved effectively by forming implementation intentions. For instance, Gollwitzer and Brandstätter (1997, Study 2) analyzed a goal intention (i.e., writing a report about how the participants spent Christmas Eve) that had to be performed at a time when people are commonly busy with other things (i.e., during the subsequent 2 days, which are family holidays in Europe). Still, research participants who had furnished their goal intention with an implementation intention that specified when, where, and how they wanted to get started on this project were about three times as likely actually to write the report as mere goal-intention participants. Similarly, Oettingen and colleagues (2000, Study 3) observed that implementation intentions helped students to act on their task goals (i.e., performing math homework) on time (e.g., at 10:00 A.M. every Wednesday over the next 4 weeks).

Other studies have examined the ability of implementation intentions to foster striving toward goals involving behaviors that are somewhat unpleasant to perform. For instance, goals to perform regular breast examinations (Orbell et al., 1997) or cervical cancer screenings (Sheeran & Orbell, 2000), to resume functional activity after joint replacement surgery (Orbell & Sheeran, 2000), to eat a low-fat diet (Armitage, 2004), to recycle (Holland, Aarts, & Langendam, 2006), and to engage in physical exercise (Milne, Orbell, & Sheeran, 2002) were all more readily acted upon when people had developed implementation intentions—even though there is an initial reluctance to execute these behaviors. Moreover, implementation intentions were associated with goal attainment in domains where it is easy to forget to act (e.g., regular intake of vitamin pills: Sheeran & Orbell, 1999; the signing of worksheets by older adults: Chasteen, Park, & Schwarz, 2001).

But many goals cannot be accomplished by a simple, discrete, one-shot action because they require that people keep striving over an extended period of time. Such *staying on track* may become very difficult when certain internal stimuli (e.g., being anxious, tired, overburdened) or external stimuli (e.g., temptations, distractions) interfere with and potentially derail ongoing goal pursuit. Implementation intentions can suppress the negative influence of interferences from outside the person (e.g., disruptions by attractive video shows; Gollwitzer & Schaal, 1998). These suppression-oriented implementation intentions may take very different forms. For instance, if a person wants to avoid being unfriendly to a friend who is known to make outrageous requests, she can form suppression-oriented implementation intentions, such as "And if my friend approaches me with an outrageous request, then I will not respond accordingly!" The then-component of suppression-oriented implementation intentions does not have to be worded in terms of not showing the critical behavior; it may alternatively specify an antagonistic behavior (" . . . , then I will respond in a friendly manner!") or focus on ignoring the critical cue (" . . . , then I'll ignore her request!").

Interestingly, suppression-oriented implementation intentions can be used not only to shield ongoing goal pursuits from disruptive external stimuli but also to curb the negative effects of interfering inner states. Achtziger, Gollwitzer, and Sheeran (2008) report two field experiments concerned with dieting (i.e., reduce snacking; Study 1) and athletic goals (i.e., win a competitive tennis match; Study 2), in which goals were shielded by suppression-oriented implementation intentions geared toward controlling potentially interfering inner states (i.e., cravings for junk food in Study 1, and disruptive thoughts, feelings, and physiological states in Study 2). An alternative way of using implementation intentions to protect ongoing goal striving from derailment is to form implementation intentions geared toward stabilizing the ongoing goal pursuit at hand (Bayer, Gollwitzer, & Achtziger, 2010). Using, again, the example of a person approached by her friend with an outrageous request, let us assume that the recipient of the request is tired or irritated, and thus particularly likely to respond in an unfriendly manner. If this person has stipulated in advance in an implementation intention what she will converse about with her friend, the interaction may come off as planned, and being tired or irritated should fail to affect the person's behavior toward her friend.

Bayer and colleagues (2010) tested this hypothesis in a series of experiments in which participants were asked to make plans (i.e., form implementation intentions) or not regarding their performance on an assigned task. Prior to beginning the task, participants' self-states were manipulated, so that the task at hand became more difficult (e.g., a state of self-definitional incompleteness prior to a task that required perspective taking: Gollwitzer & Wicklund, 1985; a good mood prior to a task that required evaluation of others nonstereotypically: Bless & Fiedler, 1995; and a state of ego depletion prior to solving difficult anagrams: Baumeister, 2000; Muraven, Tice, & Baumeister, 1998). The results suggested that the induced critical self-states negatively affected task performance only for those participants who had not planned out work on the task at hand via implementation intentions (i.e., had only set themselves the goal to come up with a great performance). In other words, implementation intentions that spelled out how to perform the task at hand were effective in protecting the individual from the negative effects associated with the induced detrimental self-states.

These findings provide a new perspective on the psychology of self-regulation. Commonly, effective self-regulation is understood in terms of strengthening the self, so that the self can meet the challenge of being a powerful executive agent (Baumeister, Heatherton, & Tice, 1994). Therefore, most research on goal-directed self-regulation focuses on strengthening the self in such a way that threats and irritations become less likely, or on restoring an already threatened or irritated self. It is important to recognize that all of these maneuvers focus on changing the self, so that it becomes a better executive. The findings of Bayer and colleagues (2010) suggest a perspective on goal-directed self-regulation that focuses on facilitating action control without changing the self. It assumes that action control becomes easier if a person's behavior is directly controlled by situational cues, and that forming implementation intentions achieves such direct action control. As this mode of action control circumvents the self, it no longer matters whether the self is threatened or secure, agitated or calm because the self is effectively disconnected from its influence on behavior. The research by Bayer and colleagues supports this line of reasoning by demonstrating that task performance (i.e., taking the perspective of another person, judging people in a nonstereotypical manner, solving difficult anagrams) does not suffer any impairment because of the respective detrimental self-states (i.e., self-definitional incompleteness, mood, and ego depletion, respectively) if performing these tasks has been planned out in advance via implementation intentions.

The self-regulatory problem of *calling a halt* to a futile goal striving (i.e., disengaging from a chosen but noninstrumental means or from a chosen goal that has become unfeasible or undesirable) can also be ameliorated by forming implementation intentions. People often fail to disengage readily from chosen means and goals that turn out to be faulty because of a strong self-justification motive (i.e., we tend to adhere to the irrational belief that decisions we have made deliberately must be good; Brockner, 1992). Such escalation effects of sticking with a chosen means or goal, even if negative feedback on goal progress mounts, are reduced effectively, however, by the use of implementation intentions. These implementation intentions only have to specify receiving negative feedback as the critical cue in the if-component and switching to available alternative means or goals as the appropriate response in the then-component (Henderson, Gollwitzer, & Oettingen, 2007).

Finally, the assumption that implementation intentions subject behavior to the direct control of situational cues (i.e., strategic automation of goal striving; Gollwitzer, 1999) implies that the person does not have to exert deliberate effort when behavior is controlled via implementation intentions. As a consequence, the self should not become depleted (Muraven & Baumeister, 2000) when task performance is regulated by implementation intentions; thus, for individuals using implementation intentions, *not overextending* themselves should become easier. Indeed, using different ego-depletion paradigms, research participants who used implementation intentions to self-regulate in one task did not show reduced self-regulatory capacity in a subsequent task (e.g., Webb & Sheeran, 2003).

WHEN THE GOING GETS TOUGH:
LIMITS OF ACTION CONTROL BY IMPLEMENTATION INTENTIONS?

As we pointed out earlier in the section on what implementation intentions are and how they work, implementation intentions can help people to overcome the common problems of goal striving (i.e., getting started, staying on track, disengage when things have been loused up, and preventing ego depletion). However, it would speak for the self-regulation strategy of if–then planning if it even fares well under conditions in which action is determined primarily by factors that do not appear to be amenable to self-regulation. This question and a respective recent line of research have been stimulated by Aristotle's concept of *akrasia* (lack of willpower) because any willful strategy of goal striving (e.g., if–then planning) has to prove itself under conditions in which people commonly fail to demonstrate willpower. Such conditions are manifold; thus, this research has focused on the following three situations: (1) situations in which a person's knowledge and skills constrain performance, such as taking academic tests; (2) situations in which an opponent's behavior limits one's performance, such as negotiation settings; and (3) situations in which the wanted behavior (e.g., no littering) runs into conflict with habits favoring an antagonistic response.

Performance on academic tests (math tests, general intelligence tests) is by design determined primarily by a person's knowledge, analytic capability, and cognitive skills. Thus, to increase test scores by willpower, a person may want to focus on motivational issues, such as concentrating on the various test items throughout the test or reducing worry cognitions (e.g., "Did I find the right answer on the last item?") and self-doubts (e.g., "Do I have the skills to find the right solution for the item at hand?"). Bayer and Gollwitzer (2007, Study 1) asked female high school students to take a math test (composed by high school math teachers) under one of two different instructions. Half of the participants were asked to form the mere achievement goal intention "I will correctly solve as many tasks as possible!" The other half of the participants had to furnish this goal intention with the self-efficacy-strengthening implementation intention "And if I start a new task, then I will tell myself: I can solve this task!" Participants in the implementation-intention group showed better performance in the math test (in terms of number of tasks solved correctly) than participants in the mere goal-intention condition, indicating that self-efficacy-strengthening implementation intentions facilitate successful goal striving in a challenging achievement situation.

Implementation intentions are usually constructed by specifying a situational cue in the if-component and linking it to goal-directed cognitive or behavioral responses in the then-component. In this study (Bayer & Gollwitzer, 2007, Study 1), a critical situational cue (i.e., starting a new test item) in the if-component was linked to a motivational response (i.e., a self-efficacy-strengthening statement) in the then-part. Interestingly, this preprogrammed, inner self-motivating speech sufficed to produce better test performance. This suggests that implementation intentions can also be used to ameliorate motivational problems of goal implementation (e.g., self-doubts), thus increasing a person's willpower (i.e., the potential to exert self-control).

This manipulation to increase willpower was particularly parsimonious because it comprised only asking participants to form a plan in respect to when they would have to execute an inner self-efficacy-strengthening statement. Still, these findings leave open a pressing question: Does this inner speech need to take the format of an implementation intention? Maybe that participants simply form a goal intention geared toward holding up self-efficacy will suffice, such as "And I will tell myself: I can solve these problems!" To explore this possibility, a follow-up study included this further control condition (i.e., a self-efficacy-strengthening goal-intention condition). Using the Raven Intelligence Test, Bayer and Gollwitzer (2007, Study 2) found that performance on the test improved only when participants were instructed to form self-efficacy-strengthening implementation intentions; self-efficacy-enhancing goal intentions did not work. This finding is important for several reasons. First, many of the field and laboratory studies investigating the benefits of implementation intentions (e.g., on health behaviors, job safety, and environment protection; see meta-analysis by Gollwitzer & Sheeran, 2006) do not use an additional condition that spells out the then-part of the implementation intention in terms of a goal intention (for an exception, see Oettingen et al., 2000). Therefore, in these studies, the benefits of implementation intentions compared to mere goal intentions could potentially be based on having access to additional information on how to act. With this study, however, we can confidently rule out this alternative account because specifying the strategy of strengthening one's self-efficacy in terms of forming a goal intention did not lead to higher test scores. Only when this strategy was suggested to participants in the format of an if–then plan did positive effects on test performance emerge.

Often our *performances are constrained by others* who are competing with us for positive outcomes. Typical examples are negotiations in which a common good has to be shared between two opposing parties. In such situations, exerting willpower involves effectively protecting one's goal striving from unwanted influences generated by the competitive situation. Negotiations are cognitively very demanding tasks in which a large amount of information has to be processed online and the course of events is hard to predict because one is performing a task not alone but conjointly with an opponent. Thus, negotiations can be understood as the prototype of a complex situation in which striving for desired goals can easily become derailed. Therefore, analyzing whether the beneficial effects of implementation intentions found in previous research also hold true in negotiations is of great interest to assess whether needed willpower accrues from if–then planning (see also Martin, Sheeran, Slade, Wright, & Dibble, 2009).

In their negotiation research, Trötschel and Gollwitzer (2007) explored whether the self-regulation strategy of forming implementation intentions enables negotiators to reach agreement even if they have to operate under the adverse conditions of a *loss frame* (i.e., participants see how many points they lose rather than win during each round and are thus reluctant to make concessions; e.g., Bottom & Studt, 1993). In one of their experiments, pairs of negotiators were assigned roles as representatives of two neighboring countries (i.e., the blue and the orange nations) and asked to negotiate the distribution of a disputed island (i.e., its regions, villages, and towns). One group of pairs of negotiators was asked to form the mere prosocial goal "I want to cooperate with my counterpart!" and the other group to furnish this goal with the respective implementation intention "And if I receive a proposal on how to share the island, then I will make a cooperative counterproposal!" Both groups were then subjected to a frame manipulation, whereby both members of the pairs received a loss frame manipulation (i.e., each region's value is expressed in points lost when the region is given away). In addition, two control conditions were established: A first control condition contained pairs of negotiators who were not assigned prosocial goals and were asked to negotiate under a loss frame; the second control condition's pairs of negotiators who were not assigned prosocial goals but were asked to negotiate under a *gain frame* (i.e., each region's value is expressed in points won when the region is kept). These two control conditions were used to establish the negative influence of loss versus gain frames on joint profits. In addition, the loss frame control condition served as a comparison group for the two critical experimental groups (i.e., the prosocial goal group and the prosocial goal plus implementation-intention group).

In the agreements achieved (i.e., level of joint outcomes), Trötschel and Gollwitzer (2007) observed that pairs of loss frame negotiators with a prosocial goal intention managed to reduce somewhat the resistance to concession making that arose from the loss frame negotiation context, but only negotiators who furnished their prosocial goal intentions with respective implementation intentions were successful in completely abolishing the negative impact of the loss frame negotiation context (i.e., showed a negotiation performance that did not differ from that of gain frame negotiators). In addition, action control via implementation intentions was found to be very efficient (i.e., implementation intentions abolished the negative effects of loss framing by leaving the negotiators' cognitive capacity intact); negotiators who had formed implementation intentions were more likely to use the cognitively demanding integrative negotiation strategy of *logrolling* (i.e., making greater concessions on low- rather than high-priority issues).

The self-regulation of one's goal striving becomes difficult when *habitual responses* conflict with initiating and executing the needed goal-directed responses that are instrumental to goal attainment (e.g., Wood & Neal, 2007). In such cases, having willpower means asserting one's will to attain the chosen goal against unwanted habitual responses. But can the self-regulation strategy of forming if–then plans help people to let their goals win out over their habitual responses? By assuming that action control by implementation intentions is immediate and efficient, and adopting a simple racehorse model of action control (Gurney, Prescott, & Redgrave, 2001a, 2001b), people might be in a position to break habitualized responses by forming implementation intentions (e.g., if–then plans that spell out a response contrary to the habitualized response to the critical situation; Holland et al., 2006).

Cohen, Bayer, Jaudas, and Gollwitzer (2008, Study 2; see also Miles & Proctor, 2008) explored the suppression of habitual responses by implementation intentions in a laboratory experiment using the Simon task. In this paradigm, participants are asked to respond to a nonspatial aspect of a stimulus (i.e., whether a presented tone is high or low) by pressing a left or right key, and to ignore the location of the stimulus (i.e., whether it is presented on one's left or right side). The difficulty of this task is in ignoring the spatial location (left or right) of the tone in one's classification response (i.e., pressing a left or right response key; Simon, 1990). The cost in reaction times is seen when the location of the tone (e.g., right) and required key press (e.g., left) are incongruent because people habitually respond to stimuli presented at the right or left side with the corresponding hand. Cohen and colleagues (2008, Study 2) found that implementation intentions eliminated the Simon effect for the stimulus that was specified in the if-component of the implementation intention. Reaction times for this stimulus did not differ between the congruent and incongruent trials (i.e., they were fast throughout).

Automatic cognitive biases, such as stereotyping, represent another type of habitualized responses that can be in opposition to one's goals. Although one may have the goal to be egalitarian, automatic stereotyping happens quickly and unintentionally; some attempts to control automatic stereotyping have even resulted in backfire effects. Extending earlier work by Gollwitzer and Schaal (1998), Stewart and Payne (2008) examined whether implementation intentions designed to counter automatic stereotypes (e.g., "When I see a black face, I will then think 'safe' ") could reduce stereotyping towards a category of individuals (versus a single exemplar). They used the process dissociation procedure (PDP; Jacoby, 1991) to estimate whether the reduction in automatic stereotyping came about by reducing automatic stereotyping, increasing control, or a combination of these two processes. It was found that implementation intentions reduced stereotyping in a weapon identification task (Studies 1 and 2) and an Implicit Association Test (IAT) (Study 3) by reducing automatic effects of the stereotype (without increasing conscious control). This reduction in automatic race bias held even for new members of the category (Study 2). These studies suggest that implementation intentions are an efficient way to overcome automatic stereotyping. Recent research by Mendoza, Gollwitzer, and Amodio (2010) has added to this insight that implementation intentions can also be used to suppress the behavioral expression of implicit stereotypes. In their research, Mendoza and colleagues examined whether two different types of implementation intentions could improve response accuracy on the shooter task (Correll, Park, Judd, & Wittenbrink, 2002), a reaction time measure of implicit stereotyping. In Study 1, participants used a distraction-inhibiting implementation intention designed to engage control over the perception of goal-irrelevant stimuli (e.g., race). In Study 2, participants used a response-facilitating implementation intention designed to promote goal-directed action (i.e., to shoot people carrying a weapon but not those carrying a tool). Across studies, implementation intentions improved accuracy, thereby limiting the behavioral expression of implicit stereotypes. Furthermore, process dissociation analyses indicated that the distraction-inhibiting implementation intention increased controlled processing, while reducing automatic stereotype activation, whereas the response-facilitating implementation intention increased only controlled processing.

Still, one wonders whether forming implementation intentions will always block habitual responses. Using a racehorse metaphor, the answer has to be "no." Whether the habitual response or the if–then guided response will win the race depends on the relative strength of the two behavioral orientations. If the habitual response is based on strong habits (Webb, Sheeran, & Luszczynska, 2009) and the if–then guided response is based on weak implementation intentions, then the habitual response should win over the if–then planned response; and the reverse should be true when weak habits are sent into a race with strong implementation intentions.

This implies that controlling behavior based on strong habits requires the formation of strong implementation intentions. Such enhancement of if–then plans can be achieved by various measures. One pertains to creating particularly strong links between situational cues (if-component) and goal-directed responses (then-component). A promising strategy has been suggested by Knäuper, Roseman, Johnson, and Krantz (2009; see also Papies et al., 2009). They asked participants to use mental imagery when linking situational cues to goal-directed responses in their if–then plans, and found that the rate of initiation of the planned response increased by almost 50%. Alternatively, Adriaanse, de Ridder, and de Wit (2009) suggested tailoring the critical cue specified in the if-part of an implementation intention to personally relevant reasons for the habitual behavior one wants to overcome, then link this cue to an antagonistic response. In their research, they asked participants who wanted to stop eating unhealthy snacks to form implementation intentions that used either situational cues (e.g., at home, at school, with friends) or motivational cues (to be social, feeling bored, distraction) in the if-part, and taking a healthy snack in the then-part. They found that the latter implementation intentions had a stronger effect on behavior change than did the former.

Also, it seems possible that certain formats of implementation intentions are better suited to fight habits than others. For instance, an implementation intention that specifies the *critical cue* (i.e., one or many features of the context that commonly elicit the habitual behavior) in its if-part and an ignore response in its then-part should have a good change to break even strong habits because the *specified response* (i.e., ignoring the critical cue) already fights the detection of the critical cue—the trigger of the habitual response (Schweiger Gallo et al., 2009). An implementation intention that specifies the critical cue and links it to an antagonistic response, on the other hand, sends this response into competition with the habitual response; here, it seems possible that a very strong habitual response could potentially outrun the antagonistic response specified in the implementation intention if participants are not strongly committed to the if–then plan and the respective goal intention. The worst format of an implementation intention for fighting habits seems to be the following: The if-part specifies the critical cue, whereas the then-part specifies the negation of the habitual behavior. Here, it seems possible that monitoring processes associated with the suppression of the habitual response may even lead to ironic effects (Wegner, 1994) in the sense that the habitual response gets strengthened.

So far, there is no systematic research on the effects of the format of implementation intentions on their potential to fight habits of different strengths. Such research is definitely needed. On the other hand, one should not forget that behavior change is possible also without changing bad habits; one can focus as well on the building of new habits in new situational contexts. With respect to this latter approach, implementation intentions can guide goal striving without having to outrun habitual responses. The "delegation of control to situational cues principle," on which implementation intention effects are based, can unfold its facilitative effects on goal striving in an undisturbed manner.

MODERATORS OF IMPLEMENTATION INTENTION EFFECTS

Whenever people set out to use implementation intentions to improve goal striving, it is important to be aware of the moderators of implementation intention effects discovered so far. These pertain to commitment to the respective goal intention and the if–then plan at hand, self-efficacy, and the personality attributes of socially prescribed perfectionism and conscientiousness.

Commitment

For implementation intention effects to occur, people need to be strongly committed to the superordinate goal intention (e.g., Gollwitzer 1999; Orbell et al., 1997; Sheeran et al., 2005, Study 1; Verplanken & Faes, 1999); also, the goal should be self-concordant (Koestner, Lekes, Powers, & Chicoine, 2002) and the goal needs to be in a state of activation (e.g., Sheeran et al., 2005, Study 2). These prerequisites help to prevent mechanistic plan enactment when people have already disengaged from the respective goal or find themselves pursuing different goals; in other words, the automaticity achieved by implementation intentions is a goal-dependent automaticity (Bargh, 1989). For example, in a puzzle task on the goal-dependence of implementation intentions (Sheeran et al., 2005, Study 2), implementation intentions that specified how to be fast in solving the puzzles did not lead to faster responses when the goal to be accurate rather than fast was being activated. However, when the goal to be fast rather than accurate was activated, these implementation intentions in fact did produce faster responses.

Moreover, the commitment to the formed implementation intention needs to be strong (e.g., Achtziger et al., 2010, Study 2) as well. When one doubts the appropriateness of the formed implementation intentions, no implementation intention effects can be expected. In line with this assumption, Achtziger and colleagues (2010, Study 2) observed weaker implementation intention effects in participants who had been told they had the type of personality that facilitates goal attainment by staying flexible (low plan commitment) compared to participants who had been told that they had the type of personality that facilitates goal attainment by sticking to one's plans (high plan commitment). There may also be ways the individual can increase the commitment to an if–then plan he or she has already made (e.g., making one's if–then plans public; Deutsch & Gerard, 1955); future research needs to explore such ways and their moderators. In any case, the requirement of commitment to the if–then plan supports the effectiveness of implementation intentions, by ensuring that incidental if–then plans do not impair flexibility for goal attainment (e.g., Gollwitzer, Parks-Stamm, Jaudas, & Sheeran, 2008).

Self-Efficacy

Perceived *self-efficacy* is also found to moderate implementation intention effects; it is defined as "the belief in one's capabilities to organize and execute the courses of action required to produce given attainments" (Bandura, 1997, p. 3). Koestner and colleagues (2006) asked whether the effects of implementation intentions on the attainment of self-generated personal goals can be bolstered for the long haul by simultaneously boosting self-efficacy. In this study, participants were randomly assigned to one of three treatment conditions. In the control condition, they completed an irrelevant goal task. In the implementation-intention condition, participants planned when, where, and how to pursue their most important New Year's resolution. In the implementation-intention plus self-efficacy boost condition, participants were additionally required to reflect on their actual New Year's resolutions using three different tasks designed to boost their self-efficacy: They had to think of past mastery experiences (i.e., situations in which they achieved a similar goal), vicarious experiences (i.e., situations in which a similar individual attained a similar goal), and means of social support (i.e., an individual who encouraged their goal). Measuring goal progress via questionnaires e-mailed 20 weeks later, participants reported a significantly higher level of goal progress in the implementation-intention plus self-efficacy boosting condition compared to the control condition, as well as to the mere implementation-intention condition. In a recent study by Wieber, Odenthal, and Gollwitzer (2010), high versus low self-efficacy was manipulated by asking participants to solve low- or high-difficulty goal-relevant tasks. It was observed that high-self-efficacy participants showed stronger implementation intention effects than low-self-efficacy participants, and this was true in particular when goal striving was difficult rather than easy.

Personal Attributes

Socially Prescribed Perfectionism

In the first set of studies (Powers, Koestner, & Topciu, 2005) on the interaction between personality traits and if–then planning, perfectionism was examined such that socially prescribed perfectionism was distinguished from self-oriented perfectionism. Similar to self-oriented perfectionism, socially prescribed perfectionism entails setting high personal standards and evaluating oneself stringently. But whereas the standards for self-oriented perfectionists are set by the people themselves, socially prescribed perfectionists try to conform to standards and expectations that are prescribed by others. A high level of socially prescribed perfectionism is related to depression, anxiety disorders, and obsessive–compulsive symptoms (e.g., Powers, Zuroff, & Topciu, 2004). It was observed that participants who scored high on the Socially Prescribed Perfectionism subscale of the Multidimensional Perfectionist Scale (MPS; Hewitt, Flett, Turnbull-Donovan, & Mikail, 1991) reported poorer progress after 2 and 4 weeks on their New Year's resolutions (i.e., three personal goals) when they formed implementation intentions rather than receiving control instructions. Participants with high scores on socially prescribed perfectionism who formed implementation intentions also reported lower levels of satisfaction with goal progress (as perceived in their own view and in the presumed view of others) than participants who formed implementation intentions but scored low on this subscale. Importantly, for participants who scored high on self-oriented perfectionism, forming implementation intentions actually did improve goal progress (Powers et al., 2005). Possibly, social perfectionists fail to commit to implementation intentions because they may feel that the expectations and standards prescribed by others often change unexpectedly, and flexibly responding to such changes may be hindered by strong commitments to a given if–then plan.

Conscientiousness

A second line of research on personal attributes examined conscientiousness (Webb, Christian, & Armitage, 2007). In an experimental study using undergraduate students, attendance in class was studied as a function of conscientiousness, openness to experience, goal intentions, and implementation intentions. Most importantly, the implementation intention effects were moderated by participants' personality trait of conscientiousness. While class attendance of highly conscientious students was not changed by the formation of implementation intentions because it was high to begin with and stayed high, low and moderately conscientious people significantly benefited from planning when, where, and how they would attend class (their class attendance rates were low to begin with and increased to high when implementation intentions were formed). If one assumes that being on time is easy for people with high conscientiousness but difficult for people who are low on this personal attribute, this finding is in line with the general observation (Gollwitzer & Sheeran, 2006) that in particular it is the difficult goals that benefit from the formation of implementation intentions; easy goals can be striven for effectively without having to prepare goal striving by forming implementation intentions.

IMPLEMENTATION INTENTIONS: PAST AND FUTURE

Past: Conceptual Roots

The concept of implementation intentions grew out of a more comprehensive approach to goal pursuit: the mindset theory of action phases (Gollwitzer, 1990). The mindset model of action phases sees successful goal pursuit as solving a series of successive tasks: deliberating on wishes (potential goals) and choosing between them; planning and initiating goal-directed actions; bringing goal pursuit to a successful end; and evaluating its outcome. This task notion implies that people can activate cognitive procedures (*mindsets*) that facilitate task completion simply by getting heavily involved with the task at hand. Whereas deliberating between potential goals (i.e., wishes) activates cognitive procedures (i.e., a *deliberative mindset*) that facilitate decision making, engaging in planning activates those procedures (i.e., an *implemental mindset*) that support the implementation of goals.

Researchers have found that when participants are asked to plan the implementation of a set goal, an implemental mindset with the following attributes develops (review by Gollwitzer, in press). Participants become closed-minded to distracting, goal-irrelevant information while processing information related to implementing goals more effectively (e.g., information on the sequencing of actions). Moreover, relevant desirability-related information is processed in a partial manner, favoring pros over cons, and relevant feasibility-related information is analyzed in a manner that favors illusory optimism. Self-perception of possessing important personal attributes (e.g., cheerfulness, smartness, social sensitivity) is strengthened, whereas perceived vulnerability to both controllable and uncontrollable risks is lowered (e.g., developing an addiction to prescription drugs or losing a partner to an early death, respectively). Thus, the implemental mindset facilitates goal attainment by focusing individuals on implementation-related information and by preventing the waning of commitment to the chosen goal.

Traditionally, implemental mindsets have been analyzed primarily in terms of their cognitive features, without direct testing of these features' effects on actual implementation of goals. Armor and Taylor (2003), however, reported that an implemental mindset facilitates better task performance (in a scavenger hunt to be performed on campus), and that this effect is mediated by the cognitive features of the implemental mindset (e.g., enhanced self-efficacy, optimistic outcome expectations, perceiving the task as easy). This finding suggests that the positive expectations associated with the implemental mindset do indeed lead to more effective self-regulation and better outcomes. Participants' performance expectations in the Armor and Taylor study, however, were for an immediate, imminent task. One wonders, therefore, whether the temporal distance of the performance at issue may moderate the beneficial effects of the implemental mindset. This assumption is supported by long-term performance data collected by Gagné and Lydon (2001). In their study, long-term relationship survival was not affected by implemental mindset participants' optimistic predictions of a stable relationship. It appears, then, that whenever actual goal implementation is assessed further and further away from the induction of the implemental mindset, the positive effects of its various cognitive features on goal implementation may no longer be observed. From a self-regulation point of view, it seems wise therefore not to rely on the beneficial effects of getting involved with planning in general when the goal that is striven for demands acting on the goal in not only the near but also the distant future; rather, one should resort to the self-regulation strategy of making specific if–then plans (i.e., form implementation intentions) because the beneficial effects of such plans on goal attainment have been found to accrue over vast periods of time (i.e., several months; see the meta-analysis by Gollwitzer & Sheeran, 2006).

Future: Intervention Research

In everyday life, people may not succeed in forming effective implementation intentions for various reasons related to putting the wrong critical situation into the if-part of the plan and specifying a response that is not very instrumental to goal attainment in the then-part. Moreover, people may forget about the preliminaries of implementation intention effects, such as a strong commitment to the superordinate goal and a strong willingness to commit to a possible if–then plan. It seems appropriate, therefore, that research turns to the question of how the self-regulation strategy of forming implementation intentions is taught best in interventions geared at helping people to strive for their goals more effectively.

There is a way of thinking about the future that prepares people maximally for forming implementation intentions. This mental strategy, spelled out in Oettingen's (2000; Oettingen et al., 2001) theory of fantasy realization, has been referred to as *mental contrasting*. It works like this: If, for instance, a person has the wish of "getting to know someone I like" or of "improving the relationship to my partner," mental contrasting requires that one first mentally elaborate the positive future of having successfully solved this issue, and right after that elaborate the negative reality impeding the attainment of the positive future. As a result, when forming goal commitments, people discriminate according to their expectations of success: They arrive at strong goal commitments when expectations of success are high, and they refrain from such commitments when expectations of success are low. Moreover, mental contrasting allows insights on what stands in the way of reaching the desired future, thus preparing one to plan how to overcome these obstacles. In other words, mental contrasting not only provides the commitment for the pursuit of promising goals but it also puts into people's heads the intricacies of striving for goal attainment. Not surprisingly, then, Oettingen and colleagues (2001, Study 3) found that research participants who were led to contrast a desired future outcome mentally subsequently engaged in more if–then planning than control participants—that is, participants who only dwelled on obstacles of reality or only indulged in the desired positive future.

That mental contrasting is indeed a sophisticated problem-solving strategy is attested by a recent study using continuous magnetoencephalography (MEG), a brain imaging technique measuring magnetic fields produced by electrical activity in the brain (Achtziger, Fehr, Oettingen, Gollwitzer, & Rockstroh, 2009). Mental contrasting as compared to indulging in a desired positive future or simply resting produced heightened brain activity in areas associated with working memory, episodic memory, intention maintenance, action preparation, and vivid visualization. That is, mental contrasting implied vividly imagining a desired future and contrasting it with the reality that stands in the way of realizing this future. The brain activity associated with indulging, on the other hand, did not differ from resting.

Recent research has also discovered a further mediating process pertaining to the energization of effort (Oettingen, Mayer, Sevincer, et al., 2009). Specifically, mentally contrasting an achievable desired future with obstacles of present reality leads to energization, which in turn creates goal commitments strong enough to lead to effective goal striving and successful goal attainment. These mediating effects of energization on goal commitment are shown on physiological indicators of energization (i.e., systolic blood pressure), as well as experiential indicators (self-report of feeling energized). Moreover, mental contrasting does not have to pertain to the attainment of a positive future; people can also fantasize about a negative future, then contrast it with elaborations of the positive reality. Oettingen, Mayer, Thorpe, Janetzke, and Lorenz (2005) created tolerance and support toward foreigners in a group of xenophobic high school students by having them elaborate on their fears that social conflicts would arise if foreign youths moved into their neighborhood and contrast these fears with positive aspects of present reality standing in the way of the feared future.

It appears, then, that mental contrasting prepares people cognitively and motivationally to engage in if–then planning for the purpose of making goal striving more effective. Oettingen and colleagues (Adriaanse et al., in press; Christiansen, Oettingen, Dahme, & Klinger, 2010; Oettingen & Gollwitzer, 2010; Oettingen & Stephens, 2009; Stadler, Oettingen, & Gollwitzer, 2009, 2010) thus developed an intervention that combines mental contrasting and formation of implementation intentions into one meta-cognitive strategy called MCII (i.e., mental contrasting with implementation intentions). In order to unfold their beneficial effects, implementation intentions require that strong goal commitments be in place (Sheeran et al., 2005, Study 1), and mental contrasting creates such strong commitments (Oettingen et al., 2001, 2009; Oettingen, Mayer, Stephens, & Brinkmann, in press; Oettingen, Mayer, & Thorpe, in press). Additionally, mental contrasting guarantees the identification of those critical obstacles that do indeed hinder goal striving. These very obstacles can then be addressed with if–then plans by specifying them as critical situations in the if-component that link them to goal-directed responses specified in the then-component. In this way, the idiosyncratic critical obstacle will be linked to an idiosyncratic, instrumental goal-directed response.

Indeed, in a recent intervention study with middle-aged women (Stadler, Oettingen, & Gollwitzer, 2009), participants were taught only the individual steps and cognitive principles of the MCII self-regulation strategy, and to apply it by themselves whenever possible to the wish of exercising more (hence, MCII is referred to as a meta-cognitive self-regulation strategy). Participants were free to choose whatever form of exercising they wished and were encouraged to anticipate exactly those obstacles that were personally most relevant and link them to exactly those goal-directed responses that personally appeared to be most instrumental. As dependent measures, participants maintained daily behavioral diaries to keep track of the amount of time they exercised every day. Overall, participants using the MCII technique exercised more than control participants given information on the beneficial health effects of exercising; this effect showed up immediately after the intervention and remained stable throughout the entire period of the study (16 weeks after the intervention). More specifically, participants in the MCII group exercised nearly twice as much: an average of 1 hour more per week than participants in the information-only control group.

Conducting the same MCII intervention to promote healthy eating in middle-aged women (i.e., eating more fruits and vegetables) also produced the desired behavior change effects, and these persisted even over the extensive time period of 2 years (Stadler, Oettingen, & Gollwitzer, 2010). Moreover, an MCII study by Adriaanse and colleagues (in press) targeted the negative eating habit of unhealthy snacking in college students. MCII worked for students with both weak and strong habits, and it was more effective than mental contrasting or formulating implementation intentions alone.

Finally, MCII seems to facilitate behavior change even when there is an initial reluctance to engage in the targeted behavior. Christiansen and colleagues (2010) promoted physical mobility in chronic back pain outpatients from a rehabilitation center in Germany by teaching them MCII. Participants were randomly assigned to either a control group (i.e., outpatient cognitive-behavioral therapy back pain program) or an intervention group (i.e., this program plus MCII intervention). The MCII intervention improved physical mobility more than the standard treatment only as observed 2 weeks and 3 months after the intervention, and as assessed by subjective and objective measures. These effects were independent of participants' experienced pain, which did not differ between conditions during and after treatment. In summary, research suggests that MCII interventions are a very useful self-regulation technique when it comes to meeting one's goals.

REFERENCES

Aarts, H., Dijksterhuis, A., & Midden, C. (1999). To plan or not to plan?: Goal achievement or interrupting the performance of mundane behaviors. *European Journal of Social Psychology, 29,* 971–979.

Achtziger, A., Bayer, U. C., & Gollwitzer, P. M. (2010). *Committing to implementation intentions: Attention and memory effects for selected situational cues.* Manuscript submitted for publication.

Achtziger, A., Fehr, T., Oettingen, G., Gollwitzer, P. M., & Rockstroh, B. (2009). Strategies of intention formation are reflected in continuous MEG activity. *Social Neuroscience, 4,* 11–27.

Achtziger, A., Gollwitzer, P. M., & Sheeran, P. (2008). Implementation intentions and shielding goal striving from unwanted thoughts and feelings. *Personality and Social Psychology Bulletin, 34,* 381–393.

Adriaanse, M. A., de Ridder, D. T. D., & de Wit, J. B. F. (2009). Finding the critical cue: Implementation intentions to change one's diet work best when tailored to personally relevant reasons for unhealthy eating. *Personality and Social Psychology Bulletin, 35,* 60–71.

Adriaanse, M. A., Oettingen, G., Gollwitzer, P. M., Hennes, E. P., de Ridder, D. T. D., & de Witt,

J. B. F. (in press). When planning is not enough: Fighting unhealthy snacking habits by mental contrasting with implementation intentions (MCII). *European Journal of Social Psychology.*

Ajzen, I. (1985). From intentions to actions: A theory of planned behavior. In J. Kuhl & J. Beckmann (Eds.), *Action control: From cognition to behavior* (pp. 11–39). Berlin: Springer-Verlag.

Armitage, C. J. (2004). Evidence that implementation intentions reduce dietary fat intake: A randomized trial. *Health Psychology, 23,* 319–323.

Armor, D. A., & Taylor, S. E. (2003). The effects of mindset on behavior: Self-regulation in deliberative and implemental frames of mind. *Personality and Social Psychology Bulletin, 29,* 86–95.

Bandura, A. (1997). *Self-efficacy: The exercise of control.* New York: Freeman.

Bargh, J. A. (1989). Conditional automaticity: Varieties of automatic influence in social perception and cognition. In J. S. Uleman & J. A. Bargh (Eds.), *Unintended thought* (pp. 3–51). New York: Guilford Press.

Bargh, J. A., & Chartrand, T. L. (2000). The mind in the middle: A practical guide to priming and automaticity research. In H. T. Reis & C. M. Judd (Eds.), *Handbook of research methods in social and personality psychology* (pp. 253–285). New York: Cambridge University Press.

Bargh, J. A., Gollwitzer, P. M., & Oettingen, G. (2010). Motivation. In S. Fiske, D. T. Gilbert, & G. Lindzey (Eds.), *Handbook of social psychology* (5th ed., Vol. 1, pp. 268–316). New York: Wiley.

Baumeister, R. E. (2000). Ego-depletion and the self's executive function. In A. Tesser, R. B. Felson, & J. M. Suls (Eds.), *Psychological perspectives on self and identity* (pp. 9–33). Washington, DC: American Psychological Association.

Baumeister, R. E., Heatherton, T. E., & Tice, D. M. (1994). *Losing control: How and why people fail at self-regulation.* San Diego, CA: Academic Press.

Bayer, U. C., Achtziger, A., Gollwitzer, P. M., & Moskowitz, G. (2009). Responding to subliminal cues: Do if–then plans cause action preparation and initiation without conscious intent? *Social Cognition, 27,* 183–201.

Bayer, U. C., & Gollwitzer, P. M. (2007). Boosting scholastic test scores by willpower: The role of implementation intentions. *Self and Identity, 6,* 1–19.

Bayer, U. C., Gollwitzer, P. M., & Achtziger, A. (2010). Staying on track: Planned goal striving is protected from disruptive internal states. *Journal of Experimental Social Psychology, 146,* 505–514.

Bless, H., & Fiedler, K. (1995). Affective states and the influence of activated general knowledge. *Personality and Social Psychology Bulletin, 21,* 766–778.

Bottom, W. P., & Studt, A. (1993). Framing effects and the distributive aspect of integrative bargaining. *Organizational Behavior and Human Decision Processes, 56,* 459–474.

Brandstätter, V., Lengfelder, A., & Gollwitzer, P. M. (2001). Implementation intentions and efficient action initiation. *Journal of Personality and Social Psychology, 81,* 946–960.

Brockner, J. (1992). The escalation of commitment to a failing course of action: Toward theoretical progress. *Academy of Management Review, 17,* 39–61.

Burgess, P. W., Dumontheil, I., & Gilbert, S. J. (2007). The gateway hypothesis of rostral PFC (Area 10) function. *Trends in Cognitive Sciences, 11,* 290–298.

Carver, C. S., & Scheier, M. E. (1998). *On the self-regulation of behavior.* New York: Cambridge University Press.

Chasteen, A. L., Park, D. C., & Schwarz, N. (2001). Implementation intentions and facilitation of prospective memory. *Psychological Science, 12,* 457–461.

Christiansen, S., Oettingen, G., Dahme, B., & Klinger, R. (2010). A short goal-pursuit intervention to improve physical capacity: A randomized clinical trial in chronic back pain patients. *Pain, 149,* 444–452.

Cohen, A.-L., Bayer, U. C., Jaudas, A., & Gollwitzer, P. M. (2008). Self-regulatory strategy and executive control: Implementation intentions modulate task switching and Simon task performance. *Psychological Research, 72,* 12–26.

Correll, J., Park, B., Judd, C. M., & Wittenbrink, B. (2002). The police officer's dilemma: Using ethnicity to disambiguate potentially threatening individuals. *Journal of Personality and Social Psychology, 83,* 1314–1329.

Deutsch, M., & Gerard, H. B. (1955). A study of normative and informational social influences upon individual judgment. *Journal of Abnormal and Social Psychology, 51,* 629–636.

Elliot, A. J. (2008). *Handbook of approach and avoidance motivation.* Mahwah, NJ: Erlbaum.

Eriksen, B. A., & Eriksen, C. W. (1974). Effects of noise letters upon the identification of a target letter in a nonsearch task. *Perception and Psychophysics, 16,* 143–149.

Gagné, E. M., & Lydon, J. E. (2001). Mindset and close relationships: When bias leads to (in) accurate predictions. *Journal of Personality and Social Psychology, 81,* 85–96.

Gawrilow, C., & Gollwitzer, P. M. (2008). Implementation intentions facilitate response inhibition in ADHD children. *Cognitive Therapy and Research, 32,* 261–280.

Gilbert, S., Gollwitzer, P. M., Cohen, A.-L., Oettingen, G., & Burgess, P. W. (2009). Separable brain systems supporting cued versus self-initiated realization of delayed intentions. *Journal of Experimental Psychology: Learning, Memory, and Cognition, 35,* 905–915.

Gollwitzer, P. M. (1990). Action phases and mind-sets. In T. E. Higgins & R. M. Sorrentino (Eds.), *Handbook of motivation and cognition: Foundations of social behavior* (Vol. 2, pp. 53–92). New York: Guilford Press.

Gollwitzer, P. M. (1993). Goal achievement: The role of intentions. *European Review of Social Psychology, 4,* 141–185.

Gollwitzer, P. M. (1999). Implementation intentions: Strong effects of simple plans. *American Psychologist, 54,* 493–503.

Gollwitzer, P. M. (in press). Mindset theory of action phases. In P. Van Lange, A. W. Kruglanski, & E. T. Higgins (Eds.), *Handbook of theories of social psychology.* London: Sage.

Gollwitzer, P. M., & Brandstätter, V. (1997). Implementation intentions and effective goal pursuit. *Journal of Personality and Social Psychology, 73,* 186–199.

Gollwitzer, P. M., & Moskowitz, G. B. (1996). Goal effects on action and cognition. In E. T. Higgins & A. W. Kruglanski (Eds.), *Social psychology: Handbook of basic principles* (pp. 361–399). New York: Guilford Press.

Gollwitzer, P. M., Parks-Stamm, E. J., Jaudas, A., & Sheeran, P. (2008). Flexible tenacity in goal pursuit. In J. Y. Shah & W. L. Gardner (Eds.), *Handbook of motivation science* (pp. 325–341). New York: Guilford Press.

Gollwitzer, P. M., & Schaal, B. (1998). Metacognition in action: The importance of implementation intentions. *Personality and Social Psychology Review, 2,* 124–136.

Gollwitzer, P. M., & Sheeran, P. (2006). Implementation intentions and goal achievement: A meta-analysis of effects and processes. *Advances in Experimental Social Psychology, 38,* 69–119.

Gollwitzer, P. M., & Wicklund, R. A. (1985). Self-symbolizing and the neglect of others' perspectives. *Journal of Personality and Social Psychology, 56,* 531–715.

Gurney, K., Prescott, T. J., & Redgrave, P. (2001a). A computational model of action selection in the basal ganglia I: A new functional anatomy. *Biological Cybernetics, 84,* 401–410.

Gurney, K., Prescott, T. J., & Redgrave, P. (2001b). A computational model of action selection in the basal ganglia II: Analysis and simulation of behaviour. *Biological Cybernetics, 84,* 411–423.

Henderson, M. D., Gollwitzer, P. M., & Oettingen, G. (2007). Implementation intentions and disengagement from a failing course of action. *Journal of Behavioral Decision Making, 20,* 81–102.

Hewitt, P. L., Flett, G. L., Turnbull-Donovan, W., & Mikail, S. F. (1991). The Multidimensional Perfectionism Scale: Reliability, validity, and psychometric properties in psychiatric samples. *Psychological Assessment, 3,* 464–468.

Holland, R. W., Aarts, H., & Langendam, D. (2006). Breaking and creating habits on the working floor: A field experiment on the power of implementation intentions. *Journal of Experimental Social Psychology, 42*, 776–783.

Jacoby, L. L. (1991). A process dissociation framework: Separating automatic from intentional uses of memory. *Journal of Memory and Language, 30*, 513–541.

Knäuper, B., Roseman, M., Johnson, P., & Krantz, L. (2009). Using mental imagery to enhance the effectiveness of implementation intentions. *Current Psychology, 28*, 181–186.

Koestner, R., Horberg, E. J., Gaudreau, P., Powers, T. A., Di Dio, P., Bryan, C., et al. (2006). Bolstering implementation plans for the long haul: The benefits of simultaneously boosting self-concordance or self-efficacy. *Personality and Social Psychology Bulletin, 32*(11), 1547–1558.

Koestner, R., Lekes, N., Powers, T. A., & Chicoine, E. (2002). Attaining personal goals: Self-concordance plus implementation intentions equals success. *Journal of Personality and Social Psychology, 83*, 231–244.

Lengfelder, A., & Gollwitzer, P. M. (2001). Reflective and reflexive action control in patients with frontal brain lesions. *Neuropsychology, 15*, 80–100.

Locke, E. A., & Latham, G. P. (2006). New directions in goal-setting theory. *Current Directions in Psychological Science, 15*, 265–268.

Martin, J., Sheeran, P., Slade, P., Wright, A., & Dibble, T. (2009). Implementation intention formation reduces consultations for emergency contraception and pregnancy testing among teenage women. *Health Psychology, 28*, 762–769.

Mendoza, S. A., Gollwitzer, P. M., & Amodio, D. M. (2010). Reducing the expression of implicit stereotypes: Reflexive control through implementation intentions. *Personality and Social Psychology Bulletin, 36*, 512–523.

Miles, J. D., & Proctor, R. W. (2008). Improving performance through implementation intentions: Are preexisting response biases replaced? *Psychonomic Bulletin and Review, 15*, 1105–1110.

Milne, S., Orbell, S., & Sheeran, P. (2002). Combining motivational and volitional interventions to promote exercise participation: Protection motivation theory and implementation intentions. *British Journal of Health Psychology, 7*, 163–184.

Molden, D. C., & Dweck, C. S. (2006). Finding "meaning" in psychology: A lay theories approach to self-regulation, social perception, and social development. *American Psychologist, 61*, 192–203.

Muraven, M., & Baumeister, R. F. (2000). Self-regulation and depletion of limited resources: Does self-control resemble a muscle? *Psychological Bulletin, 126*, 247–259.

Muraven, M., Tice, D. M., & Baumeister, R. F. (1998). Self-control as a limited resource: Regulatory depletion pattern. *Journal of Personality and Social Psychology, 74*, 774–789.

Oettingen, G. (2000). Expectancy effects on behavior depend on self-regulatory thought. *Social Cognition, 18*, 101–129.

Oettingen, G., & Gollwitzer, P. M. (2001). Goal setting and goal striving. In A. Tesser & N. Schwarz (Eds.), *The Blackwell handbook of social psychology* (pp. 329–347). Oxford, UK: Blackwell.

Oettingen, G., & Gollwitzer, P. M. (2010). Strategies of setting and implementing goals: Mental contrasting and implementation intentions. In J. E. Maddux & J. P. Tangney (Eds.), *Social psychological foundations of clinical psychology* (pp. 114–135). New York: Guilford Press.

Oettingen, G., Hönig, G., & Gollwitzer, P. M. (2000). Effective self-regulation of goal attainment. *International Journal of Educational Research, 33*, 705–732.

Oettingen, G., Mayer, D., Sevincer, A. T., Stephens, E. J., Pak, H., & Hagenah, M. (2009). Mental contrasting and goal commitment: The mediating role of energization. *Personality and Social Psychology Bulletin, 35*, 608–622.

Oettingen, G., Mayer, D., Stephens, M. E. J., & Brinkmann, B. (in press). Mental contrasting and the self-regulation of helping relations. *Social Cognition*.

Oettingen, G., Mayer, D., & Thorpe, J. (in press). Self-regulation of commitment to reduce ciga-rette consumption: Mental contrasting of future and reality. *Psychology and Health.*

Oettingen, G., Mayer, D., Thorpe, J. S., Janetzke, H., & Lorenz, S. (2005). Turning fantasies about positive and negative futures into self-improvement goals. *Motivation and Emotion, 29,* 237–267.

Oettingen, G., Pak, H.-J., & Schnetter, K. (2001). Self-regulation of goal setting: Turning free fantasies about the future into binding goals. *Journal of Personality and Social Psychology, 80,* 736–753.

Oettingen, G., & Stephens, E. J. (2009). Fantasies and motivationally intelligent goal setting. In G. B. Moskowitz & H. Grant (Eds.), *The psychology of goals* (pp. 135–178). New York: Guilford Press.

Orbell, S., Hodgkins, S., & Sheeran, P. (1997). Implementation intentions and the theory of planned behavior. *Personality and Social Psychology Bulletin, 23,* 945–954.

Orbell, S., & Sheeran, P. (2000). Motivational and volitional processes in action initiation: A field study of the role of implementation intentions. *Journal of Applied Social Psychology, 30,* 780–797.

Papies, E., Aarts, H., & de Vries, N. K. (2009). Grounding your plans: Implementation intentions go beyond the mere creation of goal-directed associations. *Journal of Experimental Social Psychology, 45,* 1148–1151.

Parks-Stamm, E., Gollwitzer, P. M., & Oettingen, G. (2007). Action control by implementation intentions: Effective cue detection and efficient response initiation. *Social Cognition, 25,* 248–266.

Paul, I., Gawrilow, C., Zech, F., Gollwitzer, P. M., Rockstroh, B., Odenthal, G., Kratzer, W., et al. (2007). If–then planning modulates the P300 in children with attention deficit hyperactivity disorder. *NeuroReport, 18,* 653–657.

Powers, T. A., Koestner, R., & Topciu, R. A. (2005). Implementation intentions, perfectionism, and goal progress: Perhaps the road to hell is paved with good intentions. *Personality and Social Psychology Bulletin, 31,* 902–912.

Powers, T. A., Zuroff, D. C., & Topciu, R. A. (2004). Covert and overt expressions of self-criticism and perfectionism and their relation to depression. *European Journal of Personality, 18,* 61–72.

Schweiger Gallo, I., Keil, A., McCulloch, K. C., Rockstroh, B., & Gollwitzer, P. M. (2009). Stra-tegic automation of emotion control. *Journal of Personality and Social Psychology, 96,* 11–31.

Sheeran, P., & Orbell, S. (1999). Implementation intentions and repeated behavior: Augmenting the predictive validity of the theory of planned behavior. *European Journal of Social Psychol-ogy, 29,* 349–369.

Sheeran, P., & Orbell, S. (2000). Using implementation intentions to increase attendance for cervi-cal cancer screening. *Health Psychology, 19,* 283–289.

Sheeran, P., Webb, T. L., & Gollwitzer, P. M. (2005). The interplay between goal intentions and implementation intentions. *Personality and Social Psychology Bulletin, 31,* 87–98.

Simon, J. R. (1990). The effects of an irrelevant directional cue on human information process-ing. In R. W. Proctor & T. G. Reeve (Eds.), *Stimulus–response compatibility: An integrative perspective* (pp. 31–86). Amsterdam: North Holland.

Stadler, G., Oettingen, G., & Gollwitzer, P. M. (2009). Physical activity in women. Effects of a self-regulation intervention. *American Journal of Preventive Medicine, 36,* 29–34.

Stadler, G., Oettingen, G., & Gollwitzer, P. M. (2010). Intervention effects of information and self-regulation on eating fruits and vegetables over two years. *Health Psychology, 29,* 274–283.

Stewart, B. D., & Payne, B. K. (2008). Bringing automatic stereotyping under control: Implemen-tation intentions as efficient means of thought control. *Personality and Social Psychology Bulletin, 34,* 1332–1345.

Trötschel, R., & Gollwitzer, P. M. (2007). Implementation intentions and the willful pursuit of prosocial goals in negotiations. *Journal of Experimental Social Psychology, 43,* 579–589.

Verplanken, B., & Faes, S. (1999). Good intentions, bad habits, and effects of forming implementation intentions on healthy eating. *European Journal of Social Psychology, 29,* 591–604.

Webb, T. L., Christian, J., & Armitage, C. J. (2007). Helping students turn up for class: Does personality moderate the effectiveness of an implementation intention intervention? *Learning and Individual Differences, 17,* 316–327.

Webb, T. L., & Sheeran, P. (2003). Can implementation intentions help to overcome ego-depletion? *Journal of Experimental Social Psychology, 39,* 279–286.

Webb, T. L., & Sheeran, P. (2004). Identifying good opportunities to act: Implementation intentions and cue discrimination. *European Journal of Social Psychology, 34,* 407–419.

Webb, T. L., & Sheeran, P. (2006). Does changing behavioural intentions engender behavior change?: A meta-analysis of the experimental evidence. *Psychological Bulletin, 132,* 249–268.

Webb, T. L., & Sheeran, P. (2007). How do implementation intentions promote goal attainment?: A test of component processes. *Journal of Experimental Social Psychology, 43,* 295–268.

Webb, T. L., & Sheeran, P. (2008). Mechanisms of implementation intention effects: The role of intention, self-efficacy, and accessibility of plan components. *British Journal of Social Psychology, 47,* 373–395.

Webb, T. L., Sheeran, P., & Luszczynska, A. (2009). Planning to break unwanted habits: Habit strength moderates implementation intention effects on behavior change. *British Journal of Social Psychology, 48,* 507–523.

Wegner, D. M. (1994). Ironic processes of mental control. *Psychological Review, 101,* 34–52.

Wieber, F., Odenthal, G., & Gollwitzer, P. M. (2010). Self-efficacy feelings moderate implementation intention effects. *Self and Identity, 9,* 177–194.

Wieber, F., & Sassenberg, K. (2006). I can't take my eyes off of it: Attention attraction effects of implementation intentions. *Social Cognition, 24,* 723–752.

Wood, W., & Neal, D. T. (2007). A new look at habits and the habit–goal interface. *Psychological Review, 114,* 842–862.

CHAPTER 10

The Reason in Passion
A Social Cognitive Neuroscience Approach to Emotion Regulation

KATERI McRAE
KEVIN N. OCHSNER
JAMES J. GROSS

Emotional responses are often quick, adaptive responses that help us successfully address challenges that arise in our environments. However, in some contexts, otherwise adaptive emotional responses may be inappropriate because they are either ill-timed or are of the wrong type or intensity for the particular situation at hand. Healthy adaptation therefore requires the ability to regulate our emotions, so that our emotional behavior is a joint function of rapidly triggered emotional impulses on the one hand, and effortfully applied self-control on the other. Drawing on an array of emotion regulatory strategies, we thus at times may wish to accentuate the positive, remain calm in the face of danger, or productively channel our anger.

One particularly powerful emotion regulation strategy involves changing the way we think in order to change the way we feel. Known as *reappraisal*, this capacity to control emotion cognitively has been recognized for many centuries. In William Shakespeare's *Henry VIII*, the king's respected advisor offers this advice:

> Be advised:
> I say again, there is no English soul
> More stronger to direct you than yourself,
> If with the sap of reason you would quench,
> Or but allay, the fire of passion. (Act I, Scene i, 144–148; Shakespeare/Garrick, 1970)

Today, reappraisal is widely used in everyday emotion regulation (Totterdell & Parkinson, 1999), as well as in structured interventions that target clinical disorders characterized by overwhelming amounts of negative emotion (Beck, Rush, Shaw, & Emery, 1979).

In the past few decades, researchers have systematically begun to investigate how reappraisal can harness reason to quench, allay, or otherwise modulate the fire of passion. Our goal in this chapter is to refine a framework for understanding the mechanisms by which reappraisal changes the trajectory of an emotional response. Toward that end, the chapter is divided into four parts. In the first, we outline a modal model of emotion and a process model of emotion regulation that can be used to place reappraisal in the context of other types of emotion regulation strategies. In the second part, we present our social cognitive neuroscience approach, which proposes neural targets of and mechanisms for reappraisal. In the third part, we present several functional magnetic resonance imaging (fMRI) studies designed to provide empirical bases for the neural model presented previously. In the last part, we consider implications for individual and group differences in emotion regulation, uninstructed emotion regulation, and the role of emotion regulation in clinical disorders.

EMOTION AND EMOTION REGULATION

Scientific conceptions of emotion take as their starting point the tension between processes that generate emotions and those that regulate them. In this section, we first outline the *modal model* of emotion, which describes the way emotions unfold over time. We then describe a *process model* of emotion regulation that uses the modal model to define points in the emotion-generative process at which regulation strategies can intervene. In the following section, we then use neuroscience data to flesh out and constrain this model.

Emotion-Generative Processes

Emotion researchers now generally agree that emotions are biologically based and socially elaborated responses that help an organism meet challenges and opportunities, and involve changes in several response channels (Levenson, 1994; Smith & Ellsworth, 1985). In our view, emotions arise when an individual encounters a situation that is potentially relevant to his or her personal goals, when attention is drawn to the goal-relevant aspects of that situation, and then the situation is appraised by the individual as having goal relevance. This often leads to behavior, facial and vocal expression, and physiological changes. However, this sequence does not end when emotional responses are produced. Instead, the expression of an emotional response immediately creates a new situation, which is then attended to and appraised, and new responses emerge. Real-life emotional experience can be characterized by extremely rapid iterations of this cycle. This *modal model* of emotion generation is depicted in Figure 10.1.

Emotion Regulatory Processes

Emotion regulation refers to any process that influences the onset, offset, magnitude, duration, intensity, or quality of one or more aspects of the emotional response (Gross,

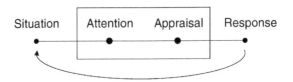

FIGURE 10.1. The modal model of emotion. From Gross and Thompson (2007). Copyright 2007 by The Guilford Press. Reprinted by permission.

1998b; Gross & Thompson, 2007; see Koole, van Dillen, & Sheppes, Chapter 2, this volume). It is now clear that effective emotion regulation is essential for mental and physical health, and that emotion dysregulation lies at the heart of mood and anxiety disorders (Campbell-Sills & Barlow, 2007; Davidson, Putnam, & Larson, 2000).

There is accumulating evidence that many strategies may be used to regulate emotions, and that these strategies have very different consequences for emotional experience, behavior, and physiology (Gross, 1998a). This led us to develop a framework for categorizing the loose-knit families of cognitive and neural processes that support different kinds of emotion regulation. We have called this framework the *process model of emotion regulation* (Gross, 1998a). According to this model, we may distinguish among emotion regulation strategies on the basis of the primary point in the emotion-generative process at which they have their effects.

Using the *modal model* of emotion as a guide, we have described five families of emotion regulation strategies. In the first, which we refer to as *situation selection*, a person can control the appraisal process before it ever begins by actively choosing to place him- or herself in particular contexts and not others. The second family of emotion regulation strategy—*situation modification*—involves direct efforts to change the situation to modify its emotional impact. Once the particular context has been set, a third strategy may direct attention to environmental cues that promote desired emotions, while ignoring cues that promote undesired emotions. *Attentional deployment* gates particular cues into the appraisal process, allowing some aspects of the situation to become the focus of attention, while excluding others from it. A fourth family of strategies, referred to as *cognitive change*, allows a person to modify the meaning of particular cues once those cues have gained access to the appraisal process. One kind of cognitive change—reappraisal—is our primary focus in this chapter. The fifth family of emotion regulation strategies, *response modulation*, affects only the outputs of reappraisal process. Using this strategy, control processes can suppress or augment behavioral manifestations of one's emotional state, such as smiles, frowns, or tendencies to approach or withdraw. The modal model of emotion is redrawn in Figure 10.2, with each of the five families of emotion regulation strategies positioned to demonstrate where in the emotion-generation process it intervenes.

These strategies are derived theoretically from their point of intervention in the emotion generation process. Empirical work initially focused on whether these strategies had differential effects on various aspects of the emotional response: subjective experience, emotional expression, and peripheral physiology. Much of this work is focused on cognitive reappraisal. In the next section, we review experimental studies on the effects of reappraisal and show how these findings prepared the ground for a neurofunctional model of reappraisal.

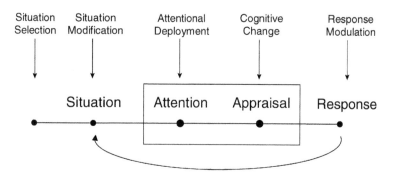

FIGURE 10.2. A process model of emotion regulation that highlights five families of emotion regulation strategies. From Gross and Thompson (2007). Copyright 2007 by The Guilford Press. Reprinted by permission.

TOWARD A NEUROFUNCTIONAL MODEL OF REAPPRAISAL

One major focus of emotion regulation research has been assessing whether explicit instructions to reappraise potentially emotional material modulates the emotional response, as evidenced by changes in self-reported negative affect and peripheral physiology. Reappraisal has been of particular focus for at least two reasons. First, initial studies showed that it is a powerful, effective way for individuals to control their emotions. Second, reappraisal surfaces as a core skill taught in cognitive-behavioral therapy (CBT; Beck et al., 1979), and CBT is one of the most commonly used treatments for mood and anxiety disorders. Although reappraisal can be used to increase or decrease positive or negative emotions, the primary focus of this research has been on the down-regulation of negative emotion.

Behavioral and Peripheral Findings

Early studies using films that elicit negative emotions demonstrated that self-reported negative affect could be modulated by the interpretation, or appraisal, given by the experimenter (Koriat, Melkman, Averill, & Lazarus, 1972). From there, investigators asked individuals to generate their own reinterpretations, or reappraisals, of negative films (Gross, 1998a). These studies demonstrated that participants could successfully decrease their self-reported negative affect when instructed to reinterpret films using reappraisal. A series of studies has shown that, compared to unregulated responding, participants instructed to reappraise report feeling less negative in response to films (Goldin, McRae, Ramel, & Gross, 2009; Gross, 1998a), pictures (Jackson, Malmstadt, Larson, & Davidson, 2000; Ochsner, Bunge, Gross, & Gabrieli, 2002), anticipation of painful shock (Kalisch et al., 2005), negative autobiographical memories (Kross, Davidson, Weber, & Ochsner, 2009), and a stressful speech task (Lam, Dickerson, Zoccola, & Zaldivar, 2009).

Reappraisal has successfully decreased and increased startle eyeblink magnitude (Dillon & LaBar, 2005; Eippert et al., 2007; Jackson et al., 2000) and corrugator muscle activity (Deveney & Pizzagalli, 2008; Jackson et al., 2000) in accordance with regulatory goals. Reappraisal also has been shown to reduce the cortisol response to a stressor (Lam et al., 2009), to reduce event-related potentials associated with emotional arousal

(Deveney & Pizzagalli, 2008; Foti & Hajcak, 2008; Hajcak & Nieuwenhuis, 2006), and to enhance memory for the emotional material that is reappraised (Dillon, Ritchey, Johnson, & LaBar, 2007; Richards & Gross, 2000). Reappraisal, therefore, has remained a focus of empirical investigation, and has been a focal point in the investigation of the neural underpinnings of emotion regulation. Below, we outline a neural model for reappraisal and review functional neuroimaging studies that have added to our knowledge of the cognitive and neural mechanisms that comprise reappraisal.

Deriving a Neurofunctional Model

In the past decade or so, functional neuroimaging has significantly advanced conceptualizations of emotion regulation (Ochsner & Gross, 2008). One way that it has done this is by adding a measure of central nervous system activity to the multimeasure approach that emotion scientists have used for decades to measure emotional responding. Because no single measure serves as a "gold standard" for measuring the presence or absence of an emotion, previous studies have measured self-reports of emotional experience alongside peripheral physiological measures associated with sympathetic nervous system activity. Noninvasive neuroimaging techniques add another level of measurement: activation from emotion-generative regions.

One emotion-generative region that has received much research attention is the amygdala (see Figure 10.3). Although activation in the amygdala was first thought to be a neural marker of fear and negative emotion, it is now thought to process both positive and negative arousal (Hamann, Ely, & Grafton, 1999). The amygdala is anatomically situated to receive multimodal sensory input and to coordinate several aspects of the emotional response (Phelps & LeDoux, 2005). The amygdala has a role in the formation of emotional memory; the direction of attention toward novel, arousing, or emotional aspects of the environment; and the modulation of physiological responses (Cahill & McGaugh, 1998; Phelps & LeDoux, 2005; Williams et al., 2001). The amygdala responds to perception of arousing and novel stimuli, even when presented below the threshold of conscious awareness (Whalen et al., 1998). Therefore, amygdala activation is thought to be a measure of emotional responding that is not necessarily dependent on consciously available subjective report. There are many reasons to believe that self-reported experience, peripheral physiology, and amygdala activation are not always redundant but sometimes coordinated measures of emotional responding (Anderson & Phelps, 2002; Ochsner et al., 2004; Wager, Davidson, Hughes, Lindquist, & Ochsner, 2008). Because these measures are vulnerable to different types of bias, assessing more than one measure at a time increases the interpretability of the data.

Neuroimaging also has allowed for a richer conceptualization of the emotion regulatory processes that are engaged when regulation strategies are used. Previously, emotion regulation strategies could only be evaluated by their effect on emotional response systems. This made it difficult to separate the effort associated with attempted regulation from the effects of successful regulation. Until the last decade, very little neuroscience research had addressed this topic directly, so insights regarding the neural bases of cognitive emotion regulation were gleaned by analogy and inference from networks identified in studies of "cold" forms of cognitive control.

Some cognitive control processes that are associated with activation in these regions are goal maintenance (dorsolateral prefrontal cortex; DLPFC), generation of verbal mate-

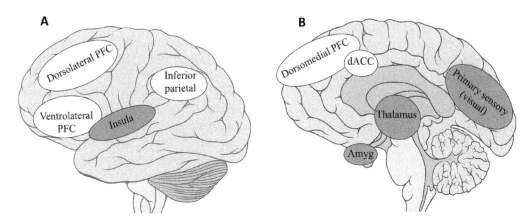

FIGURE 10.3. A representation of the cognitive down-regulation of emotion. An encounter with an emotional stimulus triggers a response in both emotional reactivity systems (gray) and emotion regulation systems (white). With successful regulation, the response in the emotional reactivity system can be substantially decreased. PFC, prefrontal cortex; Amyg, amygdala; dACC, dorsal anterior cingulate cortex. Brain sections by Patrick J. Lynch, medical illustrator, and C. Carl Jaffe, MD, cardiologist.

rial (left ventrolateral prefrontal cortex; VLPFC), maintenance and manipulation components of working memory (lateral prefrontal cortex; LPFC), response inhibition and controlled selection of appraisals (right VLFPC), conflict detection and monitoring (dorsal anterior cingulate cortex; dACC) and the direction of attention in space (inferior parietal regions; Aron, Robbins, & Poldrack, 2004; Carter & van Veen, 2007; Miller & Cohen, 2001; Ochsner & Gross, 2005; Smith & Jonides, 1999; Wager et al., 2008; see Figure 10.3). Although it is inappropriate to deduce which processes are crucial for emotion regulation based on which neural regions are activated during a regulation task, these previously established relationships mean that it is possible to generate hypotheses that lead to more specific research questions about neural bases. In addition, identifying the subsets of these regions that are engaged during different types of regulation provides a new way to compare different types of regulation, and a new basis for interpretation regarding the processes that are shared or that distinguish between different types of regulation.

TESTING A NEUROFUNCTIONAL MODEL OF REAPPRAISAL

To translate these neuroscientific predictions into testable hypotheses, we and others have conducted fMRI studies of reappraisal, whose design allowed us to make direct inferences regarding the roles that cognitive- and emotion-processing systems play in the reappraisal process.

Initial Studies of the Neural Bases of Reappraisal

Several initial studies used fMRI to address the general question of how reappraisal exerts its emotion-modulatory effects. More specifically, these studies first addressed the neural substrates of emotional responding that are modulated by reappraisal, and second, they identified what types of cognitive processes may support reappraisal. Most of these initial studies employed variations on an event-related picture-viewing paradigm that allows us to separate emotional reactivity from the effects of reappraisal (Jackson et al., 2000; Ochsner & Gross, 2008). In this task, participants view a series of negative images that are commonly used in experimental investigations of emotion (Lang, Bradley, & Cuthbert, 2001). Before performing the task, participants are trained to respond to an instruction to reappraise (commonly cued by the words *decrease, reframe,* or *think differently*). During this training for the down-regulation of negative affect, the experimenter guides them through appropriate reappraisals, in which the emotional meaning of a negative picture is changed to be less negative. For example, appropriate reappraisals of a man lying in a hospital bed include considering that he is not very seriously ill, he is being well taken care of, or that he will soon recover. During the task itself, trials with the reappraisal instruction are pseudorandomly mixed with trials in which participants are asked to look and respond naturally to negative pictures (a nonregulation instruction).

Two comparisons are typically performed to identify brain regions modulated by, and involved with, reappraisal: To characterize the effect of reappraisal on emotion processing, we identified regions more active on the nonregulation than on reappraise trials. These should be regions involved in the generation of an emotional response. To identify regions that are recruited during the cognitive control of emotion, we looked for regions in which activation was greater during reappraisal than during the nonregulation trials. Results on this task in healthy controls have been remarkably consistent across studies, laboratory groups, and variations on timing and structure of the picture-based task (Eippert et al., 2007; Gross, 1998a; Harenski & Hamann, 2006; Herwig et al., 2007; Kim & Hamann, 2007; Kross et al., 2009; Mak, Hu, Zhang, Xiao, & Lee, 2009; McRae, Hughes, et al., 2010; McRae, Ochsner, Mauss, Gabrieli, & Gross, 2008; Ochsner et al., 2002, 2004; Ohira et al., 2006; Phan et al., 2005; Schaefer et al., 2002; Urry et al., 2006; Wager et al., 2008; for a review, see Ochsner & Gross, 2005).

Across studies, the emotion-processing contrast shows modulation of visual cortex, thalamic regions, and although sometimes requiring a region-of-interest analysis, modulation of the amygdala. The cognitive control contrast shows activation primarily in left prefrontal regions implicated in working memory and response selection. The left lateralized nature of these activations is consistent with the idea that participants use verbal strategic processes to construct novel reframes of the evocative photos they viewed. Activation is also observed in medial PFC and DACC during reappraisal, which implicates self-related processing, likely related to the monitoring of one's own emotional state (Hutcherson et al., 2005; Van Overwalle, 2008). Last, bilateral activation is observed in the inferior parietal cortex during reappraisal, which indicates the involvement of the attentional control system (Wager, Jonides, & Reading, 2004). These findings are consistent with the idea that reappraisal can influence regions involved in the generation of an emotion, and does so using regions that are thought to be involved in cognitive control more generally. As our model of the neural bases of reappraisal would predict, activation in some reappraisal-related regions is negatively correlated with activation in the amygdala, a relationship that has been directly demonstrated across studies (Ochsner et al., 2002; Urry et al., 2006; but see Banks, Eddy, Angstadt, Nathan, & Phan, 2007; Wager et al., 2008).

These studies have identified the emotional outcomes of reappraisal and hinted at the cognitive control processes operating during reappraisal. These studies focused on the use of reappraisal to down-regulate negative affect. This was an important first step, but it illuminates only one of the ways reappraisal can influence emotional responding. In the next section, we broaden our focus to several types of reappraisal, and compare reappraisal to other types of emotion regulation strategies.

Types of Reappraisal and Other Emotion Regulation Strategies

In the initial fMRI experiments described earlier, reappraisal was used only to attenuate, or down-regulate, negative emotion. The use of reappraisal to decrease negative emotion might be the most relevant to process related to mood and anxiety disorders, so this was a reasonable starting point. However, many questions about reappraisal are unanswered by this narrow definition of reappraisal. First, it is important to consider that reappraisal can enhance rather than diminish the emotional impact of a situation. In the service of up-regulation, can reappraisal be used to increase, as well as decrease, responses in emotion-generative regions? Does using reappraisal for up-regulation engage the same control circuitry as that for down-regulation? Second, it is important to consider that reappraisal can also be used to modulate emotional responding to positive stimuli. It is common to try to enhance the amusement we feel in a vibrant social setting, or to increase the joy we feel at a wedding. Last, it is important to distinguish reappraisal from other types of emotion regulation. Some neural processes engaged during reappraisal might be common to all types of regulation, but others may be unique to the reconsideration of meaning that occurs during reappraisal.

Increasing and Decreasing Negative Affect

To investigate reappraisal for the purpose of increasing as well as decreasing, we used fMRI to compare directly the use of reappraisal to either down- or up-regulate negative emotional responses (Ochsner et al., 2004). We employed a variant of the experimental method in our initial study. This time, on each trial, participants first were cued either to increase or decrease their negative affect in response to a subsequently presented photo.

On the emotion-generation side of the reappraisal equation, we hypothesized that down-regulating negative affect should once again decrease activation in the amygdala, but that up-regulating negative affect should increase it. We observed this very pattern in amygdala activity, showing that individuals can both amplify and diminish their amygdala response in accordance with their emotion regulatory goals. Turning next to the control side of the reappraisal equation, our basic hypothesis was that changing the goal of reappraisal from the down-regulation to the up-regulation of emotion should not change many of the essential processes used to generate a verbal strategy for reinterpreting an event. In both cases, a common set of control systems used to generate the stories should be recruited. However, generating stories that make us feel worse or better about negative events may also recruit some distinct control systems.

To identify regions associated with the up- or down-regulation of negative emotion, we contrasted activation on increase or decrease trials with activation on baseline trials, when participants were instructed to respond naturally. Results provided support for our hypothesis that these two uses of reappraisal should involve some common and some distinct control systems. Both up- and down-regulating negative emotion engaged left lateral prefrontal control systems implicated in verbal strategic processes, such as the maintenance and manipulation of verbal information in working memory processes essential to reappraisal.

We identified regions unique to each form of reappraisal by directly comparing activation on increase and decrease trials. In keeping with predictions, up-regulating negative affect uniquely recruited a region of left rostral LPFC previously implicated in self-generating negative words to emotional category cues (Cato et al., 2004; Lane & McRae, 2004), whereas down-regulating negative affect recruited right LPFC and lateral orbitofrontal cortex regions previously implicated in inhibiting prepotent responses and altering emotional associations. These patterns of similarities and differences between up- and down-regulation have been replicated several times (Eippert et al., 2007; Kim & Hamann, 2007; Mak et al., 2009), leading to the overall conclusion that many cognitive control processes are engaged regardless of the regulatory goal, but that some processes are unique to increasing or decreasing negative affect.

Reappraising Positive Stimuli

These studies provide a strong foundation for understanding the neural bases for using reappraisal to up- and down-regulate negative emotion when presented with inherently negative pictures. Our next goal was to understand whether reappraisal could be used in another important emotional context: to up- or down-regulate positive emotion, such as amusement. There are many professional or somber moments in which the experience or display of strong positive emotion may be unhelpful or inappropriate, and must be down-regulated. In addition, the up-regulation of positive affect is useful to navigate social situations, in which those around one are more mirthful than one might feel, as well as to counteract negative emotion, when one is less mirthful than one might wish to be.

A behavioral and psychophysiological study indicated that individuals could increase and decrease their self-reported negative affect and sympathetic nervous system activation in accordance with reappraisal instructions to increase and decrease amusement (Giuliani, McRae, & Gross, 2008). However, the degree to which the reappraisal of positive and negative emotion relies on the same neural networks was until recently unknown. Kim and Hamann (2007) performed this comparison when they used a complete factorial design to investigate the neural bases of up- and down-regulating positive and negative stimuli. They observed reappraisal-related modulation of the amygdala in accordance with the regulation goal. For the first time, they reported increases in striatal activation in accordance with the increase instruction for positive pictures. Like the regulation of negative emotion, they found dorsomedial PFC, LPFC, and ACC regions that were activated during up- and down-regulation of positive pictures. In addition, they identified medial prefrontal and cingulate regions that showed greater activation while using reappraisal to up-regulate positive affect than to down-regulate positive affect.

Comparing Different Types of Emotion Regulation

To this point, investigations of the neural basis of emotion regulation have focused on cognitive reappraisal. However, several other regulation strategies outlined by the process model of emotion regulation are also commonly used. We sought to compare reappraisal to the two strategies that precede and follow it in the process model: attentional deployment and response modulation. Our goal was to compare and contrast the emotional effects of these different strategies, to see which strategies resulted in greater down-regulation of (1) self-reported negative affect and (2) amygdala activation. In addition, we wanted to examine the degree to which these different strategies employed overlapping or distinct neural networks related to cognitive control more generally.

Reappraisal and Distraction

We compared reappraisal with an attentional deployment strategy, distraction, by using a slight modification of the reappraisal task described earlier (McRae, Hughes, et al., 2010). Like previous studies, we used the instruction to look and respond naturally, or to reappraise negative pictures. To study distraction, we used a working memory task to direct attention away from the emotional content of the picture. Participants were asked to maintain six letters during picture presentation and were tested on this maintenance after the picture went off the screen.

We first examined the success with which these two regulation strategies reduced different aspects of the emotional response. We saw that both regulation strategies resulted in a significant decrease in self-reported negative affect in response to the pictures. However, the decrease due to reappraisal was significantly greater than the decrease due to distraction. In terms of neural indices of negative affect, we also observed significant down-regulation of amygdala activation for both strategies. However, distraction resulted in a more significant decrease in amygdala activation than reappraisal.

In terms of the control networks engaged by these two strategies, we observed a network of overlapping regions that included bilateral DLPFC, VLPFC, and inferior parietal cortices. However, we also saw that many of these regions showed greater activation during reappraisal than during distraction. In addition, we noticed several regions showing greater activation for reappraisal than for distraction, including anterior temporal cortices and medial PFC. We interpreted these activations as representing the processing of emotional meaning, which occurs to a greater extent during reappraisal than distraction. In comparison to the regions that were more active during reappraisal than distraction, very few regions were more active for distraction than for reappraisal. Only inferior parietal cortex and a small prefrontal region were more active during distraction.

We interpreted these findings to indicate that reappraisal is more effective at reducing the subjective experience of emotion, but that it is a relatively complex cognitive process that involves maintaining and manipulating the affective meaning of the negative stimulus. Distraction, on the other hand, is more effective at reducing amygdala activation, and may be a simpler cognitive process. We think that these distinctions help to delineate the situations in which it might be more effective to use distraction or reappraisal.

Reappraisal and Suppression

We also compared cognitive reappraisal with expressive suppression, one of the frequently studied strategies that falls under the category of response modulation (Goldin et al., 2009). In this study, participants viewed 15-second disgusting film clips while following instructions to use a distancing reappraisal to decrease their experience of negative emotion (reappraisal), or to inhibit their facial expressions in such a way that no one could tell how they were feeling (*expressive suppression*). As with distraction, we were interested in the relative success of both strategies at reducing self-reported negative affect, as well as activity in the amygdala. Additionally, we measured facial expressive behavior while participants completed the task and investigated the effects of both strategies on the expressive component of the emotional response.

We observed significant down-regulation of emotional experience when participants were reappraising, and when they were using expressive suppression. However, this difference was significantly greater when participants were reappraising. As with the studies mentioned earlier, we observed significant down-regulation of amygdala activation when individuals were reappraising. However, we observed an *increase* in amygdala activation when individuals were asked to suppress their facial expressions. This is consistent with previous reports that suppression results in greater sympathetic activation than does responding naturally to a negative stimulus (Gross, 1998a). Finally, both reappraisal and suppression resulted in decreased facial expressive behavior, but this difference was greatest when individuals were asked to suppress.

In terms of the neural networks involved in these emotion regulation strategies, we considered two important aspects of overlap and difference. First, as with previous reports, we examined differences in which regions were recruited by each of the strategies. However, because we used 15-second film clips, we were also able to investigate differences in the temporal dynamics of these different strategies. Both levels of analysis proved informative: We observed activation in bilateral DLPFC and VLPFC (stronger on the left) and bilateral parietal cortices during reappraisal. These regions were active very early in the film clip, and then activation trailed off to nonsignificant levels by the last 5 seconds of the clip. By contrast, suppression uniquely recruited areas of right VLPFC that have been previously implicated in motor inhibition tasks. Interestingly, activation in this region became stronger over the 15-second film clip, reaching its highest levels during the last 5 seconds. We interpreted these differences as indicating that the cognitive processes required for reappraisal are relatively "front-loaded," but continue to have an effect on emotional experience and amygdala activation throughout the duration of the negative stimulus. The processes recruited by suppression, by contrast, became increasingly active as the negative stimulus endured, but paradoxically resulted in increased amygdala activation by the end of the clip.

Summary of Neural Findings to Date

Together with the previous work, this series of studies of the neurocognitive bases of reappraisal have identified several important properties of the mechanism by which reappraisal can modulate emotion. The first is that reappraisal successfully modulates emotion-processing regions such as the amygdala and the striatum in accordance with the regulatory goal. The second is that reappraisal depends on prefrontal systems implicated more broadly in other forms of cognitive control. Depending on the goal of reappraisal, to up- or down-regulate negative emotion, similar and overlapping but distinct networks of prefrontal control systems will be recruited to make one feel better or worse.

Studies comparing reappraisal to other strategies indicate that different emotion regulation strategies have some elements in common but are also different in important ways. Distraction, reappraisal, and suppression reduced self-reported negative affect, but reappraisal consistently resulted in the greatest decrease in this measure of emotion. In terms of amygdala activation, distraction resulted in the greatest decrease, and reappraisal resulted in a significant, but smaller, decrease. Suppression, however, resulted in an increase in amygdala activation. This pattern of amygdala activation is consistent with the claim that emotion regulation strategies gain more commanding control over emotion the earlier they intervene in the emotion-generation process. Some of the regions involved in reappraisal are also recruited during the use of other regulation strategies, such as distraction and expressive suppression. However, there are also distinct regions whose activation distinguishes reappraisal from these other strategies, and the timing of these regions further distinguishes these regulation strategies. The processes reflected by the activation in these regions should inform the contexts in which it is most adaptive to use reappraisal or another type of strategy.

IMPLICATIONS AND FUTURE DIRECTIONS

Our working model of the cognitive control of emotion necessarily simplifies matters, and much work remains to further test the model and extend it to other types of emotion regulatory phenomena. In this section, we use the model to help generate hypotheses concerning emotion and emotion regulation in a series of domains to illustrate how neurocognitive analyses could develop our model and deepen our understanding of emotion regulation processes.

Individual Differences in Reappraisal

Just as there is considerable variation across individuals and groups in emotional reactivity, there is also variation across individuals and groups in the frequency and skill with which they use different emotion regulation strategies. Several studies have examined group differences related to the capacity to use emotion regulation when trained to do so. For example, according to self-reported negative affect reports, adolescents become more successful at reappraisal throughout development, and improvements in reappraisal are mediated by increases in cognitive functioning during development (McRae, Gross, et al., 2010). Limited neuroimaging evidence hints that both young adolescents and older adults can successfully modulate amygdala activity in accordance with an explicitly stated emotion regulation goal (Levesque et al., 2003; Urry et al., 2006). However, adult men and women show interesting differences on this task: Although they show no differences in self-reported reappraisal success, men show greater reduction in amygdala activity than do women (McRae et al., 2008).

In addition to age and gender, personality and cognitive variables influence success when using a given strategy. One important source of individual variation is thought to be the frequency with which different strategies are used in everyday life. In the case of reappraisal, those who use reappraisal more frequently seem to enjoy long-term benefits that are conceptual extensions of the short-term benefits observed in laboratory studies. Frequent reappraisers report greater well-being, greater positive affect, lesser negative affect, and fewer depressive symptoms than infrequent reappraisers (Gross & John, 2003). More frequent use of reappraisal has also been associated with lesser amygdala activity when individuals are viewing emotional faces (Drabant, McRae, Manuck, Hariri, & Gross, 2009). Therefore, those who use reappraisal frequently appear somewhat buffered from their negative emotional encounters. Although this relationship is important to document, the mechanism by which these long-term habits influence online emotional processing is unknown. One possibility is that these individuals engage in reappraisal even when not explicitly instructed to do so, an idea we develop further in the next section.

Uninstructed Emotion Regulation

The experimental literature reviewed earlier examines the effects of reappraisal when participants are trained in reappraisal and instructed to use it during certain parts of an experimental task. However, this capacity to use reappraisal may not be the only predictor of real-life reappraisal use. It is possible that some individuals engage in emotion regulation without being trained or instructed, and so many have become interested in what has been called spontaneous, automatic, implicit, or *uninstructed emotion regulation*.

Many investigations into the use of uninstructed emotion regulation infer the use of regulation based on two observations. The first, as mentioned earlier, is covariation with an individual-difference measure that sensibly relates to emotion regulation. For example, one study found that resting EEG asymmetry predicted uninstructed emotional responding to negative pictures, and inferred that this biologically based individual difference reflected spontaneous engagement of emotion regulation processes (Jackson et al., 2003). The second is the inference of regulation from diminished emotional responding. Although many studies conclude that regulation might have been used if responding is lessened, it is also possible to bias individuals' likelihood of using a strategy without explicitly instructing them to do so. One investigation of automatic emotion regulation used an implicit priming task that manipulated whether participants were exposed to regulation-related words (e.g., *contain, calm*, and *cool*) as opposed to expression-related words (e.g., *explode, hot*, and *burst*). This study found diminished anger reactivity following the regulation prime (Mauss, Evers, Wilhelm, & Gross, 2006).

These initial studies are exciting in that they indicate there may be less direct, conscious, and effortful ways that individuals influence their own emotional responding. However, there are some challenges in studying implicit or automatic emotion regulation. In the case of individual differences, it is impossible to tell which processes are occurring to a greater or lesser degree in those individuals who show less emotional responding in these tasks. Are these individuals just less emotionally responsive to begin with, and have therefore developed a sense of great success regulating their emotions, along with experience-based biological changes? Or are they engaging in a quick and effective reappraisal that occurs so quickly they do not even think of it as requiring effort? More broadly, what processes are included under this umbrella of implicit emotion regulation? Would covert shifts in attention, or implicit cognitive biases, be included in the definition of spontaneous emotion regulation, or are these more aptly considered part of unregulated emotional responding?

Emotion Regulation in Clinical Disorders

Emotion regulation is thought to play a role in most mood and anxiety disorders. The DSM-IV descriptions of major depressive disorder, anxiety disorders, and posttraumatic stress disorder include the mention of exaggerated, overwhelming, or uncontrollable negative affect (American Psychiatric Association, 2000). Recently, the same paradigm used to study emotional reactivity and regulation in healthy controls has been used to determine the degree to which these disorders are characterized by a decreased capacity to use cognitive reappraisal to decrease negative emotion. Neuroimaging evidence indicates that the inverse relationship between reappraisal-related prefrontal regions and amygdala activity is not as strong or effective in those with these clinical disorders. Those with posttraumatic stress disorder are less successful when using reappraisal to reduce self-reported negative affect, and fail to recruit prefrontal regions that healthy controls use to reappraise (New et al., 2009). Several disordered populations, including those with major depressive disorder, social anxiety disorder, specific phobia, and borderline personality disorder, show less activation in regulation-related regions, or diminished functional connectivity between the regulation-related regions and the amygdala that is observed in healthy controls (Goldin, Manber-Ball, Werner, Heimberg, & Gross, 2009; Hermann et al., 2009; Johnstone, van Reekum, Urry, Kalin, & Davidson, 2007; Koenigsberg et al., 2009). These deficits in emotion regulation are important aspects of these disorders and offer promising avenues for intervention that may correct or reverse these difficulties in emotion regulation in clinical disorders.

CONCLUSIONS

The ability to modify our emotional responses is a core feature of self-regulation. In this chapter, we have used the process model of emotion regulation to group emotion regulation strategies into loose-knit families. Using this framework as a backdrop, we have focused primarily on cognitive reappraisal, a powerful way to use cognition to change the emotion that follows. We have discussed reappraisal as an effective way to modulate many aspects of the emotional response. In addition, we have identified cognitive processes that constitute reappraisal. These include language generation, internal state monitoring, working memory, attentional control, and goal pursuit. These cognitive processes are engaged when reappraisal is used to increase or decrease positive, negative, or neutral emotional targets. Some of these processes are specific to reappraisal, and others are engaged during other types of regulation. This provides us with a better basis for determining which strategies are maximally adaptive in different situations. Finally, we have outlined three important directions for future on emotion regulation research: identifying individual differences in emotion regulation, distinguishing between implicit and explicit regulation, and characterizing the role of emotion regulation in clinical disorders.

REFERENCES

American Psychiatric Association. (2000). *Diagnostic and statistical manual of mental disorders* (4th ed., text rev.). Washington, DC: Author.

Anderson, A. K., & Phelps, E. A. (2002). Is the human amygdala critical for the subjective experience of emotion?: Evidence of intact dispositional affect in patients with amygdala lesions. *Journal of Cognitive Neuroscience, 14,* 709–720.

Aron, A. R., Robbins, T. W., & Poldrack, R. A. (2004). Inhibition and the right inferior frontal cortex. *Trends in Cognitive Sciences, 8,* 170–177.

Banks, S. J., Eddy, K. T., Angstadt, M., Nathan, P. J., & Phan, K. L. (2007). Amygdala frontal connectivity during emotion regulation. *Social Cognitive and Affective Neuroscience, 2,* 303–312.

Beck, A. T., Rush, A. J., Shaw, P. F., & Emery, G. (1979). *Cognitive therapy of depression*. New York: Guilford Press.

Cahill, L., & McGaugh, J. L. (1998). Mechanisms of emotional arousal and lasting declarative memory. *Trends in Neuroscience, 21*, 294–299.

Campbell-Sills, L., & Barlow, D. H. (2007). Incorporating emotion regulation into conceptualizations and treatments of anxiety and mood disorders. In J. J. Gross (Ed.), *Handbook of emotion regulation* (pp. 542–559). New York: Guilford Press.

Carter, C. S., & van Veen, V. (2007). Anterior cingulate cortex and conflict detection: An update of theory and data. *Cognitive, Affective and Behavioral Neuroscience, 7*, 367–379.

Cato, M. A., Crosson, B., Gökçay, D., Soltysik, D., Wierenga, C., Gopinath, K., et al. (2004). Processing words with emotional connotation: An fMRI study of time course and laterality in rostral frontal and retrosplenial cortices. *Journal of Cognitive Neuroscience, 16*, 167–177.

Davidson, R. J., Putnam, K. M., & Larson, C. L. (2000). Dysfunction in the neural circuitry of emotion regulation—a possible prelude to violence. *Science, 289*, 591–594.

Deveney, C. M., & Pizzagalli, D. A. (2008). The cognitive consequences of emotion regulation: An ERP investigation. *Psychophysiology, 45*, 435–444.

Dillon, D. G., & LaBar, K. S. (2005). Startle-modulation during conscious emotion regulation is arousal-dependent. *Behavioral Neuroscience, 119*, 1118–1124.

Dillon, D. G., Ritchey, M., Johnson, B. D., & LaBar, K. S. (2007). Dissociable effects of conscious emotion regulation strategies on explicit and implicit memory. *Emotion, 7*, 354–365.

Drabant, E. M., McRae, K., Manuck, S. B., Hariri, A. R., & Gross, J. J. (2009). Individual differences in typical reappraisal use predict amygdala and prefrontal responses. *Biological Psychiatry, 65*, 367–373.

Eippert, F., Veit, R., Weiskopf, N., Erb, M., Birbaumer, N., & Anders, S. (2007). Regulation of emotional responses elicited by threat-related stimuli. *Human Brain Mapping, 28*, 409–423.

Foti, D., & Hajcak, G. (2008). Deconstructing reappraisal: Descriptions preceding arousing pictures modulate the subsequent neural response. *Journal of Cognitive Neuroscience, 20*, 977–988.

Giuliani, N. R., McRae, K., & Gross, J. J. (2008). The up- and down-regulation of amusement: Experiential, behavioral, and autonomic consequences. *Emotion, 8*, 714–719.

Goldin, P. R., Manber-Ball, T., Werner, K., Heimberg, R., & Gross, J. J. (2009). Neural mechanisms of cognitive reappraisal of negative self-beliefs in social anxiety disorder. *Biological Psychiatry, 66*, 1091–1099.

Goldin, P. R., McRae, K., Ramel, W., & Gross, J. J. (2009). The neural bases of emotion regulation: Reappraisal and suppression of negative emotion. *Biological Psychiatry, 65*, 170–180.

Gross, J. J. (1998a). Antecedent- and response-focused emotion regulation: Divergent consequences for experience, expression, and physiology. *Journal of Personality and Social Psychology, 74*, 224–237.

Gross, J. J. (1998b). The emerging field of emotion regulation: An integrative review. *Review of General Psychology, 2*, 271–299.

Gross, J. J., & John, O. P. (2003). Individual differences in two emotion regulation processes: Implications for affect, relationships, and well-being. *Journal of Personality and Social Psychology, 85*, 348–362.

Gross, J. J., & Thompson, R. A. (2007). Emotion regulation: Conceptual foundations. In J. J. Gross (Ed.), *Handbook of emotion regulation* (pp. 3–24). New York: Guilford Press.

Hajcak, G., & Nieuwenhuis, S. (2006). Reappraisal modulates the electrocortical response to unpleasant pictures. *Cognitive, Affective, and Behavioral Neuroscience, 6*, 291–297.

Hamann, S., Ely, T. D., & Grafton, S. (1999). Amygdala activity related to enhanced memory for pleasant and aversive stimuli. *Nature Neuroscience, 2*, 289–293.

Harenski, C. L., & Hamann, S. (2006). Neural correlates of regulating negative emotions related to moral violations. *NeuroImage, 30,* 313–324.

Hermann, A., Schafer, A., Walter, B., Stark, R., Vaitl, D., & Schienle, A. (2009). Emotion regulation in spider phobia: Role of the medial prefrontal cortex. *Social Cognitive and Affective Neuroscience, 4,* 257–267.

Herwig, U., Baumgartner, T., Kaffenberger, T., Brühl, A., Kottlow, M., Schreiter-Gasser, U., et al. (2007). Modulation of anticipatory emotion and perception processing by cognitive control. *NeuroImage, 37,* 652–662.

Hutcherson, C. A., Goldin, P. R., Ochsner, K. N., Gabrieli, J. D. E., Feldman Barrett, L., & Gross, J. J. (2005). Attention and emotion: Does rating emotion alter neural responses to amusing and sad films? *NeuroImage, 27,* 656–668.

Jackson, D. C., Malmstadt, J. R., Larson, C. L., & Davidson, R. J. (2000). Suppression and enhancement of emotional responses to unpleasant pictures. *Psychophysiology, 37,* 515–522.

Jackson, D. C., Mueller, C. J., Dolski, I., Dalton, K. M., Nitschke, J. B., Urry, H. L., et al. (2003). Now you feel it, now you don't: Frontal brain electrical asymmetry and individual differences in emotion regulation. *Psychological Science, 14,* 612–617.

Johnstone, T., van Reekum, C. M., Urry, H. L., Kalin, N. H., & Davidson, R. J. (2007). Failure to regulate: Counterproductive recruitment of top-down prefrontal-subcortical circuitry in major depression. *Journal of Neuroscience, 27,* 8877–8884.

Kalisch, R., Wiech, K., Critchley, H. D., Seymour, B., O'Doherty, J. B., Oakley, D. A., et al. (2005). Anxiety reduction through detachment: Subjective, physiological, and neural effects. *Journal of Cognitive Neuroscience, 17,* 874–883.

Kim, S. H., & Hamann, S. (2007). Neural correlates of positive and negative emotion regulation. *Journal of Cognitive Neuroscience, 19,* 776–798.

Koenigsberg, H. W., Fan, J., Ochsner, K. N., Liu, X., Guise, K. G., Pizzarello, S., et al. (2009). Neural correlates of the use of psychological distancing to regulate responses to negative social cues: A study of patients with borderline personality disorder. *Biological Psychiatry, 66*(9), 854–863.

Koriat, A., Melkman, R., Averill, J. R., & Lazarus, R. S. (1972). The self-control of emotional reactions to a stressful film. *Journal of Personality, 40,* 601–619.

Kross, E., Davidson, M., Weber, J., & Ochsner, K. (2009). Coping with emotions past: The neural bases of regulating affect associated with negative autobiographical memories. *Biological Psychiatry, 65,* 361–366.

Lam, S., Dickerson, S. S., Zoccola, P. M., & Zaldivar, F. (2009). Emotion regulation and cortisol reactivity to a social-evaluative speech task. *Psychoneuroendocrinology, 34,* 1355–1362.

Lane, R. D., & McRae, K. (2004). Neural substrates of conscious emotional experience: A cognitive-neuroscientific perspective. In M. Beauregard (Ed.), *Consciousness, emotional self-regulation and the brain* (pp. 87–122). Amsterdam: Benjamins.

Lang, P. J., Bradley, M. M., & Cuthbert, B. N. (2001). International Affective Picture System (IAPS): Instruction manual and affective ratings [Technical report]. Gainesville: University of Florida, Center for Research in Psychophysiology, Gainesville.

Levenson, R. W. (1994). Human emotions: A functional view. In P. Ekman & R. J. Davidson (Eds.), *The nature of emotion: Fundamental questions* (pp. 123–126). New York: Oxford University Press.

Levesque, J., Eugene, F., Joanette, Y., Paquette, V., Mensour, B., Beaudoin, G., et al. (2003). Neural circuitry underlying voluntary suppression of sadness. *Biological Psychiatry, 53,* 502–510.

Mak, A. K. Y., Hu, Z.-G., Zhang, J. X., Xiao, Z.-W., & Lee, T. M. C. (2009). Neural correlates of regulation of positive and negative emotions: An fMRI study. *Neuroscience Letters, 457,* 101–106.

Mauss, I. B., Evers, C., Wilhelm, F. H., & Gross, J. J. (2006). How to bite your tongue without blowing your top: Implicit evaluation of emotion regulation predicts affective responding to anger provocation. *Personality and Social Psychology Bulletin, 32*, 589–602.

McRae, K., Gross, J. J., Robertson, E. R., Sokol-Hessner, P., Ray, R. D., Gabrieli, J. D. E., et al. (2010). *The development of the cognitive control of emotion.* Manuscript in preparation.

McRae, K., Hughes, B., Chopra, S., Gabrieli, J. D. E., Gross, J. J., & Ochsner, K. N. (2010). The neural correlates of cognitive reappraisal and distraction: An fMRI study of emotion regulation. *Journal of Cognitive Neuroscience, 22*, 248–262.

McRae, K., Ochsner, K. N., Mauss, I. B., Gabrieli, J. D. E., & Gross, J. J. (2008). Gender differences in emotion regulation: An fMRI study of cognitive reappraisal. *Group Processes and Intergroup Relations, 11*, 143–162.

Miller, E. K., & Cohen, J. D. (2001). An integrative theory of prefrontal cortex function. *Annual Review of Neuroscience, 24*, 167–202.

New, A. S., Fan, J., Murrough, J. W., Liu, X., Liebman, R. E., Guise, K. G., et al. (2009). A functional magnetic resonance imaging study of deliberate emotion regulation in resilience and posttraumatic stress disorder. *Biological Psychiatry, 66*, 656–664.

Ochsner, K. N., Bunge, S. A., Gross, J. J., & Gabrieli, J. D. E. (2002). Rethinking feelings: An fMRI study of the cognitive regulation of emotion. *Journal of Cognitive Neuroscience, 14*, 1215–1229.

Ochsner, K. N., & Gross, J. J. (2005). The cognitive control of emotion. *Trends in Cognitive Sciences, 9*, 242–249.

Ochsner, K. N., & Gross, J. J. (2008). Cognitive emotion regulation: Insights from social cognitive and affective neuroscience. *Current Directions in Psychological Science, 17*, 153–158.

Ochsner, K. N., Ray, R. D., Cooper, J. C., Robertson, E. R., Chopra, S., Gabrieli, J. D. E., et al. (2004). For better or for worse: Neural systems supporting the cognitive down- and up-regulation of negative emotion. *NeuroImage, 23*, 483–499.

Ohira, H., Nomura, M., Ichikawa, N., Isowa, T., Iidaka, T., Sato, A., et al. (2006). Association of neural and physiological responses during voluntary emotion suppression. *NeuroImage, 29*, 721–733.

Phan, K. L., Fitzgerald, D. A., Nathan, P. J., Moore, G. J., Uhde, T. W., & Tancer, M. E. (2005). Neural substrates for voluntary suppression of negative affect: A functional magnetic resonance imaging study. *Biological Psychiatry, 57*, 210–219.

Phelps, E. A., & LeDoux, J. E. (2005). Contributions of the amygdala to emotion processing: From animal models to human behavior. *Neuron, 48*, 175–187.

Richards, J. M., & Gross, J. J. (2000). Emotion regulation and memory: The cognitive costs of keeping one's cool. *Journal of Personality and Social Psychology, 79*, 410–424.

Schaefer, S. M., Jackson, D. C., Davidson, R. J., Aguirre, G. K., Kimberg, D. Y., & Thompson-Schill, S. L. (2002). Modulation of amygdalar activity by the conscious regulation of negative emotion. *Journal of Cognitive Neuroscience, 14*, 913–921.

Shakespeare, W., & Garrick, D. (1970). *King Henry VIII/[by William Shakespeare; with alterations by] David Garrick.* London: Cornmarket Press.

Smith, C. A., & Ellsworth, P. C. (1985). Patterns of cognitive appraisal in emotion. *Journal of Personality and Social Psychology, 48*, 813–838.

Smith, E. E., & Jonides, J. (1999). Storage and executive processes in the frontal lobes. *Science, 283*, 1657–1661.

Totterdell, P., & Parkinson, B. (1999). Use and effectiveness of self-regulation strategies for improving mood in a group of trainee teachers. *Journal of Occupational Health Psychology, 4*, 219–232.

Urry, H. L., van Reekum, C. M., Johnstone, T., Kalin, N. H., Thurow, M. E., Schaefer, H. S., et al. (2006). Amygdala and ventromedial prefrontal cortex are inversely coupled during regulation of negative affect and predict the diurnal pattern of cortisol secretion among older adults. *Journal of Neuroscience, 26*, 4415–4425.

Van Overwalle, F. (2008). Social cognition and the brain: A meta-analysis. *Human Brain Mapping, 30*(3), 829–858.

Wager, T. D., Davidson, M. L., Hughes, B. L., Lindquist, M. A., & Ochsner, K. N. (2008). Prefrontal-subcortical pathways mediating successful emotion regulation. *Neuron, 59*, 1037–1050.

Wager, T. D., Jonides, J., & Reading, S. (2004). Neuroimaging studies of shifting attention: A meta-analysis. *NeuroImage, 22*, 1679–1693.

Whalen, P. J., Rauch, S. L., Etcoff, N. L., McInerney, S. C., Lee, M. B., & Jenike, M. A. (1998). Masked presentations of emotional facial expressions modulate amygdala activity without explicit knowledge. *Journal of Neuroscience, 18*, 411–418.

Williams, L. M., Phillips, M. L., Brammer, M. J., Skerrett, D., Logopoulos, J., Rennie, C., et al. (2001). Arousal dissociates amygdala and hippocampal fear responses: Evidence from simultaneous fMRI and skin conductance recording. *NeuroImage, 14*, 1070–1079.

CHAPTER 11

Working Memory and Self-Regulation

WILHELM HOFMANN
MALTE FRIESE
BRANDON J. SCHMEICHEL
ALAN D. BADDELEY

The purpose of this chapter is to apply insights from cognitive psychology on working memory to everyday self-regulation. We first introduce contemporary views surrounding the multicomponent view of working memory. Our emphasis is on the central executive as the component that is assumed to orchestrate perceptual, cognitive, and motor processes in the service of goal pursuit. We then spell out in more detail how working memory may benefit self-regulation. Research pertaining to momentary fluctuations in working memory capacity are reviewed, as well as research highlighting the role of working memory capacity in the control of attention, thought, emotion, and action. We conclude by discussing why, in our view, there is no simple mapping of working memory operations on the distinction between conscious and nonconscious processing.

WHAT IS WORKING MEMORY?

Current frameworks of working memory (for an overview, see Miyake & Shah, 1999) originated from earlier models of short-term memory (e.g., Broadbent, 1958). Contemporary models typically go beyond these earlier models by assuming a multicomponent cognitive architecture rather than a unitary storage system. They also emphasize the function of such an architecture in complex cognition, such as the control of attention and the manipulation of information—hence, the term *working* memory—rather than information storage per se. One of the most influential frameworks for working memory in cognitive science is the multicomponent model proposed by Baddeley and Hitch (1974). The updated model (Baddeley, 2000, 2007) assumes an attentional control system, the *central executive*, and three storage subsystems, the *phonological loop*, the *visuospatial sketchpad*, and the *episodic buffer*. The phonological loop holds verbal and acoustic information. The sketchpad holds visual and spatial information. The *episodic buffer* forms an interface between long-term memory, the other storage systems, and the central executive. It is assumed to provide a common coding mechanism (i.e., a common "language") for the exchange and manipulation of information from different modalities. It thus may serve as a basis for a temporary and flexible *workspace* in which diverse information can be combined into meaningful chunks under the attentional control of the central executive. The episodic buffer, like the phonological loop and the visuospatial sketchpad, is limited by the number of chunks of information it can maintain (Baddeley, 2007).

The Central Executive

The central executive is the most elusive and difficult component to conceptualize (e.g., Baddeley, 2003; Miyake & Shah, 1999). Even though there is no generally agreed upon definition of the *central executive* to date, most researchers regard it as a broad system (or collection of subsystems) that has evolved to allow the flexible, controlled processing of information in the service of one's goals. More specifically, the central executive is often thought to subsume a number of executive functions or capacities: (1) to allocate attention to task- or goal-relevant information, thus keeping this information in an active state; (2) to enable the flexible, context-relevant manipulation and updating of the contents of working memory; and (3) to inhibit prepotent, irrelevant responses that interfere with the present task or goal at hand (Smith & Jonides, 1999). The debate surrounding the central executive is in no way finished (Miyake & Shah, 1999). Yet from the broader perspective of this chapter, one can state that at least some consensus has been reached regarding the conceptualization, underlying neurological substrates, development, and assessment of central executive functions.

First, most researchers would agree that executive control involves the flexible allocation of "top-down" or "endogenous" attentional resources in a goal-directed manner. This view is perhaps most prominently endorsed by Engle and colleagues, who use the term *executive attention* to emphasize this contention and have provided convincing evidence for the close connection between the control of attention and central executive working memory operations (Engle, Kane, & Tuholski, 1999; Kane, Bleckley, Conway, & Engle, 2001; see also Knudsen, 2007).

A second issue concerns whether the central executive is a unitary construct, or whether it can be decomposed/fractionated into more specialized subfunctions. Probably the best-known decompositional approach is Miyake, Friedman, Emerson, Witzki, and Howerter's (2000) attempt to isolate such subfunctions on the level of latent variables. Administering a large battery of executive tasks to a larger sample, Miyake et al. identified three latent factors of central executive functioning, *shifting* between task sets, *updating* (including maintaining) relevant information in working memory, and *inhibiting* prepotent responses (see Shimamura, 2000, for a related distinction). However, these three latent factors all shared considerable overlap in variance (i.e., latent correlations between .40 and .60). Although distinguishable, these factors therefore seem to share considerable underlying commonality. Moreover, little is known yet about how these discernible subfunctions interact in complex task performance or goal pursuit.

Third, with the advent of neuroscientific methods of inquiry, researchers have begun to explore the neural subsystems underlying working memory (Baddeley, 2007; Kane & Engle, 2002; see Wager & Smith, 2003, for a meta-analysis). There is no doubt that the frontal lobes are the primary region involved in central executive function (Miller & Cohen, 2001; Smith & Jonides, 1999; Stuss & Knight, 2002) or dysfunction (Baddeley & Wilson, 1988). Mirroring the previously discussed three-factor distinction, Collete and colleagues (2005) found that shifting, updating, and inhibiting involve both factor-specific brain regions and common areas of activation. However, common activity was not restricted to regions in the frontal cortex alone but was also present in more parietal regions (see also Wager & Smith, 2003). This finding suggests that central executive functions involve the orchestration of more widely distributed areas than the frontal lobes alone.

Fourth, there is converging evidence from developmental psychology that executive functioning undergoes marked developmental changes over the lifespan. Improvements during childhood and adolescence are paralleled by growth spurts in the development of the frontal lobes. Full maturation is reached only at around age 19 (see Jurado & Rosselli, 2007, for a review). Conversely, there is a decline in executive functioning at the other end of the lifespan (Hasher & Zacks, 1988; von Hippel, 2007). It has been associated with, among other things, anatomical changes (e.g., volume reductions) in the frontal lobes due to normal aging (West, 1996). However, age declines may not be inevitable because recent research suggests that working memory functions can still be trained in older adults (Dahlin, Nyberg, Backman, & Neely, 2008).

Fifth, there is wide consensus that individuals differ with regard to the effectiveness of their central executive (Barrett, Tugade, & Engle, 2004; Engle et al., 1999). Individual differences in central executive functioning are often referred to under the label of *working memory capacity* (WMC), and the assessment of these differences has been a major research enterprise over the last decades. Special attention should be allocated to the meaning of the word *capacity* as we use it here: WMC is not so much about memory capacity in terms of storage volume per se, which may be primarily determined by the storage capacity of the phonological loop, the visuospatial sketchpad, and the episodic buffer. Rather, WMC is about the capacity (in terms of effectiveness) with which the central executive can perform task-relevant operations on the stored information, in the service of the task or goal at hand. WMC limitations may therefore primarily reflect resource limitations rather than information storage limitations (Engle et al., 1999). To be sure, resource limitations can in turn lead to subsequent loss of information. For instance, information may be lost due to the inability to shield task-relevant information from interference. Given that these individual differences in WMC are likely to relate to important real-world outcomes, we now turn to the question of how such differences in WMC can be adequately assessed.

Measuring WMC

Cognitive psychologists have put a lot of effort into developing good measures of WMC, and a wide range of tests has been suggested. However, it is not always clear what exactly is measured by these tests (for a summary and critique, see Jurado & Rosselli, 2007). There will probably never be a single test of WMC because it is notoriously difficult to map the complex nature of central executive functions onto structured tests or test batteries. Nevertheless, the last decades have seen considerable advances in the development and validation of such measures. For instance, one widely used method to assess WMC is operation span (OSPAN; see Conway et al., 2005, for a review). In OSPAN tasks, participants have to engage in a primary processing task (e.g., memorizing presented information). At the same time, they have to engage in an interfering secondary processing task (e.g., indicating via keypress whether a presented equation is true or false). Participants taking an OSPAN task would see items such as: IS 3 + 5 = 9? (keypress) "HOUSE." After three to eight items are presented in a sequence, the participant would then be asked to recall the words in their serial order. Hence, participants have to update the information relevant to the primary task (i.e., the words) and shield this task-relevant information from interfering information imposed by the secondary task. The number of trial items correctly solved, weighted by trial length, serves as a measure of WMC. Individual differences measured with OSPAN tasks have been shown to predict performance on a wide range of real-world, higher-order cognitive abilities, such as reading comprehension, language comprehension, reasoning abilities, and lecture note taking (e.g., Daneman & Carpenter, 1980; Kiewra & Benton, 1988; for a review, see Barrett et al., 2004).

From a decompositional perspective (e.g., Miyake et al., 2000), one could say that most specialized experimental tasks primarily tap into one of the three executive functions identified earlier. OSPAN measures, for instance, have been found to load primarily on the updating factor, which is consistent with the high task demands of maintaining and updating task-relevant information (Miyake et al., 2000). Conversely, Stroop (1935) or stop-signal task performance (Logan, Cowan, & Davis, 1984) is typically more strongly associated with the inhibition factor, as would be expected given that participants have to inhibit a prepotent response. More complex executive tasks, however, such as the Wisconsin Card Sorting Test (Berg, 1948) or the Tower of London (Shallice, 1982), appear to tap into a combination of factors (Jurado & Rosselli, 2007; Miyake et al., 2000).

BRIDGING WMC AND SELF-REGULATION RESEARCH

In our view, the working memory literature from cognitive psychology and the social and personality psychological literature on self-regulation have largely led separate lives (Baddeley, 2007; for a notable exception, see Barrett et al., 2004). This is regrettable since both fields may benefit greatly from each other's insights and expertise. Although recent years have seen significant advances in bridging the two areas, much work needs to be done. The purpose of this section is to spell out how working memory may aid self-regulatory goal pursuit. To build such a bridge, two pillars need to be constructed. First, we propose that the working memory mechanisms identified in basic cognitive research relate directly to the mechanisms involved in self-regulatory goal pursuit. Second, we attempt to explain how working memory—traditionally a "cool" cognitive concept—may be involved in the regulation of "hot" processes. Such hot processes make up an essential part of everyday self-regulation, especially the regulation of emotions, desires, and cravings. In the following we first explore this latter question of how cold and hot cognition might meet. We then highlight several working memory mechanisms that we believe are central to the self-regulation of everyday behavior.

Hot Cognition: Working Memory and the Regulation of Emotions and Desires

The main line of thinking we adopt here is that emotions, desires, urges, and cravings all initiate as phenomenal *primitives*, that is, relatively automatic processing outcomes that typically involve bodily sensations and crude feelings or "core affect" (Frijda, 2005; Hofmann & Wilson, 2010; Russell, 2003). The extent to which such basic phenomenal experiences gain access to working memory and its resources may depend (1) on the strength of bottom-up activation (i.e., the strength of the initial signal produced by affective and reward-related processing modules in lower regions of the brain) and (2) on whether the "spotlight" of (top-down) attention is allocated to the signal, thereby amplifying and maintaining it above a critical threshold necessary for its mental representation in working memory (Dehaene & Naccache, 2001; Hofmann & Wilson, 2010). Once in the focus of executive attention, immediate affective reactions may develop into more full-blown emotions because they are endowed with a richer set of cognitions generated by attribution and appraisal processes (Baumeister, Vohs, DeWall, & Zhang, 2007; Russell, 2003). These accompanying cognitions in working memory may help to shape, sustain, or even amplify the emotional experience at hand (Bradley, Cuthbert, & Lang, 1996). However, the effective deployment of working memory resources away from phenomenal cues, such as through distraction, may prevent the development of affective reactions into full-blown emotional episodes (Van Dillen & Koole, 2007; see also Koole, Van Dillen, & Sheppes, Chapter 2, this volume). In a similar vein, the flexible cognitive (re-)appraisal of affective information may help to alter significantly how an emotional episode unfolds over time (Gross, 1998).

Special consideration in the context of self-regulation should be given to an important class of hot cognition, desires (see also Herman & Polivy, Chapter 28, this volume). A *desire* can be defined as "an affectively charged cognitive event in which an object or activity that is associated with pleasure or relief of discomfort is in focal attention" (Kavanagh, Andrade, & May, 2005, p. 447). As Kavanagh and colleagues (2005) pointed out in their elaborated *intrusion theory of desire*, external (e.g., tempting objects in the environment) and internal factors (e.g., deprivation) may trigger desire-related thoughts and emotional reactions in a spontaneous, bottom-up fashion. Such automatically driven reactions are transitory events. Once in the focus of attention, however, they may receive additional elaboration in working memory and develop into "elaborated desires" (Kavanagh et al., 2005). Such elaborations may include processes of motivated reasoning (e.g., why it may be a good idea to smoke a "last" cigarette; see Sayette & Griffin, Chapter 27, this volume) and planning (e.g., how to get to the next cigarette dispenser even though it is miles away). Due to their effortful nature, elaborated desires usurp considerable working memory resources (Kemps, Tiggemann, & Grigg, 2008; Zwaan & Truitt, 1998) and may finally drive self-regulatory goal representations out of working memory (and sometimes, as the saying goes, "common sense out the window").

Working Memory Mechanisms and Self-Regulatory Goal Pursuit

A quick browse through the chapters of this handbook shows that one of the central foci of self-regulation research is how well people manage to pursue personally endorsed, long-term goals, such as getting good grades, maintaining a healthy diet, remaining faithful to one's partner, or staying clean of drugs in the presence of tempting alternatives. There is no a priori reason why the working memory operations involved in the performance of simple experimental rules, task sets, or processing goals should not also be crucial for the effective pursuit of everyday self-regulatory goals. We do not tackle here the difficult question of where these self-regulatory goals actually stem from or what determines whether or not they are personally endorsed. However, given a personally endorsed self-regulatory goal, a number of key features can be derived from the perspective of a working memory framework as to when and how self-regulatory goal pursuit may be successful.

Active Representation of Goal-Relevant Information in Working Memory

First, successful self-regulation involves the active representation of goals and goal-relevant information in working memory (Kane et al., 2001; Kuhl, 1983; Miller & Cohen, 2001; Smith & Jonides, 1999). This point is related to what has been referred to as the *standards* ingredient of self-regulation (Baumeister & Heatherton, 1996; Carver & Scheier, 1981). Goals involve a mental representation of the desired end state (i.e., the goal standard), and, typically, also a mental representation of the means by which and the circumstances under which the goal can be attained (Kruglanski et al., 2002; Miller & Cohen, 2001). Without a clear goal standard as a reference point, self-regulation is directionless and doomed to fail.

Clarity of goal standards can refer to a number of parameters. We focus here on accessibility and duration as the most central ones: The more accessible the mental representation of a goal in working memory and the longer a sufficiently high level of accessibility is maintained over time, the more likely it is that the goal can exert its "biasing" influence in the top-down control of behavior (Miller & Cohen, 2001). However, powerful distractions and temptations may cause a self-regulatory goal to drift out of working memory, thereby losing its biasing influence on attention, thought, and action (Duncan, 1995; Kavanagh et al., 2005). By directing attention to the goal, goal representations may receive renewed activation, thereby forestalling the natural decay to which all representations in working memory are subject. This is what seems to happen when people "remind" themselves (or are reminded by contextual or social cues) about their self-regulatory goals.

Directing and redirecting executive attention to goal-relevant information may be the primary mechanism by which self-regulatory goals are "shielded" from competing goals or other distractions in working memory (Shah, Friedman, & Kruglanski, 2002). In this view, goal shielding is the "passive" consequence of sustained attention to a goal or task (see also Dreisbach & Haider, 2009). Its effects are akin to the way a flashlight illuminates the particular objects at which it is pointed and at the same time leaving all other things in the dark. As a consequence of sustained attention, access to working memory may be directed toward highly goal-relevant information and divorced from possible distractions. Such a working memory state may closely correspond to what has been called an *implementation mindset* (Gollwitzer & Bayer, 1999; see Gollwitzer & Oettingen, Chapter 9, this volume). A second mechanism that may contribute to goal-shielding effects is the active inhibition of mental contents or behavioral schemas that are unrelated or incompatible with the focal goal in working memory. These inhibitory mechanisms are discussed in more detail below.

Flexible Updating of Goal Representations

Self-regulatory success may also depend on the context-relevant, flexible updating of goal representations in working memory. Updating of goal representations refers to the "monitoring" ingredient of self-regulation (Baumeister & Heatherton, 1996; Carver & Scheier, 1981). Monitoring involves the analysis of the current context, one's inner states, and one's actions. Discrepancies between the actual state and one's goal standards can thus be detected, and working memory resources can be allocated to solve the conflict at hand (Botvinick, Braver, Carter, Barch, & Cohen, 2001)—for instance, when realizing that drinking the cocktail one was just handed at a party is not a good idea in light of one's intention to drive home safely.

However, this type of conflict monitoring is probably only half the story of the updating mechanism subserved by working memory. At least as important for self-regulatory success is the capacity to adjust one's goal representation flexibly as new information about the current state keeps coming in. Whereas it is generally beneficial for one's goal persistence to actively maintain the respective goal standards in working memory, it is counterproductive to set rigidly the *means* (i.e., the plans) by which one expects to attain the goal. As one navigates through the (social) world in space and time, unforeseen obstacles may suddenly block the planned course of action, or new opportunities may present themselves. Intelligent self-regulation may benefit from the capacity to adjust plans flexibly to the changing circumstances (Vallacher & Wegner, 1987). To be sure, there is a practical question—with philosophical undertones—about the point at which, instead of adjusting means, it may be better to adjust one's standards or to disengage from the goal altogether (as when the person with whom one has always wanted to be marries someone else). Hence, goal adjustment or goal disengagement will become increasingly functional as the perceived chances for success fall below a certain threshold (Jostmann & Koole, 2009; Wrosch, Scheier, Miller, Schulz, & Carver, 2003).

Inhibition of Interfering Thoughts and Emotions

Earlier, we discussed a passive form of inhibition through attention. Self-regulation may also involve active attempts at suppressing unwanted thoughts and emotional reactions. For example, to maintain a harmonious relationship with one's partner, it may occasionally be necessary to suppress one's immediate anger to a level at which constructive responses are possible (Finkel & Campbell, 2001). The need to fence off interfering thoughts and emotions may be particularly relevant for the regulation of desires and cravings, which typically combine intrusive thoughts and hedonic feelings (Kavanagh et al., 2005).

Research by Wegner and colleagues, however, suggests that the active suppression of mental contents is a risky self-regulatory enterprise (for a review, see Wegner, 1994). First, active suppression may bring the very target of suppression into the focus of a monitoring process searching for goal-inconsistent information (Wegner, 1994). Ironically, being the focus of the current attentional task set may give the critical information an accessibility advantage in the competition for access to working memory and result in further intrusions that need to be suppressed. Second, even though it can be successful in the short run, active suppression may result in rebound effects (Wenzlaff, Wegner, & Roper, 1988) and create physiological and psychological side effects, such as increased somatic arousal and negative affect (Gross & Levenson, 1993; Polivy, 1998). Third, active suppression is a highly effortful process that saps available resources (e.g., Baumeister, Bratslavsky, Muraven, & Tice, 1998; Vohs & Heatherton, 2000). Active inhibition of mental contents may therefore be inferior to passive inhibition through selective attention, and only work reasonably well among high WMC individuals—those who have ample resources.

Behavioral Inhibition (Impulse Control)

A final hallmark of successful self-regulation is the inhibition or overriding of unwanted behavioral responses, such as habits and impulses. Although habits and impulses can be differentiated in terms of their affective qualities or "hotness" (e.g., Hofmann, Friese, & Strack, 2009), both concepts are typically used to denote prepotent behavioral responses that are activated automatically given certain context and stimulus configurations in the environment. Habits and impulses presumably activate behavioral motor schemas. These may be expressed in behavior given that a certain threshold of activation is reached (Norman & Shallice, 1986; Strack & Deutsch, 2004). However, habitual and impulsive behavioral schemas (e.g., picking one's nose) may often be incompatible with a given self-regulatory goal (e.g., appearing intelligent to others). A supervisory attentional system (SAS; Norman & Shallice, 1986) may provide a "last resort" control of behavior by inhibiting task-irrelevant or goal-incompatible schemas. At the same time, the SAS may direct extra activation to behavioral schemas that are compatible with the task or goal at hand but not yet sufficiently activated (e.g., scratching one's head instead). Baddeley (1986) and others have assigned the SAS an integral part of the central executive. It is not entirely clear, though, whether working memory should be best seen (1) as fully supervising the voluntary control of motor behavior or (2) as a mediator of behavioral control in the prefrontal cortex that closely communicates with a more specialized (and potentially separable) behavioral inhibition system at the late-output stage of information processing (e.g., McNab et al., 2008). For the sake of parsimony we do not make a distinction here and include behavioral inhibition as one of the primary functions subserved by the central executive.

Whether attempts at impulse control are successful depends on the *relative* strength of impulsive and inhibitory mechanisms (see also Herman & Polivy, Chapter 28, this volume). As William James (1890/1950; citing Clouston) put it, impulse control may fail because either "the driver may be so weak that he cannot control well-broken horses, or the horses may be so hard-mouthed that no driver can pull them up" (p. 540). In some rare cases, such as extreme temptation or compulsive disorders, impulses may simply be too strong to be controlled, even with inhibitory mechanisms fully intact. More probably, impulses that are normally held in check may break through when WMC is temporarily or dispositionally reduced (Hofmann, Friese, & Strack, 2009).

Summary

In summary, working memory processes appear to be involved in a host of mechanisms that may promote successful self-regulation. Specifically, working memory may be involved in directing and maintaining attention to goal-directed processing (thus shielding the goal from interference), in flexibly updating goal representations in accordance with changing states of the environment, and in the inhibition of interfering thoughts and emotions, as well as prepotent behavioral tendencies (Barrett et al., 2004).

In specifying the interplay between hot cognition and working memory, special consideration has been given to the idea that self-regulation often involves the regulation of desires. We have discussed two main mechanisms by which desires may influence behavior. First, tempting stimuli in the environment may often automatically activate impulsive behavioral tendencies (e.g., approaching or consuming an object of desire). What may be most needed in such circumstances is the capacity for conflict monitoring (i.e., becoming aware of potentially goal-incompatible behavior) and behavioral inhibition (i.e., stopping the problematic act). A second, perhaps more insidious route by which desires may compromise self-regulation is by "hijacking" working memory in the service of short-term hedonic fulfillment. Via this route (automatically triggered), desire-related thoughts and feelings may develop into elaborated desires that commandeer considerable working memory resources (Kavanagh et al., 2005). This case is trickier because, although desire springs from genuinely automatic processes, it may seize the control processes of planning and behavior execution that were originally harnessed by one's long-term self-regulatory goal.

It should be noted that we did not emphasize the switching component of the central executive in our discussion (Miyake et al., 2000). From the perspective of everyday self-regulation, quickly switching between two or more task sets appears to be less important for goal pursuit than maintaining and updating one's long-term goals and inhibiting distraction. We would, however, be ready to switch over to another opinion in case this factor proves to be important in explaining variance in everyday self-regulatory behavior—for instance, with regard to the balancing of multiple self-regulatory goals.

EMPIRICAL EVIDENCE

In the following, we review empirical evidence that has directly addressed the relationship between working memory and self-regulation. We start with evidence supporting the limited and fluctuating nature of WMC. Subsequently, we review research on the relationship between individual differences in WMC and the regulation of attention, thought, emotion, and action.

WMC as a Limited Resource: Cognitive Load and Depleting Aftereffects

One of the basic assumptions of the working memory model is that the capacity of the central executive is severely limited (Baddeley, 2007). Such resource limitations may manifest in two ways. A first way, primarily investigated by cognitive psychology, is related to the idea that central executive functioning is compromised by secondary task loads because the attentional resources of the central executive have to be shared between the primary and the secondary tasks. In support, numerous studies show that imposing a secondary (or dual) task reduces performance on tasks of executive control (e.g., Baddeley, Emslie, Kolodny, & Duncan, 1998; Lavie, Hirst, de Fockert, & Viding, 2004). Cognitive load manipulations have also been fruitfully applied to study the degree to which certain types of cognition and behaviors depend on cognitive control (e.g., Gilbert & Hixon, 1991; Ward & Mann, 2000). A number of "risk" situations in which people's success at self-regulation is often at stake, among them stress (Schoofs, Preuss, & Wolf, 2008), stereotype threat (Schmader & Johns, 2003), or alcohol intoxication (Saults, Cowan, Sher, & Moreno, 2007), may be functionally equivalent to cognitive load effects due to the preoccupation with task-irrelevant thoughts that they produce; that is, their documented detrimental impact on self-regulation may be mediated by temporary reductions in WMC.

A second way by which the limited capacity of the central executive may manifest itself has been illuminated by the seminal research program on ego depletion by Baumeister and colleagues (1998; for a review, see Bauer & Baumeister, Chapter 4, this volume), who argued that self-regulatory capacity may be akin to a muscle. The exertion of self-control depletes self-regulatory resources temporarily, which may compromise *subsequent* efforts at self-control (e.g., Baumeister et al., 1998; Vohs & Heatherton, 2000). Because self-regulatory resources are assumed to be domain-independent, any act of self-control may negatively affect any subsequent act of self-control. The depletion effect has been replicated with regard to a broad range of depletion manipulations and self-regulatory domains, including eating (Vohs & Heatherton, 2000), drinking (Muraven, Collins, & Neinhaus, 2002), sexual behavior (Gailliot & Baumeister, 2006), and aggression (Dewall, Baumeister, Stillman, & Gailliot, 2007). It was first conceptually related to central executive functioning in a series of studies by Schmeichel, Vohs, and Baumeister (2003), who showed that only complex, higher-order cognitive activities are negatively affected by prior depletion, such as taking the Analytical subtest of the Graduate Record Exam—a test many of us still remember with horror. In contrast, simple cognitive activities involving only information retrieval from long-term memory are unaffected by resource depletion (Schmeichel et al., 2003). These findings yielded clear evidence that ego depletion primarily drains the type of mental resources underpinning the central executive. Subsequent research has taken this idea one step further into the cognitive domain. If different facets of central executive functioning, such as shifting, updating, and response inhibition, all draw on a general resource, Schmeichel (2007) argued, each of these forms of executive control may have negative aftereffects on each other. Four experiments involving different executive tests supported this general prediction (Schmeichel, 2007). The finding that a common depletable resource may underlie all tasks of executive control may be one explanation for the relatively high degree of commonality among the subcomponents of the central executive identified by Miyake et al. (2000).

In sum, both the work in the cognitive load tradition and more recent work on the depleting aftereffects of prior self-control point to the importance of the central executive in mediating the controlled expression of behavior. Both lines of work also attest to the fluctuating nature of available WMC. Such fluctuations can result either from secondary task load or preceding demands on central executive processing.

WMC and the Self-Regulation of Attention, Thought, Emotion, and Action

There is abundant literature on the relationship between WMC and indicators of cognitive task performance, such as reading comprehension, writing (e.g., taking lecture notes), and reasoning (e.g., Barrett et al., 2004; Daneman & Merikle, 1996). However, research that relates these measures to the types of everyday self-regulatory outcomes that are the focus of this handbook appears to be still in its infancy. In reviewing this intersecting area here, we focus on studies that assessed individual differences in WMC and related these differences to the everyday self-regulation of attention, thought, emotion, and action. These four areas can be assigned to three different stages of information processing: (1) early attentional processing, (2) the regulation of internal states via thought control and emotion regulation, and (3) the control of behavior, especially the control of prepotent impulses.

WMC and the Top-Down Regulation of Attention

Attention can be regarded as an important first "battlefield" of self-regulation: Whatever grabs our attention will have a chance to plant the seeds for later behavior by gaining privileged access to working memory. The regulation of attention is assumed to be subject to a tug-of-war between stimulus-driven (bottom-up) influences and the goal-directed (top-down) allocation of attention (Corbetta & Shulman, 2002; Knudsen, 2007; Pashler, Johnston, & Ruthruff, 2001). In such a conception, the bottom-up allocation of attention is assumed to occur automatically and to be determined by stimulus properties, such as salience and motivational relevance (e.g., Knudsen, 2007). In contrast, the top-down allocation of attention is biased by goal representations in working memory (Corbetta & Shulman, 2002; Folk, Remington, & Johnston, 1992; Knudsen, 2007); that is, our current goals (e.g., shopping for healthy food) can selectively bias which incoming stimulus information receives a processing advantage in the competition for access to working memory (e.g., when entering the supermarket, the vegetable section visually "pops out" in the distance). Although goals greatly influence what we attend to, this does not mean that goal-irrelevant or competing stimuli cannot grab our attention at all. Specifically, certain stimuli in our environment may gain access to working memory because they are detected by automatic salience filters (Knudsen, 2007). The salience of stimuli can simply be the result of unexpectedness. More importantly, stimuli may be flagged as motivationally salient by reward-processing systems in the brain, which are fine-tuned to biological and learned needs of the organism (e.g., Field & Cox, 2008; Knudsen, 2007). Thus, despite an active self-regulatory goal, attention can be attracted by motivationally salient cues such as high-caloric foods (in the supermarket example, halfway to the cabbage shelf, our gaze gets diverted by the confectionery aisle to the side). To stay on track of one's self-regulatory goals, top-down attentional control is needed (1) to prevent attentional capture by distracting or irrelevant cues and (2) to disengage and redirect attention if it has been grabbed by these cues (e.g., Mischel & Ayduk, Chapter 5, this volume).

Corroborating the role of the central executive in allocating top-down attention, cognitive research has established that WMC is positively related to performance in the antisaccade task (Kane et al., 2001, Study 1). This task requires the participant to respond as quickly as possible to a target stimulus that is presented in the opposite location to an initial orienting cue (i.e., the "distractor"). A subsequent study using eye-tracking technology showed that high-WMC individuals were considerably less likely to make reflexive saccades to the orienting cue than were low-WMC individuals (Kane et al., 2001, Study 2). In other words, high-WMC individuals are better at resisting the attention-grabbing power of distracting stimuli (see also Fukuda & Vogel, 2009; Unsworth, Schrock, & Engle, 2004).

Two recent studies (Friese, Bargas-Avila, Hofmann, & Wiers, 2010; Hofmann, Gschwendner, Friese, Wiers, & Schmitt, 2008, Study 3) applied this line of reasoning to investigate attention regulation in the domains of sex and drugs (rock'n'roll is still miss-ing from that research agenda). In both of these studies, automatic affective reactions toward the stimuli of interest (pictures of seminude women or alcohol stimuli, respec-tively) were assessed with a version of the Implicit Association Test (IAT; Greenwald, McGhee, & Schwartz, 1998). WMC was assessed with an OSPAN task. In the Hofmann and colleagues (2008) study, heterosexual male participants' viewing time of sexual pic-tures relative to control pictures served as the dependent variable. Results indicated that automatic affect toward sexual stimuli predicted actual viewing time well for low- (but not high-) WMC individuals. This pattern of findings suggests that low-WMC individu-als may have had more difficulties to overcome attentional biases triggered by the affec-tive processing of the sexual material.

Friese and colleagues (2010) adopted the eye-tracking method for a more fine-grained analysis of attentional processes in the context of alcohol stimuli. The authors expected that WMC may be crucial for counteracting the bottom-up orienting and main-tenance mechanisms triggered by automatic affect. Again, automatic affect was assessed with an IAT, and WMC with an OSPAN task. Then participants were presented with a series of slides depicting one alcoholic drink and one soft drink each, and their eye-gaze behavior was tracked. In line with the predictions, only the gaze behavior of those low in WMC was influenced by automatic affect: Low-WMC individuals fixated on the alco-hol pictures quicker and spent more time fixating on them (in comparison to soft drink pictures), to the extent that they had more positive automatic affective reactions toward alcohol. In contrast, no relationship between affective reactions and attentional behavior emerged for high-WMC individuals. This finding suggests that the latter group may have successfully counteracted the influence of prepotent automatic associations at the early stage of attention orientation and maintenance.

WMC and Thought Suppression

Wegner's (1994) influential theory of thought suppression distinguishes between an automatic, resource-independent thought-monitoring process and a controlled, resource-dependent operating (suppression) process. Given the resource-dependent character of WMC, it is plausible to assume that WMC may relate directly to the capacity to sup-press irrelevant thoughts once they are detected. A study by Brewin and Beaton (2002) tested this hypothesis with the white bear paradigm that has often been used to investi-gate thought intrusions (Wegner, Schneider, Carter, & White, 1987). Participants were instructed either *not* to think of a white bear (suppression) or to think of a white bear (expression). They found a significant negative correlation between OSPAN and the num-ber of white bear occurrences in the thought suppression condition, indicating that high-WMC individuals more capably suppressed thoughts of a white bear when instructed to do so. No such association was obtained in the thought expression condition. A similar pattern of results was obtained in an extension in which the content of the thoughts was tailored to the personally most relevant intrusive thoughts of participants (Brewin & Smart, 2005).

Inadequate suppression or inhibition of irrelevant thoughts is also assumed to be a major component underlying mind wandering. In an experience sampling study, Kane and colleagues (2007) prompted their participants eight times a day over a period of 1 week to report whether their thoughts had wandered from their current activity. The results indicated that pretested WMC moderated the degree of mind wandering for challenging activities: High-WMC individuals maintained task-relevant thoughts better and mind-wandered less than low-WMC individuals in circumstances of high attentional demands.

The capacity to suppress interfering thoughts may be particularly relevant in the context of temptation. "Hot" thoughts about the object of desire ("This double cheeseburger looks delicious!") may intrude into consciousness and use up precious WMC resources (Kavanagh et al., 2005). Individuals able to purge working memory quickly from such tempting thoughts may have better chances to attain their self-regulatory goals ("I want to eat healthily"). We know of no research that has directly tested this assumption yet. However, data from one of our studies may speak to this idea (Hofmann et al., 2008, Study 2). At the beginning of the study, participants' automatic affect toward M&Ms candy was assessed with an IAT, and individual differences in WMC were measured with an OSPAN task. Participants were then given 5 minutes to taste a sample of M&Ms and to self-report the perceived tastiness and likability of the candy. It was found that automatic affect predicted the explicit liking of the candy more strongly for low- (than for high-) WMC individuals (Hofmann et al., 2008). This finding tentatively suggest that low-WMC individuals may have had more difficulties at suppressing or discounting intrusive, hot thoughts in response to the immediate hedonic properties of the candy during the product test.

The studies reviewed so far have shown how individual differences relate to thought suppression. A somewhat different research strategy has been pursued with regard to establishing WMC's role as a mediating factor of stereotype threat. *Stereotype threat* is the tendency of individuals to perform worse in intellectual tests after a negative stereotype about their ingroup has been made salient. Schmader and Johns (2003) hypothesized that stereotype threat may sap WMC resources because test takers must allocate parts of their resources to the suppression of negative thoughts and anxiety evoked by the stereotype threat. As a consequence, fewer working memory resources are left to be allocated to the test itself. In support of this hypothesis, participants under stereotype threat showed situationally reduced OSPAN scores in two studies (Schmader & Johns, 2003). A third study established that the reduction in WMC fully mediated the effects of stereotype threat on test performance.

WMC and Emotion Regulation

Recalling our earlier claim that working memory may also provide a mental workspace for emotion, there are a number of interesting possibilities as to how WMC may modulate the regulation of emotional experiences (see also Wranik, Barrett, & Salovey, 2007). First, high-WMC individuals may show a greater flexibility in antecedent-focused emotion regulation. Antecedent-focused emotion regulation takes place before an emotional response is fully generated. It includes strategies such as attentional deployment and cognitive change (Gross, 1998). Regarding attentional deployment, high- (as compared to low-) WMC individuals may be better at distracting themselves from an emotional aspect of a given situation or at attending only to selective parts of the emotional episode at hand. However, even though the above findings on attention regulation point in this direction, to our knowledge, no research thus far has directly tested this assumption in the emotion domain.

Regarding cognitive change, high-WMC individuals may have a greater variety and flexibility of strategies at their disposal. Such strategies shape the cognitive framing or appraisal of an emotional episode. In support, two recent studies showed that, compared to low-WMC individuals, those high in WMC were better at appraising emotional stimuli in an unemotional manner and thereby experienced less intense emotional responses to those stimuli (Schmeichel, Volokhov, & Demaree, 2008, Studies 2 and 3). These findings support WMC's assumed role for shaping the degree of emotional responses in an antecedent manner.

WMC may also aid response-focused emotion regulation, that is, the modulation of a full-blown emotional response once it has been elicited (Gross, 1998). Specifically, high-WMC individuals may be better at suppressing or inhibiting unwanted experiential, cognitive, and behavioral emotional responses when these responses are in conflict with the endorsed self-regulatory goal. To test this conjecture, Schmeichel and colleagues (2008) instructed their participants to suppress either negative emotions in response to a disgusting film clip (Study 1) or positive emotions in response to a comical film clip (Study 2). Results revealed that high-WMC participants were better at suppressing the expression of emotions in both studies. This indicates that WMC can be harnessed for the suppression of emotion, irrespective of the specific valence of the emotional experience. Based on these findings, it is tempting to conclude that people high in WMC may generally display less intense emotions than low-WMC individuals. Additional research has shown, however, that response amplification draws on working memory resources as well (Schmeichel, 2007; Schmeichel, Demaree, Robinson, & Pu, 2006; Study 4). Thus, the crucial difference between high- and low-WMC individuals may not so much lie in emotional intensity per se but rather in the *flexibility* with which emotional responding is fine-tuned to the context and the regulatory goal at hand.

The studies reviewed thus far all imposed self-regulatory goals (suppression or exaggeration) by instruction. However, in their daily lives, people may differ with regard to the degree to which they endorse certain emotion regulation goals. For instance, people differ in how strongly they are motivated to control their anger (Spielberger, Jacobs, Russell, & Crane, 1983). A recent study (Hofmann et al., 2008, Study 3) investigated the interplay between goal standards to control anger and WMC on anger expression upon social provocation. At one point during the study, participants were provoked through negative social feedback from an anonymous interaction partner. Subsequently, they were provided with a chance to retaliate to the provocation. It was found that, on average, high-anger-control participants retaliated significantly less than low-anger-control participants. However, this main effect was qualified by a significant anger control × WMC interaction, indicating that only participants both high in anger control and high in WMC effectively controlled their anger (Hofmann et al., 2008). In contrast, participants high in anger control but low in WMC did not differ in their reactions from participants low in anger control. Hence, having the self-regulatory goal to control anger is not enough. In order for it to effectively guide one's behavior, working memory resources are required.

WMC and Impulse Control

Self-regulation may go awry because people fail to inhibit their impulses. However, a close look at self-regulation research reveals that this conclusion is often inferred indirectly from group differences in behavior (e.g., participants in the alcohol condition consumed more sweets—so they must have acted more strongly on impulse). It has been suggested recently that more direct demonstrations should involve the assessment of markers for impulsive precursors, such as automatic affective reactions toward tempting stimuli (Hofmann, Friese, & Strack, 2009). The predictive validity of impulsive precursors may then illustrate how strongly individuals acted on impulse in a given situation of interest. Using such an approach, it has been found that the impact of impulses on behavior tends to increase under situations such as cognitive load (Friese, Hofmann, & Wänke, 2008), ego depletion (Hofmann, Rauch, & Gawronski, 2007), alcohol consumption (Hofmann & Friese, 2008), or mortality salience (Friese & Hofmann, 2008). Conversely, the consistency between self-regulatory goal standards and actual behavior was reduced under these circumstances.

Just as situational boundary conditions appear to shift the relative influence of impulsive versus reflective determinants on behavior, individual differences in control capacities may moderate predictive validities. Adopting such a dispositional perspective, two studies showed that individual differences in WMC moderate the relationship between automatic affect and eating behavior (Hofmann, Friese, & Roefs, 2009; Hofmann et al., 2008; Study 2): Low-WMC individuals acted more strongly in line with their automatic affective reactions, whereas high-WMC individuals acted more strongly in line with their goal to forego sweets (Hofmann et al., 2008). Analogous findings have been reported with regard to smoking behavior (Grenard et al., 2008), alcohol use among at-risk adolescents (Thush et al., 2008), aggressive behavior after alcohol intake in men (Wiers, Beckers, Houben, & Hofmann, 2009), and when using Stroop performance (Houben & Wiers, 2009) or stop-signal task performance (Hofmann, Friese, & Roefs, 2009) was employed as a more proximal measure of inhibitory control. The latter study also demonstrated that both an OSPAN and a stop-signal task interacted independently with automatic affective reactions in predicting impulsive behavior. This finding suggests that both tasks tap into separable executive components that contribute independently to impulse control (Hofmann, Friese, & Roefs, 2009). Taken together, these findings converge well on the idea that WMC is strongly involved in the "biasing" of behavior in accordance with self-regulatory goals, and in the inhibition of desire-related impulsive action tendencies that are incompatible with these goals.

WORKING MEMORY AND NONCONSCIOUS PROCESSES

Throughout this chapter, we have purposely avoided attaching the labels *conscious* and *unconscious* to the mechanisms of working memory. This decision was motivated by three main reasons that, in our view, complicate the use of these labels. First, the conception of working memory as a multicomponent system for storing and manipulating information (e.g., Baddeley, 2007) entails components such as the phonological loop and the visuospatial sketchpad, whose operations are almost certainly not explicitly conscious. Rather, they provide information that eventually becomes conscious through attentional amplification (Dehaene & Naccache, 2001). Only information in the current focus of selective attention is fully conscious, whereas, according to the flashlight metaphor introduced earlier, a great deal of information remains in an *active* but unattended state at the fringe of consciousness. Hence, whether a goal in working memory is currently available to consciousness may fluctuate considerably from moment to moment, even though by virtue of its accessible state it may nevertheless exert a biasing influence on information processing (Miller & Cohen, 2001). Thus, sustained accessibility rather than conscious availability should be the primary determinant of goal impact, even though the two dimensions may often be quite strongly correlated.

Second, nonconscious processes may often be the direct consequence of *conscious* goal setting (not just a long-term consequence of habit formation). Specifically, goals can be viewed as devices for "self-programming," such that conscious goal intentions configure or bias parameters in a whole range of lower-order subsystems involved in, for instance, attention allocation, stimulus encoding, response selection, and response execution (Dreisbach & Haider, 2009; Folk et al., 1992; Miller & Cohen, 2001). Hence, conscious intentions are typically translated into automatic and potentially nonconscious processes at a lower level but in a way these nonconscious processes still represent the overarching goal. From such a hierarchical perspective, the distinction between conscious and unconscious processing depends on the level of analysis, and the idea of conscious goal pursuit without supporting nonconscious processes does not seem to make much sense. However, the reverse seems probable. Recent research has shown that, given the right triggering conditions (e.g., Custers & Aarts, 2005), the nonconscious apparatus that supports goal pursuit can be set in motion even in the absence of conscious intentions (for a review, see Papies & Aarts, Chapter 7, this volume).

Third, some of the working memory mechanisms aiding self-regulatory goal pursuit may be more accessible to consciousness than others. For instance, the active suppression of consciousness-intruding thoughts or emotions appears, by definition, to be contingent on conscious awareness. Other mechanisms, such as goal shielding (Shah et al., 2002), the tuning of attention to goal-relevant information (Dreisbach & Haider, 2009), or simple updating processes (Hassin, Bargh, Engell, & McCulloch, 2009), may work just as well in the absence of conscious awareness. One possible agenda for future research is to delineate the exact features of these component processes more clearly. For instance, there is evidence that nonconscious goal priming, though completely inaccessible to conscious awareness, may nevertheless involve the allocation of WMC to the primed goal (Hassin, Bargh, & Zimerman, 2009). Although speculative at this point, one common denominator of working memory operations in goal pursuit may thus lie in their resource-consuming character, irrespective of whether the goal that is subserved by these processes is conscious or not (Aarts, Custers, & Veltkamp, 2008).

CONCLUSION

To conclude, working memory appears to be a central component in people's everyday attempts at self-regulation. Its resource-dependent character and its demonstrated involvement in the regulation of attention, thought, emotion, and behavior render working memory a prime candidate for the limited-capacity aspect of self-regulation. Important as WMC may be, it is not everything: To self-regulate, people must form self-regulatory goals in the first place, and they must be motivated to do so. Even high-WMC individuals will fail to self-regulate in the absence of goal standards and motivation. Keeping these limitations of working memory in our limited working memories, we look forward to seeing what insights future research on the intersection of cognition and self-regulation will bring.

ACKNOWLEDGMENTS

We thank Katie Lancaster, Lotte van Dillen, and Claire Zedelius for valuable comments.

REFERENCES

Aarts, H., Custers, R., & Veltkamp, M. (2008). Goal priming and the affective-motivational route to nonconscious goal pursuit. *Social Cognition, 26,* 555–577.

Baddeley, A. (2000). The episodic buffer: A new component of working memory? *Trends in Cognitive Sciences, 4,* 417–423.

Baddeley, A., Emslie, H., Kolodny, J., & Duncan, J. (1998). Random generation and the executive control of working memory. *Quarterly Journal of Experimental Psychology A: Human Experimental Psychology, 51,* 819–852.

Baddeley, A., & Wilson, B. (1988). Frontal amnesia and the dysexecutive syndrome. *Brain and Cognition, 7,* 212–230.

Baddeley, A. D. (1986). *Working memory.* Oxford, UK: Clarendon Press.

Baddeley, A. D. (2003). Working memory: Looking back and looking forward. *Nature Reviews Neuroscience, 4,* 829–839.

Baddeley, A. D. (2007). *Working memory, thought, and action.* Oxford, UK: Oxford University Press.

Baddeley, A. D., & Hitch, G. J. (1974). Working memory. In G. A. Bower (Ed.), *The psychology of learning and motivation* (Vol. 8, pp. 47–90). New York: Academic Press.

Barrett, L. F., Tugade, M. M., & Engle, R. W. (2004). Individual differences in working memory capacity and dual-process theories of the mind. *Psychological Bulletin, 130,* 553–573.

Baumeister, R. F., Bratslavsky, M., Muraven, M., & Tice, D. M. (1998). Ego depletion: Is the active self a limited resource? *Journal of Personality and Social Psychology, 74,* 1252–1265.

Baumeister, R. F., & Heatherton, T. F. (1996). Self-regulation failure: An overview. *Psychological Inquiry, 7,* 1–15.

Baumeister, R. F., Vohs, K. D., DeWall, N., & Zhang, L. (2007). How emotion shapes behavior: Feedback, anticipation, and reflection, rather than direct causation. *Personality and Social Psychology Review, 11,* 167–203.

Berg, E. A. (1948). A simple objective technique for measuring flexibility in thinking. *Journal of General Psychology, 39,* 15–22.

Botvinick, M. M., Braver, T. S., Carter, C. S., Barch, D. M., & Cohen, J. D. (2001). Conflict monitoring and cognitive control. *Psychological Review, 108,* 624–652.

Bradley, M. M., Cuthbert, B. N., & Lang, P. J. (1996). Picture media and emotion: Effects of a sustained affective content. *Psychophysiology, 33,* 662–670.

Brewin, C. R., & Beaton, A. (2002). Thought suppression, intelligence, and working memory capacity. *Behaviour Research and Therapy, 40,* 923–930.

Brewin, C. R., & Smart, L. (2005). Working memory capacity and suppression of intrusive thoughts. *Journal of Behavior Therapy and Experimental Psychiatry, 36,* 61–68.

Broadbent, D. E. (1958). *Perception and communication.* Elmsford, NY: Pergamon Press.

Carver, C. S., & Scheier, M. F. (1981). *Attention and self-regulation: A control-theory approach to human behavior.* New York: Springer.

Collette, F., Van der Linden, M., Laureys, S., Delfiore, G., Degueldre, C., Luxen, A., et al. (2005). Exploring the unity and diversity of the neural substrates of executive functioning. *Human Brain Mapping, 25,* 409–423.

Conway, A. R. A., Kane, M. J., Bunting, M. F., Hambrick, D. Z., Wilhelm, O., & Engle, R. W. (2005). Working memory span tasks: A methodological review and user's guide. *Psychonomic Bulletin and Review, 12,* 769–786.

Corbetta, M., & Shulman, G. L. (2002). Control of goal-directed and stimulus-driven attention in the brain. *Nature Reviews Neuroscience, 3,* 201–215.

Custers, R., & Aarts, H. (2005). Positive affect as implicit motivator: On the nonconscious operation of behavioral goals. *Journal of Personality and Social Psychology, 89,* 129–142.

Dahlin, E., Nyberg, L., Backman, L., & Neely, A. S. (2008). Plasticity of executive functioning in young and older adults: Immediate training gains, transfer, and long-term maintenance. *Psychology and Aging, 23,* 720–730.

Daneman, M., & Carpenter, P. A. (1980). Individual differences in working memory and reading. *Journal of Verbal Learning and Verbal Behavior, 19,* 450–466.

Daneman, M., & Merikle, P. M. (1996). Working memory and language comprehension: A meta-analysis. *Psychonomic Bulletin and Review, 3,* 422–433.

Dehaene, S., & Naccache, L. (2001). Towards a cognitive neuroscience of consciousness: Basic evidence and a workspace framework. *Cognition, 79,* 1–37.

Dewall, C. N., Baumeister, R. F., Stillman, T. F., & Gailliot, M. T. (2007). Violence restrained: Effects of self-regulation and its depletion on aggression. *Journal of Experimental Social Psychology, 43,* 62–76.

Dreisbach, G., & Haider, H. (2009). How task representations guide attention: Further evidence for the shielding function of task sets. *Journal of Experimental Psychology: Learning, Memory, and Cognition, 35,* 477–486.

Duncan, J. (1995). Attention, intelligence, and the frontal lobes. In M. S. Gazzaniga (Ed.), *The cognitive neurosciences* (pp. 721–733). Cambridge, MA: MIT Press.

Engle, R. W., Kane, M. J., & Tuholski, S. W. (1999). Individual differences in working memory capacity and what they tell us about controlled attention, general fluid intelligence, and functions of the prefrontal cortex. In A. Miyake & P. Shah (Eds.), *Models of working memory: Mechanisms of active maintenance and executive control* (pp. 102–134). New York: Cambridge University Press.

Field, M., & Cox, W. M. (2008). Attentional bias in addictive behaviors: A review of its development, causes, and consequences. *Drug and Alcohol Dependence, 97,* 1–20.

Finkel, E. J., & Campbell, W. K. (2001). Self-control and accommodation in close relationships: An interdependence analysis. *Journal of Personality and Social Psychology, 81,* 263–277.

Folk, C. L., Remington, R. W., & Johnston, J. C. (1992). Involuntary covert orienting is contingent on attentional control settings. *Journal of Experimental Psychology: Human Perception and Performance, 18,* 1030–1044.

Friese, M., Bargas-Avila, J., Hofmann, W., & Wiers, R. W. (2010). Here's looking at you, Bud: Alcohol-related memory structures predict eye movements for social drinkers with low executive control. *Social and Personality Psychology Science, 7,* 743–757.

Friese, M., & Hofmann, W. (2008). What would you have as a last supper?: Thoughts about death influence evaluation and consumption of food products. *Journal of Experimental Social Psychology, 44,* 1388–1394.

Friese, M., Hofmann, W., & Wänke, M. (2008). When impulses take over: Moderated predictive validity of implicit and explicit attitude measures in predicting food choice and consumption behaviour. *British Journal of Social Psychology, 47,* 397–419.

Frijda, N. H. (2005). Emotion experience. *Cognition and Emotion, 19,* 473–497.

Fukuda, K., & Vogel, E. K. (2009). Human variation in overriding attentional capture. *Journal of Neuroscience, 29,* 8726–8733.

Gailliot, M. T., & Baumeister, R. F. (2006). Self-regulation and sexual restraint: Dispositionally and temporarily poor self-regulatory abilities contribute to failures at restraining sexual behavior. *Personality and Social Psychology Bulletin, 33,* 173–186.

Gilbert, D. T., & Hixon, J. G. (1991). The trouble of thinking: Activation and application of stereotypic beliefs. *Journal of Personality and Social Psychology, 60,* 509–517.

Gollwitzer, P. M., & Bayer, U. (1999). Deliberative versus implemental mindsets in the control of action. In S. Chaiken & Y. Trope (Eds.), *Dual-process theories in social psychology* (pp. 403–422). New York: Guilford Press.

Greenwald, A. G., McGhee, D. E., & Schwartz, J. L. K. (1998). Measuring individual differences in implicit cognition: The Implicit Association Test. *Journal of Personality and Social Psychology, 74,* 1464–1480.

Grenard, J. L., Ames, S. L., Wiers, R. W., Thush, C., Sussman, S., & Stacy, A. W. (2008). Working memory capacity moderates the predictive effects of drug-related associations on substance use. *Psychology of Addictive Behaviors, 22,* 426–432.

Gross, J. J. (1998). The emerging field of emotion regulation: An integrative review. *Review of General Psychology, 2,* 271–299.

Gross, J. J., & Levenson, R. W. (1993). Emotional suppression: Physiology, self-report, and expressive behavior. *Journal of Personality and Social Psychology, 64,* 970–986.

Hasher, L., & Zacks, R. T. (1988). Working memory, comprehension, and aging: A review and a new view. In G. H. Bower (Ed.), *The psychology of learning and motivation: Advances in research and theory* (Vol. 22, pp. 193–225). San Diego, CA: Academic Press.

Hassin, R. R., Bargh, J. A., Engell, A. D., & McCulloch, K. C. (2009). Implicit working memory. *Consciousness and Cognition, 18,* 665–678.

Hassin, R. R., Bargh, J. A., & Zimerman, S. (2009). Automatic and flexible: The case of nonconscious goal pursuit. *Social Cognition, 27,* 20–36.

Hofmann, W., & Friese, M. (2008). Impulses got the better of me: Alcohol moderates the influence of implicit attitudes toward food cues on eating behavior. *Journal of Abnormal Psychology, 117,* 420–427.

Hofmann, W., Friese, M., & Roefs, A. (2009). Three ways to resist temptation: The independent contributions of executive attention, inhibitory control, and affect regulation to the impulse control of eating behavior. *Journal of Experimental Social Psychology, 45,* 431–435.

Hofmann, W., Friese, M., & Strack, F. (2009). Impulse and self-control from a dual-systems perspective. *Perspectives on Psychological Science, 4,* 162–176.

Hofmann, W., Gschwendner, T., Friese, M., Wiers, R. W., & Schmitt, M. (2008). Working memory capacity and self-regulatory behavior: Toward an individual differences perspective on behavior determination by automatic versus controlled processes. *Journal of Personality and Social Psychology, 95,* 962–977.

Hofmann, W., Rauch, W., & Gawronski, B. (2007). And deplete us not into temptation: Automatic attitudes, dietary restraint, and self-regulatory resources as determinants of eating behavior. *Journal of Experimental Social Psychology, 43,* 497–504.

Hofmann, W., & Wilson, T. D. (2010). Consciousness, introspection, and the adaptive unconscious. In B. Gawronski & B. K. Payne (Eds.), *Handbook of implicit social cognition: Measurement, theory, and applications* (pp. 197–215). New York: Guilford Press.

Houben, K., & Wiers, R. W. (2009). Response inhibition moderates the relationship between implicit associations and drinking behavior. *Alcoholism: Clinical and Experimental Research, 33,* 1–8.

James, W. (1950). *The principles of psychology.* New York: Dover. (Original work published 1890)

Jostmann, N. B., & Koole, S. L. (2009). When persistence is futile: A functional analysis of action orientation and goal disengagement. In G. B. Moskowitz & H. Grant (Eds.), *The psychology of goals* (pp. 337–361). New York: Guilford Press.

Jurado, M. B., & Rosselli, M. (2007). The elusive nature of executive functions: A review of our current understanding. *Neuropsychology Review, 17,* 213–233.

Kane, M. J., Bleckley, M. K., Conway, A. R. A., & Engle, R. W. (2001). A controlled-attention view of working-memory capacity. *Journal of Experimental Psychology: General, 130,* 169–183.

Kane, M. J., Brown, L. H., McVay, J. C., Silvia, P. J., Myin-Germeys, I., & Kwapil, T. R. (2007).

For whom the mind wanders, and when: An experience-sampling study of working memory and executive control in daily life. *Psychological Science, 18*, 614–621.

Kane, M. J., & Engle, R. W. (2002). The role of prefrontal cortex in working-memory capacity, executive attention, and general fluid intelligence: An individual-differences perspective. *Psychonomic Bulletin and Review, 9*, 637–671.

Kavanagh, D. J., Andrade, J., & May, J. (2005). Imaginary relish and exquisite torture: The elaborated intrusion theory of desire. *Psychological Review, 112*, 446–467.

Kemps, E., Tiggemann, M., & Grigg, M. (2008). Food cravings consume limited cognitive resources. *Journal of Experimental Psychology: Applied, 14*, 247–254.

Kiewra, K. A., & Benton, S. L. (1988). The relationship between information-processing and ability in notetaking. *Contemporary Educational Psychology, 13*, 33–44.

Knudsen, E. I. (2007). Fundamental components of attention. *Annual Review of Neuroscience, 30*, 57–78.

Kruglanski, A. W., Shah, J. Y., Fishbach, A., Friedman, R., Chun, W. Y., & Sleeth-Keppler, D. (2002). A theory of goal systems. In M. P. Zanna (Ed.), *Advances in experimental social Psychology* (Vol. 34, pp. 331–378). San Diego, CA: Academic Press.

Kuhl, J. (1983). *Motivation, Konflikt und Handlungskontrolle* [Motivation, conflict, and action control]. Berlin: Springer.

Lavie, N., Hirst, A., de Fockert, J. W., & Viding, E. (2004). Load theory of selective attention and cognitive control. *Journal of Experimental Psychology: General, 133*, 339–354.

Logan, G. D., Cowan, W. B., & Davis, K. A. (1984). On the ability to inhibit responses in simple and choice reaction time tasks: A model and a method. *Journal of Experimental Psychology: Human Perception and Performance, 10*, 276–291.

McNab, F., Leroux, G., Strand, F., Thorell, L., Bergman, S., & Klingberg, T. (2008). Common and unique components of inhibition and working memory: An fMRI, within-subjects investigation. *Neuropsychologia, 46*, 2668–2682.

Miller, E. K., & Cohen, J. D. (2001). An integrative theory of prefrontal cortex function. *Annual Review of Neuroscience, 24*, 167–202.

Miyake, A., Friedman, N. P., Emerson, M. J., Witzki, A. H., & Howerter, A. (2000). The unity and diversity of executive functions and their contributions to complex "frontal lobe" tasks: A latent variable analysis. *Cognitive Psychology, 41*, 49–100.

Miyake, A., & Shah, P. (Eds.). (1999). *Models of working memory: Mechanisms of active maintenance and executive control.* Cambridge, UK: Cambridge University Press.

Muraven, M., Collins, R. L., & Neinhaus, K. (2002). Self-control and alcohol restraint: An initial application of the self-control strength model. *Psychology of Addictive Behavior, 16*, 113–120.

Norman, D. A., & Shallice, T. (1986). Attention to action. Willed and automatic control of behavior. In R. J. Davidson, G. E. Schwartz, & D. Shapiro (Eds.), *Consciousness and self regulation: Advances in research* (pp. 1–18). New York: Plenum Press.

Pashler, H., Johnston, J. C., & Ruthruff, E. (2001). Attention and performance. *Annual Review of Psychology, 52*, 629–651.

Polivy, J. (1998). The effects of behavioral inhibition: Integrating internal cues, cognition, behavior, and affect. *Psychological Inquiry, 9*, 181–204.

Russell, J. A. (2003). Core affect and the psychological construction of emotion. *Psychological Review, 110* 145–172.

Saults, J. S., Cowan, N., Sher, K. J., & Moreno, M. V. (2007). Differential effects of alcohol on working memory: Distinguishing multiple processes. *Experimental and Clinical Psychopharmacology, 15*, 576–587.

Schmader, T., & Johns, M. (2003). Converging evidence that stereotype threat reduces working memory capacity. *Journal of Personality and Social Psychology, 85*, 440–452.

Schmeichel, B. J. (2007). Attention control, memory updating, and emotion regulation temporarily reduce the capacity for executive control. *Journal of Experimental Psychology: General, 136,* 241–255.

Schmeichel, B. J., Demaree, H. A., Robinson, J. L., & Pu, J. (2006). Ego depletion by response exaggeration. *Journal of Experimental Social Psychology, 42,* 95–102.

Schmeichel, B. J., Vohs, K. D., & Baumeister, R. F. (2003). Intellectual performance and ego depletion: Role of the self in logical reasoning and other information processing. *Journal of Personality and Social Psychology, 85,* 33–46.

Schmeichel, B. J., Volokhov, R. N., & Demaree, H. A. (2008). Working memory capacity and the self-regulation of emotional expression and experience. *Journal of Personality and Social Psychology, 95,* 1526–1540.

Schoofs, D., Preuss, D., & Wolf, O. T. (2008). Psychosocial stress induces working memory impairments in an *n*-back paradigm. *Psychoneuroendocrinology, 33,* 643–653.

Shah, J. Y., Friedman, R. S., & Kruglanski, A. W. (2002). Forgetting all else: On the antecedents and consequences of goal shielding. *Journal of Personality and Social Psychology, 83,* 1261–1280.

Shallice, T. (1982). Specific impairments of planning. *Philosophical Transactions of the Royal Society, 298,* 199–209.

Shimamura, A. P. (2000). The role of the prefrontal cortex in dynamic filtering. *Psychobiology, 28,* 207–218.

Smith, E. E., & Jonides, J. (1999). Storage and executive processes in the frontal lobes. *Science, 283,* 1657–1661.

Spielberger, C. D., Jacobs, G., Russell, S. F., & Crane, R. S. (1983). Assessment of anger: The State–Trait Anger Scale. In J. N. Butcher & C. D. Spielberger (Eds.), *Advances in personality assessment* (Vol. II, pp. 159–187). Hillsdale, NJ: Erlbaum.

Strack, F., & Deutsch, R. (2004). Reflective and impulsive determinants of social behavior. *Personality and Social Psychology Review, 8,* 220–247.

Stroop, C. D. (1935). Studies of interference in serial verbal reactions. *Journal of Experimental Psychology, 18,* 643–662.

Stuss, D. T., & Knight, R. T. (2002). *Principles of frontal lobe function.* New York: Oxford University Press.

Thush, C., Wiers, R. W., Ames, S. L., Grenard, J. L., Sussman, S., & Stacy, A. W. (2008). Interactions between implicit and explicit cognition and working memory capacity in the prediction of alcohol use in at-risk adolescents. *Drug and Alcohol Dependence, 94,* 116–124.

Unsworth, N., Schrock, J. C., & Engle, R. W. (2004). Working memory capacity and the antisaccade task: Individual differences in voluntary saccade control. *Journal of Experimental Psychology: Learning, Memory, and Cognition, 30,* 1302–1321.

Vallacher, R. R., & Wegner, D. M. (1987). What do people think they're doing?: Action identification and human behavior. *Psychological Review, 94,* 3–15.

Van Dillen, L. F., & Koole, S. L. (2007). Clearing the mind: A working memory model of distraction from negative mood. *Emotion, 7,* 715–723.

Vohs, K. D., & Heatherton, T. F. (2000). Self-regulatory failure: A resource-depletion approach. *Psychological Science, 11,* 249–254.

von Hippel, W. (2007). Aging, executive functioning, and social control. *Current Directions in Psychological Science, 16,* 240–244.

Wager, T. D., & Smith, E. E. (2003). Neuroimaging studies of working memory: A meta-analysis. *Cognitive, Affective and Behavioral Neuroscience, 3,* 255–274.

Ward, A., & Mann, T. (2000). Don't mind if I do: Disinhibited eating under cognitive load. *Journal of Personality and Social Psychology, 78,* 753–763.

Wegner, D. M. (1994). Ironic processes of mental control. *Psychological Review, 101,* 34–52.

Wegner, D. M., Schneider, D. J., Carter, S. R., & White, T. L. (1987). Paradoxical effects of thought suppression. *Journal of Personality and Social Psychology, 53*, 5–13.

Wenzlaff, R. M., Wegner, D. M., & Roper, D. W. (1988). Depression and mental control: The resurgence of unwanted negative thoughts. *Journal of Personality and Social Psychology, 55*, 882–892.

West, R. L. (1996). An application of prefrontal cortex function theory to cognitive aging. *Psychological Bulletin, 120*, 272–292.

Wiers, R. W., Beckers, L., Houben, K., & Hofmann, W. (2009). A short fuse after alcohol: Implicit power associations predict aggressiveness after alcohol consumption in young heavy drinkers with limited executive control. *Pharmacology Biochemistry and Behavior, 93*, 300–305.

Wranik, T., Barrett, L. F., & Salovey, P. (2007). Intelligent emotion regulation: Is knowledge power? In J. J. Gross (Ed.), *Handbook of emotion regulation* (pp. 393–428). New York: Guilford Press.

Wrosch, C., Scheier, M. F., Miller, G. E., Schulz, R., & Carver, C. S. (2003). Adaptive self-regulation of unattainable goals: Goal disengagement, goal reengagement, and subjective well-being. *Personality and Social Psychology Bulletin, 29*, 1494–1508.

Zwaan, R. A., & Truitt, T. P. (1998). Smoking urges affect language processing. *Experimental and Clinical Psychopharmacology, 6*, 325–330.

CHAPTER 12

Local and Global Evaluations
Attitudes as Self-Regulatory Guides
for Near and Distant Responding

ALISON LEDGERWOOD
YAACOV TROPE

lthough we often think of our attitudes and beliefs as inherent and enduring aspects of ourselves, we also find that they fail to guide us in many everyday social situations. At times, we act in accordance with our core values and ideals. Often, however, our behavior seems to be far more strongly shaped by the particularities of the current context. Building on a wealth of past research that has examined issues related to evaluative consistency and inconsistency, this chapter examines the question of when and why evaluative responses might be more or less consistent across contexts from a self-regulatory perspective. Specifically, we propose that evaluations can serve as self-regulatory guides for action either within the current context or outside of it. Whereas flexible action guides that incorporate local details in the current context tend to be useful for responding appropriately to proximal objects, consistent action guides that globally generalize across contexts are more useful for responding to distant objects. From this perspective, cues about distance should functionally influence the extent to which evaluative responses fluctuate or remain consistent across different contexts. This issue is important for understanding self-control, since local and global evaluations may have conflicting action implications, and distance may therefore play a key role in resolving such self-control dilemmas. More broadly, our goal in this chapter is to form a bridge between the literatures on attitudes and self-regulation to improve our understanding of how these often separate fields of research can each elucidate the other.

We begin by briefly reviewing some of the ways that attitudes have been assumed to promote consistency or flexibility in the literature, and then describe why evaluative flexibility, as well as consistency, might be functional from a self-regulatory perspective.

Next we discuss in more detail the notion that evaluations can either summarize information from the current context, thereby promoting evaluative flexibility, or summarize information that is consistent across contexts, thereby promoting evaluative consistency. We propose that distance plays a key role in determining which form of evaluative summary is used to guide behavior, and draw on construal level theory to delineate the cognitive process by which this could occur. After describing a series of empirical studies that provide support for several of our hypotheses, we discuss points of interface with other theories of self-regulation and self-control, and highlight some implications of the present perspective for understanding the role of evaluation in regulating action.

CONCEPTUALIZING ATTITUDES

The study of attitudes has long been motivated by the assumption that attitudes play a key role in regulating behavior. In other words, attitudes guide action: They serve to provide a quick summary of whether an attitude object is positive or negative, which facilitates approach or avoidance of that object (Fazio, 1989; Katz, 1960; M. B. Smith, Bruner, & White, 1956; Wilson, Lindsey, & Schooler, 2000). Furthermore, attitudes can function to regulate social action and interaction by summarizing information from the social environment (e.g., other people's opinions) that helps individuals create and maintain a shared view of the world with those around them (Echterhoff, Higgins, & Levine, 2009; C. D. Hardin & Higgins, 1996; Jost, Ledgerwood, & Hardin, 2008; Smith et al., 1956). Thus, attitudes help guide action and interaction by providing efficient, valenced summaries of a large amount of evaluative information that would be difficult to process piece by piece before each behavior we undertake in daily life.

Despite widespread consensus that an important function of attitudes is to guide behavior, researchers have conceptualized the fundamental nature of that behavioral guide in somewhat different ways. Historically, attitudes have often been characterized as dispositional evaluative tendencies toward a given attitude object that are relatively consistent across situations, unless (or until) a successful persuasion attempt changes the first attitude into a new one (Ajzen, 1988; Allport, 1935; D. T. Campbell, 1950; Krech & Crutchfield, 1948; Tourangeau & Rasinski, 1988). Indeed, there is good evidence to suggest attitudes can at least sometimes display a high level of stability across times and contexts (e.g., A. Campbell, Converse, Miller, & Stokes, 1960; Krosnick, 1988; see Eagly & Chaiken, 1995, for a review). Furthermore, stability has frequently been equated with importance or consequentiality, whereas instability in evaluative responding has been assumed to reflect inconsequential attitudes or even just error in measurement (e.g., Bassili, 1996; Converse, 1964, Schuman & Presser, 1981). Attitudes are thus often assumed to be relatively static, schematic mental representations, and to therefore guide evaluative responding in a fairly consistent way.

Meanwhile, however, other researchers conceptualize attitudes as intrinsically malleable representations or even de novo constructions that flexibly incorporate the particular information that happens to be activated in a given context (Conrey & Smith, 2007; Lord & Lepper, 1999; Schwarz, 2007). These perspectives fit particularly well with research demonstrating that attitudes often fluidly shift in response to other people in the immediate social situation, including conversation partners, significant others, salient social groups, and incidentally encountered strangers (Baldwin & Holmes, 1987; Davis

& Rusbult, 2001; Higgins & Rholes, 1978; Ledgerwood & Chaiken, 2007; Sinclair, Lowery, Hardin, & Colangelo, 2005). From this view, attitudes naturally fluctuate from situation to situation, and evaluative consistency arises only when the evaluative implications of inputs activated in one setting happen to match those activated in another.

LOCAL AND GLOBAL ACTION GUIDES

To some extent, these different conceptualizations of attitudes as stable versus shifting may reflect differences in assumptions about the functionality or usefulness of flexibility versus consistency in guiding action. On the one hand, consistent evaluations should often be effective for regulating behavior, given that local information is frequently irrelevant for evaluative responding. If someone is voting for the next president, for instance, it does not seem particularly useful for variations in the weather, or who happens to be waiting in line at the polling station, to influence her evaluative responses toward the candidates. From this perspective, action would ideally be based on a summary guide of whether a person, object, or event tends to be positive or negative across situations. Thus, a global evaluative response that remains consistent in the face of contextual fluctuation would seem particularly functional in some cases. Such global evaluations could provide a relatively stable summary guide for engaging with an attitude object by taking into account general information from multiple contexts. They might incorporate what is consistently relevant for action toward an attitude object across different situations, including broad principles and values, the opinions of significant others or groups, societal norms, long-term goals, and central and enduring features of the attitude object.

On the other hand, it seems equally plausible that a flexible evaluative response that allows a person to adapt fluidly to his current social environment would be helpful in guiding behavior (see also Schwarz, 2007). Different contexts call for different responses: If someone needs to slice an apple, for example, he might approach a paring knife if it is sitting peacefully on the counter but jump away if it slides off and clatters to the floor. Furthermore, flexible evaluative responses facilitate the creation of socially shared viewpoints, which are a necessary basis of communication, relationships, and the regulation of social action (see, e.g., Festinger, 1950; C. D. Hardin & Higgins, 1996; Ledgerwood & Liviatan, 2010). From this perspective, local evaluations that flexibly tune to the current situation might be optimal for regulating action. These local evaluations could incorporate details of the current context, including the presumed attitudes of others who happen to be in the immediate social situation, as well as nonsocial aspects of the current context, short-term concerns, and unique details of a particular instantiation of the attitude object.

Although both types of evaluations seem potentially useful, it seems possible to distinguish situations in which each form of evaluation would be more or less effective for regulating behavior. After all, in the present moment, individuals need to be able to regulate their actions flexibly to pursue their immediate goals, coordinate action with others around them, and interact effectively with their local environment. Local evaluations could serve to guide action effectively toward objects within the current situation because they are sensitive to specific contextual information. However, humans are also able to transcend their immediate situation to plan for the future, coordinate action at a distance, and predict other people's behaviors. Thus, they must be able to regulate their actions for not only the here and now but also the there and then. Global evaluations could serve to guide action appropriately toward objects *outside* of the present situation by drawing on evaluation-relevant information that is consistent across contexts.

Importantly, then, information about the proximity of an attitude object should play a key role in determining which form of evaluation arises in a given setting. Specifically, we suggest that cues about distance will set into motion a self-regulatory evaluative system geared toward guiding action either within the current context or outside of it. Responses to proximal objects should be guided by local evaluations that incorporate information relevant for action in the current situation, whereas responses to distal objects should be guided by global evaluations that summarize context-independent information.

How exactly might such a process play out? To better delineate both the construct of distance and the cognitive process by which it could influence evaluative responding, we next describe construal level theory.

DISTANCE AND LEVEL OF CONSTRUAL

According to construal level theory, psychological distance plays a key role in determining how we subjectively represent an object or event (N. Liberman & Trope, 2008; Trope & Liberman, 2003). There are different dimensions of psychological distance: An object can be removed from us in time (the future or the past) as well as space, social distance (e.g., others vs. ourselves, us vs. them), and hypotheticality (e.g., a counterfactual alternative vs. reality, a distant chance vs. a near certainty). Interestingly, however, these different dimensions of distance converge in their effects on mental representation (e.g., Fujita, Henderson, Eng, Trope, & Liberman, 2006; Wakslak, Trope, Liberman, & Aloni, 2006; see N. Liberman & Trope, 2008, for a review). As an object or event grows increasingly distant, we tend to mentally represent it more in terms of its essential, superordinate, and stable characteristics. These *high-level construals* are abstract and structured; they extract gist information and leave out irrelevant details that could vary without changing the core meaning we have assigned to the object. In contrast, we tend to subjectively represent psychologically proximal objects in terms of their detailed, subordinate, and contextualized features. These *low-level construals* are more concrete and lack a clear structure separating important from peripheral and irrelevant features.

Consider, for instance, the impact of psychological distance on perception. Researchers have found that participants were better able to visually abstract the big picture from a set of fragments in the Gestalt Completion Test when they imagined working on the task in the distant future (on a day 1 year from now) versus the near future (tomorrow), or when the task was psychologically distant in probability (i.e., when they thought they were unlikely vs. likely to actually receive the task in a later session) (Forster, Friedman, & Liberman, 2004, Study 3; Wakslak et al., 2006, Study 5). Distance has a similar impact on cognition: For example, individuals grouped objects into fewer, broader categories when they imagined using the objects in the distant (vs. near) future, and they predicted that people's behaviors would be more dispositionally driven (and less susceptible to situational variation) at a temporally distant versus proximal time point (Nussbaum, Trope, & Liberman, 2003). Likewise, psychological distance increases the extent to which people focus on superordinate ends versus subordinate means. When an activity was expected occur in the distant (vs. near) future or in a spatially remote (vs. close) location, participants were more likely to describe it in terms of its abstract purpose; when the activity was psychological closer, participants used more concrete descriptions that emphasized the means by which the activity was performed (Fujita, Henderson, et al., 2006, Study 1; N. Liberman & Trope, 1998, Study 1).

Importantly, this relationship between psychological distance and construal level elucidates a key mechanism by which distance could influence evaluative action guides. By highlighting the central and defining features of an attitude object, high-level construals could enable relatively global evaluations that integrate what is consistent about the object across contexts. Evaluations of psychologically distant attitude objects could therefore be based on information relevant for evaluating the object's superordinate and central features, and would appear relatively stable in the face of shifting contextual details. For example, a dieter's global evaluation of a piece of cake might screen out situation-specific information (the enticing chocolate icing, the fact that it is served at a birthday party) and focus instead on context-independent information, such as the negative impact of high-calorie foods on his goal to lose weight. In contrast, by including the concrete, contextual aspects of an attitude object, low-level construals could enable more local evaluations that integrate the unique details of the present situation. Because they incorporate evaluative information from specific contextual details that often change across situations, these local action guides would appear relatively malleable. For instance, a dieter's local evaluation of a cake might fluctuate depending on whether the cake looks moist or dry, or whether a stranger happens to like it, or whether the situation seems to call for eating cake (e.g., a birthday party vs. chatting with a friend at a coffee shop).

Thus, we postulate that distance directs the self-regulatory system via its impact on the mental representation of an attitude object, which determines the basis or form of evaluation (i.e., a more global or more local integration of evaluative information). This pattern should therefore generalize beyond any particular dimension of distance. Any variable that influences the level at which an attitude object is mentally construed should be sufficient to trigger these self-regulatory effects.

MENTALLY REPRESENTING THE ATTITUDE OBJECT

The notion that psychological distance might influence evaluative responding by changing the way an attitude object is mentally construed fits well with other perspectives that have emphasized the importance of subjective representation in guiding evaluative consistency. Echoing Asch's (1940) distinction between "a change in the object of judgment, rather than in the judgment of the object" (p. 458), theorists have examined the notion that inconsistency in evaluative responding can arise when the mental representation of an attitude object changes (e.g., Ferguson & Bargh, 2007; Lord & Lepper, 1999; Lord, Lepper, & Mackie, 1984; Schwarz, 2007). For instance, attitude representation theory (Lord & Lepper, 1999) suggests that a person's evaluation of an attitude object depends on his or her subjective representation of that object, and that inconsistency in evaluative responding will arise when a person's subjective representations differ between contexts. Thus, a person's evaluation of the same social category (e.g., politicians) can shift when different category exemplars are activated (e.g., a liked vs. disliked politician) (Sia, Lord, Blessum, Ratcliff, & Lepper, 1997; see also Asch, 1948; Bodenhausen, Schwarz, Bless, & Wanke, 1995).

Similarly, constructionist approaches suggest that attitudes can be best understood as spontaneous integrations across relevant and activated evaluative information (e.g., Ferguson & Bargh, 2007; Schwarz, 2007; E. R. Smith & Conrey, 2007). From this perspective, evaluative responses depend on momentarily activated patterns of information in response to a set of inputs, which can vary from one situation to another. Building on this notion, Ferguson and Bargh (2007) proposed that attitudes might best be conceptualized as evaluations of "object-based contexts" (p. 232)—a phrase that helps to highlight the idea that a person's subjective representation of a given object includes the context in which the object is encountered. According to this perspective, then, variations in the context actually change the target of evaluation. Thus, for example, a person might evaluate a salty pretzel when she is hungry or a salty pretzel when she is thirsty, or a pretzel on a plate versus a pretzel on the ground, rather than evaluating just the pretzel in the absence of its context. The context is thus inextricably bound up with the object of evaluation.

Our approach similarly suggests that variations in subjective representation can give rise to inconsistencies in evaluative responding, and that evaluations can flexibly tune to the current context. However, we also suggest that the extent to which a mental representation of an object includes the immediate context can vary depending on the *level* at which the object is construed. Concrete mental representations include aspects of the immediate context and give rise to local evaluations of the "object-centered context." Abstract representations, on the other hand, screen out peripheral and contextual details, and therefore give rise to global evaluations of the object's central and enduring aspects.

EMPIRICAL EVIDENCE

The notion that attitudes can summarize evaluative information in different ways depending on the psychological distance of the attitude object (or, more broadly, the level at which that object is mentally represented) suggests a number of intriguing predictions that are important for understanding when individuals will regulate their action to meet the demands of their local social environment, or to transcend the current context in favor of long-term and cross-situational concerns. In the first research to test this model, we examined the implications of a global–local perspective for understanding when people will be susceptible versus resistant to incidental social influences (Ledgerwood, Trope, & Chaiken, 2010). As guides to action and interaction in the current situation, local evaluations should flexibly adapt to the immediate social context. Therefore, evaluations of psychologically close (vs. distant) attitude objects should show greater malleability in response to the attitudes of an incidentally encountered stranger.

However, although global (vs. local) evaluations should be less influenced by contextual factors, they should still relate to other attitude-relevant variables. Specifically, as guides to action and interaction that must transcend the present situation, global evaluations should reflect factors that relate to the core, enduring features of an attitude object. For example, ideological values can be considered broad principles that apply to attitude objects across situations, relate to their central and defining features, and tend to be socially shared within ongoing and important relational contexts (see, e.g., Conover & Feldman, 1981; Jost et al., 2008; Rokeach, 1968). Thus, although evaluations of psychologically distant or abstractly construed attitude objects (vs. near or concretely construed objects) should be less influenced by the immediate social context, they should still strongly reflect an individual's ideological values.

We tested these predictions in a series of five studies. The first study focused on temporal distance and examined whether attitude alignment with an incidental stranger would be greater when a policy was set to be implemented in the near (vs. distant) future. In Studies 2 and 3, we used more direct manipulations of construal level to determine whether our hypothesized mechanism was really responsible for the effects observed in Study 1. Our fourth and fifth studies were designed to show that temporal distance and level of construal do not merely attenuate the relationship between evaluation and any potential predictor, but instead differentially moderate this relationship depending on whether the predictor is contextual or central to the attitude object. We predicted that whereas temporal distance or a direct manipulation of construal would weaken the relationship between evaluative responding and an incidental stranger's views, it would leave unchanged—or even increase—the consistency between participants' evaluations and their previously reported ideological values.

Local Action Guides Facilitate Incidental Social Alignment

Our first study was designed to test the basic notion that evaluative responses toward psychologically near objects would indeed show greater context dependence than evaluative responses toward psychologically distant objects. Drawing on our self-regulatory perspective, we hypothesized that participants would align their attitudes with those of an incidental stranger when contemplating an attitude object that was temporally close, but not one that was temporally distant. Participants took part in an anticipated interaction paradigm (adapted from Chen, Shechter, & Chaiken, 1996), in which they expected to discuss a proposed policy on organ donation with another person in the study. They learned that the policy would be implemented either next week (near-future condition) or next year (distant-future condition), and that their discussion partner was either in favor of or against the issue. Distance to the partner and the length of time until the ostensible conversation were always held constant; the only difference between conditions was therefore whether the attitude object itself was close or distant in time.[1] Participants then privately reported how likely they would be to vote for the described policy (i.e., they did not expect their responses to be shared with their partner). In actuality, this attitude measure was our variable of interest and, ultimately, no discussion took place.

As predicted, participants' voting intentions aligned with those of their interaction partner when the policy was going to be implemented in the near future: When the partner supported (vs. opposed) the near-future policy, participants expressed a greater likelihood of supporting it as well. In contrast, participants were unaffected by their partners' views when the policy was going to be implemented in the distant future. Moreover, these findings were obtained despite participants in the two conditions reporting equal motivation to get along with their discussion partner, suggesting that the distance manipulation was not simply changing the extent to which they were focused on agreeing or affiliating with other people. This is consistent with our suggestion that although local and global evaluations may be particularly useful for facilitating certain types of social coordination, they arise in response to cues about distance rather than in response only to explicit affiliative goals. Study 1 therefore provided intriguing initial support for the idea that responses to near attitude objects are guided by a local evaluative summary that integrates information from the current social context, whereas responses to distant attitude objects are guided by a global summary that is less context-dependent.

In our next two studies, we zeroed in on the mechanism hypothesized to underlie the distance–evaluation link observed in Study 1. In other words, instead of indirectly manipulating level of construal by varying the temporal distance of the attitude object, these studies directly induced participants to adopt an abstract or concrete processing orientation using a procedural priming technique. Research has shown that when participants are led to adopt a particular processing orientation on one task, the primed cognitive procedures then transfer to subsequent, seemingly unrelated activities (e.g., Freitas, Gollwitzer, & Trope, 2004; Fujita, Trope, Liberman, & Levin-Sagi, 2006).

One way to procedurally prime abstract or concrete thinking is to lead participants to focus either on the superordinate, goal-related aspects of activities or else on more subordinate, concrete means. Thus in Study 2, we adapted a procedure developed by Freitas and colleagues (2004) that manipulates level of construal by asking participants to generate either more and more superordinate goals (abstract construal condition) or else more and more subordinate means (concrete construal condition). In Study 3, we sought to conceptually replicate these results by using an alternative manipulation of construal level. Past research has shown that abstract construals can also be procedurally primed by asking participants to generate category labels, whereas concrete construals can be procedurally primed by asking participants to generate exemplars (Fujita & Han, 2009; Fujita, Trope, et al., 2006).

Insofar as our effects truly reflect differences in level of construal, such diverse manipulations of processing orientation should produce results that mirror those obtained in our first experiment. In Studies 2 and 3, therefore, participants first completed one of these two priming procedures designed to induce abstract or concrete thinking. Next, they learned that an anticipated interaction partner was either in favor of or against doctor-assisted suicide. Finally, they completed a 7-item measure of their attitudes toward euthanasia.

As predicted, social alignment was moderated by level of construal. Participants' attitudes aligned with those of their partner when they had been led to think concretely, but not when they had been led to think abstractly. These findings thus supported the notion that people form local action guides when responding to a concretely represented attitude object, but form global action guides when responding to an object that has been construed more abstractly.

Global Action Guides Preserve Ideological Consistency

Importantly, our perspective predicts not only that local action guides will tune to a particular situation, but also that global action guides will show stability across time and contexts. Although the studies reported thus far provide important support for a global–local model, it is unclear whether the lack of a social alignment effect in the distant future or abstract construal conditions truly reflects attitude stability. It is possible, for example, that such an effect could result from apathy engendered by time discounting. If evaluative responding at a distance is truly directed by global action guides that summarize context-independent information, then temporal distance should decrease the extent to which a contextual, but *not* a central, factor predicts evaluation of an attitude object. Thus, responses to psychologically distant attitude objects should still be predicted by people's overarching, decontextualized ideological values.

In Studies 4 and 5, we assessed participants' ideological support for the societal status quo (one of two key elements of left–right ideologies; see Jost, Banaji, & Nosek, 2004; Jost, Glaser, Kruglanski, & Sulloway, 2003) as a potential predictor of evaluation that should relate to the central features of a number of different political issues. Study 4 again manipulated temporal distance, and measured participants' attitudes toward a policy on deporting illegal immigrants. In Study 5, we directly manipulated level of construal using the procedural priming manipulation from our second study, and measured participants' voting intentions and attitudes toward universal health care. We reasoned that insofar as an influx of illegal immigrants (Study 4) and a radical change to the health care system at the time (Study 5) both threaten to disrupt the status quo, the extent to which people value preserving the status quo should predict their evaluations of such policies. In both studies, each participant expected to interact with another student who seemed to support or oppose the policy in question.

The results supported our predictions. When participants were led to think concretely, their attitudes were predicted by their partner's attitude, and not by their previously reported ideological values. In both studies, individuals' evaluative responses toward a political policy were more positive when their partner was in favor of rather than against the policy, regardless of their previously reported ideological values. However, after being led to think abstractly, participants' attitudes were predicted by their ideological values rather than by their partners' views. In Study 3, the extent to which participants valued preserving the societal status quo at time 1 significantly predicted their support for a policy that would increasingly deport illegal immigrants at time 2, regardless of their partner's attitudes on the topic. Likewise, in Study 4, the greater participants' ideological support for protecting the status quo, the more they opposed radically revamping the health care system, whereas the opinions of an incidental stranger had no effect on their evaluative responses.

Taken together, then, these findings provide considerable initial support for the global–local model of evaluation proposed here. When participants construed an attitude object concretely, whether because it was close to them in time or they had been led to adopt a concrete processing orientation, their attitudes fluidly incorporated the opinions of an incidental stranger with whom they expected to have a fleeting interaction. However, when participants construed that same object more abstractly, because it was distant in time or they had been led to adopt an abstract processing orientation, their attitudes were less susceptible to incidental social influence. Instead, these global evaluations incorporated elements of participants' previously reported ideological values that related to the central and defining features of the attitude object.

CONNECTIONS AND IMPLICATIONS

The notion that evaluations can serve to guide action at local and global levels fits well with existing theory and research on self-control that distinguishes between immediate and long-range implications of behavior. In this section, we discuss several ways in which the global–local perspective proposed here can both complement and extend existing research, and highlight one way in which our approach provides a unique perspective on the issue of self-regulation.

Social Dilemmas

Research on social dilemmas has examined how people behave in situations that involve a trade-off between local (individual and/or short-term) concerns on the one hand, and global (collective and/or long-term) concerns on the other. For instance, in his 1973 discussion of social dilemmas, John Platt defined *social traps* as situations in which behavior leading to a short-term or individual gain simultaneously contributes to a long-term or collective loss. In counterpoint, *social fences* referred to situations in which behavior that would produce positive long-term or collective gains also led to negative short-term personal outcomes.

Classically, researchers have sought to explain and predict behavior in social dilemma situations from a rational choice perspective, which assumes that individuals decide whether to cooperate or compete based on the expected utility of each behavioral option (e.g., G. R. Hardin, 1968; Platt, 1973; for reviews, see Dawes, 1980; Weber, Kopelman, & Messick, 2004). For instance, Kelley and Grzelak (1972) showed that increasing the size of short-term, individual consequences versus long-term, collective consequences led participants increasingly to choose actions that improved their own individual outcomes at the expense of the collective. Likewise, a rational choice model suggests that individual differences in the tendency for individuals to focus on the self versus others should predict competitive versus cooperative responding in social dilemma situations. Research confirms that social value orientation (individual differences in proself vs. prosocial orientation) can predict choice in social dilemmas: Proself individuals tend to take more of a shared resource in a commons dilemma and to defect more often in a prisoner's dilemma game than do prosocial individuals (Gärling, 1999; Kramer, McClintock, & Messick, 1986; Parks, 1994).

A global–local model of attitudes suggests additional hypotheses about evaluative responding in social dilemmas that a rational choice model would not necessarily predict. For instance, it implies that the extent to which individuals value cooperation versus competition (e.g., as measured by their social value orientation) should more strongly predict evaluations of cooperative versus competitive options in social dilemmas when respondents construe these dilemmas in abstract terms. In contrast, low-level construals of social dilemmas should increase the extent to which individuals align with the social context, and might therefore lead people increasingly to match their opponent's behavior rather than responding in line with their overarching values.

Put more broadly, a global–local perspective suggests that varying cues related to psychological distance should engender changes in the extent to which people's responses are driven by more global or more local evaluations, even when such cues have no bearing on the expected utility of cooperative or competitive behavior. For example, when long-standing social norms promote fairness or public welfare, distance should increasingly lead participants to rely on global evaluations that draw on these cooperative norms. Interestingly, a public goods dilemma study that found above-average levels of cooperative behavior (Marwell & Ames, 1979) also incorporated two aspects of distance often absent from such research: time (participants made their decisions over the course of a few days rather than immediately; see also Dawes, 1980) and spatial distance (participants reported their decisions to an experimenter in a different location, over the phone, rather than to someone in the same laboratory room). From a global–local perspective, increasing psychological distance in these ways, as well as others, should lead individuals to base their responses increasingly on global rather than local evaluations in various social dilemmas.

Intertemporal Choice

Our focus on psychological distance as a critical dimension in guiding self-regulation echoes the role accorded to temporal distance in research on intertemporal choice and time discounting. This literature suggests that individuals tend to underestimate the value of future rewards, such that as temporal distance to the reward increases, value decreases at a decelerating rate (Ainslie, 2001; Chapman, 1996; Green, Fry, & Myerson, 1994; Kirby, 1997; for reviews, see Frederick, Loewenstein, & O'Donoghue, 2002; Green & Myerson, 2004). Whether this tendency reflects an inability to delay gratification or a rational accounting for the risk inherent in far-off rewards (see, e.g., Kagel, Green, & Caraco, 1986; Mischel, Shoda, & Rodriguez, 1989), the prediction is the same: Individuals will often choose short-term gains (e.g., $10 now; a short-term improvement in health that will begin immediately) over long-term rewards of objectively greater value (e.g., $100 later; a long-term improvement in health that will begin 2 years from now).

A global–local model of attitudes likewise predicts that when individuals make decisions in the here and now, their responses will be guided by local (immediate) rather than global (long-term) information. However, increasing psychological distance (from the attitude object, or even from another, unrelated aspect of the situation) should lead people increasingly to rely on global action guides that incorporate information about long-term rewards. For instance, individuals should be more likely to choose $100 later over $10 today when reporting their decision to a dissimilar (i.e., socially distant) other rather than to someone who is similar.

A global–local perspective also makes predictions for decision making beyond situations involving intertemporal choice (see also Fujita, Trope, & Liberman, 2010). For example, a patient deciding between two medications might consider whether to choose the one favored anecdotally by an acquaintance versus the one favored by statistics across thousands of trials. In such a situation, a local action guide should incorporate information about the acquaintance's opinion in the present social context, whereas a global action guide should summarize information that is consistent across multiple contexts, such as statistical evidence based on many different patients in many different settings. Thus, a global–local model would predict that psychological distance should increase the extent to which patients' choices are influenced by global statistical information (vs. an acquaintance's opinion) in such a situation, even though both types of information are equally proximal in time. Indeed, recent results support this prediction (Ledgerwood, Wakslak, & Wang, 2010).

Construal-Level Analysis of Self-Control

Most obviously, the current perspective relates to a construal level analysis of self-control, which proposes that self-control conflicts develop when low-level and high-level construals of the same object or event prompt opposing behavioral responses (see Fujita, 2008; Fujita, Trope, et al., 2006). According to this perspective, self-control increases when individuals mentally represent an object in terms of its high-level (vs. low-level) features. For example, when participants were led to construe a scene in a broad (high-level) or specific (low-level) way, they reported that they would feel more negatively about succumbing to a temptation within the described setting (e.g., cheating during an exam; Fujita, Trope, et al., 2006, Study 5).

Similarly, a global–local model of attitudes suggests that level of construal plays an important role in determining behavior. According to this perspective, high-level construals should increase the extent to which evaluative action guides draw on global information that applies to an attitude object across situations. Thus, while a person might positively evaluate cheating on an exam in one particular situation (because it will lead to a higher test grade, or because one's classmates approve of it), a global evaluation is more likely to incorporate negative information about cheating that exists across situations (it conflicts with one's core values of honesty and integrity; it would disappoint one's parents or others with whom one has long-term, important relationships). Because high-level construals lead people to rely more on global rather than local action guides, they increase the extent to which self-control conflicts of this type are resolved in favor of global (rather than local or impulsive) concerns. In this way, global evaluations confer value to exercising self-control by emphasizing what is long-term and context-independent, while screening out the evaluative implications of context-specific temptations.

Global evaluations may also be necessary to recognize that the presence of a temptation poses a self-control problem, which represents a critical first step in exercising self-control (Myrseth & Fishbach, 2009). Because local evaluations tune to the current situation, a locally evaluated temptation is perceived as simply a desirable object. A temptation's negativity comes from the fact that it detracts from an overarching, long-term goal: evaluative information that will be included in a global evaluation. Likewise, global evaluations should help to promote counteractive control operations, such as devaluating temptations and precommitment, by highlighting positive evaluative information related to a long-term, context-independent goal and deemphasizing the positivity of local temptations (e.g., Fishbach & Trope, 2005; Fujita & Han, 2009; Trope & Fishbach, 2000).

One important way that this perspective differs from previous construal-level analyses of self-control is in its emphasis on the potential impact of irrelevant, contextual features on evaluative responding. Thus, we propose that people's responses are critically influenced by not only low-level, peripheral features of an attitude object, but also incidental, situational details external to the object itself (like a stranger's opinion).

In addition, our model suggests that global attitudes might play an interesting role in overcoming temptation in situations where temporarily succumbing to a temptation has a relatively low cost. Consider, for example, a dieter at a party, who wonders whether to indulge in just one small piece of chocolate cake. In such a case, past behavior (e.g., successfully following the diet for the last week) and/or future plans (e.g., deciding to be especially good about following the diet starting tomorrow) might help to justify a temporary indulgence. However, a global evaluation of the indulgence should be negative, insofar as it summarizes information that is consistent across contexts; thus, if the dieter forms a global evaluation of indulging in the cake, he should view it negatively and successfully resist the temptation. Indeed, research shows that high-level construals can increase the extent to which participants implicitly associate temptations with negativity (Fujita & Han, 2009), consistent with the notion that global evaluations integrate context-independent, negative information about a temptation, while screening out temporary positive details.

The Functionality of Local Action Guides

Importantly, this perspective also differs from many theories of self-regulation in suggesting that behaving in accord with short-term and situation-specific cues can be quite functional. Whereas self-control has most typically been conceptualized as a conflict between undesired short-term impulses and desirable long-term consequences (see, e.g., Fujita et al., 2010; Mead, Alquist, & Baumeister, in press; Trope & Fishbach, 2000; von Hippel & Ronay, 2009), a global–local model suggests that at times, flexibly acting in accord with the demands of the present social context is both desirable and beneficial, so that it makes sense for humans to be able to regulate their behavior both locally, in the present situation, and globally, across different situations. Although certainly it is often true that controlling local impulses to behave in line with global concerns is beneficial (e.g., Ainslie, 1975; Duckworth & Seligman, 2005; Fujita, Trope, et al., 2006; Mischel et al., 1989), it is also the case that flexibly tuning one's behavior to the current context (even at the expense of long-term goals or normative standards) can have important positive consequences, such as maintaining and improving social bonds.

For instance, behavioral mimicry has been shown to facilitate interpersonal relationships by improving liking and rapport (e.g., Bernieri, 1988; Lakin & Chartrand, 2003). Research on social tuning suggests that participants' racial attitudes shift to align with the presumed attitudes of an experimenter; such shifts in cognition should theoretically help to regulate positive interpersonal interactions (Sinclair et al., 2005; see also C. D. Hardin & Higgins, 1996; Jost et al., 2008). Finally, one might argue that a plethora of context effects—including automatic effects of context on attitudes and behavior, as well as situationally activated goals—represent key components of an important and adaptive *local* self-regulatory process, allowing individuals to adjust their behavior automatically to the specific requirements and affordances of the immediate social situation (see, e.g., Aarts, Gollwitzer, & Hassin, 2004; Bargh, 1997; Cesario, Plaks, & Higgins, 2006; Fishbach, Friedman, & Kruglanski, 2003; Fitzsimons & Bargh, 2003; Kay, Wheeler, Bargh, & Ross, 2004; Ledgerwood & Chaiken, 2007; Shah, 2003).

CONCLUSION

In summary, we have proposed that people must be able to regulate their behavior both within and outside the present context. To do so, they rely on evaluative action guides that can integrate across activated information in two different ways. Local evaluations serve to guide behavior in the here and now by integrating specific details of the present context. They can therefore fluidly incorporate the views of incidental others and tend to look relatively malleable. Global evaluations, on the other hand, enable individuals to transcend the here and now to act on the "there and then." They summarize what is invariant about an attitude object across contexts and therefore tend to reflect people's core values and ideals, and appear relatively stable in the face of changing contextual details. We believe this perspective has the potential to integrate the literatures on attitudes and self-regulation to shed light on the self-regulatory functions of evaluation and the importance of evaluation in guiding effective self-control.

NOTE

1. It is important to distinguish between the manipulation of temporal distance used in this research and one of the classic manipulations of involvement used in persuasion research. Time has often been used in conjunction with a carefully selected issue to manipulate involvement by changing whether a participant will be personally affected by the issue (e.g., whether a university policy change will be instituted next year, while participants are still attending the university, or 10 years from now, after participants have graduated; A. Liberman & Chaiken, 1996; Petty, Cacioppo, & Goldman, 1981). However, in many cases—as with the national policies used in the studies described here—the applicability of a policy to a particular individual does not change over time; thus, manipulating the date of a policy's implementation should not change the extent to which people are motivated to think about it. This theoretical and methodological point has been confirmed empirically: Data collected in our laboratory show that whereas a manipulation of involvement increased the number of thoughts participants listed and the amount of time they spent elaborating on a political policy, our manipulation of temporal distance had no such effect (Ledgerwood et al., 2010).

REFERENCES

Aarts, H., Gollwitzer, P. M., & Hassin, R. R. (2004). Goal contagion: Perceiving is for pursuing. *Journal of Personality and Social Psychology, 87*, 23–37.

Ainslie, G. (1975). Specious reward: A behavioral theory of impulsiveness and impulse control. *Psychological Bulletin, 82*, 463–496.

Ainslie, G. (2001). *Breakdown of will*. Cambridge, UK: Cambridge University Press.

Ajzen, I. (1988). *Attitudes, personality, and behavior*. Buckingham, UK: Open University Press.

Allport, G. W. (1935). Attitudes. In C. Murchison (Ed.), *A handbook of social psychology* (pp. 798–844). Worcester, MA: Clark University Press.

Asch, S. E. (1940). Studies in the principles of judgments and attitudes: II. Determination of judgments by group and by ego standards. *Journal of Social Psychology; Political, Racial, and Differential Psychology, 12*, 433–465.

Asch, S. E. (1948). The doctrine of suggestion, prestige, and imitation in social psychology. *Psychological Review, 55*, 250–276.

Baldwin, M. W., & Holmes, J. G. (1987). Salient private audiences and awareness of the self. *Journal of Personality and Social Psychology, 52*, 1087–1098.

Bargh, J. A. (1997). The automaticity of everyday life. In J. R. S. Wyer (Ed.), *Advances in social cognition* (Vol. 10, pp. 1–61). Mahwah, NJ: Erlbaum.

Bassili, J. N. (1996). Meta-judgmental versus operative indexes of psychological attributes: The case of measure of attitude strength. *Journal of Personality and Social Psychology, 71*, 637–653.

Bernieri, F. J. (1988). Coordinated movement and rapport in teacher–student interactions. *Journal of Nonverbal Behavior, 12*, 120–138.

Bodenhausen, G. V., Schwarz, N., Bless, H., & Wanke, M. (1995). Effects of atypical exemplars on racial beliefs: Enlightened racism or generalized appraisals? *Journal of Experimental Social Psychology, 31*, 48–63.

Campbell, A., Converse, P. E., Miller, W. E., & Stokes, D. E. (1960). *The American voter*. New York: Wiley.

Campbell, D. T. (1950). The indirect assessment of social attitudes. *Psychological Bulletin, 47,* 15–38.

Cesario, J., Plaks, J. E., & Higgins, E. T. (2006). Automatic social behavior as motivated preparation to interact. *Journal of Personality and Social Psychology, 90,* 893–910.

Chapman, G. B. (1996). Temporal discounting and utility for health and money. *Journal of Experimental Psychology: Learning, Memory, and Cognition, 22,* 771–791.

Chen, S., Shechter, D., & Chaiken, S. (1996). Getting at the truth or getting along: Accuracy-versus impression-motivated heuristic and systematic processing. *Journal of Personality and Social Psychology, 71,* 262–275.

Conover, P. J., & Feldman, S. (1981). The origins and meaning of liberal/conservative self identification. *American Journal of Political Science, 25,* 617–645.

Conrey, F. R., & Smith, E. R. (2007). Attitude representation: Attitudes as patterns in a distributed, connectionist representational system. *Social Cognition, 25,* 718–735.

Converse, P. E. (1964). The nature of belief systems in mass politics. In D. E. Apter (Ed.), *Ideology and discontent* (pp. 206–261). New York: Free Press.

Davis, J. L., & Rusbult, C. E. (2001). Attitude alignment in close relationships. *Journal of Personality and Social Psychology, 81,* 65–84.

Dawes, R. M. (1980). Social dilemmas. *Annual Review of Psychology, 31,* 169–193.

Duckworth, A. L., & Seligman, M. E. P. (2005). Self-discipline outdoes IQ in predicting academic performance of adolescents. *Psychological Science, 16,* 939–944.

Eagly, A. H., & Chaiken, S. (1995). Attitude strength, attitude structure, and resistance to change. In R. E. Petty & J. A. Krosnick (Eds.), *Attitude strength: Antecedents and consequences* (Vol. 4, pp. 413–432). Hillsdale, NJ: Erlbaum.

Echterhoff, G., Higgins, E. T., & Levine, J. M. (2009). Shared reality: Experiencing commonality with others' inner states about the world. *Perspectives on Psychological Science, 4,* 496–521.

Fazio, R. H. (1989). On the power and functionality of attitudes: The role of attitude accessibility. In A. R. Pratkanis, S. J. Breckler, & A. G. Greenwald (Eds.), *Attitude structure and function* (pp. 153–179). Hillsdale, NJ: Erlbaum.

Ferguson, M. J., & Bargh, J. A. (2007). Beyond the attitude object: Implicit attitudes spring from object-centered contexts. In B. Wittenbrink & N. Schwarz (Eds.), *Implicit measures of attitudes* (pp. 216–246). New York: Guilford Press.

Festinger, L. (1950). Informal social communication. *Psychological Review, 57,* 271–282.

Fishbach, A., Friedman, R. S., & Kruglanski, A. W. (2003). Leading us not into temptation: Momentary allurements elicit overriding goal activation. *Journal of Personality and Social Psychology, 84,* 296–309.

Fishbach, A., & Trope, Y. (2005). The substitutability of external control and self-control in overcoming temptation. *Journal of Experimental Social Psychology, 41,* 256–270.

Fitzsimons, G. M., & Bargh, J. A. (2003). Thinking of you: Nonconscious pursuit of interpersonal goals associated with relationship partners. *Journal of Personality and Social Psychology, 84,* 148–163.

Forster, J., Friedman, R. S., & Liberman, N. (2004). Temporal construal effects on abstract and concrete thinking: Consequences for insight and creative cognition. *Journal of Personality and Social Psychology, 87,* 177–189.

Frederick, S., Loewenstein, G., & O'Donoghue, T. (2002). Time discounting and time preference: A critical review. *Journal of Economic Literature, 40,* 351–401.

Freitas, A. L., Gollwitzer, P. M., & Trope, Y. (2004). The influence of abstract and concrete mindsets on anticipating and guiding others' self regulatory efforts. *Journal of Experimental Social Psychology, 40,* 739–752.

Fujita, K. (2008). Seeing the forest beyond the trees: A construal level approach to self-control. *Social and Personality Psychology Compass, 2,* 1475–1496.

Fujita, K., & Han, H. A. (2009). Moving beyond deliberative control of impulses: The effect of construal levels on evaluative associations in self-control conflicts. *Psychological Science, 20,* 799–804.

Fujita, K., Henderson, M. D., Eng, J., Trope, Y., & Liberman, N. (2006). Spatial distance and mental construal of social events. *Psychological Science, 17,* 278–282.

Fujita, K., Trope, Y., & Liberman, N. (2010). Seeing the big picture: A construal level analysis of self-control. In R. Hassin, K. Ochsner, & Y. Trope (Eds.), *From society to brain: The new sciences of self-control.* New York: Oxford University Press.

Fujita, K., Trope, Y., Liberman, N., & Levin-Sagi, M. (2006). Construal levels and self-control. *Journal of Personality and Social Psychology, 90,* 351–367.

Gärling, T. (1999). Value priorities, social value orientations and cooperation in social dilemmas. *British Journal of Social Psychology, 38,* 397–408.

Green, L., Fry, A., & Myerson, J. (1994). Discounting of delayed rewards: A life-span comparison. *Psychological Science, 5,* 33–36.

Green, L., & Myerson, J. (2004). A discounting framework for choice with delayed and probabilistic rewards. *Psychological Bulletin, 130,* 769–772.

Hardin, C. D., & Higgins, E. T. (1996). Shared reality: How social verification makes the subjective objective. In R. M. Sorrentino & E. T. Higgins (Eds.), *Handbook of motivation and cognition: Vol. 3. The interpersonal context* (pp. 28–84). New York: Guilford Press.

Hardin, G. R. (1968). The tragedy of the commons. *Science, 162,* 1243–1248.

Higgins, E. T., & Rholes, W. S. (1978). "Saying is believing": Effects of message modification on memory and liking for the person described. *Journal of Experimental and Social Psychology, 14,* 363–378.

Jost, J. T., Banaji, M. R., & Nosek, B. A. (2004). A decade of system justification theory: Accumulated evidence of conscious and unconscious bolstering of the status quo. *Political Psychology, 25,* 881–919.

Jost, J. T., Glaser, J., Kruglanski, A. W., & Sulloway, F. (2003). Political conservatism as motivated social cognition. *Psychological Bulletin, 129,* 339–375.

Jost, J. T., Ledgerwood, A., & Hardin, C. D. (2008). Shared reality, system justification, and the relational basis of ideological beliefs. *Social and Personality Psychology Compass, 2*(1), 171–186.

Kagel, J. H., Green, L., & Caraco, T. (1986). When foragers discount the future: Constraint or adaptation? *Behaviour, 34,* 271–283.

Katz, D. (1960). The functional approach to the study of attitudes. In R. H. Fazio & R. E. Petty (Eds.), *Public opinion quarterly* (pp. 163–204). New York: Psychology Press.

Kay, A. C., Wheeler, S. C., Bargh, J. A., & Ross, L. (2004). Material priming: The influence of mundane physical objects on situational construal and competitive behavioral choice. *Organizational Behavior and Human Decision Processes, 95*(1), 83–96.

Kelley, H. H., & Grzelak, J. (1972). Conflict between individual and common interest in an N-person relationship. *Journal of Personality and Social Psychology, 21,* 190–197.

Kirby, K. N. (1997). Bidding on the future: Evidence against normative discounting of delayed rewards. *Journal of Experimental Psychology: General, 126,* 54–70.

Kramer, R. M., McClintock, C. G., & Messick, D. M. (1986). Social values and cooperative response to a simulated resource conservation crisis. *Journal of Personality, 54,* 576–592.

Krech, D., & Crutchfield, R. S. (1948). *Theory and problems of social psychology.* New York: McGraw-Hill.

Krosnick, J. A. (1988). Attitude importance and attitude change. *Journal of Experimental Social Psychology, 24,* 240–255.

Lakin, J., & Chartrand, T. L. (2003). Increasing nonconscious mimicry to achieve rapport. *Psychological Science, 27,* 145–162.

Ledgerwood, A., & Chaiken, S. (2007). Priming us and them: Automatic assimilation and contrast in group attitudes. *Journal of Personality and Social Psychology, 93*, 940–956.

Ledgerwood, A., & Liviatan, I. (2010). The price of a shared vision: Group identity goals and the social creation of value. *Social Cognition, 28*, 401–421.

Ledgerwood, A., Trope, Y., & Chaiken, S. (2010). Flexibility now, consistency later: Psychological distance and construal shape evaluative responding. *Journal of Personality and Social Psychology, 99*, 32–51.

Ledgerwood, A., Wakslak, C. J., & Wang, M. K. (2010). Differential information use for near and distant decisions. *Journal of Experimental Social Psychology, 46*, 638–642.

Liberman, A., & Chaiken, S. (1996). The direct effect of personal relevance on attitudes. *Personality and Social Psychology Bulletin, 22*, 269–279.

Liberman, N., & Trope, Y. (1998). The role of feasibility and desirability considerations in near and distant future decisions: A test of temporal construal theory. *Journal of Personality and Social Psychology, 75*, 5–18.

Liberman, N., & Trope, Y. (2008). The psychology of transcending the here and now. *Science, 322*, 1201–1205.

Lord, C. G., & Lepper, M. (1999). Attitude representation theory. In M. Zanna (Ed.), *Advances in experimental social psychology* (pp. 265–343). San Diego, CA: Academic Press.

Lord, C. G., Lepper, M. R., & Mackie, D. M. (1984). Attitude prototypes as determinants of attitude–behavior consistency. *Journal of Personality and Social Psychology, 46*, 1254–1266.

Marwell, G., & Ames, R. E. (1979). Experiments on the provision of public goods: I. Resources, interest, group size, and the free-rider problem. *American Journal of Sociology, 84*, 1335–1360.

Mead, N. L., Alquist, J. L., & Baumeister, R. F. (in press). Ego depletion and the limited resource model of self-regulation. In R. Hassin, K. Ochsner, & Y. Trope (Eds.), *From society to brain: The new sciences of self-control.* New York: Oxford University Press.

Mischel, W., Shoda, Y., & Rodriguez, M. L. (1989). Delay of gratification in children. *Science, 244*, 933–938.

Myrseth, K. O. R., & Fishbach, A. (2009). Self-control: A function of knowing when and how to exercise restraint. *Current Directions in Psychological Science, 18*, 247–252.

Nussbaum, S., Trope, Y., & Liberman, N. (2003). Creeping dispositionism: The temporal dynamics of behavioral prediction. *Journal of Personality and Social Psychology, 84*, 485–497.

Parks, C. D. (1994). The predictive ability of social values in resource dilemmas and public goods games. *Personality and Social Psychology Bulletin, 20*, 431–438.

Petty, R. E., Cacioppo, J. T., & Goldman, R. (1981). Personal involvement as a determinant of argument-based persuasion. *Journal of Personality and Social Psychology, 41*, 847–855.

Platt, J. (1973). Social traps. *American Psychologist, 28*(8), 641–651.

Rokeach, M. (1968). *Beliefs, attitudes, and values: A theory of organization and change.* San Francisco: Jossey-Bass.

Schuman, H., & Presser, S. (1981). *Questions and answers: Experiments on question form, wording, and context in attitude surveys.* New York: Academic Press.

Schwarz, N. (2007). Attitude construction: Evaluation in context. *Social Cognition, 25*, 638–656.

Shah, J. (2003). Automatic for the people: How representations of significant others implicitly affect goal pursuit. *Journal of Personality and Social Psychology, 84*, 661–681.

Sia, T. L., Lord, C. G., Blessum, K., Ratcliff, C. D., & Lepper, M. R. (1997). Is a rose always a rose?: The role of social category exemplar-change in attitude stability and attitude–behavior consistency. *Journal of Personality and Social Psychology, 72*, 501–514.

Sinclair, S., Lowery, B. S., Hardin, C. D., & Colangelo, A. (2005). Social tuning of automatic racial attitudes: The role of affiliative motivation. *Journal of Personality and Social Psychology, 89,* 583–592.

Smith, E. R., & Conrey, F. R. (2007). Mental representations as states not things: Implications for implicit and explicit measurement. In B. Wittenbrink & N. Schwarz (Eds.), *Implicit measures of attitudes* (pp. 247–264). New York: Guilford Press.

Smith, M. B., Bruner, J. S., & White, R. W. (1956). *Opinions and personality.* New York: Wiley.

Tourangeau, R., & Rasinski, K. A. (1988). Cognitive processes underlying context effects in attitude measurement. *Psychological Bulletin, 103,* 299–314.

Trope, Y., & Fishbach, A. (2000). Counteractive self-control in overcoming temptation. *Journal of Personality and Social Psychology, 79,* 493–506.

Trope, Y., & Liberman, N. (2003). Temporal construal. *Psychological Review, 110,* 403–421.

von Hippel, W., & Ronay, R. (2009). Executive functions and self-control. In J. P. Forgas, R. F. Baumeister, & D. Tice (Eds.), *The psychology of self regulation: Cognitive, affective, and motivational processes* (pp. 303–318). New York: Psychology Press.

Wakslak, C. J., Trope, Y., Liberman, N., & Aloni, R. (2006). Seeing the forest when entry is unlikely: Probability and the mental representation of events. *Journal of Experimental Psychology: General, 135,* 641–653.

Weber, J. M., Kopelman, S., & Messick, D. M. (2004). A conceptual review of decision making in social dilemmas: Applying a logic of appropriateness. *Personality and Social Psychology Review, 8,* 281–304.

Wilson, T., Lindsey, S., & Schooler, T. Y. (2000). A model of dual attitudes. *Psychological Review, 107,* 101–126.

CHAPTER 13

Identifying and Battling Temptation

AYELET FISHBACH
BENJAMIN A. CONVERSE

Despite knowing well that "you can't have your cake and eat it too," people still want many conflicting things at once; that is, people want to fulfill short-term desires, and they want to do so without obstructing their long-term interests. Thus, weight watchers wish to eat many delicious cakes, and they also wish not to look like they have eaten many delicious cakes. Similarly, professionals wish for early leave on Friday afternoon, and they also wish for early promotions at year-end reviews. And feuding partners want to have the last word in every battle, and they also want to maintain their relationship through every battle. In a world where people want to have it both ways—to enjoy the moment and to prosper in the long run, how do they protect long-term interests from the allure of short-term desires?

An individual faces a self-control dilemma whenever the attainment of an alluring desire or temptation would conflict with more important, longer-term goals (Ainslie, 1992; Loewenstein, 1996; Rachlin, 2000; Thaler, 1991; Trope & Fishbach, 2000). Despite the pervasiveness of self-control dilemmas, identifying that a situation poses such a dilemma can be surprisingly difficult. Thus, when people choose to pursue short-term desires, it is not always as a result of bad judgment defeating good judgment in the archetypal battle. In many cases, people choose the tempting option because they do not realize it will hurt them in the long run. For example, the professional may leave work early because she does not consider that leaving early on a single Friday afternoon will put her promotion at risk, just as the smoker may light up without considering that a single cigarette poses a health risk. It is only when one has identified a potential conflict that resolution in favor of higher-order goals hinges on effective employment of self-control strategies.

This chapter reviews our research on identifying and counteracting temptations. First, it is useful to define *temptations* versus *goals*. We define these conflicting motivations within a given context and with respect to each other (Fishbach & Shah, 2006; Leander, Shah, & Chartrand, 2009). A stimulus can only represent a temptation with respect to another, higher-order goal, which the individual believes is more important. According to this definition, temptations do not have specific content. Rather, any personal motivation can potentially constitute an interfering temptation with respect to a higher-level goal, or it can constitute an overriding goal with respect to a lower-level temptation. For example, "making friends" may be perceived as a temptation that interferes with the pursuit of "going to class," and it may be perceived as a goal with which the pursuit of "being competitive" interferes. Similarly, drinking and smoking interfere with the pursuit of a healthy lifestyle (hence, they are temptations), but at the same time they promote social acceptance to certain social groups (hence, they are goals). Effective self-control operates on the focal activity in a way that depends on its relative status in the present motivational conflict. Self-control increases the strength of goals and decreases the strength of competing impulses or temptations.

CONFLICT IDENTIFICATION

Success at self-control depends first on identifying a conflict. When observing a single behavior that resembles self-control failure, it is safe to assume that a conflict is identified only if the long-term costs of indulgence are clear and high. Cheating on one's spouse, for example, may carry extreme long-term costs, such that a person choosing this path has likely considered the possible devastating consequences and tried, but failed, to resist. As the long-term costs of a single temptation indulgence decrease, however, it becomes less certain that one will identify a potential self-control conflict. For example, the net impact of a single jelly donut is probably negligible to a person's overall health. Temptations like this one, for which a single consumption experience has negligible negative consequences, are pervasive. We term them *epsilon-cost temptations* (as opposed to *clear-cost temptations*; Myrseth & Fishbach, 2009). It is only through repeated consumption that the cost of these kinds of indulgences becomes consequential.

The question of conflict identification further becomes trivial whenever external agents (e.g., parents, educators, experimenters) identify the conflict for the individual and explicitly demand restraint. For example, in ego-depletion research, participants are specifically instructed to avoid some impulse (e.g., to eat radishes rather than cookies, to suppress emotions in response to some evocative stimulus; Baumeister, Bratslavsky, Muraven, & Tice, 1998). And in delay-of-gratification paradigms, children are explicitly told to resist short-term rewards in favor of long-term payoff (e.g., one marshmallow now in favor of two marshmallows later; Mischel & Baker, 1975). In these situations the researchers identify the conflict for the individual, so any success or failure necessarily reflects the person's attempts to resist that temptation.

What then facilitates identification of conflict for epsilon-cost temptations? We suggest that viewing an action opportunity with *width*—that is, in relation to future opportunities—facilitates conflict identification. Framing a single opportunity to act in isolation may not cue the presence of a conflict, whereas framing the opportunity in relation to other opportunities is more likely to cue conflict. The person who says "One jelly donut won't kill me," perceives the temptation in isolation, notes that there are trivial costs associated with eating it, and likely does not experience a conflict between this breakfast and his more important health goals. The person who is planning a new morning routine, however, may be more likely to perceive today's choice of a donut in relation to many future breakfast choices, and may be more likely to identify a self-control conflict.

In addition, conflict identification also requires *consistency*. The individual must expect the present decision to be replayed in future opportunities. When setting a morning routine, for example, the diner will only feel conflicted about his donut if he expects it to set a precedent for future mornings. If today is a special donut day, whereas future days will be fruit days instead, then the donut will not pose a threat to long-term health goals, and conflict will not be identified. We next summarize the evidence that the frame necessary for conflict identification is one that meets conditions of both *width* and *consistency*.

Width: Perceiving Current Choices in Relation to Future Choices

A failure to identify a self-control conflict occurs when individuals respond to contextual cues or opportunities rather mindlessly, without considering a pattern of responses or a large "bracket" (Rachlin, 2000; Read, Loewenstein, & Rabin, 1999). For example when habitual smokers light up a cigarette in response to contextual cues (e.g., "gin and tonic") they often fail to consider a pattern of behaviors that would undermine their long-term interests (Wood & Neal, 2007). Making decisions within wider brackets, in contrast, encourages people to consider multiple opportunities together, thus increasing the likelihood of identifying a potential self-control conflict. In one illustrative study (Read, Loewenstein, & Kalyanaraman, 1999), students who chose three video rentals simultaneously chose more highbrow over lowbrow movies (e.g., *Schindler's List* over *My Cousin Vinny*) than did students who chose each video on the day they would watch it. The simultaneous condition induced students to consider a choice pattern, thus making self-control conflicts between pleasurable but not thought-provoking lowbrow movies and difficult but enriching highbrow movies more salient, and leading students to choose more highbrow movies.

In our research, we find that even subtle cues for a wide versus narrow frame are sufficient to influence conflict identification and success at self-control. For example, in one study, we (Myrseth & Fishbach, 2009) set up a free food stand in an area of campus that commonly provides such amenities. The stand featured an assortment of carrots and chocolates, and a large sign invited passersby to help themselves "in celebration of the lighter and warmer times ahead." In the wide-frame condition, the sign indicated this was the "Spring Food Stand," whereas in the narrow-frame condition, the sign indicated it was the "April 12th Food Stand." Accordingly, participants consumed fewer chocolates and more carrots when the sign implied wide versus narrow framing.

Extant work on choice bracketing and more recent work exploring the conflict experience thus illustrate the first necessary condition for self-control conflict identification. Low-cost temptations do not seem problematic in narrow frames or on special occasions: They only introduce conflict when they are considered in relation to future choices because only the accumulated cost of these temptations undermines goal attainment. Wide frames therefore promote conflict identification.

Consistency: Expecting Future Choices to Be Similar to Current Choices

Even when one considers current and future choices in relation to each other, conflict identification further requires that one expects current choices to be consistent with future choices. This depends on which of two dynamics, or choice patterns, an individual expects to follow when considering a sequence of actions. Our research has helped to draw the distinction between sequences that balance goals and temptations over time, and sequences that highlight goals (Fishbach, Dhar, & Zhang, 2006; Fishbach & Zhang, 2008; Koo & Fishbach, 2008). In a *balancing* dynamic, individuals plan to alternate between goals and temptations in successive choices. One can therefore give in to temptation without identifying a conflict if she expects that tomorrow she will switch to pursuing the goal instead. If one plans to choose fruit tomorrow, then choosing cake over fruit today does not pose a threat to long-term health goals. This pattern of behaviors contrasts with a choice dynamic of *highlighting*. In a highlighting dynamic, individuals plan to pursue the same motive on each opportunity. In this dynamic, a choice between cake and fruit arouses the conflict that is characteristic of a self-control dilemma.

In one study of the consequences of these opposing choice dynamics (Fishbach & Zhang, 2008), healthy versus unhealthy food choices were presented to participants in one of two formats. Some participants encountered one bowl with packets of baby carrots and a separate bowl with chocolates. Presenting these options apart induced a sense of competition between them, which was expected to invoke a highlighting dynamic (eat healthy now and later). Other participants encountered one big bowl with carrots and chocolates interspersed. Presenting these options together induced a sense of complementarity, which was expected to invoke a *balancing* dynamic (eat unhealthy now and compensate later). Accordingly, participants chose carrots more frequently when the items were presented apart than when they were presented together. We assumed that the highlighting dynamic increased the likelihood of identifying a self-control conflict and therefore led participants in this condition to exercise self-control. Indeed, consistent with our interpretation, individual differences in the strength of the weight-watching goal (i.e., how much participants wanted to lose weight) predicted healthy food choices when the options were presented apart but not when they were presented together. We can therefore conclude that presenting options apart helped individuals identify a self-control problem and, as a result, their actions were more closely associated with the strength of their desire to eat healthy.

The balancing dynamic threatens the engagement of self-control because choices consistent with short-term rather than long-term goals can be made at each opportunity, without the experience of conflict. When one plans to switch between goals and temptations, this tends to promote a "temptation now, goal later" plan, which provides instant gratification and continually postpones goal pursuit. Temptation indulgence thus ensues not as a result of self-control failure but as a repeated failure to identify self-control conflict in the first place.

This inconsistent pattern of choices is illustrated in full by another study of immediate and delayed choices. In that study, we (Fishbach & Zhang, 2008) asked participants to choose a full two-course meal consisting of an entrée (immediate choice) and a dessert (delayed choice). Some participants chose from a menu that presented the unhealthier fare on one page and the healthier fare on a separate page to induce a sense of competition and a highlighting dynamic. Other participants chose from a menu that presented the unhealthy and healthy fare mixed together across the two pages to induce complementarity and a balancing dynamic. As expected, those who chose from separate menus were better able to identify and resolve the self-control conflict: They tended to prefer healthy entrees and desserts. Those who chose from one menu, in comparison, planned to choose healthy desserts for later but opted to indulge in more unhealthy entrees up front. We can thus conclude that perceiving multiple action opportunities (*width*) is a necessary but insufficient condition for identifying a self-control conflict. In addition, one must see the potential for consistent actions that correspond to either temptation or the more important goal.

Given that conflict has been identified upon encountering temptation, the individual is likely to exert self-control efforts. In what follows, we address our research on counteractive control, which describes the process by which individuals offset the influence of temptation on goal pursuit.

COUNTERACTIVE CONTROL: ASYMMETRIC RESPONSES TO GOALS AND TEMPTATIONS

Self-control works to resolve the tension between goals and temptations. According to *counteractive control theory* (Fishbach & Trope, 2005; Trope & Fishbach, 2000), the essence of this process involves asymmetrically shifting the motivational strengths of conflicting motivations. High-order goals are strengthened so they may override low-order temptations. Low-order temptations are weakened so they may be overridden by high-order goals. These asymmetric shifts in motivational strength may be achieved by modulating the situation (e.g., imposing penalties, rewards) or by modulating mental representations of the situation (e.g., devaluing or bolstering the value of activities). These shifts may further involve explicit operations that require conscious awareness and planning, or implicit processes that operate with minimal awareness and conscious planning. Regardless of the specific type of self-control operation, its function is similar: It either increases the tendency to operate on a personal motive or decreases the tendency to operate on it, depending on the status of the motive as a goal or temptation. We summarize the various self-control operations in Table 13.1 and elaborate on them in this section.

Importantly, each operation increases proportionally, as the strength of the temptation increases, to diminish the impact of temptation on one's behavior. Thus, when people anticipate strong (vs. weak) temptation, they increase their self-control efforts pro-

TABLE 13.1. Self-Control Strategies That Create Asymmetric Change in Motivational Strength of Goals and Temptations

	Temptations	Goals
Changing the choice situation	• Precommitment to forego • Self-imposed penalties • Avoidance	• Precommitment to pursue • Self-imposed rewards • Approach
Changing the psychological meaning of choice options	• Inhibit • Devalue • Setting low expectations • Cool and abstract construal	• Activate • Bolster • Setting high expectations • Hot and concrete construal

portionally. As a result, their likelihood of adhering to their long-term interests remains intact despite the presence of strong temptations. Notably, there can also be variation in the degree to which individuals expect particular temptations to pose a risk. Thus, two individuals can face the same temptation and vary in their successful self-control toward the temptation depending on expectations. The person who expects strong interference will be more likely to exercise self-control and adhere to her goals than will the person who does not anticipate such strong interference. In these situations, the anticipation of a temptation not only counteracts its impact on behavior but further improves goal adherence because those who expect interference counteract it and work harder to pursue their long-term goals.

To demonstrate the impact of anticipated obstacles or temptations, we (Sheldon & Fishbach, 2009) studied people's cooperation in mixed-motive interactions (e.g., social dilemmas; Dawes, 1980; Messick & Brewer, 1983). Mixed-motive interactions pose a self-control conflict because people recognize that the long-term benefits of cooperation outweigh the short-term payoffs of competition but nonetheless feel tempted to compete for an immediate benefit (Dewitte & De Cremer, 2001). In our studies, participants were more tempted to compete when they anticipated barriers to successful outcomes (e.g., when they expected doing well to be difficult) than when they did not anticipate barriers. They in turn counteracted the increasing temptation by cooperating more when expecting strong (vs. weak) barriers to success, but only as long as they were imbued with a strong sense of personal control. This pattern is indicative of counteractive self-control.

Modulating Choice Situations

If people identify a potential conflict in advance, they can essentially resolve it before it occurs by changing the choice set, so it no longer presents a conflict. This precommitment strategy restricts their options but increases goal-consistent behavior. Alternatively, people may strategically affect the value of available options. By attaching bonuses to goals or penalties to temptations, they can tip the value scales to favor goal-consistent behavior. In addition, people may distance themselves from temptations and approach goals. Implicit dispositions toward goals and away from temptations that develop over time can increase the probability of goal pursuit. In this section, we explicate each of these strategies.

Precommitment

When potential conflicts between goals and temptations loom in the future, proactive self-regulators may diverge from the common pattern of seeking to maintain available options (Brehm, 1966), and instead restrict future choice sets to favor goal pursuit (Ainslie, 1992; Schelling, 1984; Strotz, 1956; Thaler & Shefrin, 1981; Wertenbroch, 1998). Specifically, self-regulators eliminate tempting alternatives and increase the share of goal alternatives in future choice sets. Many gamblers, for example, leave their wallets in the hotel room, taking only a set amount of cash into the casino with them. When the money is gone, the temptation to gamble more has already been eliminated. Similarly, grocery-shopping dieters may fill their carts with only healthy foods, limiting their own (and their unsuspecting families) snacking options later. In one illustrative study (Ariely & Wertenbroch, 2002), students committed themselves to earlier-than-necessary class deadlines when given the option to set them in advance. By precommitting, these students not only took on unnecessary potential costs, such as grade penalties for late submissions, but also limited their pursuit of temptations and increased the motivational strength of their academic pursuits.

Penalties and Rewards

Another way to change the situation in favor of goals is to affect the relative value of goals and temptations asymmetrically. One way people can proactively stack the deck against temptations is to bolster the value of goal pursuit by attaching contingent bonuses. When people wager with friends that they can finish a marathon, promise themselves a new outfit for losing 10 pounds, or let themselves leave an hour early from work if they can complete their to-do list, they are using contingent bonuses to make their goals more valuable. In one experimental demonstration of this behavior (Trope & Fishbach, 2000), students were given the opportunity to receive reliable and accurate feedback about their future health risks. Some of the students learned that the necessary medical test would be highly uncomfortable, thus making it tempting to avoid the test and lose the long-term benefits of receiving the results. Other students learned that the medical test would be very easy, thus posing no risk to deter them from pursuing the long-term benefits. Students who faced an uncomfortable (vs. easy) medical test, and who thought the feedback was important, more frequently opted to make their study compensation contingent on completing the exam. By self-imposing this contingency, they were exercising self-control, risking their compensation, but making it more likely that they would follow through on the action providing long-term benefits.

The asymmetry of counteractive control suggests that people can similarly stack the deck against temptations using self-imposed penalties. This popular self-control tool recently became available at stickK (*www.stickk.com*), a website that relies primarily on the principle of self-imposed penalties. Here, people can write contracts to help them stick to their goals, preauthorizing certain punishments for temptation indulgence. An extra hour of sleep might seem less appealing to an aspiring marathoner, for example, if she has contracted to forfeit money to a despised charity for missing her workout. In support of this principle, one study demonstrated that the strong temptation to interrupt a 3-day glucose fast (compared with the weaker temptation of interrupting a 6-hour glucose fast) led people to set higher monetary penalties for themselves (Trope & Fishbach, 2000). By agreeing to penalize themselves, these people increased their likelihood of persisting through the long-term fast despite the strong temptation to give in. When there is tension between the value of goals and competing temptations, contingent bonuses tip the scales toward goals, and contingent penalties tip the scales away from temptations. Both changes to the choice situation increase the relative value and, therefore, the pursuit of higher-order goals.

Approach and Avoidance

When choice sets feature goals and formidable temptations, people might increase the motivational strength of high-order goals by keeping their distance from the temptations and establishing their proximity to objects associated with their goals (Ainslie, 1992; Schelling, 1984; Thaler & Shefrin, 1981). Diners often ask waiters to clear their half-eaten plates, just to help them stop picking at meals that have already satisfied them. Motivated students may deliberately select rooms that are closer to the library and further from fraternity row to facilitate studying and avoid partying. And on the interpersonal level, people keep a distance from those who are believed to exert "bad influence" (e.g., an ex-boyfriend), while maintaining proximity to those who help them pursue long-term interests (Fitzsimons & Shah, 2008). Actions like these, by which effective self-regulators explicitly and routinely resist temptations, may develop into implicit dispositions to approach goals and avoid temptations. These dispositions can be acted on effortlessly upon encountering temptation.

Self-control research has investigated a variety of implicit self-control strategies that often accompany, or sometimes replace, explicit, deliberative control (e.g., Fishbach, Friedman, & Kruglanski, 2003; Fishbach & Shah, 2006; Fishbach & Trope, 2007; Fujita & Han, 2009; Gollwitzer, Bayer, & McCulloch, 2004; Moskowitz, Gollwitzer, Wasel, & Schaal, 1999). Implicit self-control differs from other mechanisms of unconscious goal pursuit (Aarts & Dijksterhuis, 2000; Bargh, Gollwitzer, Lee-Chai, Barndollar, & Troetschel, 2001; Shah & Kruglanski, 2003; see also Papies & Aarts, Chapter 7, this volume) in that it counteracts the influence of situationally primed goals that conflict with other, higher-order goals. For example, according to unconscious goal priming, cues about one's boyfriend (e.g., seeing his name) can activate the goal to think carefully about the behavior of social targets (Fitzsimons & Bargh, 2003). To the extent, however, that this goal to think about others' behavior conflicts with a higher-order goal (e.g., when trying to pay attention in class rather than check for Twitter updates), according to work on implicit self-control, this same prime could increase efforts to ignore this social target.

In a series of studies, we (Fishbach & Shah, 2006) examined the implicit analogue to explicit approach and avoidance self-control strategies. The main prediction was that participants would adopt an automatic approach tendency to goal-related stimuli and an avoidance tendency to temptation-related stimuli. In one study, participants completed a lexical decision task, deciding whether letter strings represented words or nonwords. On some trials, they indicated words by pushing a joystick away from themselves, and on others they indicated words by pulling the joystick toward themselves. An approach orientation enables faster pulling of a lever, whereas an avoidance orientation enables faster pushing away of a lever (Chen & Bargh, 1999; Markman & Brendl, 2005; Solarz, 1960). Embedded in the words were participants' own idiosyncratic goals (e.g., *exercise*), temptations (e.g., *alcohol*), and control activities (e.g., *internship*). This study found that participants were faster to pull goal-related (than temptation-related) words, and faster to push temptation-related (than goal-related) words. A follow-up study found that a tendency to approach academic goals and avoid nonacademic temptations related to higher grade point averages. Thus, this very simple implicit action disposition is associated with real self-regulatory benefits.

When self-control changes the situation, people are affecting objective features of the choice sets available to them. Contingent bonuses actually make goal pursuit more attractive, and contingent penalties actually increase the objective price of indulgence. Precommitment works by increasing the availability of goal-relevant options and decreasing the availability of options that could tempt one away. And by approaching goals and avoiding temptations, people physically draw closer to goal-relevant objects and create distance from tempting objects. In the next section, we discuss how self-control can operate without exerting an objective influence on the choice set or the environment.

Modulating Mental Representations

Self-control strategies can also operate purely through mental representations. By bringing goal-related options and actions to mind, and inhibiting thoughts about temptations, people increase the likelihood of goal pursuit. By focusing on the positive aspects of goal-related objects and the negative aspects of temptation-related objects, people can inflate the subjective value of goals and increase the likelihood of their pursuit. Similarly, reflecting on the cool, abstract features of a temptation rather than the hot, concrete features affects the motivational strength in favor of goal pursuit. Additionally, people can modulate their future plans to increase goal pursuit. By setting optimistic expectations for future choices (i.e., more goal engagement, less temptation engagement), people can motivate increased goal pursuit. We discuss each of these changing mental representations in turn.

Activation/Inhibition

Earlier, we discussed self-control strategies that operate by changing relative availabilities in the choice situation. Expecting future self-control conflict, people precommit to choice sets that have more goal-related options and fewer temptation-related options, like the dieter who stocks the house with fruit and strips the house of cookies. Our research suggests that people have developed other strategies that similarly affect availability, but solely at the level of mental representations (Fishbach et al., 2003); that is, counteractive control also entails changes in the activation level of goal- and temptation-related constructs. By activating constructs related to high-order goals in response to reminders of interfering temptations, people increase the relative mental "availability" of goal-consistent behavior. Alternatively, by inhibiting temptation-related constructs in response to reminders of overriding goals, people decrease the relative mental "availability" of temptation-related behavior. These asymmetric mental operations on goal and temptation constructs increase the likelihood that one will secure high-order goals.

Specifically, we found that subliminal presentation of a temptation-related construct facilitated the activation of constructs related to a potentially threatened goal. In one study, participants first indicated their own goal-temptation pairs (e.g., *class–sleep*, *save–spend*). In a sequential priming paradigm, goal-related words (*class*) were more quickly recognized following subliminal presentation of relevant temptation-related words (*sleep*) than irrelevant temptation-related words (*spend*). Consistent with work on *goal shielding* (Shah, Friedman, & Kruglanski, 2002), we also documented the asymmetric effect on temptations. In particular, we found that it took longer for participants to recognize temptation-related words (*sleep*) following subliminal presentation of relevant goals (*class*) than irrelevant goals (*save*). Thus, counteractive control influenced mental availability in favor of goals (by activating them in response to temptations) and against temptations (by inhibiting them in response to goals). The resource independence of this strategy was demonstrated in a subsequent study, which found these same effects even under cognitive load.

Similar strategies can be set in motion by supraliminal primes as well. In another study (Fishbach et al., 2003), dieters were influenced by (supposedly) incidental aspects of the situation in which they made food choices. Specifically, the dieters either spent time in a room scattered with fatty food items and gourmet magazines, or with health magazines and dieting fliers, or with general interest magazines, before completing a lexical decision task. Those who spent time in the temptation-related food room were faster to recognize the word *diet* and, later, were more likely to choose apples than chocolates as a free gift. Thus, the presence of temptations in the environment activated concepts associated with overriding goals and affected subsequent choice consistently. As with implicit activation and inhibition, the presence of these implicit responses characterizes successful self-regulators more than unsuccessful self-regulators (Papies, Stroebe, & Aarts, 2008).

Value

Self-control strategies affect the objective value of options in the choice situation, such that in anticipation of a self-control conflict, people often bundle goal pursuit with bonuses and temptation indulgence with penalties. While these contingent bonuses and penalties change objective features of the choice situation, people can also alter the perceived value of goals and temptations simply through changing mental representations. People may bolster the value of high-order goals by linking the attainment of these goals to their self standards (Bandura, 1989) or by elaborating on what makes them positive (e.g., important, appealing, attractive, etc.; Beckmann & Kuhl, 1985; Fishbach, Shah, & Kruglanski, 2004; Kuhl, 1984). They may further devalue temptations by disassociating these motives from the self, or ignoring aspects that make temptations positively valued. This asymmetric bolstering and devaluation may then take an explicit or implicit form.

The availability of temptations should then affect judgments of their subjective value. When available, potential temptations pose a threat to higher-order goals. The Atkins diet devotee, for instance, will experience great conflict upon wandering by the wafting fragrance of a bakery. Assuming the dieter identifies this threat, he should engage counteractive control processes to protect the long-term goal. One way to protect the diet is to devalue the bread ("The bread in the window doesn't look very good today"). However, if the temptations are not available (if the bakery is closed for the day) there is no need for self-control, and their perceived value should not be impacted ("That bread in the window looks delicious"). Thus, because of counteractive control, making temptations available should make them less tempting.

Our research (Myrseth, Fishbach, & Trope, 2009) put this hypothesis to the test by presenting exercisers on their way out of the gym with a choice between health bars and chocolate bars. Almost everybody chose a health bar to take home, and we examined how they evaluated their two available options. Specifically, one group evaluated the foods before choosing the health bar. For these people, the chocolate bars represented a tempting alternative to the food option that was consistent with their long-term health goals. As predicted, they counteracted this temptation by dampening their positive evaluations of the chocolate bars relative to the health bars. A separate group evaluated the foods after choosing the health bar. Once this choice was made, the chocolates no longer represented a threat to long-term goals. For these people, there was no evidence of counteractive evaluation—the health bars and chocolate bars were evaluated as equally attractive. The dampened evaluations were in the service of promoting higher-order goals, and they followed a pattern opposite to that of the "sour grapes" effect (i.e., devaluation of unavailable options) that dissonance theory would predict (Festinger, 1957). Instead, they reflected a "reverse" spreading of alternatives (Aronson, 1997; Brehm, 1956). Rather than preserving the integrity of one's decision by increasing postchoice evaluations of the chosen option, counteractive control led people to protect their high-order goals from alluring temptations by increasing the chosen option's evaluation before choice.

Notably, these counteractive evaluations manifest in implicit judgments as well. In one study (Fishbach, Zhang, & Trope, 2010), participants completed an evaluative priming procedure (Bargh, Chaiken, Govender, & Pratto, 1992; Fazio, Jackson, Dunton, & Williams, 1995), in which they categorized affective words as positive (e.g., *peace, love*) or negative (e.g., *evil, cancer*). Subliminal primes preceded the affective target words. Sometimes the primes were healthy foods (e.g., *apple, broccoli*), and other times they were unhealthy foods (e.g., *bacon, fries*). Evaluations of the healthy and unhealthy food primes were thus indexed by the relative facility of categorizing the positive versus negative words that followed them. For example, more positive evaluations of healthy foods would be reflected by subsequently faster categorization of *peace* and *love*, and slower categorization of *evil* and *cancer*.

Importantly, before beginning the evaluative priming task, all participants first viewed a series of images as part of an ostensible visual perception task. In the high-accessibility temptation condition, a number of the images were of unhealthy temptations, such as fried chicken and ice cream. In the low accessibility condition, these images were replaced with mundane control images, such as hammers and lamps. This study found that healthy concepts were evaluated more positively and unhealthy concepts more negatively in the high-accessibility than the low-accessibility condition. Thus, only when people considered the various foods that threatened to tempt them away from their goals did they counteractively devalue unhealthy foods and bolstered healthy foods.

Levels of Construal

Another mental operation that people employ strategically to shift the motivational strength of goals and temptations is to change the processing level at which these competing motivations are construed. A tempting double-mocha latte with extra whipped cream, for example, can be viewed in a "cool," abstract, psychologically distanced way or in a "hot," concrete, psychologically proximal way. A cooler, abstract, and more distanced view of this temptation should attenuate its threat to overriding goals (Fujita & Han, 2009; Fujita, Trope, Liberman, & Levin-Sagi, 2006; Kross, Ayduk, & Mischel, 2005; Metcalfe & Mischel, 1999; see also Ledgerwood & Trope, Chapter 12, this volume). Consistent with this logic, children who were striving to avoid eating marshmallows now (in favor of more marshmallows later), were more successful at waiting if they thought of the marshmallows in cool, nonappetitive terms, such as "white, puffy clouds" or "round, white moons" rather than as "sweet and chewy and soft" (Mischel & Baker, 1975). In another study (Fujita et al., 2006), adults who construed a temptation in a high-level, abstract fashion (rather than a low-level, concrete fashion) were willing to pay a smaller premium to receive attractive gifts sooner rather than later.

The asymmetry assumption of counteractive control suggests that goal-congruent choice could also be increased by forming a "hot," concrete, or psychologically proximal representation of the benefits of goal pursuit. This hypothesis is consistent with the demonstrated benefits of concrete implementation intentions (Gollwitzer, 1999). For example, in a study on the regulation of academic goals, students formed concrete behavioral plans to facilitate pursuit of their academic goals (Gollwitzer & Brandstätter, 1997).

Expectations

The mental operations we have discussed so far act directly on representations of the goals and temptations that are in competition. Representations of goal constructs are increasingly activated, their values are bolstered, and they are considered in more hot, concrete or proximal ways. Similarly, representations of temptation constructs are inhibited, their values are undermined, and they are construed in more cool, abstract, or distanced ways. The mental representations of goal pursuit, however, include constructs other than those directly related to the motivation itself or to related objects. Mental representations also include, for instance, plans of action (e.g., implementation intentions; Gollwitzer, 1999) and performance standards (Locke & Latham, 1990; Wright & Brehm, 1989). Indeed, research has identified counteractive control strategies that operate on these aspects of goal representations as well.

The strategy of counteractive optimism asymmetrically affects people's anticipated goal and temptation pursuits, which in turn influence their actual motivation to pursue goals or give in to temptations (Zhang & Fishbach, 2010). Specifically, *counteractive optimism* refers to a tendency to provide optimistic predictions of future engagement with goals and disengagement from temptations. These optimistic predictions act as higher performance standards that elicit greater motivation than lower performance standards because people adjust their effort to match their anticipated level of performance (Atkinson & Feather, 1966; Brehm & Self, 1989; Heath, Larrick, & Wu, 1999; Locke & Latham, 1990; Oettingen & Mayer, 2002; Taylor & Brown, 1988).

For example, in one study (Zhang & Fishbach, 2010), participants predicted their performance on a task that they were to complete either in the presence or absence of clear obstacles to goal attainment. Specifically, they were asked to predict how well they would do on an anagram task to be completed while listening to music. The music was portrayed as either potentially helpful or potentially harmful to performance. Participants who were motivated to perform well made predictions that would counteract the obstacle to their goal attainment: They predicted better performance when they thought the music would hurt rather than help their performance. Thus, when needed to overcome a performance obstacle, people set higher standards to motivate more goal striving.

Notably, this pattern of optimism resembles prediction effects attributed to other nonmotivational mechanisms, such as the planning fallacy (Buehler, Griffin, & Ross, 1994), or general optimism biases (Brown, 1986; Chambers & Windschitl, 2004; Kruger & Dunning, 1999; Kunda, 1987). Predictions that result from counteractive optimism, however, would have motivationally functional origins and would therefore result only when high-order goals are threatened by low-order temptations. Demonstrating this point, another study (Zhang & Fishbach, 2010) found that optimistic predictions in the face of more (vs. less) challenging tasks actually led to increased effort investment on the more challenging task. Anticipated obstacles alone, without an opportunity for participants to make performance predictions, did not increase effort investment. Specifically, participants in this study expected to complete an anagram task that was presented as either difficult or easy. Those who stated performance predictions expected to do better when they anticipated a difficult rather than easy task. Consequently, they persisted longer. As in previous studies, we found that participants who anticipated obstacles actually improved their performance compared to participants facing the same level of challenge but without anticipating an obstacle (or temptation) in advance.

In another study, we examined whether counteractive optimism would manifest when predicting risk likelihoods in the same way it did when setting performance standards. To the extent that more optimistic predictions (i.e., lower subjective risk levels) motivate prevention behaviors that can reduce objective risk levels, they could be instrumental in counteracting temptation-related behavior and encouraging goal-related behavior. In this study, participants estimated their likelihood of suffering from high cholesterol, with the "knowledge" that their gender was either at a lower risk (no obstacle) or higher risk (obstacle) of having high cholesterol. When high cholesterol was described as an acquired, relatively controllable disease, participants made more optimistic predictions in the presence of obstacles. Those who "learned" that their sex was at a higher risk than the opposite sex, rather than a lower risk, predicted that their own likelihood of ending up with high cholesterol was lower.

Taken together, the strategies described in this section reveal an asymmetric process of counteractive control. These strategies generate an increase in the motivational strength of goals and a decrease in the motivational strength of temptations. They can operate by modulating the actual choice situation or mental representations of the choice situation. They involve explicit, more planned, and effortful processes (see also Muraven & Baumeister, 2000; Trope & Neter, 1994; Vohs, Baumeister, & Ciarocco, 2005), as well as an implicit mode of operations that is nonconscious and requires fewer psychological resources.

CONCLUSIONS

Self-control is a two-stage process. To succeed at goal pursuit, individuals facing temptations must first identify the conflict between those temptations and their goals. If, and only if, they have identified the conflict, they then have the opportunity to draw on self-control strategies to promote goal pursuit. We have described the conditions for identifying a self-control conflict, namely, width and consistency. Conflict identification is more likely when a person considers multiple opportunities to act and expects to make consistent choices at each opportunity. We further portrayed the process of self-control as an asymmetric response to goals and temptations, such that self-control strategies either increase the motivational strength of goals or decrease that of temptations.

One implication of our model is the etiological distinction between the failure to identify a self-control problem and the failure to exercise self-control. One can only fail at exercising self-control per se if one attempts to resist temptation. We believe that a large proportion of the variance in apparent self-control success depends on whether the individual was able to identify a problem in the first place. We therefore call for a more thorough investigation of the variables that influence identification. Our model further offers remedies for overindulgence and lack of self-control employment. We suggest that individuals should strive to identify potential self-control conflicts even before exercising self-control strategies. For example, the dieter faced with the opportunity to indulge should think about similar, future consumption opportunities and avoid thinking about the opportunity as unique or special. Similarly, the smoker should not consider the question of having one cigarette alone but consider instead the prospect of regularly smoking, to activate self-control strategies associated with quitting. In addition, educators and policymakers should consider measures that promote interrelated decision frames, and that discourage the presentation of potential temptations as special opportunities.

In terms of exercising self-control, it is useful to consider how each self-control operation can act on both the goals and the temptations. It is possible that acting on one of these elements is at times more adaptive and executable than acting on the other. For example, research on thought suppression (e.g., Wegner, 1989) suggests that inhibiting temptations may be a harder task overall than activating concepts related to the overriding goals. It follows then that self-regulators may be better off directing efforts toward focusing on their goals rather than inhibiting temptations. It is also possible that making penalties contingent on giving in to temptations is more effective than making rewards contingent on goal adherence because people are more averse to prospective losses than to gains (e.g., Kahneman & Tversky, 1979). Our research on implicit self-control strategies further raises the questions of when implicit strategies accompany more explicit ones, when they substitute for explicit strategies, and which tend to be more effective. Finally, given the richness of self-control operations that individuals display and that we have documented in this review, it would be beneficial to study what enables self-control success as a path to better understanding why people so often fail.

REFERENCES

Aarts, H., & Dijksterhuis, A. (2000). Habits as knowledge structures: Automaticity in goal-directed behavior. *Journal of Personality and Social Psychology, 78*(1), 53–63.

Ainslie, G. (1992). *Picoeconomics: The strategic interaction of successive motivational states within the person.* Cambridge, UK: Cambridge University Press.

Ariely, D., & Wertenbroch, K. (2002). Procrastination, deadlines, and performance: Self control by precommitment. *Psychological Science, 13*(3), 219–224.

Aronson, E. (1997). The theory of cognitive dissonance: The evolution and vicissitudes of an idea. In C. McGarty & S. A. Haslam (Eds.), *The message of social psychology: Perspectives on mind in society* (pp. 20–35). Cambridge, MA: Blackwell.

Atkinson, J. W., & Feather, N. T. (1966). *A theory of achievement motivation.* New York: Wiley.

Bandura, A. (1989). Self-regulation of motivation and action through internal standards and goal systems. In L. A. Pervin (Ed.), *Goal concepts in personality and social psychology* (pp. 19–85). Hillsdale, NJ: Erlbaum.

Bargh, J. A., Chaiken, S., Govender, R., & Pratto, F. (1992). The generality of the automatic attitude activation effect. *Journal of Personality and Social Psychology, 62*(6), 893–912.

Bargh, J. A., Gollwitzer, P. M., Lee-Chai, A., Barndollar, K., & Troetschel, R. (2001). The automated will: Unconscious activation and pursuit of behavioral goals. *Journal of Personality and Social Psychology, 81*(6), 1014–1027.

Baumeister, R. F., Bratslavsky, E., Muraven, M., & Tice, D. M. (1998). Ego-depletion: Is the active self a limited resource? *Journal of Personality and Social Psychology, 74*(5), 1252–1265.

Beckmann, J., & Kuhl, J. (1985). *Action control: From cognition to behavior.* Berlin: Springer-Verlag.

Brehm, J. W. (1956). Postdecision changes in the desirability of alternatives. *Journal of Abnormal and Social Psychology, 52*, 384–389.

Brehm, J. W. (1966). *A theory of psychological reactance.* New York: Academic Press.

Brehm, J. W., & Self, E. A. (1989). The intensity of motivation. *Annual Review of Psychology, 40*, 109–131.

Brown, J. D. (1986). Evaluations of self and others: Self-enhancement biases in social judgments. *Social Cognition, 4,* 353–376.

Buehler, R., Griffin, D., & Ross, M. (1994). Exploring the "planning fallacy": Why people underestimate their task completion times. *Journal of Personality and Social Psychology, 67*(3), 366–381.

Chambers, J. R., & Windschitl, P. D. (2004). Biases in social comparative judgments: The role of nonmotivated factors in above-average and comparative-optimism effects. *Psychological Bulletin, 130,* 813–838.

Chen, M., & Bargh, J. A. (1999). Consequences of automatic evaluation: Immediate behavioral predispositions to approach or avoid the stimulus. *Personality and Social Psychology Bulletin, 25*(2), 215–224.

Dawes, R. M. (1980). Social dilemmas. *Annual Review of Psychology, 31,* 169–193.

Dewitte, S., & De Cremer, D. (2001). Self-control and cooperation: Different concepts, similar decisions?: A question of the right perspective. *Journal of Psychology, 135*(2), 133–153.

Fazio, R. H., Jackson, J. R., Dunton, B. C., & Williams, C. J. (1995). Variability in automatic activation as an unobstrusive measure of racial attitudes: A bona fide pipeline? *Journal of Personality and Social Psychology, 69*(6), 1013–1027.

Festinger, L. (1957). *A theory of cognitive dissonance.* Evanston, IL: Row, Peterson.

Fishbach, A., Dhar, R., & Zhang, Y. (2006). Subgoals as substitutes or complements: The role of goal accessibility. *Journal of Personality and Social Psychology, 91*(2), 232–242.

Fishbach, A., Friedman, R. S., & Kruglanski, A. W. (2003). Leading us not unto temptation: Momentary allurements elicit overriding goal activation. *Journal of Personality and Social Psychology, 84*(2), 296–309.

Fishbach, A., & Shah, J. Y. (2006). Self control in action: Implicit dispositions toward goals and away from temptations. *Journal of Personality and Social Psychology, 90*(5), 820–832.

Fishbach, A., Shah, J. Y., & Kruglanski, A. W. (2004). Emotional transfer in goal systems. *Journal of Experimental Social Psychology, 40,* 723–738.

Fishbach, A., & Trope, Y. (2005). The substitutability of external control and self-control in overcoming temptation. *Journal of Experimental Social Psychology, 41,* 256–270.

Fishbach, A., & Trope, Y., (2007). Implicit and explicit mechanisms of counteractive self-control. In J. Y. Shah & W. L. Gardner (Eds.), *Handbook of motivation science* (pp. 281–294). New York: Guilford Press.

Fishbach, A., & Zhang, Y. (2008). Together or apart: When goals and temptations complement versus compete with each other. *Journal of Personality and Social Psychology, 94*(4), 547–559.

Fishbach, A., Zhang, Y., & Trope, Y. (2010). Counteractive evaluation: Asymmetric shifts in the implicit value of conflicting motivations. *Journal of Experimental Social Psychology, 46,* 29–38.

Fitzsimons, G. M., & Bargh, J. A. (2003). Thinking of you: Nonconscious pursuit of interpersonal goals associated with relationship partners. *Journal of Personality and Social Psychology, 84*(1), 148–164.

Fitzsimons, G. M., & Shah, J. (2008). How goal instrumentality shapes relationship evaluations. *Journal of Personality and Social Psychology, 95*(2), 319–337.

Fujita, K., & Han, H. A. (2009). Moving beyond deliberative control of impulses: The effect of construal levels on evaluative associations in self-control conflicts. *Psychological Science, 20*(7), 799–804.

Fujita, K., Trope, Y., Liberman, N., & Levin-Sagi, M. (2006). Construal levels and self control. *Journal of Personality and Social Psychology, 90*(3), 351–367.

Gollwitzer, P. M. (1999). Implementation intentions: Strong effects of simple plans. *American Psychologist, 54,* 493–503.

Gollwitzer, P. M., Bayer, U. C., & McCulloch, K. C. (2004). The control of the unwanted. In J. A.

Bargh, J. Uleman, & R. Hassin (Eds.), *The new unconscious*. New York: Oxford University Press.

Gollwitzer, P. M., & Brandstätter, V. (1997). Implementation intentions and effective goal pursuit. *Journal of Personality and Social Psychology, 73*, 186–199.

Heath, C., Larrick, R. P., & Wu, G. (1999). Goals as reference points. *Cognitive Psychology, 38*(1), 79–109.

Kahneman, D., & Tversky, A. (1979). Prospect theory: An analysis of decisions under risk. *Econometrica, 47*(2), 313–327.

Koo, M., & Fishbach, A. (2008). Dynamics of self-regulation: How (un)accomplished goal actions affect motivation. *Journal of Personality and Social Psychology, 94*(2), 183–195.

Kross, E., Ayduk, O., & Mischel, W. (2005). When asking "why" does not hurt: Distinguishing rumination from reflective processing of negative emotions. *Psychological Science, 16*(9), 709–715.

Kruger, J., & Dunning, D. (1999). Unskilled and unaware of it: How difficulties in recognizing one's own incompetence lead to inflated self-assessments. *Journal of Personality and Social Psychology, 77*(6), 1121–1134.

Kuhl, J. (1984). Volitional aspects of achievement motivation and learned helplessness: Toward a comprehensive theory of action control. In B. A. Maher (Ed.), *Progress in experimental personality research* (Vol. 13, pp. 99–171). New York: Academic Press.

Kunda, Z. (1987). Motivated inference: Self-serving generation and evaluation of causal theories. *Journal of Personality and Social Psychology, 53*(4), 636–647.

Leander, N. P., Shah, J., & Chartrand, T. L. (2009). Moments of weakness: The implicit context dependencies of temptations. *Personality and Social Psychology Bulletin, 35*(7), 853–866.

Locke, E. A., & Latham, G. P. (1990). *A theory of goal setting and task performance*. Upper Saddle River, NJ: Prentice-Hall.

Loewenstein, G. (1996). Out of control: Visceral influences on behavior. *Organizational Behavior and Human Decision Processes, 65*(3), 272–292.

Markman, A. B., & Brendl, C. (2005). Constraining theories of embodied cognition. *Psychological Science, 16*(1), 6–10.

Messick, D. M., & Brewer, M. B. (1983). Solving social dilemmas: A review. *Review of Personality and Social Psychology, 4*, 11–44.

Metcalfe, J., & Mischel, W. (1999). A hot/cool-system analysis of delay of gratification: Dynamics of willpower. *Psychological Review, 106*(1), 3–19.

Mischel, W., & Baker, N. (1975). Cognitive appraisals and transformations in delay behavior. *Journal of Personality and Social Psychology, 31*(2), 254–261.

Moskowitz, G. B., Gollwitzer, P. M., Wasel, W., & Schaal, B. (1999). Preconscious control of stereotype activation through chronic egalitarian goals. *Journal of Personality and Social Psychology, 77*(1), 167–184.

Muraven, M., & Baumeister, R. F. (2000). Self-regulation and depletion of limited resources: Does self-control resemble a muscle? *Psychological Bulletin, 126*, 247–259.

Myrseth, K. O. R., & Fishbach, A. (2009). Self-control: A function of knowing when and how to exercise restraint. *Current Directions in Psychological Science, 18*, 247–252.

Myrseth, K. O. R., Fishbach, A., & Trope, Y. (2009). Counteractive self-control: When making temptation available makes temptation less tempting. *Psychological Science, 20*(2), 159–163.

Oettingen, G., & Mayer, D. (2002). The motivating function of thinking about the future: Expectations versus fantasies. *Journal of Personality and Social Psychology, 83*(5), 1198–1212.

Papies, E. K., Stroebe, W., & Aarts, H. (2008). The allure of forbidden food: On the role of attention in self-regulation. *Journal of Experimental Social Psychology, 44*, 1283–1292.

Rachlin, H. (2000). *The science of self control*. Cambridge, MA: Harvard University Press.

Read, D., Loewenstein, G., & Kalyanaraman, S. (1999). Mixing virtue and vice: Combining the immediacy effect and the diversification heuristic. *Journal of Behavioral Decision Making, 12*(4), 257–273.

Read, D., Loewenstein, G., & Rabin, M. (1999). Choice bracketing. *Journal of Risk and Uncertainty, 19*(1–3), 171–197.

Schelling, T. C. (1984). Self-command in practice, in policy, and in a theory of rational choice. *American Economic Review, 74*(2), 1–11.

Shah, J. Y., Friedman, R., & Kruglanski, A. W. (2002). Forgetting all else: On the antecedents and consequences of goal shielding. *Journal of Personality and Social Psychology, 83*(6), 1261–1280.

Shah, J. Y., & Kruglanski, A. W. (2003). When opportunity knocks: Bottom-up priming of goals by means and its effects on self-regulation. *Journal of Personality and Social Psychology, 84*(6), 1109–1122.

Sheldon, O. J., & Fishbach, A. (2009). *Resisting the temptation to retaliate: Self-control in overcoming barriers to cooperation.* Unpublished manuscript, University of Chicago.

Solarz, A. K. (1960). Latency of instrumental responses as a function of compatibility with the meaning of eliciting verbal signs. *Journal of Experimental Psychology, 59*, 239–245.

Strotz, R. H. (1956). Myopia and inconsistency in dynamic utility maximization. *Review of Economic Studies, 23*, 166–180.

Taylor, S. E., & Brown, J. D. (1988). Illusion and well-being: A social psychological perspective on mental health. *Psychological Bulletin, 103*(2), 193–210.

Thaler, R. H. (1991). *Quasi rational economics.* New York: Russell Sage Foundation.

Thaler, R. H., & Shefrin, H. M. (1981). An economic theory of self-control. *Journal of Political Economy, 89*, 392–406.

Trope, Y., & Fishbach, A. (2000). Counteractive self-control in overcoming temptation. *Journal of Personality and Social Psychology, 79*(4), 493–506.

Trope, Y., & Neter, E. (1994). Reconciling competing motives in self-evaluation: The role of self-control in feedback seeking. *Journal of Personality and Social Psychology, 66*, 646–657.

Vohs, K. D., Baumeister, R. F., & Ciarocco, N. J. (2005). Self-regulation and self-presentation: Regulatory resource depletion impairs impression management and effortful self-presentation depletes regulatory resources. *Journal of Personality and Social Psychology, 88*, 632–657.

Wegner, D. M. (1989). *White bears and other unwanted thoughts: Suppression, obsession, and the psychology of mental control.* New York: Viking.

Wertenbroch, K. (1998). Consumption self-control by rationing purchase quantities of virtue and vice. *Marketing Science, 17*(4), 317–337.

Wood, W., & Neal, D. T. (2007). A new look at habits and the habit-goal interface. *Psychological Review, 114*(4), 843–863.

Wright, R. A., & Brehm, J. W. (1989). Energization and goal attractiveness. In L. A. Pervin (Ed.), *Goal concepts in personality and social psychology* (pp. 169–210). Hillsdale, NJ: Erlbaum.

Zhang, Y., & Fishbach, A. (2010). Counteracting obstacles with optimistic predictions. *Journal of Experimental Psychology: General, 139*, 16–31.

PART III

DEVELOPMENT OF SELF-REGULATION

CHAPTER 14

Effortful Control

Relations with Emotion Regulation, Adjustment, and Socialization in Childhood

NANCY EISENBERG
CYNTHIA L. SMITH
TRACY L. SPINRAD

Our purpose in this chapter is to discuss the construct of effortful control and review literature relevant to its importance, development, and significance for optimal development in childhood. First, we review important definitional and conceptual issues. Then we review literature on the emergence of effortful control in childhood. Next we consider the issue of its role in development—for example, its associations with emotionality, moral development, empathy, adjustment, and social competence. Finally, we consider what is known about the socialization of effortful control, especially in the family.

THE DEFINITION OF EFFORTFUL CONTROL

Temperamental self-regulatory capacities are often called *effortful control*, defined as "the efficiency of executive attention—including the ability to inhibit a dominant response and/or to activate a subdominant response, to plan, and to detect errors" (Rothbart & Bates, 2006, p. 129). Effortful control pertains to the ability to willfully or voluntarily inhibit, activate, or change (modulate) attention and behavior, as well as executive functioning tasks of planning, detecting errors, and integrating information relevant to selecting behavior. As a component of temperament, it is viewed as having some constitutional basis and as being an individual-difference variable that is relatively stable across time and contexts. Measures of effortful control often include indices of *attentional regulation* (e.g., the ability to voluntarily focus or shift attention as needed, called *attentional control*) and/or *behavioral regulation* (e.g., the ability to inhibit behavior effortfully as appropriate, called *inhibitory control*). Investigators sometimes have included measures of the ability to activate behavior when needed (even if someone does not feel like doing so; called *activation control*), for example, when needed to complete a task or to persist on a task (e.g., Eisenberg, Spinrad, et al., 2004; Kochanska, Murray, & Harlan, 2000). Effortful control, as part of executive attention, is viewed as involved in the awareness of one's planned behavior (Posner & DiGirolamo, 2000) and subjective feelings of voluntary control of thoughts and feelings, and is believed to come into play when resolving conflict (e.g., in regard to discrepant information), correcting errors, and planning new actions (Posner & Rothbart, 1998).

THE ROLE OF EFFORTFUL CONTROL
IN EMOTION REGULATION AND SOCIAL FUNCTIONING: CONCEPTUAL ISSUES

Effortful control plays a central role in the self-regulation of emotion and related processes. For example, when people are experiencing (or are likely to experience) negative emotions, they may often use attentional processes such as distracting themselves by shifting their attention to something else, or simply breaking off input from the fear-inducing stimuli. They also may use inhibitory control, for example, to mask the expression of negative emotion or to inhibit aggressive impulses when angered. Moreover, the planning capacities linked to effortful control (or executive attention) can be viewed as contributing to attempts to cope actively with stress—that is, active coping or engagement coping (Compas, Connor-Smith, & Saltzman, 2001). In stressful situations or when people are experiencing negative emotion, they also may need to force themselves to take action that will ameliorate the situation—that is, they may use activational control.

Eisenberg and colleagues (e.g., Eisenberg, Spinrad, et al., 2004; Valiente et al., 2003) have attempted to differentiate effortful or willful regulation of emotion, emotion-relevant motivation and cognitions, and related behavior—largely accomplished through effortful control—from less voluntary, reactive control-related processes. They have argued that effortful self-regulation should be differentiated from the general construct of *control*, defined in the dictionary as inhibition or restraint. Although voluntarily managed inhibition (or control) is part of effortful control (i.e., what Rothbart has labeled *inhibitory control*), inhibition often may be involuntary or so automatic that it usually is not under voluntary control. For example, behaviorally inhibited children, who are wary and overly constrained in novel or stressful contexts, seem to have difficulty modulating their inhibition. Similarly, the impulse to activate behavior and approach people or things in the environment often may be relatively nonvoluntary—for example, people may be "pulled" toward rewarding or positive situations, with little ability to inhibit themselves (i.e., they are impulsive and exhibit surgent, approach behaviors). Optimal emotion-related regulation, which generally involves effortful control, is believed to be flexible and willfully modulated so a person is not overly controlled or out of control. Regulated individuals are expected to be able to respond in a spontaneous manner when in contexts where such reactions are acceptable, and also to effortfully inhibit their approach or avoidant tendencies when appropriate.

Effortful control is believed to be grounded primarily in processes in the anterior cingulate gyrus and regions of the prefrontal cortex (e.g., Posner & Rothbart, 2007;

Rothbart & Bates, 2006). In contrast, Pickering and Gray (1999), among others, have argued that approach and avoidance motivational systems related to impulsive and overly inhibited behaviors, respectively, are centered in subcortical systems. Although these sub-cortical bases are intimately associated in complex ways with cortical functioning (see Goldsmith, Pollak, & Davidson, 2008), the neural bases of reactive systems appear to be somewhat different than those involved in effortful control.

Effortful control and reactive control are conceptually and statistically inversely related (e.g., Eisenberg, Spinrad, et al., 2004). However, they tend to load on different latent constructs in structural equation models (e.g., Eisenberg, Spinrad, et al., 2004; Valiente et al., 2003). In this chapter, we focus primarily on effortful control, not reactive control.

DEVELOPMENT OF EFFORTFUL CONTROL

In tracing the development of executive attention and effortful control, Rothbart and colleagues (Posner & Rothbart, 1998; Rothbart & Bates, 2006) have differentiated between attentional systems that are largely reactive and those that appear to denote self-regulatory mechanisms (i.e., effortful processes). The former system is present very early in life and is evident in behaviors such as infants' orienting responses to novelty, early attentional persistence, duration and latency of orienting, and early state control. This early attentional system is thought to be controlled by posterior orienting systems in the brain, which are involved in orienting to sensory stimuli.

Posner and Rothbart (1998) have proposed that the attentional processes involved in effortful control (i.e., executive attention) develop later than the posterior attentional system. Executive attention is viewed as involved in not only the abilities to willfully focus and shift attention as needed to adapt, but also inhibitory control and activational control (i.e., the abilities to inhibit or activate behavior as needed, especially when one is not inclined to do so). As already noted, this second system is thought to be centered primarily in anterior cingulate gyrus.

Posner and Rothbart (1998) believe there is modest development in the anterior attentional system around the second half of the first year of life, although this system is believed to be quite immature in the first couple of years of life. Indeed, the capacity for effortful control is believed to increase markedly in the preschool years and may continue to develop into adulthood (Carlson, 2005; Leon-Carrion, García-Orza, & Pérez-Santamaría, 2004; Mezzacappa, 2004; Murphy, Eisenberg, Fabes, Shepard, & Guthrie, 1999; Rueda et al., 2004; Williams, Ponesse, Schachar, Logan, & Tannock, 1999).

In fact, executive attention, which is a large part of effortful control, has been demonstrated in infancy and toddlerhood, and improves throughout the toddler and preschool period. Between 9 and 18 months of age, attention becomes more voluntary (Ruff & Rothbart, 1996) as infants learn to resolve conflicts (e.g., when processing information), correct errors, and plan new actions (Posner & Rothbart, 1998). Diamond (1991), for example, has shown that 12-month-olds are able to reach for a target not in their line of sight, demonstrating the ability to coordinate reach and vision, and attend to both. Moreover, infants' performance on visual sequencing tasks to assess anticipatory looking also demonstrates rudimentary executive functioning skills. For example, Sheese,

Rothbart, Posner, White, and Fraundorf (2008) found that anticipatory looking (i.e., looking to the location of a target prior to its appearance in that location) was observable in 6- and 7-month-old infants. Moreover, anticipatory looking in 24- and 30-month-old children has been related to better conflict resolution in a visuospatial conflict task and parent-report of child effortful control (Rothbart, Ellis, Rueda, & Posner, 2003).

According to Posner and Rothbart (1998), another transition in the development of executive attention (and inhibition of related behavior) can be seen around 30 months of age. Using a Stroop-like task that requires toddlers to switch attention and inhibit behavior accordingly, Posner and Rothbart reported that children showed significant improvement in performance by 30 months of age and performed with high accuracy by 36–38 months of age. Moreover, toddlers' ability on this sort of task, which improved from 24 to 36 months, was positively related to parents' ratings of attention-shifting abilities at 30 and 36 months of age (Gerardi-Caulton, 2000; also see Garon, Bryson, & Smith, 2008).

The ability to inhibit behavior upon command also appears to improve across the toddler and preschool years (Rothbart & Bates, 2006). Kochanska and colleagues (2000) developed a battery of effortful control tasks designed to measure five components of effortful control: delaying, slowing down motor activity, suppressing or initiating activity to signal, lowering voice, and effortful attention. Kochanska and colleagues demonstrated significant improvement in children's effortful control between 22 and 33 months of age. Other researchers have shown that the ability to inhibit behavior effortfully on tasks such as Simon Says appears to improve between 36 and 48 months of age (Jones, Rothbart, & Posner, 2003; Posner & Rothbart, 1998).

There is also evidence that effortful control or components of effortful control show interindividual (i.e., correlational) stability in the early years of life. Stability of attention span has been observed in young toddlers (Gaertner, Spinrad, & Eisenberg, 2008; Kannass, Oakes, & Shaddy, 2006), and parental reports of attentional regulation are correlated across infancy and toddlerhood (Gaertner et al., 2008; Putnam, Rothbart, & Gartstein, 2008). In terms of the broader construct of effortful control, Kochanska and colleagues found that effortful control observed at 22 months substantially predicted effortful control at both 33 months (Kochanska et al., 2000) and 45 months (Kochanksa & Knaack, 2003; also see Li-Grining, 2007; Spinrad et al., 2007). Moreover, early focused attention has been shown to predict later effortful control (Kochanska et al., 2000), although Putnam and colleagues (2008) found that orienting in infancy was not related to effortful control at age 2.

Stability in effortful control has also been found in early childhood to adolescence. For example, teachers' and parents' reports of aspects of effortful control have been found to be relatively stable over 4, or sometimes 6, years during childhood (especially for attention focusing and inhibitory control; less so for attention shifting; Eisenberg, Zhou, et al., 2005; Murphy et al., 1999; Valiente et al., 2006). Given her longitudinal findings of stability from toddlerhood through preschool and into early school age years (Kochanska & Knaack, 2003; Kochanska, Murray, & Coy, 1997), Kochanska has compared the stability of effortful control to the stability of IQ. According to Kochanska and colleagues (2000), the robust stability findings in their work indicate a trait-like quality of effortful control and support Rothbart and Bates's (2006) view of effortful control as a temperamental construct.

RELATIONS OF EFFORTFUL CONTROL TO DEVELOPMENTAL OUTCOMES

Effortful control is believed to play an important role in the development of a wide range of socioemotional outcomes, including negative emotionality, the development of a conscience, prosocial behavior, empathy-related responding, social competence, and adjustment. Due to space limitations, our review is illustrative rather than exhaustive, and we review only studies with children.

Relations to Emotionality

Effortful control generally has been associated with low levels of children's negative emotionality. For example, 4-month-old infants who demonstrated high levels of refocusing attention away from one location to another were less distressed in laboratory situations (Rothbart, Ziaie, & O'Boyle, 1992). Moreover, 18-month-olds who showed relatively high distress during a frustration task were less likely than their peers to use adaptive regulation strategies, which included distracting their attention away from the source of the frustration (Calkins & Johnson, 1998). Similarly, Calkins, Dedmon, Gill, Lomax, and Johnson (2002) found that compared to infants who were not easily frustrated (as assessed with laboratory tasks and mothers' reports), easily frustrated 6-month-olds exhibited less focused attention during an attention task and showed less attentional regulation during frustration tasks (i.e., they were less likely to shift their attention away from the focal object). Gaertner and colleagues (2008) found that toddlers' observed attention was negatively related to negative emotionality at both 18 and 30 months of age; in longitudinal analyses, early negative emotionality predicted less focused attention over time when researchers controlled for initial levels of attention, suggesting that negative affect may have a negative impact on children's capacity to learn to sustain attention.

Other measures of regulation (besides attentional control) or composite indices of effortful control also seem to be related to young children's emotionality. For example, Gerardi-Caulton (2000) found that 30- and 36-month-olds' delay scores on a spatial conflict (Stroop-like) task were negatively related to parents' ratings of the toddlers' anger and frustration. Hill-Sonderlund and Braungart-Rieker (2008) found that increases in fear reactivity in infancy predicted low effortful control in early childhood, suggesting that bidirectional relations between emotion and EC may exist (see, however, Aksan & Kochanska, 2004). Kochanska and Knaack (2003) noted that toddlers who were more emotionally intense (more prone to display anger and joy at 14 and 22 months of age) scored lower on a composite measure of effortful control tasks at 22, 33, and 45 months of age. Not only were there concurrent associations between emotional intensity and effortful control, but the toddlers' emotional intensity also predicted effortful control at ages 22–45 months. Effortful control may help children to regulate emotions, and/or children high in negative emotionality may have more difficulty than their more placid peers in developing effortful control.

Similar finding have been obtained in studies of preschoolers and school-age children (Eisenberg et al., 1993; Eisenberg, Fabes, Nyman, Bernzweig, & Pinuelas, 1994). Hanish and colleagues (2004) found that teacher-reported EC was inversely related to parents' and another teacher's reports of children's anger and observed anger at preschool (similar relations with anxiety were not significant). In a different sample, Fabes and colleagues

(1999) found that preschoolers who were high in effortful control were relatively unlikely to experience strong negative emotional arousal in response to peer interactions, but this relation held only for moderate- to high-intensity interactions (there was no differ-ent for mild-intensity interactions). Gilliom, Shaw, Beck, Schonberg, and Lukon (2002) reported that shifting attention away from sources of frustration and seeking informa-tion about situational constraints were associated with decreased anger for 3½-year-olds. Similar patterns of inverse relations between schoolchildren's adult-reported effortful control and their negative emotionality have been found in non-Western samples, includ-ing patterns for anger or negative emotional intensity in China (Eisenberg, Ma, et al., 2007; Zhou, Eisenberg, Wang, & Reiser, 2004) and in Indonesia (Eisenberg, Liew, & Pidada, 2004; Eisenberg, Pidada, & Liew, 2001). Moreover, delay of gratification in pre-school has predicted the ability to deal with frustration in adolescence (Mischel, Shoda, & Peake, 1988).

Moral Development

Measures of effortful control or related constructs have been linked to the development of conscience, empathy-related responding, and prosocial behavior.

Conscience

Measures of children's internalized, committed compliance with adults' wishes, a cor-relate precursor or correlate of early conscience (Kochanska, Coy, & Murray, 2001), has been associated with the observed effortful control in the toddler and preschool years (Kochanska et al., 1997, 2001). Moreover, Kochanska and colleagues (1997) found that children's effortful control and conscience were positively related at each age (i.e., in con-current analyses at toddler, preschool, and early school age), and that effortful control at all three ages predicted early school-age conscience. Measures of conscience included rat-ings on items reflecting dimensions of the moral self (e.g., concern about others' wrong-doing, apology, and empathy), responses to hypothetical moral dilemmas, internalization of mother's rules, internalization of the experimenter's rules (not cheating at a game while the experimenter was not in the room), and internalization of experimenter's rules in a peer context (not cheating on a game while the experimenter was not in the room but two other children were also present). Kochanska and Knaack (2003) were able to repli-cate the results of Kochanska and colleagues and found that effortful control at 22, 33, and 45 months, as well as the composite score of effortful control across those ages, pre-dicted a more internalized conscience at 56 months. In this study, measures of conscience included ratings of moral self, internalization of the mother's rules, and internalization of the experimenter's rules. Moreover, Rothbart, Ahadi, and Hershey (1994) found that parents' reports of children's effortful control were associated with their reports of their 7-year-old children's tendencies to experience guilt. Due to a dearth of research, it is not clear whether such relations would hold in adolescence.

Empathy and Prosocial Behavior

Eisenberg, Fabes, Karbon, and colleagues (1996) hypothesized that individuals high in effortful regulation tend to experience *sympathy* (an other-oriented response to another's emotion or condition) rather than *personal distress* (a self-focused, aversive response to another's emotional state or condition) because empathic overarousal is aversive and leads to a self-focus and self-concern. Consistent with this premise, positive relations between effortful control and empathy-related responding have been found in studies with preschoolers and school-age children. For example, Guthrie and colleagues (1997) found that children rated high on adult-reported effortful regulation exhibited greater facial sadness during an empathy-inducing film than did children low in effortful control. Children's postfilm reports of sadness and sympathy to the film were also positively correlated with parents' ratings of regulation. Conversely, children low in parent-rated effortful regulation were prone to experience personal distress (e.g., anxiety, tension) during the film. In another study, children's reports of sympathy when viewing an empathy-inducing film were related to adult-reported high effortful control (Valiente et al., 2004).

Effortful control also has been positively related to self- or other-report measures of empathy/sympathy. Eisenberg, Fabes, Murphy, and colleagues (1996), Eisenberg, Fabes, and colleagues (1998), and Rothbart et al. (1994) all found associations between children's effortful control (as assessed through parents' and teachers' reports) and parents' or teachers' reports of sympathy or children's self-reported empathy or sympathy. In some studies, effortful control (or a composite comprised mostly of effortful control and low impulsivity) predicted sympathy over 2, 4, or even 6–8 years (e.g., Eisenberg, Michalik, et al., 2007; Murphy et al., 1999).

Consistent with the relation between effortful control and sympathy/empathy, adults' ratings of elementary schoolchildren's effortful attentional control and/or a behavioral measure assessing effortful control (and perhaps impulsivity, to some degree) have been correlated with peers' (Eisenberg, Fabes, Karbon, et al., 1996; Eisenberg, Guthrie, et al., 1997) or teachers' ratings (Diener & Kim, 2004, for effortful and reactive control combined) of prosocial behavior. Thus, individuals who can regulate their emotion and behavior are more likely not only to experience sympathy but also to act in morally desirable ways with others.

Social Competence and Adjustment

In general, measures that likely tap effortful control have been positively related to children's adjustment and social competence (see Eisenberg, Spinrad, & Eggum, 2010, for a more detailed review). In one of the most relevant longitudinal studies to examine this issue, children's lack of control at age 3 and 5—likely a combination of effortful control, low reactive control, and negative emotionality (e.g., variables such as fleeting attention, emotional lability)—were rated on their behaviors when performing a variety of tasks (e.g., Henry, Caspi, Moffitt, Harrington, & Silva, 1999). In addition, at age 3, children were classified into various personality types based in part on this index of lack of control (the undercontrolled group was characterized primarily by lack of control). Lack of control at age 3 or age 5 was positively associated with parents' and/or teachers' reports of externalizing problems (e.g., hyperactive behavior, inattention, antisocial behavior or conduct disorder), and internalizing problems (anxiety/fearfulness) in late childhood (age 9 and/or 11) and adolescence (age 13 and/or 15), and negatively related with the number of children's strengths (e.g., parent- and teacher-rated caring, maturity, friendliness, interest, determination, good behavior, enthusiasm, creativity, confidence, sense of humor, popularity, cooperativeness, helpfulness, ability at sports, cleanliness, activity) in adolescence (Caspi, Henry, McGee, Moffitt, & Silva, 1995). At age 18, the undercontrolled individuals scored high on measures of impulsivity, danger seeking, aggression, and interpersonal alienation (Caspi & Silva, 1995). At age 21, lack of control was related to number of criminal convictions for men and women, with this relation being stronger for men (but not women) who dropped out of school (Henry et al., 1999). In addition, undercontrolled 3-year-olds were more antisocial at age 21 and had poorer social relations and higher levels of interpersonal conflict (Newman, Caspi, Moffitt, & Silva, 1997).

Although the measure of undercontrol used in the aforementioned studies likely assessed impulsivity and emotionality as well as effortful control, other investigators have obtained similar results using somewhat purer measures of effortful control. In regard to social competence, for example, Raver, Blackburn, Bancroft, and Torp (1999) found that preschoolers who used more attentional strategies (self-distraction) during a delay task were rated by their teachers as higher in social competence, and peers tended to rate them as popular and average rather than as rejected or neglected. Furthermore, Eisenberg and colleagues (1993, 1994) reported that adults' ratings of preschoolers' and kindergarteners' effortful attention shifting and focusing were associated with children's socially appropriate behavior, boys' (but not girls') peer status, and children's constructive coping with real-life incidents involving negative emotion at preschool (also see Spinrad et al., 2004). In addition, teachers' and/or mothers' reports of attentional control at this age often predicted children's social functioning and prosocial/social behavior at school 2, 4, and 6 years later (Eisenberg et al., 1995; Eisenberg, Fabes, & Shepard, 1997; Murphy, Shepard, Eisenberg, & Fabes, 2004). Moreover, Eisenberg, Guthrie, and colleagues (1997) found an association between peer nominations for social status and teachers' and parents' reports of elementary schoolchildren's attentional control, as well as a behavioral measure of persistence (rather than cheating or being off-task). In this same study, children's adult-rated effortful attentional control and performance on a behavioral task generally were related to teachers' ratings of socially appropriate behavior and popularity (Eisenberg, Fabes, Guthrie, & Reiser, 2000; Eisenberg, Guthrie, et al., 1997; Eisenberg et al., 2003). Similar relations were obtained for popularity in a different longitudinal sample (Spinrad et al., 2006).

Effortful control and related constructs have also been linked with social competence in older samples of children. For example, in the Mischel and colleagues (1988) longitudinal study, delay of gratification at age 4 or 5 predicted parent-reported social competence and coping with problems in adolescence. For vulnerable children (those who were sensitive to rejection), the ability to delay gratification predicted better peer relationships (lower peer rejection and aggression), higher self-worth in middle school children, and lower use of drugs in adulthood (Ayduk et al., 2000). In contrast, in a study of French high school students, relations between parents', teachers', and adolescents' reports of effortful control and popularity varied with the reporter, although there was an indirect positive relation between effortful control and popularity through youths' ego resiliency (Hofer, Eisenberg, & Reiser, in press).

Relations of effortful control and social competence have tended to be especially evident for children prone to negative emotion (Eisenberg, Fabes, et al., 2000; Eisenberg, Guthrie, et al., 1997; also see Belsky, Friedman, & Hsieh, 2001). In addition, relations between effortful control and social functioning often have been mediated by ego resiliency (Eisenberg, Fabes, et al., 2000; Eisenberg, Guthrie, et al., 1997; Hofer et al., in press; Spinrad et al., 2006).

Consistent with the findings of Caspi and colleagues (1995) and Henry and colleagues (1999), low effortful control has also been rather consistently linked to problems with maladjustment. This association is evident even in the toddler and preschool years (Calkins & Dedmon, 2000; Crockenberg, Leerkes, & Jó, 2008; Eiden, Colder, Edwards, & Leonard, 2009; Kochanska, Barry, Aksan, & Boldt, 2008; Olson, Sameroff, Kerr, Lopez, & Wellman, 2005; Raaijmakers et al., 2008; Spinrad et al., 2007). In a longitudinal study, Kochanska and Knaack (2003) found that children's lack of effortful control (as measured by a battery of tasks at 22, 33, and 45 months) was related to increased mother-reported behavior problems at 73 months. Similarly, Lemery, Essex, and Snider (2002) found that mothers' reports of children's attention focusing and inhibitory control (averaged across ratings provided when the children were 3.5 and 4.5 years of age) predicted mothers' and fathers' reports of externalizing problems and attention-deficit/ hyperactivity disorder at age 5.5 years. Moreover, similar findings have been obtained with school-age children, within and across time (Eisenberg et al., 1995; Eisenberg, Guthrie, et al., 1997; Murphy et al., 2004). For example, Eisenberg and colleagues (e.g., Eisenberg, Guthrie, et al., 1997; Eisenberg, Spinrad, et al., 2004; Eisenberg, Zhou, et al., 2005; Valiente et al., 2003, 2006), in several longitudinal studies, have found fairly consistent relations between measures of effortful control and children's externalizing problems. Children with teacher- and parent-reported externalizing problems (co-occurring with internalizing or not) tended to be low in adult-reported attentional effortful control and inhibitory control, and at younger ages, with behavioral measures of persistence and inhibitory control (e.g., persisting on a puzzle task rather than cheating, sitting still when asked to do so) (Eisenberg, Cumberland, et al., 2001; Eisenberg, Sadovsky, et al., 2005; Eisenberg, Valiente, et al., 2009). Converging findings have been obtained in numerous studies of effortful control/executive skills using a variety of measures of the constructs (Belsky, Fearon, & Bell, 2007; Lengua, 2006, 2008; Martel et al., 2007; see Eisenberg et al., 2010), and the association has been found in Western Europe (e.g., Hofer et al., in press; Muris, 2006; Oldehinkel, Hartman, Ferdinant, Verhulst, & Ormel, 2007; Rydell, Berlin, & Bohlin, 2003), Indonesia (Eisenberg, Pidada, & Liew, 2001), and China (Eisenberg, Ma, et al., 2007; Zhou et al., 2004), as well as in the aforementioned study in New Zealand (e.g., Caspi et al., 1995).

In longitudinal studies in which stability in both externalizing problems and in effortful control were taken into account in structural equation models, investigators have found support for the assumption that change in effortful control is related to change in externalizing problems after about age 4½ (Eisenberg, Sadovsky, et al., 2005; Kim & Brody, 2005; Valiente et al., 2006). In a study with a large sample (which makes it more likely to obtain significant bidirectional paths), Belsky and colleagues (2007) found that children's attentional regulation at 54 months, grade 1, and grade 5 predicted externalizing problems at the next assessment and vice versa (although attentional control apparently was not assessed at grade 5; also see Eisenberg et al., 1999, for evidence of bidirectional relations). In contrast, Spinrad and colleagues (2007) did not obtain similar findings longitudinally in a study of children at 18 and 30 months of age.

Supporting the distinction between reactive control and effortful control, both constructs provide some unique prediction of early to mid-elementary schoolchildren's externalizing problems (Eisenberg, Fabes, Guthrie, et al., 1996; Eisenberg, Sadovsky, et al.,

2005; Valiente al., 2003). However, by around middle to late childhood and moving into adolescence, the relation of reactive control drops to marginal significance or nonsignificance when children's effortful control is also used to predict externalizing problems (despite significant concurrent correlations between reactive impulsivity and externalizing problems; Eisenberg, Spinrad, et al., 2004; Valiente et al., 2003). In contrast, in a larger study of more high-risk youths, Martel and colleagues (2007) reported that both early reactive undercontrol and poor response inhibition provided unique prediction of externalizing problems in adolescence.

Children's negative emotionality has been found to moderate the degree of relation between effortful control/self-regulation and children's externalizing problems. In general, effortful control/self-regulation is a better negative predictor of children's and adolescents' externalizing problems if they are prone to negative emotions, especially anger (Degnan, Calkins, Keane, & Hill-Soderlund, 2008; Diener & Kim, 2004; Eisenberg, Ma, et al., 2007; Eisenberg, Spinrad, et al., 2004; Muris, 2006; Oldehinkel et al., 2007; Valiente et al., 2003; see Eisenberg, Guthrie, et al., 2000; cf. Eisenberg, Cumberland, et al., 2001), although this interaction was not found in research with infants (Belsky et al., 2001) or 3-year-olds (Olson et al., 2005). Thus, negative emotionality may start to moderate the relation of self-regulation to externalizing after the early years, possibly because of the emergence of more mature effortful self-regulation and/or more serious externalizing problems.

Findings in regard to the relation of effortful control to internalizing problems are somewhat less consistent. Attentional control might be expected to help children refocus attention from negative and threatening stimuli, and facilitate refocusing attention on neutral or positive stimuli or thoughts. In addition, activational control likely helps children with internalizing problems to approach threatening objects and situations when it is adaptive to do so. In a number of studies in which internalizing problems have been assessed without taking into account the degree of co-occurring externalizing problems, effortful control has been inversely related to children's and adolescents' internalizing problems (e.g., Buckner, Mezzacappa, & Beardslee, 2009; Silk, Shaw, Forbes, Lane, & Kovacs, 2006; Silk, Steinberg, & Morris, 2003; Spinrad et al., 2007). In some of these studies, relations were found even when overlapping or confounding items were removed from the scales (e.g., Eisenberg, Zhou, et al., 2005; Lemery et al., 2002; cf. Lengua, West, & Sandler, 1998).

The inverse relation between effortful control/self-regulation and internalizing problems may increase with age (Dennis, Brotman, Huang, & Gouley, 2007). Indeed, in the preschool years, there is some evidence that internalizing problems are positively related to effortful control (Murray & Kochanska, 2002). Reactive inhibition to novelty—often viewed as an early internalizing problem—may decrease the speed of approach responses early in life, which in turn facilitates the emerging capacity for effortful inhibitory control (Aksan & Kochanska, 2004).

In a few longitudinal studies, relations of effortful control to internalizing problems have been examined when researchers controlled for the stability of both constructs across time in models. Spinrad and colleagues (2007) found that 18-month effortful control did not relate to 30-month internalizing when they controlled for stability in internalizing. In a study including children approximately 4½–7 years of age and followed up 2 years later, Eisenberg, Spinrad, and colleagues (2004) reported that effortful control predicted internalizing indirectly through low ego resiliency. In a follow-up of this sample at three time points, Valiente and colleagues (2006) found some evidence of effortful control predicting teacher-, but not mother-reported internalizing problems across 2 years.

The relations between effortful control and internalizing problems may be much weaker, and may decrease with age when one considers internalizing problems that are not co-occurring with externalizing problems (Eisenberg, Cumberland, et al., 2001; Eisenberg, Sadovsky, et al., 2005; Eisenberg, Valiente, et al., 2009). However, although the relation between "pure" internalizing problems and effortful control dropped out for children in the United States who were approximately 7–9 years of age, the same relation was significant in a Chinese sample (Eisenberg, Ma, et al., 2007), suggesting that these relations may vary across cultures. Note, however, that Zhou, Lengua, and Wang (2009) did not find a difference between Chinese and U.S. samples in the strength of the inverse relation when using a measure of internalizing problems that did not take into account co-occurring externalizing problems.

Summary

Although the relevant literature is not entirely consistent, there is mounting evidence that individual differences in effortful control are linked to a variety of important developmental outcomes. It seems likely children's relative lack of ability to regulate their attention effectively puts them at risk for behavior problems, either directly or indirectly, through deficits in the ability to regulate negative emotions. Children high in effortful control tend to exhibit relatively low levels of negative emotion, high levels of social competence, high levels of conscience and prosocial responding, and low rates of externalizing and internalizing problem behaviors. In contrast, researchers have found that children with low effortful control tend to be at risk for social, moral, emotional, and psychological problems. Thus, it appears that effortful control contributes to the emergence of desirable patterns of behavior in the early years, and also is involved in the continued development and maintenance of positive emotional, social, and cognitive development.

THE SOCIALIZATION OF EFFORTFUL CONTROL

According to Kopp (1989; Kopp & Neufeld, 2003), successful regulation of behavior in infants and young children can be indexed by how closely children meet familial and social conventions. Infants and young children must have external support for regulating their behavior, and the development of self-regulation involves give-and-take between the children's needs and caregivers' behaviors (Calkins, 1994; Kopp, 1989). Consistent with Kopp's theorizing, although effortful control likely has relatively strong hereditary and constitutional origins, parenting styles and behaviors are believed to play an important role in children's effortful control.

Findings from several investigators (e.g., Gaertner et al., 2008; Gilliom et al., 2002; Karreman, van Tuijl, van Aken, & Dekovic, 2008; Li-Grining, 2007) suggest that responsive, supportive parenting is linked with children's effortful control abilities. Calkins and colleagues (2002) found that easily frustrated 6-month-old infants, who were not efficient at controlling their attention, had mothers who were less sensitive, more intrusive, and provided less physical stimulation to the infants than were mothers of nonfrustrated infants, who were better at controlling their attention as needed. Moreover, parental responsiveness in toddlerhood has been associated with relatively high effortful control abilities (Gilliom et al., 2002; Kochanska, Aksan, Prisco, & Adams, 2008; Kochanska & Knaack, 2003; Kochanska et al., 2000). Spinrad and colleagues (2007) found that maternal supportive behaviors (observed sensitivity and warmth and maternal report of supportive responses to children's emotions) were positively associated with children's effortful control. The associations were found concurrently at 18 and 30 months of age, and over time, even when researchers controlled for stability in the constructs.

Associations between maternal support and children's effortful control have been found beyond the toddler years as well (e.g., Eisenberg, Zhou, et al., 2005). Belsky and colleagues (2007) found that higher levels of observed maternal supportive behavior predicted higher levels of observed child attentional control. The positive associations were found across two different time series (maternal supportive behaviors at 54 months predicted attentional control in first grade, and maternal supportive behaviors at first grade predicted attentional control in fourth grade). The longitudinal associations were found when researchers controlled for the stability of the measures; thus, increases (vs. declines) in maternal support were associated with increases (vs. declines) in children's attentional control. Thus, based on this study and findings with younger children (e.g., Spinrad et al., 2007), maternal supportive parenting (including warmth and responsivity) is associated with higher effortful control both concurrently and over time.

Parental discipline and parenting styles also have been related to children's effortful control (Hofer et al., in press; Karreman et al., 2008; Xu, Farver, & Zhang, 2009). In this regard, harsh parental control or an authoritarian parenting style (characterized by low warmth and high control) is expected to result in overarousal in children, particularly for those low in regulatory abilities (Calkins, 1994). Kochanska, Aksan, and colleagues (2008) found that higher levels of observed parental (maternal and paternal) power assertion in toddlerhood were associated with lower levels of observed effortful control during the preschool years. Furthermore, in a large sample of first- and second-grade Chinese children, Zhou and colleagues (2004) found that parents who endorsed authoritarian parenting practices, particularly verbal hostility and corporal punishment, had children lower in adult-reported effortful control. On the other hand, parental report of authoritative parenting (warmth/acceptance, reasoning, and democratic policies) has been positively related to adults' reports of children's effortful control in a sample of Chinese first and second graders (Eisenberg, Chang, Ma, & Haung, 2009). Thus, these findings, along with those on parental warmth, suggest that supportive parenting is positively related to the development of effortful control from infancy into the early school-age years, and that harsh, controlling parenting may interfere with the development of effortful control.

Research on the socialization correlates of effortful control also has included parental responses to children's emotions (Eisenberg, Cumberland, & Spinrad, 1998). Parents who appropriately respond to children's emotions may be directly teaching their children effective strategies for self-regulation. Consistent with this notion, using a diverse sample of 7- to 12-year-old children, Valiente, Lemery-Chalfant, and Reiser (2007) found that high levels of positive parental (mostly mothers') reactions to children's emotions (problem-focused, emotion-focused, and expressive encouragement reactions) and low levels of negative parental reactions to children's emotions (minimization, punitive, and distress reactions) were associated with higher levels of children's effortful control, measured from children's and parents' reports. Similar findings have been obtained with younger children (e.g., Spinrad et al., 2007). These findings support the view that parents who use more effective responses to children's emotions may provide children with strategies for effortful control of emotions.

In addition to maternal responses to children's emotions, researchers have also examined how maternal emotional expressions are related to children's effortful control across childhood and into adolescence (e.g., Eisenberg, Zhou, et al., 2005). The type and intensity of emotions expressed by parents may provide children with either positive or negative models of emotional control (Eisenberg, Cumberland, et al., 1998). Valiente and colleagues (2006) found that children's effortful control (examined at three time points, spanning early childhood into early adolescence) and maternal emotional expressivity (a composite score of negative subtracted from positive expressivity) were fairly consistent over time, as was the relation between them. Thus, maternal characteristics, in this case the level of positive emotion expressed, appeared to support the development of children's effortful control.

Other parental characteristics, such as parents' own dispositions or psychopathology, also are likely to be important to children's self-regulation (Blandon, Calkins, Keane, & O'Brien, 2008; Yap, Allen, Leve, & Katz, 2008). Kochanska and colleagues (2000) found that mothers who rated themselves higher on a socialization scale (e.g., ratings of acceptance of cultural norms, patience, and persistence) had toddlers who exhibited higher effortful control. Thus, the mothers' own ability to follow rules and show patience, as well as their behavior with their children, was a predictor of effortful control. Similarly, Valiente and colleagues (2007) found that parents' reports of their own effortful control were associated with more positive and less negative parenting reactions to children's emotions. Although there were significant correlations between parents' and 7- to 12-year-old children's effortful control, the association of parental effortful control to child effortful control was mediated by parenting. Thus, parents' characteristics, such as their own regulatory capacity, are likely to have both direct and indirect associations with children's effortful control.

It is also interesting to note that there may be interactions between parenting and child characteristics that predict children's effortful control. In fact, using a candidate gene approach, Kochanksa, Philibert, and Barry (2009) found that children's genotype (serotonin transporter [5-HTTLPR] polymorphism) and infant attachment (likely related to parental responsivity) interacted to predict the children's level of effortful control. Children who were genetically at risk for problems with self-regulation only demonstrated lower levels of effortful control when they also experienced insecure attachments to their mothers during infancy. Maternal behaviors, in this case developing a secure attachment with infants, may protect children who are genetically vulnerable for problems with self-regulation.

Furthermore, the relations between parental socialization and children's effortful control are likely to be bidirectional. Supporting the idea that children's regulatory ability may elicit different parenting behaviors, Bridgett and colleagues (2009) found that steeper decreasing trajectories of regulatory capacity across infancy were associated with less maternal negative parenting at 18 months of age (also see Lengua, 2006). Moreover,

Belsky and colleagues (2007) found bidirectional associations between children's attentional control and maternal supportive behaviors over time.

The importance of the socialization of effortful control is highlighted by evidence that effortful control statistically mediates the association between parenting and child outcomes, especially behavior problems (e.g., Belsky et al., 2007; Eisenberg, Zhou, et al., 2005; Kochanska & Knaack, 2003; Spinrad et al., 2007; Valiente et al., 2006). Findings from Belsky and colleagues (2007) indicated that the children's attentional control partially mediated the across-time association between maternal behavior and behavior problems (across two time series; 54 months to first grade to third grade; first grade to third grade to fifth grade). The findings in this study provide a strong test of mediation, which was examined longitudinally with three time points in a panel design (controlling for stability of the constructs). Because effortful control appears to be a key factor in children's development of behavior problems, how parenting either enhances or interferes with effortful control is important both for understanding the development of behavior problems and targeting interventions for behavior problems.

In summary, findings are consistent with the view that environmental factors, including the quality of parenting, contribute to the development of effortful control. Parental supportive directives, behaviors, and expression of emotion have been correlated with higher levels of effortful control in children. In addition, parental attempts to scaffold children's use of effective self-regulatory strategies and of positive discipline strategies are associated with the level of children's effortful control. Thus, although effortful control has a genetic, temperamental basis (Goldsmith et al., 2008), it likely is fostered in interactions with socializers.

CONCLUSIONS

In the past decade it has become increasingly clear that effortful control is intimately related to social, emotional, moral, and cognitive development in childhood. Of course, because the research generally is correlational in design, it is very difficult to prove causal relations. Nonetheless, researchers have found that early measures of effortful control (or measures including effortful control) predict a broad range of important outcomes in childhood and beyond. Moreover, relations between effortful control and emotionality, adjustment, and social competence are evident across childhood and at older ages. Thus, self-regulation is a capacity that appears to play a major role in many aspects of development.

Findings also suggest that socialization in the home may contribute to the development of effortful control. It is possible that a number of effects of parental socialization on developmental outcomes are partly mediated through their relations to effortful control. However, experimental studies in which parents are trained to interact with their children in ways likely to foster effortful control are needed to prove a causal link. This is an important task for future study. Moreover, given the critical role of effortful control in many aspects of development, it is important that developmentalists find ways to stimulate its development outside of the home. Although some intervention/prevention researchers have designed programs to foster emotion regulation (e.g., Greenberg, Kusche, Cook, & Quamma, 1995), much more should be done in this domain.

ACKNOWLEDGMENTS

This research was supported by grants from the National Institutes of Mental Health and the National Institute of Child Health and Human Development to Nancy Eisenberg and Tracy L. Spinrad.

REFERENCES

Aksan, N., & Kochanska, G. (2004). Links between systems of inhibition from infancy to preschool years. *Child Development, 75,* 1477–1490.

Ayduk, O., Mendoza-Denton, R., Mischel, W., Downey, G., Peake, P. K., & Rodriguez, M. (2000). Regulating the interpersonal self: Strategic self-regulation for coping with rejection sensitivity. *Journal of Personality and Social Psychology, 79,* 776–792.

Belsky, J., Fearon, R. M. P., & Bell, B. (2007). Parenting, attention and externalizing problems: Testing mediation longitudinally, repeatedly and reciprocally. *Journal of Child Psychology and Psychiatry, 48,* 1233–1242.

Belsky, J., Friedman, S. L., & Hsieh, K. H. (2001). Testing a core emotion-regulation prediction: Does early attentional persistence moderate the effect of infant negative emotionality on later development? *Child Development, 72,* 123–133.

Blandon, A. Y., Calkins, S. D., Keane, S. P., & O'Brien, M. (2008). Individual differences in trajectories of emotion regulation processes: The effects of maternal depressive symptomatology and children's physiological regulation. *Developmental Psychology, 44,* 1110–1123.

Bridgett, D. J., Gartstein, M. A., Putnam, S. P., McKay, T., Iddins, E., Robertson, C., et al. (2009). Maternal and contextual influences and the effect of temperament development during infancy on parenting in toddlerhood. *Infant Behavior and Development, 32,* 103–116.

Buckner, J. C., Mezzacappa, E., & Beardslee, W. R. (2009). Self-regulation and its relations to adaptive functioning in low income youths. *American Journal of Orthopsychiatry, 79,* 19–30.

Calkins, S. D. (1994). Origins and outcomes of individual differences in emotion regulation. *Monographs of the Society for Research in Child Development, 59*(Serial No. 240), 53–72.

Calkins, S. D., & Dedmon, S. E. (2000). Physiological and behavioral regulation in two-year-old children with aggressive/destructive behavior problems. *Journal of Abnormal Child Psychology, 28,* 103–118.

Calkins, S. D., Dedmon, S. E., Gill, K. L., Lomax, L. E., & Johnson, L. M. (2002). Frustration in infancy: Implications for emotion regulation, physiological processes, and temperament. *Infancy, 3,* 175–197.

Calkins, S. D., & Johnson, M. J. (1998). Toddler regulation of distress to frustrating events: Temperamental and maternal correlates. *Infant Behavior and Development, 21*(3), 379–395.

Carlson, S. M. (2005). Developmentally sensitive measures of executive function in preschool children. *Developmental Neuropsychology, 28,* 595–616.

Caspi, A., Henry, B., McGee, R. O., Moffitt, T. E., & Silva, P. A. (1995). Temperamental origins of child and adolescent behavior problems: From age three to age fifteen. *Child Development, 66,* 55–68.

Caspi, A., & Silva, P. A. (1995). Temperamental qualities at age three predict personality traits in young adulthood: Longitudinal evidence from a birth cohort. *Child Development, 66,* 486–498.

Compas, B. E., Connor-Smith, J. K., & Saltzman, H. (2001). Coping with stress during childhood and adolescence: Problems, progress, and potential in theory and research. *Psychological Bulletin, 127,* 87–127.

Crockenberg, S. C., Leerkes, E. M., & Jó, P. S. B. (2008). Predicting aggressive behavior in the third year from infant reactivity and regulation as moderated by maternal behavior. *Development and Psychopathology, 20,* 37–54.

Degnan, K. A., Calkins, S. D., Keane, S. P., & Hill-Soderlund, A. L. (2008). Profiles of disruptive behavior across early childhood: Contributions of frustration reactivity, physiological regulation, and maternal behavior. *Child Development, 79,* 1357–1376.

Dennis, T. A., Brotman, L. M., Huang, K. Y., & Gouley, K. K. (2007). Effortful control, social competence, and adjustment problems in children at risk for psychopathology. *Journal of Clinical Child and Adolescent Psychology, 36,* 442–454.

Diamond, A. (1991). Neuropsychological insights into the meaning of object concept development. In S. Carey & R. Gelman (Eds.), *The epigensis of mind: Essays on biology and cognition.* Hillsdale, NJ: Erlbaum.

Diener, M. L., & Kim, D.-Y. (2004). Maternal and child predictors of preschool children's social competence. *Applied Developmental Psychology, 25,* 3–24.

Eiden, R. D., Colder, C., Edwards, E. P., & Leonard, K. E. (2009). A longitudinal study of social competence among children of alcoholics and nonalcoholic parents: Role of parental psychopathology, parental warmth, and self-regulation. *Psychology of Addictive Behaviors, 23,* 36–46.

Eisenberg, N., Chang, L., Ma, Y., & Haung, X. (2009). Relations of parenting style to Chinese children's effortful control, ego resilience, and maladjustment. *Development and Psychopathology, 21,* 455–477.

Eisenberg, N., Cumberland, A., & Spinrad, T. L. (1998). Parental socialization of emotion. *Psychological Inquiry, 9,* 241–273.

Eisenberg, N., Cumberland, A., Spinrad, T. L., Fabes, R. A., Shepard, S. A., Reiser, M., et al. (2001). The relations of regulation and emotionality to children's externalizing and internalizing problem behavior. *Child Development, 72,* 1112–1134.

Eisenberg, N., Fabes, R. A., Bernzweig, J., Karbon, M., Poulin, R., & Hanish, L. (1993). The relations of emotionality and regulation to preschoolers' social skills and sociometric status. *Child Development, 64,* 1418–1438.

Eisenberg, N., Fabes, R. A., Guthrie, I., Murphy, B. C., Maszk, P., Holmgren, R., et al. (1996). The relations of regulation and emotionality to problem behavior in elementary school children. *Development and Psychopathology, 8,* 141–162.

Eisenberg, N., Fabes, R. A., Guthrie, I. K., & Reiser, M. (2000). Dispositional emotionality and regulation: Their role in predicting quality of social functioning. *Journal of Personality and Social Psychology, 78,* 136–157.

Eisenberg, N., Fabes, R. A., Karbon, M., Murphy, B. C., Wosinski, M., Polazzi, L., et al. (1996). The relations of children's dispositional prosocial behavior to emotionality, regulation, and social functioning. *Child Development, 67,* 974–992.

Eisenberg, N., Fabes, R. A., Murphy, B., Karbon, M., Smith, M., & Maszk, P. (1996). The relations of children's dispositional empathy-related responding to their emotionality, regulation, and social functioning. *Developmental Psychology, 32,* 195–209.

Eisenberg, N., Fabes, R. A., Murphy, B., Maszk, P., Smith, M., & Karbon, M. (1995). The role of emotionality and regulation in children's social functioning: A longitudinal study. *Child Development, 66,* 1360–1384.

Eisenberg, N., Fabes, R. A., Nyman, M., Bernzweig, J., & Pinuelas, A. (1994). The relations of emotionality and regulation to children's anger-related reactions. *Child Development, 65,* 109–128.

Eisenberg, N., Fabes, R. A., & Shepard, S. A. (1997). Contemporaneous and longitudinal prediction of children's social functioning from regulation and emotionality. *Child Development, 68,* 642–664.

Eisenberg, N., Fabes, R. A., Shepard, S. A., Guthrie, I. K., Murphy, B. C., & Reiser, M. (1999).

Parental reactions to children's negative emotions: Longitudinal relations to quality of children's social functioning. *Child Development, 70*, 513–534.

Eisenberg, N., Fabes, R. A., Shepard, S. A., Murphy, B. C., Jones, S., & Guthrie, I. K. (1998). Contemporaneous and longitudinal prediction of children's sympathy from dispositional regulation and emotionality. *Developmental Psychology, 34*, 910–924.

Eisenberg, N., Guthrie, I. K., Fabes, R. A., Resier, M., Murphy, B. C., Holmgren, R., et al. (1997). The relations of regulation and emotionality to resiliency and competent social functioning in elementary school children. *Child Development, 68*, 367–383.

Eisenberg, N., Guthrie, I. K., Fabes, R. A., Shepard, S., Losoya, S., Murphy, B. C., et al. (2000). Prediction of elementary school children's externalizing problem behaviors from attentional and behavioral regulation and negative emotionality. *Child Development, 71*, 1367–1382.

Eisenberg, N., Liew, J., & Pidada, S. U. (2004). The longitudinal relations of regulation and emotionality to quality of Indonesian children's socioemotional functioning. *Developmental Psychology, 40*, 790–804.

Eisenberg, N., Ma, Y., Chang, L., Zhou, Q., West, S. G., & Aiken, L. (2007). Relations of effortful control, reactive undercontrol, and anger to Chinese children's adjustment. *Development and Psychopathology, 19*, 385–409.

Eisenberg, N., Michalik, N., Spinrad, T. L., Hofer, C., Kupfer, A., Valiente, C., et al. (2007). Relations of effortful control and impulsivity to children's sympathy: A longitudinal study. *Cognitive Development, 22*, 544–567.

Eisenberg, N., Pidada, S. U., & Liew, J. (2001). The relations of regulation and negative emotionality to Indonesian children's social functioning. *Child Development, 72*, 1747–1763.

Eisenberg, N., Sadovsky, A., Spinrad, T. L., Fabes, R. A., Losoya, S. H., Valiente, C., et al. (2005). The relations of problem behavior status to children's negative emotionality, effortful control, and impulsivity: Concurrent relations and prediction of change. *Developmental Psychology, 41*, 193–211.

Eisenberg, N., Spinrad, T. L., & Eggum, N. D. (2010). Emotion-related self-regulation and its relation to children's maladjustment. *Annual Review of Clinical Psychology, 6*, 495–523.

Eisenberg, N., Spinrad, T. L., Fabes, R. A., Reiser, M., Cumberland, A., Shepard, S. A., et al. (2004). The relations of effortful control and impulsivity to children's resiliency and adjustment. *Child Development, 75*, 25–46.

Eisenberg, N., Valiente, C., Fabes, R. A., Smith, C. L., Reiser, M., Shepard, S. A., et al. (2003). The relations of effortful control and ego control to children's resiliency and social functioning. *Developmental Psychology, 39*, 761–776.

Eisenberg, N., Valiente, C., Spinrad, T. L., Cumberland, A., Liew, J., Reiser, M., et al. (2009). Longitudinal relations of children's effortful control, impulsivity, and negative emotionality to their externalizing, internalizing, and co-occurring behavior problems. *Developmental Psychology, 45*, 988–1008.

Eisenberg, N., Zhou, Q., Spinrad, T. L., Valiente, C., Fabes, R. A., & Liew, J. (2005). Relations among positive parenting, children's effortful control, and externalizing problems: A three-wave longitudinal study. *Child Development, 76*, 1055–1071.

Fabes, R. A., Eisenberg, N., Jones, S., Smith, M., Guthrie, I., Poulin, R., et al. (1999). Regulation, emotionality, and preschoolers' socially competent peer interactions. *Child Development, 70*, 432–442.

Gaertner, B. M., Spinrad, T. L., & Eisenberg, N. (2008). Focused attention in toddlers: Measurement, stability, and relations to negative emotion and parenting. *Infant and Child Development, 17*, 339–363.

Garon, N., Bryson, S. E., & Smith, I. M. (2008). Executive function in preschoolers: A review using an integrative framework. *Psychological Bulletin, 134*, 31–60.

Gerardi-Caulton, G. (2000). Sensitivity to spatial conflict and the development of self-regulation in children 24–36 months of age. *Developmental Science, 3*, 397–404.

Gilliom, M., Shaw, D. S., Beck, J. E., Schonberg, M. A., & Lukon, J. L. (2002). Anger regulation in disadvantaged preschool boys: Strategies, antecedents, and the development of self-control. *Developmental Psychology, 38*, 222–235.

Goldsmith, H. H., Pollak, S. D., & Davidson, R. J. (2008). Developmental neuroscience perspectives on emotion regulation. *Child Development Perspectives, 2*, 132–140.

Greenberg, M. T., Kusche, C. A., Cook, E. T., & Quamma, J. P. (1995). Promoting emotional competence in school-aged children: The effects of the PATHS curriculum. *Development and Psychopathology, 7*, 117–136.

Guthrie, I. K., Eisenberg, N., Fabes, R. A., Murphy, B. C., Holmgren, R., Maszk, P., et al. (1997). The relations of regulation and emotionality to children's situational empathy-related responding. *Motivation and Emotion, 21*, 87–108.

Hanish, L. D., Eisenberg, N., Fabes, R. A., Spinrad, T. L., Ryan, P., & Schmidt, S. (2004). The expression and regulation of negative emotions: Risk factors for young children's peer victimization. *Development and Psychopathology, 16*, 335–353.

Henry, B., Caspi, A., Moffitt, T. E., Harrington, H., & Silva, P. (1999). Staying in school protects boys with poor self-regulation in childhood from later crime: A longitudinal study. *International Journal of Behavioral Development, 23*, 1049–1073.

Hill-Soderlund, A. L., & Braungart-Rieker, J. M. (2008). Early individual differences in temperamental reactivity and regulation: Implications for effortful control in early childhood. *Infant Behavior and Development, 31*, 386–397.

Hofer, C., Eisenberg, N., & Reiser, M. (in press). The role of socialization, effortful control and ego resiliency in French adolescents' social functioning. *Journal of Research in Adolescence.*

Jones, L. B., Rothbart, M. K., & Posner, M. I. (2003). Development of executive attention in preschool children. *Developmental Science, 6*, 498–504.

Kannass, K. N., Oakes, L. M., & Shaddy, D. J. (2006). A longitudinal investigation of the development of attention and distractibility. *Journal of Cognition and Development, 7*, 381–409.

Karreman, A., van Tuijl, C., van Aken, M. A. G., & Dekovic, M. (2008). Parenting, coparenting, and effortful control in preschoolers. *Journal of Family Psychology, 22*, 30–40.

Kim, S., & Brody, G. H. (2005). Longitudinal pathways to psychological adjustment among black youth living in single-parent households. *Journal of Family Psychology, 19*, 305–313.

Kochanska, G., Aksan, N., Prisco, T. R., & Adams, E. E. (2008). Mother–child and father–child mutually responsive orientation in the first 2 years and children's outcomes at preschool age: Mechanisms of influence. *Child Development, 79*, 30–44.

Kochanska, G., Barry, R. A., Aksan, N., & Boldt, L. J. (2008). A developmental model of maternal and child contributions to disruptive conduct: The first six years. *Journal of Child Psychology and Psychiatry, 49*, 1220–1227.

Kochanska, G., Coy, K. C., & Murray, K. T. (2001). The development of self-regulation in the first four years of life. *Child Development, 72*, 1091–1111.

Kochanska, G., & Knaack, A. (2003). Effortful control as a personality characteristic of young children: Antecedents, correlates, and consequences. *Journal of Personality, 71*, 1087–1112.

Kochanska, G., Murray, K., & Coy, K. (1997). Inhibitory control as a contributor to conscience in childhood: From toddler to early school age. *Child Development, 68*, 263–277.

Kochanska, G., Murray, K. L., & Harlan, E. T. (2000). Effortful control in early childhood: Continuity and change, antecedents, and implications for social development. *Developmental Psychology, 36*, 220–232.

Kochanska, G., Philibert, R. A., & Barry, R. A. (2009). Interplay of genes and early mother–child relationship in the development of self-regulation from toddler to preschool age. *Journal of Child Psychology and Psychiatry, 5*, 1331–1338.

Kopp, C. B. (1989). Regulation of distress and negative emotions: A developmental view. *Developmental Psychology, 25*, 343–354.

Kopp, C. B., & Neufeld, S. J. (2003). Emotional development during infancy. In R. J. Davidson, K.

R. Scherer, & H. H. Goldsmith (Eds.), *Handbook of affective sciences* (pp. 347–374). New York: Oxford University Press.

Lemery, K. S., Essex, M. J., & Snider, N. A. (2002). Revealing the relation between temperament and behavior problem symptoms by eliminating measurement confounding: Expert ratings and factor analyses. *Child Development, 73*, 867–882.

Lengua, L. J. (2006). Growth in temperament and parenting as predictors of adjustment during children's transition to adolescence. *Developmental Psychology, 42*, 819–832.

Lengua, L. J. (2008). Anxiousness, frustration, and effortful control as moderators of the relation between parenting and adjustment in middle-childhood. *Social Development, 17*, 554–577.

Lengua, L. J., West, S. G., & Sandler, I. N. (1998). Temperament as a predictor of symptomatology in children: Addressing contamination of measures. *Child Development, 69*, 164–181.

Leon-Carrion, J., García-Orza, J., & Pérez-Santamaría, F. J. (2004). Development of the inhibitory component of the executive functions in children and adolescents. *International Journal of Neuroscience, 114*, 1291–311.

Li-Grining, C. P. (2007). Effortful control among low-income preschoolers in three cities: Stability, change, and individual differences. *Developmental Psychology, 43*, 208–221.

Martel, M. M., Nigg, J. T., Wong, M. M., Fitzgerald, H. E., Jester, J. M., Puttler, L. I., et al. (2007). Childhood and adolescent resiliency, regulation, and executive functioning in relation to adolescent problems and competence in a high-risk sample. *Development and Psychopathology, 19*, 541–563.

Mezzacappa, E. (2004). Alerting, orienting, and executive attention: Developmental properties and sociodemographic correlates in an epidemiological sample of young, urban children. *Child Development, 75*, 1373–1386.

Mischel, W., Shoda, Y., & Peake, P. K. (1988). The nature of adolescent competencies predicted by preschool delay of gratification. *Journal of Personality and Social Psychology, 54*, 687–696.

Muris, P. (2006). Unique and interactive effects of neuroticism and effortful control on psychopathological symptoms in non-clinical adolescents. *Personality and Individual Differences, 40*, 1409–1419.

Murphy, B. C., Eisenberg, N., Fabes, R. A., Shepard, S., & Guthrie, I. K. (1999). Consistency and change in children's emotionality and regulation: A longitudinal study. *Merrill–Palmer Quarterly, 46*, 413–444.

Murphy, B. C., Shepard, S. A., Eisenberg, N., & Fabes, R. L. A. (2004). Concurrent and across time prediction of young adolescents' social functioning. *Social Development, 13*, 56–86.

Murray, K. T., & Kochanska, G. (2002). Effortful control: Factor structure and relation to externalizing and internalizing behaviors. *Journal of Abnormal Child Psychology, 30*, 503–514.

Newman, D. L., Caspi, A., Moffitt, T. E., & Silva, P. A. (1997). Antecedents of adult interpersonal functioning: Effects of individual differences in age 3 temperament. *Developmental Psychology, 33*, 206–217.

Oldehinkel, A. J., Hartman, C. A., Ferdinand, R. F., Verhulst, F. C., & Ormel, J. (2007). Effortful control as a modifier of the association between negative emotionality and adolescents' mental health problems. *Development and Psychopathology, 19*, 523–539.

Olson, S. L., Sameroff, A. J., Kerr, D. C. R., Lopez, N. L., & Wellman, H. M. (2005). Developmental foundations of externalizing problems in young children: The role of effortful control. *Development and Psychopathology, 17*, 25–45.

Pickering, A. D., & Gray, J. A. (1999). The neuroscience of personality. In L. A. Pervin & O. P. John (Eds.), *Handbook of personality: Theory and research* (2nd ed., pp. 277–299). New York: Guilford Press.

Posner, M. I., & DiGirolamo, G. J. (2000). Cognitive neuroscience: Origins and promise. *Psychological Bulletin, 126*, 873–889.

Posner, M. I., & Rothbart, M. K. (1998). Attention, self-regulation, and consciousness. *Transactions of the Philosophical Society of London B*, 1915–1927.

Posner, M. I., & Rothbart, M. K. (2007). Research on attention networks as a model for the integration of psychological science. *Annual Review of Psychology, 58,* 1–23

Putnam, S. P., Rothbart, M. K., & Gartstein, M. A. (2008). Homotypic and heterotypic continuity of fine-grained temperament during infancy, toddlerhood, and early childhood. *Infant and Child Development, 17,* 387–405.

Raaijmakers, M. A. J., Smidts, D. P., Sergeant, J. A., Maassen, G. H., Posthumus, J. A., van Engeland, H., et al. (2008). Executive functions in preschool children with aggressive behavior: Impairments in inhibitory control. *Journal of Abnormal Child Psychology, 36,* 1097–1107.

Raver, C. C., Blackburn, E. K., Bancroft, M., & Torp, N. (1999). Relations between effective emotional self-regulation, attentional control, and low-income preschoolers' social competence with peers. *Early Education and Development, 10,* 333–350.

Rothbart, M. K., Ahadi, S. A., & Hershey, K. L. (1994). Temperament and social behavior in childhood. *Merrill–Palmer Quarterly, 40,* 21–39.

Rothbart, M. K., & Bates, J. E. (2006). Temperament. In N. Eisenberg & W. Damon (Eds.), *Handbook of child psychology: Vol. 3. Social, emotional, and personality development* (6th ed., pp. 99–166). New York: Wiley.

Rothbart, M. K., Ellis, L. K., Rueda, M. R., & Posner, M. I. (2003). Developing mechanisms of temperamental effortful control. *Journal of Personality, 71,* 1113–1143.

Rothbart, M. K., Ziaie, H., & O'Boyle, C. G. (1992). Self regulation and emotion in infancy. *New Directions for Child Development, 55,* 7–23.

Rueda, M., Fan, J., McCandliss, B. D., Halparin, J. D., Gruber, D. B., Lercari, L. P., et al. (2004). Development of attentional networks in childhood. *Neuropsychologia, 42,* 1029–1040.

Ruff, H. A., & Rothbart, M. K. (1996). *Attention in early development.* New York: Oxford University Press.

Rydell, A.-M., Berlin, L., & Bohlin, G. (2003). Emotionality, emotion regulation, and adaptation among 5- to 8-year-old children. *Emotion, 3,* 30–47.

Sheese, B. E., Rothbart, M. K., Posner, M. I., White, L. K., & Fraundorf, S. H. (2008). Executive attention and self-regulation in infancy. *Infant Behavior and Development, 31,* 501–510.

Silk, J. S., Shaw, D. S., Forbes, E. E., Lane, T. L., & Kovacs, M. (2006). Maternal depression and child internalizing: The moderating role of child emotion regulation. *Journal of Clinical and Child Adolescent Psychology, 35,* 116–126.

Silk, J. S., Steinberg, L., & Morris, A. S. (2003). Adolescents' emotion regulation in daily life: Links to depressive symptoms and problem behavior. *Child Development, 74,* 1869–1880.

Spinrad, T. L., Eisenberg, N., Cumberland, A., Fabes, R. A., Valiente, C., Shepard, S., et al. (2006). Relation of emotion-related regulation to children's social competence: A longitudinal study. *Emotion, 6,* 498–510.

Spinrad, T. L., Eisenberg, N., Gaertner, B., Popp, T., Smith, C. L., Kupfer, A., et al. (2007). Relations of maternal socialization and toddlers' effortful control to children's adjustment and social competence. *Developmental Psychology, 43,* 1170–1186.

Spinrad, T. L., Eisenberg, N., Harris, E., Hanish, L., Fabes, R. A., Kupanoff, K., et al. (2004). The relations of children's everyday nonsocial peer play behavior to their emotionality, regulation, and social functioning. *Developmental Psychology, 40,* 67–80.

Valiente, C., Eisenberg, N., Fabes, R. A., Shepard, S. A., Cumberland, A., & Losoya, S. H. (2004). Prediction of children's empathy-related responding from their effortful control and parents' expressivity. *Developmental Psychology, 40,* 911–926.

Valiente, C., Eisenberg, N., Smith, C. L., Reiser, M., Fabes, R. A., Losoya, S., et al. (2003). The relations of effortful control and reactive control to children's externalizing problems: A longitudinal assessment. *Journal of Personality, 71,* 1171–1196.

Valiente, C., Eisenberg, N., Spinrad, T. L., Reiser, M., Cumberland, A., Losoya, S. H., et al. (2006). Relations among mothers' expressivity, children's effortful control, and their problem behaviors: A four-year longitudinal study. *Emotion, 6,* 459–472.

Valiente, C., Lemery-Chalfant, K., & Reiser, M. (2007), Pathways to problem behaviors: Chaotic homes, parent and child effortful control, and parenting. *Social Development, 16,* 249–267.

Williams, B. R., Ponesse, J. S., Schachar, R. J., Logan, G. D., & Tannock, R. (1999). Development of inhibitory control across the life span. *Developmental Psychology, 35,* 205–213.

Xu, Y., Farver, J. A. M., & Zhang, Z. (2009). Temperament, harsh and indulgent parenting, and Chinese children's proactive and reactive aggression. *Child Development, 80,* 244–258.

Yap, M. B. H., Allen, N. B., Leve, C., & Katz, L. F. (2008). Maternal meta-emotion philosophy and socialization of adolescent affect: The moderating role of adolescent temperament. *Journal of Family Psychology, 22,* 688–700.

Zhou, Q., Eisenberg, N., Wang, Y., & Reiser, M. (2004). Chinese children's effortful control and dispositional anger/frustration: Relations to parenting styles and children's social functioning. *Developmental Psychology, 40,* 352–366.

Zhou, Q., Lengua, L. J., & Wang, Y. (2009). The relations of temperament reactivity and effortful control to children's adjustment problems in China and the United States. *Developmental Psychology, 45,* 724–739.

CHAPTER 15

Attentional Control and Self-Regulation

M. ROSARIO RUEDA
MICHAEL I. POSNER
MARY K. ROTHBART

SELF-REGULATION

Self-regulation has been a central concept in developmental psychology and in the study of psychopathologies. Fonagy and Target (2002, p. 307) see *self-regulation* as "the key mediator between genetic predisposition, early experience and adult functioning." In their view, self-regulation refers to "(1) children's ability to control the reaction to stress, (2) [their] capacity to maintain focused attention and (3) the capacity to interpret mental states in themselves and others." Self-regulation is also an obvious feature of normal socialization that is apparent to caregivers, teachers, and others who work with children.

Bronson (2000) has outlined perspectives on self-regulation from psychoanalysis, social learning theory, Vygotsky, Piaget (including neo-Piagetians), and the information-processing tradition. Each of these approaches seeks to account for how children achieve the ability to regulate their emotions, and to an extent, their thought processes. The first edition of this handbook reviewed the current state of self-regulation (Baumeister & Vohs, 2004).

This chapter stresses efforts to develop a neurological basis for self-regulation based on the use of neuroimaging, studies of the assessment of attention from questionnaires (see Rothbart & Bates, 1998; Rothbart, Ellis, & Posner, Chapter 24, this volume), and individual differences in performance on attention tasks that can be used to define phenotypes for genetic analysis (Fossella, Posner, Fan, Swanson, & Pfaff, 2002; Posner, Rothbart, & Sheese, 2007). Although we discuss the neural networks related to self-regulation, our goal is not to review the field's theoretical positions as Bronson (2000) has done, but instead to provide an example of one analysis based on imaging and genetic studies of attention and self-regulation that may prove to be relevant to all of the theoretical perspectives cited by Bronson.

ATTENTION AS SELF-REGULATION

The study of attention has been a central topic from the start of human experimental psychology (Broadbent, 1958; Titchener, 1909). Generally the focus has been on probing fundamental mechanisms, by training or instructions, to perform tasks that call for various attentional functions, such as remaining vigilant to external events, selecting among concurrent information sources, processing difficult targets, or ignoring conflicting signals. A usually unstated idea in these studies is that by controlling the focus of attention through instructions, one can observe the properties of mechanisms that would also be used during self-motivated performance. Below we argue that it is now possible to see how attentional mechanisms influence other brain networks to allow people to regulate their emotions and thoughts.

INTEGRATION

Although discussion of neural networks in the human brain has the potential to link knowledge of the human brain to the efforts of educators and parents to socialize children, until recently these goals seemed remote. Two major developments changed the prospect of such integration. Neuroimaging combined with electrical or magnetic recordings from outside the skull now allow us to see in real time the circuits computing sensory, semantic, and emotional response to input (Dale et al., 2000; Posner & Raichle, 1994, 1998). Although some aspects of this technology have been around for a long time, only in the last decade has it become clear that a new era has given us the ability to create local images of human brain activity through changes in cerebral blood flow. Imaging studies have also examined how areas of the brain are functionally connected during activation (Posner, Sheese, Odludas, & Tang, 2006). The study of functional connectivity provides the opportunity to examine how attention interacts with other brain networks. The second event is the sequencing of the human genome (Venter et al., 2001). Now it is possible not only to study the functional anatomy of brain networks but also to examine how genetic differences might lead to individual variations in the potential to use these networks to acquire and perform skills.

Ruff and Rothbart (1996) attempted to integrate the study of attention and self-regulation in their volume *Attention in Early Development*. They viewed attention as "part of the larger construct of self-regulation—the ability to modulate behavior according to the cognitive, emotional and social demands of specific situations" (p. 133). They argued further that self-regulation places emphasis on attention, including inhibitory control, strategies of problem solving, memory, and self-monitoring. In addition to their argument that attention is a part of the mechanisms of self-regulation, Ruff and Rothbart discuss how individual differences in attentional efficiency play a part in successful self-regulation.

In previous work we have stressed important results showing that some brain networks provide control operations that facilitate or inhibit the functions of other networks, providing a neural basis for self-regulation (Posner & Rothbart, 1998, 2000). For example, different parts of the anterior cingulate cortex (ACC) have been involved in cognitive and emotional monitoring processes. Areas of the dorsal ACC are highly interconnected with lateral frontal and parietal structures, and become active when a task requires selection among conflicting alternatives (Botvinick, Braver, Barch, Carter, & Cohen, 2001; Bush, Luu, & Posner, 2000). More ventral areas of the ACC in conjunction with other limbic structures (e.g., the amygdala) provide a basis for regulation of emotion (Bush et al., 2000; Drevets & Raichle, 1998). Although more detailed analysis of the cingulate has revealed additional subareas, the distinction between the dorsal area involved in cognition and the ventral area involved in emotion has continued (Beckman, Johansen-Berg, & Rushworth, 2009). As neural networks responsible for self-regulation are established by neuroimaging, we are able to observe how genes and environment regulate the networks during development. We have been involved in this effort for some time (Posner & Rothbart, 1998, 2007) and provide in this chapter an overview of our approach and findings.

The approach in this chapter follows the framework of Ruff and Rothbart (1996) but involves a more detailed analysis of the links between self-regulation and attention, available from more recent studies. The functions associated with the executive attention network overlap with the more general notion of executive functions in childhood. These functions include working memory, planning, switching, and inhibitory control (Welch, 2001). For example, *working memory*, as defined by Baddeley (Hofmann, Friese, Schmeichel, & Baddeley, Chapter 11, this volume) includes both a storage component and an executive component that is the same as the one we call executive attention in this chapter. Some functions of working memory and other executive functions are self-regulatory and are carried out by brain structures that involve the executive attention network. However, we place emphasis on the monitoring and control functions of attention, without attempting to develop a strict boundary between these and other executive functions that may not emphasize attention.

ATTENTIONAL NETWORKS

Functional neuroimaging has allowed analysis of many cognitive tasks in terms of the brain areas they activate. Studies of attention have been among the most often examined in this way (Corbetta & Shulman, 2002; Driver, Eimer, Macaluso, & van Velzen, 2004; Posner & Fan, 2008; Wright & Ward, 2008). Imaging data have supported the presence of three networks related to different aspects of attention. These networks carry out the functions of alerting, orienting, and providing executive control (Posner & Fan, 2008). A summary of the anatomy and transmitters involved in the three networks is shown in Table 15.1.

Alerting is defined as achieving and maintaining a state of high sensitivity to incoming stimuli; *executive control* involves the mechanisms for monitoring and resolving conflict among thoughts, feelings, and responses. *Orienting* is the selection of information from sensory input and involves aligning attention with a source of sensory signals. The link to self-regulation, at least in older children and adults, is mediated by the executive attention network. Executive attention is most often studied by using tasks that involve conflict, such as various versions of the Stroop task. In the Stroop task, subjects must respond to the color of ink (e.g., red), while ignoring the color word name (e.g., blue) (Bush et al., 2000). Resolving conflict in the Stroop task activates midline frontal areas (anterior cingulate) and lateral prefrontal cortex (Botvinick et al., 2001; Fan, Flombaum, McCandliss, Thomas, & Posner, 2002).

TABLE 15.1. Brain Areas and Neuromodulators Involved in Attention Networks

Function	Structures	Modulator
Orienting	Superior parietal Temporal–parietal junction Frontal eye fields Superior colliculus	Acetylcholine
Alerting	Locus coeruleus Right frontal and parietal cortex	Norepinephrine
Executive attention	Anterior cingulate Lateral ventral prefrontal Basal ganglia	Dopamine

While the conflict theory involves the role of a common brain network in resolving conflict when different responses are simultaneously active, a rather different but related approach stresses that the exercise of self-control can be fatigued by use (Baumeister, Vohs, & Tice, 2007), thus reducing its role in subsequent activity. In this literature, the exercise of self-control involves a limited resource and its use results in temporary depletion. Although no studies provide an anatomical basis for this system, it seems likely that it would involve the same anatomy as the executive attention network. There is also evidence for the activation of the executive network in tasks involving conflict between a central target and surrounding flankers that may be congruent or incongruent with the target (Botvinick et al., 2001; Fan, Flombaum, et al., 2002). Experimental tasks may provide a means of identifying the functional contributions of different areas within the executive attention network (Fan et al., 2009; MacDonald, Cohen, Stenger, & Carter, 2000).

Regulatory Functions of Attention

The ACC, one of the main nodes of the executive attention network, has been linked to a variety of specific functions in attention (Posner & Fan, 2008), working memory (Duncan et al., 2000), emotion (Bush et al., 2000), pain (Rainville, Duncan, Price, Carrier, & Bushnell, 1997), monitoring for conflict (Botvinick et al., 2001), and detection of error (Holroyd & Coles, 2002). These functions have been well documented, but no single rubric seems to explain all of them. In emotional studies, the ACC is often seen as part of a network involving orbitofrontal and limbic (amygdala) structures. The frontal areas seem to have an ability to interact with the limbic system (Davidson, Putnam, & Larson, 2000) that could fit well with self-regulation.

A specific test of this idea involved exposure to erotic films, with participants instructed to regulate any resulting arousal. The cingulate activity shown by functional magnetic resonance imaging (fMRI) was found to be related to the regulatory instruction (Beauregard, Levesque, & Bourgouin, 2001). In a different study, cognitive reappraisal of photographs producing negative affect showed a relation between extent of cingulate activity and reduction in negative affect (McRae, Ochsner, & Gross, Chapter 10, this volume; Ochsner, Bunge, Gross, & Gabrieli, 2002). Studies of functional connectivity have also shown that the ACC is coupled to relevant sensory areas during the selection of auditory or visual signals (Crottaz-Herbette & Mennon, 2006) and to the limbic area during emotional control (Etkin, Egner, Peraza, Kandel, & Hirsch, 2006). Similarly, when hypnotism was used to control the perception of pain, the cingulate activity reflected the perception, not the strength, of the physical stimulus (Rainville et al., 1997). These results indicate a role for this anatomical structure in regulating limbic activity related to emotion and provide evidence for a role of the cingulate as a part of the network controlling affect (Bush et al., 2000).

In many tasks, conflict is introduced by the need to respond to one aspect of the stimulus while ignoring another (Bush et al., 2000; Fan, Flombaum, et al., 2002). Cognitive activity that involves this kind of conflict activates the dorsal ACC and lateral prefrontal cortex. Large lesions of the ACC in either adults or children (Anderson, Damasio, Tranel, & Damasio, 2000) result in great difficulty in regulating behavior, particularly in social situations. Smaller lesions may produce only a temporary inability to deal with conflict in cognitive tasks (Ochsner et al., 2001; Turken & Swick, 1999). The transient nature of the lesion data suggests that other brain areas are also involved in self-regulation. One possibility is the anterior insula. Both the cingulate and insula have large projection cells (von Economo cells) that have links to remote areas of the brain, and both areas may be related to the resolution of conflict (Sridharan, Levitin, & Menon, 2008).

DEVELOPMENT OF ATTENTIONAL SELF-REGULATION

A major advantage of viewing attention in relation to self-regulation is that it allows one to relate the development of a specific neural network to the ability of children and adults to regulate their thoughts and feelings. Over the first few years of life the regulation of emotion is a major issue of development.

The ability of attention to control distress can be traced to early infancy (Harman, Rothbart, & Posner, 1997). In infants as young as 3 months, we have found that orienting to a visual stimulus provided by the experimenter produces powerful, if only temporary, soothing of distress. One of the major accomplishments of the first few years is for infants to develop the means to achieve this regulation on their own. Recent studies have provided evidence that one of the functions of the ACC, namely, the detection of error, is present in infants by age 7 months (Berger, Tzur, & Posner, 2006). Studies of connectivity using fMRI have shown that newborns have relatively sparse connectivity of the midprefrontal cortex, but by 2 years of age, both the midprefrontal cortex and adjacent ACC show considerable connectivity (Gao et al., 2009). Connectivity continues to develop until at least late childhood (Fair et al., 2009).

Signs of the control of conflict are found in the first year of life. In A, not B, tasks, for example, children are rewarded for reaching for a hidden object at one location (A) and then tested on their ability to search for the hidden object at a new location (B). Children younger than 12 months of age tend to look to the previous location (A), even though they have seen the object disappear behind location B. After the first year, children develop the ability to inhibit the prepotent response toward the trained location A and successfully reach for the new location B (Diamond, 1991). During this period, infants also develop the ability to resolve conflict between line of sight and line of reach when retrieving an object. At 9 months of age, line of sight dominates completely. If the open side of a box is not in line with the side in view, infants will reach directly along the line of sight, striking the closed side (Diamond, 1991). In contrast, 12-month-old infants can simultaneously look at a closed side and reach through the open end to retrieve a toy.

The ability to use context to reduce conflict can be traced developmentally using the learning of sequences of locations. Infants as young as 4 months can learn to anticipate the location of a stimulus, provided that the associations in the sequence are unambiguous (Colombo, 2001; Haith, Hazan, & Goodman, 1988). In unambiguous sequences, each location is invariably associated with another location (e.g., 123123) (Clohessy, Posner, & Rothbart, 2001). Because the location of the current target is fully determined by the preceding item, only one type of information need be attended to; therefore, there is no conflict (e.g., location 3 always follows location 2). Adults can learn unambiguous sequences of spatial locations implicitly even when attention is distracted by a secondary task (Curran & Keele, 1993).

Ambiguous sequences (e.g., 121312) require attention to the current association in addition to the context in which the association occurs (e.g., location 1 may be followed by location 2, or by location 3). Ambiguous sequences pose conflict because for any association, there exist two strong candidates that can only be disambiguated by context. When distracted by counting clicks irrelevant to the main task, adults are unable to learn ambiguous sequences of length six (e.g., 123213) (Curran & Keele, 1993), a finding that demonstrates the need for higher-level attentional resources to resolve this conflict. Even simple ambiguous associations (e.g., 1213) were not performed at above chance level until infants were about 2 years of age (Clohessy et al., 2001).

Developmental changes in executive attention were found during the third year of life with use of a conflict key-pressing task (Gerardi-Caulton, 2000). Because children of this age do not read, location and identity rather than word meaning and ink color served as the dimensions of conflict (spatial conflict task). Children sat in front of two response keys, one located to the child's left and one to the right. Each key displayed a picture, and on every trial a picture identical to one of the pair appeared on either the left or right side of the screen. Children were rewarded for responding to the identity of the stimulus, regardless of its spatial compatibility with the matching response key (Gerardi-Caulton, 2000). Reduced accuracy and slowed reaction times for spatially incompatible relative to spatially compatible trials reflect the effort required to resist the prepotent response and resolve conflict between these two competing dimensions. Performance on this task produces a clear interference effect in adults and activates the anterior cingulate (Fan, Flombaum, et al., 2002). Children 24 months of age tended to perseverate on a single response, while 36-month-old children performed at high accuracy levels; like adults, they responded more slowly and with reduced accuracy to incompatible trials.

At 30 months, when toddlers were first able to perform the spatial conflict task successfully, we found that performance on this task was significantly correlated with their ability to learn the ambiguous associations in the sequence learning task described earlier (Rothbart, Ellis, Rueda, & Posner, 2003). This finding, together with the failure of 4-month-olds to learn ambiguous sequences, holds out the promise of being able to trace the emergence of executive attention during the first years of life.

The importance of being able to study the emergence of executive attention is enhanced because cognitive measures of conflict resolution in these laboratory tasks have been linked to aspects of children's temperament. Signs of the development of executive attention by cognitive tasks relate to a temperament measure called effortful control, obtained from caregiver reports (see Rothbart et al., Chapter 24, this volume, for a review). Children relatively less affected by spatial conflict received higher parental ratings of temperamental effortful control and higher scores on laboratory measures of inhibitory control (Gerardi-Caulton, 2000). We regard effortful control as reflecting the efficiency with which the executive attention network operates in naturalistic settings.

The attention network task (ANT; Fan, McCandliss, Sommer, Raz, & Posner, 2002) was developed to assess the efficiency of the three attentional networks. The task was built around the flanker task, in which conflict is introduced by surrounding the target with flankers that indicate either the opposite (incongruent) or the same (congruent) response (Eriksen & Eriksen, 1974). The child-ANT is an adaptation of this task for children in which fish are used instead of arrows (Rueda, Fan, et al., 2004).

Using the child-ANT we have studied the evolution of conflict scores from age 4½ years to adulthood, shown in Table 15.2. The conflict score is computed by taking the median reaction time (RT) for trials with congruent flankers from the median RT for incongruent flanker trials (an index of conflict resolution abilities). Conflict scores showed a marked decrease between ages 6 and 7, but above age 7 there was remarkably little difference in conflict scores (as measured by both RT and errors) up to and including adults (Rueda, Fan, et al., 2004). This result is surprising given the general expectation that the executive network would improve until adulthood, as children are able to solve more difficult problems. A previous developmental study of the flanker task (Ridderinkhof, van der Molen, Band, & Bashore, 1997) showed improvement in conflict from ages 5 to 10, then little difference between this age and adulthood. Ridderinkhof and colleagues (1997) concluded that the major problem for children in flanker tasks is in the translation of the input code into an appropriate response code, particularly when there are incompatible responses. It seems likely that such a transformation would involve cingulate activity in monitoring the possible conflict.

Diamond and Taylor (1996) carried out a study in which they used the tapping test to evaluate performance of children between 3½ and 7 years of age. In this test children are asked to tap once when the experimenter taps twice, and to tap twice when the experimenter taps once. Correct performance of this test is thought to require certain aspects of executive control, such as the ability to hold two rules in mind and to inhibit the tendency to imitate the experimenter. Diamond and Taylor found a steady improvement in both accuracy and speed on the tapping test in children ages 3½ to 7 years. However,

TABLE 15.2. Conflict Resolution as a Function of Age in the Attention Network Task

	Overall performance		Conflict scores	
Age	Overall RT (msec)	Overall accuracy (% errors)	RT (msec)	Accuracy (% errors)
4.5	1,599	12.79	207	5.8
6	931	15.8	115	15.6
7	833	5.7	63	0.7
8	806	4.9	71	−0.3
9	734	2.7	67	1.6
10	640	2.2	69	2.1
Adults	483	1.2	61	1.6

Note. RT, reaction time.

consistent with our result, most of the improvement occurred by 6 years of age, with the 7-year-old group demonstrating an accuracy rate close to 100%.

Our findings of little or no development in the executive network for the resolution of conflict after age 7 may not extend to more difficult executive tasks (e.g., those involving strategic decisions). A recent imaging study found a common network of brain areas involved in the arrow version of the flanker task (similar to the adult version of the ANT), the Stroop color task, and a task involving a conflict between location and identity (Fan, McCandliss, et al., 2002). Of these tasks the flanker had the largest conflict effect as measured by RT difference and the strongest activation within the ACC. The fish and arrow ANTs differ a great deal in level of difficulty, yet they showed about the same developmental trend (Rueda, Fan, et al., 2004). These findings suggest earlier than might be expected development of neural areas related to the resolution of conflict, but this needs to be tested more directly in future work.

Using the child version of the ANT while recording brain activity with a high-density scalp electrode array, we compared 4-year-olds and adults (Rueda, Posner, Rothbart, & Davis-Stober, 2004). Despite dramatically different RTs and conflict resolution scores (see Table 15.2), the event-related potentials (ERPs) differences between incongruent and congruent trials were strikingly similar. Consistent with other studies (Kopp, Rist, & Mattler, 1996; van Veen & Carter, 2002), adults showed differences in the brain waves for congruent and incongruent conditions around 300 ms after the presentation of the target in both child and adult versions of the task. This effect is related to action monitoring processes (Botvinick et al., 2001) and has been associated with differences in activation localized in the anterior cingulate (van Veen & Carter, 2002). Electrophysiological measures can be relatively easily used with young children and are useful in linking behavioral changes in development of attention with the underlying brain networks involved.

Above the age of 6, children are more amenable to study using fMRI. In children ages 5–16, there is a significant relation between the volume of the area of the right anterior cingulate and the ability to perform tasks requiring focal attention (Casey, Trainor, Giedd, et al., 1997). In an fMRI study, performance of children ages 7–12 and adults was studied in a go/no-go task. In comparison with a control (go) condition, where children responded to all stimuli, the condition requiring inhibitory control (no-go) activated prefrontal cortex in both children and adults. The number of false alarms in this condition also correlated significantly with the extent of cingulate activity (Casey, Trainor, Orendi, et al., 1997).

We may consider two major changes in brain activity that seem to occur with development. One is a focalization of activity, so that fewer brain areas are active, and often those that are active are smaller in size (Durston & Casey, 2006). This leads to a view of more localized activity occurring with age. At the same time, the connectivity also changes from stronger local connections to more long-range or global connections (Fair et al., 2009). This leads to a somewhat opposite view of more distributed networks with age. Thus, activity seems more local with development, but connectivity seems more global. By adulthood, a small number of quite localized nodes are active in many tasks, but these can be highly distributed across the brain, most often involving both posterior and frontal sites (Posner & Rothbart, 2007). Development seems to be somewhat like practice on a single task, which often produces a reduction in both the number and size of overall brain activity, while enhancing connectivity between remote sites, thus achieving an efficient but distributed network.

These studies provide evidence for the development of an executive network during early childhood. The development of executive attention contributes to the socialization process by increasing the likelihood of learning important behaviors related to self-regulation, and understanding the cognition and emotion of others. Fostering the understanding of normal development of this system is also likely to illuminate the comprehension of some pathologies (Rothbart & Posner, 2006).

ROLE OF GENES AND ENVIRONMENT

The specification of development of a specific neural network related to self-regulation is only one step toward a biological understanding. It is also important to know the genetic and environmental influences that work together to produce the neural network.

Candidate Genes

To determine whether the executive network is likely to be under genetic control, we conducted a small-scale twin study to determine its heritability (Fan, Wu, Fossella, & Posner, 2001). The study showed substantial heritability for the conflict network. These results encourage the search for candidate genes related to the executive network. Links between specific neural networks of attention and chemical modulators allow one to investigate the genetic basis of normal attention (Fossella et al., 2002; Green et al., 2008). Green and colleagues (2008) argue that the three networks measured by the ANT involve different neuromodulators and are thus influenced by genes related to these modulators. Alerting appears to involve genes related to the norepinephrine system, orienting to cholinergic genes, and executive attention to dopaminergic genes. As one example, in our work on 200 subjects, we found that measures of the executive attention network were specifically related to the dopamine 4 receptor gene (*DRD4*) and three other dopaminergic genes. Subsequently, we found that when participants carried out the ANT during an fMRI scan, different alleles of the *DRD4* gene differentially activated the anterior cingulate gyrus (Fan, Fosella, Summer, Wu, & Posner, 2003).

In our longitudinal study, we found that the 7-repeat allele of the *DRD4* gene interacted with the quality of parenting to influence temperamental variables in the child such as activity level, sensation seeking, and impulsivity (Sheese, Voelker, Rothbart, & Posner, 2007). With high-quality parenting, 2-year-old children with the 7-repeat allele showed average levels of these temperamental traits, while those with poorer quality parenting showed much higher levels, and individuals without the 7-repeat allele were not influenced by parenting. Other research has shown similar findings for the effect of parenting on the externalizing behavior of the child, as rated by the parents in the Child Behavior Checklist (Bakermans-Kranenburg & van IJzendoorn, 2006).

There is evidence that the 7-repeat allele of the *DRD4* gene is under positive selective pressure, which means it is increasing in frequency during human evolution (Ding et al., 2002). Our results suggest a possible reason for this, in that genetic variation makes it more likely that children are influenced by their culture through parenting style. This idea could be important for understanding why the frequency of genetic alleles has changed during human evolution. In accord with this idea, a recent study showed that only those children with the 7-repeat allele of the *DRD4* gene showed the influence of a parent training intervention (Bakersman-Kranenburg, van IJzendoorn, Pijlman, Mesman, & Juffer, 2008).

In other work we have found a gene × environment interaction that clearly works by changes in attention. One of the strongest links between adult individual differences in executive attention and genes is for the catechol-O-methyltransferase (*COMT*) gene (Blasi et al., 2005), and a study of 7- to 14-year-old children (Diamond, Briand, Fosella, & Gehlbach, 2004) found a similar effect. In most studies one genotype (valine; Val/Val) shows better performance in a variety of tasks than does the other (methionine; Met/Met). Another approach to the gene has been to construct a haplotype that comprises three different polymorphisms in the gene. Versions of this haplotype are closely related to the perception of pain (Diatchenko et al., 2005), and executive attention and pain have both been shown to involve the anterior cingulate gyrus.

In both 7-month-olds and 2-year-olds in our longitudinal study, the genotype and the haplotypes were related to aspects of performance in the visual sequence task and, overall, the haplotype was more strongly linked to performance. At 2 years of age it was possible to examine the relation between observed parenting and variations in the *COMT* gene (Voelker, Sheese, Rothbart, & Posner, 2009). An interaction was found between the genetic variation and parenting quality in determining performance in the visual sequence task. Those 2-year-olds with higher quality parenting and the haplotype that included the Val/Val genotype were superior in the task. This confirms that, even during infancy, both genetic variation and parenting can influence the executive attention network.

FOSTERING SELF-REGULATION

The strong emphasis on genetic influences on neural networks may lead the reader to think that these networks are not amenable to interventions involving training or other behavioral therapies, although our interaction findings argue otherwise. It is not our intention to leave the impression that attention networks cannot be changed. Indeed, we think that normal socialization is important for the development of these networks, and that specific training may well be an effective way of fostering them at particular stages of development.

As noted earlier, the executive attention network appears to show substantial development between ages 2 and 7. In studies of monkeys trained for space flight, a series of training programs has been found to be very appealing to the primates and to result in general improvements in aggression, social relations, and hyperactivity (Rumbaugh & Washburn, 1995). We tested the effects of training on 4- and 6-year-old children using programs adapted from the monkey studies (Rueda, Rothbart, McCandliss, Saccomanno, & Posner, 2005). The training began with the children learning to use a joystick. This skill was then used to teach target tracking and spatial prediction, to exercise working memory, and finally to practice resolving conflict. Children who went through the training were compared with a randomly selected control group engaged with interactive videos.

Before and after training the children performed the ANT while their brain waves were recorded. Children who had undergone attention training showed clear evidence of improvement in the executive attention network following training in comparison with the control children. The N2 component of the scalp's recorded average electrical potential has been shown to arise in the anterior cingulate and is related to monitoring or resolving conflict (Jonkman, Sniedt, & Kemner, 2007; van Veen & Carter, 2002). We found N2 differences between congruent and incongruent trials of the ANT in trained 6-year-olds that resembled differences found in adults. In the 4-year-olds, the training seemed to influence more anterior electrodes, which are related to emotional control areas of the cingulate (Bush et al., 2000). These data suggest that training altered the network for the resolution of conflict in the direction of being more like that found in adults. We also found a significantly greater improvement in a measure of intelligence in the trained group compared to the control group. This finding suggests that training effects had generalized to a measure of cognitive processing that is far removed from the training exercises (Rueda et al., 2005).

A replication and extension of this study was carried out for 5-year-olds in a Spanish preschool (Rueda, Checa, & Santonja, 2008). Several additional exercises were added, and 10 days of training were provided for both experimental and control groups. As in the previous study, the randomly assigned control group viewed child-appropriate videos for the same amount of time as the training group. A follow-up session for all children was also given 2 months after the training. Unlike the control group, trained children showed improvement in intelligence scores, as measured by the Matrices scale of the Kaufman Brief Intelligence Test (K-BIT) following training. In addition, whereas the trained group held sustained improvement over a 2-month follow-up without further training, the control group did not. The training of attention also produced beneficial effects in task performance involving affective regulation, such as the Children's Gambling Task (Hongwanishkul, Happaney, Lee, & Zelazo, 2005).

A number of other reports have shown that aspects of attention can be trained in preschool children (Diamond, Barnett, Thomas, & Munro, 2007; Klingberg, Forssberg, & Westerberg, 2002). We hope our training method can be evaluated, along with other such methods, as possible means of improving attention of preschoolers and children diagnosed with attention-related disorders. However, we do not have any expectation that our exercises are optimal or even better than other methods. The study of attention training as a whole suggests that networks can be shaped by various methods of training.

Psychologists have often argued that learning must involve domain specificity (Simon, 1969; Thorndike, 1903). However, viewing attention as an organ system closely related to self-regulation, as we have done in this chapter, suggests a somewhat different view. Attention is domain-general in the sense that any content area can be the subject of modification through attention. If the appropriate methods for training attention in young children can be identified, systematic training of attention would be an important addition to preschool education.

ACKNOWLEDGMENTS

The research reported in this chapter was supported by the James S. McDonnell Foundation through a grant to the University of Oregon in support of research on training of attention. M.

Rosario Rueda was supported by a grant from La Caixa Foundation–USA Program and the Spanish Ministry of Science and Innovation (Ref. No. SEJ2005-01473).

REFERENCES

Anderson, S. W., Damasio, H., Tranel, D., & Damasio, A. R. (2000). Long-term sequelae of prefrontal cortex damage acquired in early childhood. *Developmental Neuropsychology, 18*(3), 281–296.

Bakermans-Kranenburg, M. J., & van IJzendoorn, M. H. (2006). Gene–environment interaction of the dopamine D4 receptor (DRD4) and observed maternal insensitivity predicting externalizing behavior in preschoolers. *Developmental Psychobiology, 48*, 406–409.

Bakermans-Kranenburg, M. J., van IJzendoorn, M. H., Pijlman, F. T. A., Mesman, J., & Juffer, F. (2008). Experimental evidence for differential susceptibility: Dopamine D4 receptor polymorphism (DRD4 VNTR) moderates intervention effects on toddlers' externalizing behavior in a randomized controlled trial. *Developmental Psychology, 44*(1), 293–300.

Baumeister, R. F., & Vohs, K. D. (Eds.). (2004) *Handbook of self-regulation: Research, theory, and applications.* New York: Guilford Press.

Baumeister, R. F., Vohs, K. D., & Tice, D. M. (2007). The strength model of self control. *Current Directions in Psychological Science*, 16, 351–355.

Beauregard, M., Levesque, J., & Bourgouin, P. (2001). Neural correlates of conscious self-regulation of emotion. *Journal of Neuroscience, 21*, 165.

Beckman, M., Johansen-Berg, H., & Rushworth, M. F. S. (2009). Connectivity based parcellation of human cingulate cortex and its relation to functional specialization. *Journal of Neuroscience, 29*, 1175–1190.

Berger, A., Tzur, G., & Posner, M. I. (2006). Infant babies detect arithmetic error. *Proceeding of the National Academy of Science USA, 103*, 12649–12553.

Blasi, G., Mattay, V. S., Bertolino, A., Elvevåg, B., Callicott, J. H., Das, S., et al. (2005). Effect of catechol-O-methyltransferase *val^{158} met* genotype on attentional control. *Journal of Neuroscience, 25*(20), 5038–5045.

Botvinick, M. M., Braver, T. S., Barch, D. M., Carter, C. S., & Cohen, J. D. (2001). Conflict monitoring and cognitive control. *Psychological Review, 108*, 624–652.

Broadbent, D. E. (1958). *Perception and communication.* London: Pergamon.

Bronson, M. B. (2000). *Self-regulation in early childhood: Nature and nurture.* New York: Guilford Press.

Bush, G., Luu, P., & Posner, M. I. (2000). Cognitive and emotional influences in the anterior cingulate cortex. *Trends in Cognitive Science, 4/6*, 215–222.

Casey, B. J., Trainor, R., Giedd, J., Vauss, Y., Vaituzis, C. K., Hamburger, S., et al. (1997). The role of the anterior cingulate in automatic and controlled processes: A developmental neuroanatomical study. *Developmental Psychobiology, 3*, 61–69.

Casey, B. J., Trainor, R. J., Orendi, J. L., Schubert, A. B., Nystrom, L. E., Giedd, J. N., et al. (1997). A developmental functional MRI study of prefrontal activation during performance of a go/no-go task. *Journal of Cognitive Neuroscience, 9*, 835–847.

Clohessy, A. B., Posner, M. I., & Rothbart, M. K. (2001). Development of the functional visual field. *Acta Psychologica, 106*, 51–68.

Colombo, J. (2001). The development of visual attention in infancy. *Annual Review of Psychology, 52*, 337–367.

Corbetta, M., & Shulman, G. L. (2002). Control of goal-directed and stimulus-driven attention in the brain. *Nature Neuroscience Reviews, 3*, 201–215.

Crottaz-Herbette, S., & Mennon, V. (2006). Where and when the anterior cingulate cortex modulates attentional response: Combined fMRI and ERP evidence. *Journal of Cognitive Neuroscience, 18, 766–780.*

Curran, T., & Keele, S. W. (1993). Attentional and non-attentional forms of sequence learning. *Journal of Experimental Psychology: Learning, Memory and Cognition, 19,* 189–202.

Dale, A. M., Liu, A. K., Fischi, B. R., Ruckner, R., Beliveau, J. W., Lewine, J. D., et al. (2000). Dynamic statistical parameter mapping: Combining fMRI and MEG for high resolution cortical activity. *Neuron, 26,* 55–67.

Davidson, R. J., Putnam, K. M., & Larson, C. L. (2000). Dysfunction in the neural circuitry of emotion regulation: A possible prelude to violence. *Science, 289,* 591–594.

Diamond, A. (1991). Neuropsychological insights into the meaning of object concept development. In S. Carey & R. Gelman (Eds.), *The epigenesis of mind: Essays on biology and cognition* (pp. 67–110). Hillsdale, NJ: Erlbaum.

Diamond, A., Barnett, S., Thomas, J., & Munro, S. (2007). Preschool improves cognitive control. *Science, 138,* 1387–1388.

Diamond, A., Briand, L., Fossella, J., & Gehlbach, L. (2004). Genetic and neurochemical modulation of prefrontal cognitive functions in children. *American Journal of Psychiatry, 161,* 125–132.

Diamond, A., & Taylor, C. (1996). Development of an aspect of executive control: Development of the abilities to remember what I said and "do as I say, not as I do." *Developmental Psychobiology, 29*(4), 315–334.

Diatchenko, L., Slade, G. D., Nackley, A. G., Bhalang, K., Sigurdsson, A., Belfer, I., et al. (2005). Genetic basis for individual variations in pain perception and the development of a chronic pain condition. *Human Molecular Genetics, 14*(1), 135–143.

Ding, Y. C., Chi, H. C., Grady, D. L., Morishima, A., Kidd, J. R., Kidd, K. K., et al. (2002). Evidence of positive selection acting at the human dopamine receptor D4 gene locus. *Proceedings of the National Academy of Sciences USA, 99*(1), 309–314.

Drevets, W. C., & Raichle, M. E. (1998). Reciprocal suppression of regional blood flow during emotional versus higher cognitive processes: Implications for interactions between emotion and cognition. *Cognition and Emotion, 12,* 285–353.

Driver, J., Eimer, M., van Velzen, J., & Macaluso, E. (2004). Neurobiology of human spatial attention: Modulation, generation, and integration. In N. Kanwisher & J. Duncan (Eds.), *Attention and performance XX: Functional brain imaging of visual cognition* (pp. 267–300). Oxford, UK: Oxford University Press.

Duncan, J., Seitz, R. J., Kolodny, J., Bor, D., Herzog, H., Ahmed, A., et al. (2000). A neural basis for general intelligence. *Science, 289,* 457–460.

Durston, S., & Casey, B. J. (2006). What have we learned about cognitive development from neuroimaging? *Neuropsychologia, 44,* 2149–2157.

Eriksen, B. A., & Eriksen, C. W. (1974). Effects of noise letters upon the identification of a target letter in a nonsearch task. *Perception and Psychophysics, 16,* 143–149.

Etkin, A., Egner, T., Peraza, D. M., Kandel, E. R., & Hirsch, J. (2006). Resolving emotional conflict: A role for the rostral anterior cingulate cortex in modulating activity in the amygdala. *Neuron, 51,* 871–882.

Fair, D. A., Cohen, A. L., Power, J. D., Dosenbach, N. U. F., Church, J. A., Meizin, F. M., et al. (2009). Functional brain networks develop from a "local to distributed" organization. *PLoS Computational Biology, 5/5,* e1000381.

Fan, J., Flombaum, J. I., McCandliss, B. D., Thomas, K. M., & Posner, M. I. (2002). Cognitive and brain mechanisms of conflict. *NeuroImage, 18,* 42–57.

Fan, J., Fossella, J. A., Summer, T., Wu, Y., & Posner, M. I. (2003). Mapping the genetic variation of executive attention onto brain activity. *Proceedings of the National Academy of Science USA, 100,* 7406–7411.

Fan, J., Gu, X., Guise, K. G., Liu, X., Fossella, J., Wang, H., et al. (2009). Testing the behavior interaction and integration of attentional networks. *Brain and Cognition, 70*, 209–220.

Fan, J., McCandliss, B. D., Sommer, T., Raz, M., & Posner, M. I. (2002). Testing the efficiency and independence of attentional networks. *Journal of Cognitive Neuroscience, 14*, 340–347.

Fan, J., Wu, Y., Fossella, J., & Posner, M. I. (2001). Assessing the heritability of attentional networks. *BioMed Central Neuroscience, 2*, 14.

Fonagy, P., & Target, M. (2002). Early intervention and the development of self-regulation. *Psychoanalytic Quarterly, 22*, 307–335.

Fossella, J., Posner, M. I., Fan, J., Swanson, J. M., & Pfaff, D. M. (2002). Attentional phenotypes for the analysis of higher mental function. *Scientific World Journal, 2*, 217–223.

Gao, W., Zhu, H., Giovanello, K. S., Smith, J. K., Shen, D., Gilmore, J. H., et al. (2009). Evidence on the emergence of the brain's default network from 2-week-old to 2-year-old healthy pediatric subjects. *Proceedings of the National Academy of Sciences USA, 106*, 6790–6795.

Gerardi-Caulton, G. (2000). Sensitivity to spatial conflict and the development of self-regulation in children 24–36 months of age. *Developmental Science, 3/4*, 397–404.

Green, A. E., Munafo, M. R., DeYoung, C. G., Fossella, J. A., Fan, J., & Grey, J. R. (2008). Using genetic data in cognitive neuroscience: From growing pains to genuine insights. *Nature Neuroscience Reviews, 9*, 710–719.

Haith, M. M., Hazan, C., & Goodman, G. S. (1988). Expectation and anticipation of dynamic visual events by 3.5 month-old babies. *Child Development, 59*, 467–479.

Harman, C., Rothbart, M. K., & Posner, M. I. (1997). Distress and attention interactions in early infancy. *Motivation and Emotion, 21*, 27–43.

Holroyd, C. B., & Coles, M. G. H. (2002). The neural basis of human error processing: Reinforcement learning, dopamine and the error related negativity. *Psychological Review, 109*, 679–709.

Hongwanishkul, D., Happaney, K. R., Lee, W. S., & Zelazo, P. D. (2005). Assessment of hot and cool executive function in young children: Age-related changes and individual differences. *Developmental Neuropsychology, 28*(2), 617–644.

Jonkman, L. M., Sniedt, F. L., & Kemner, C. (2007). Source localization of the Nogo-N2: A developmental study. *Clinical Neurophysiology, 118*(5), 1069–1077.

Klingberg, T., Forssberg, H., & Westerberg, H. (2002). Training of working memory in children with ADHD. *Journal of Clinical and Experimental Neuropsychology, 24*, 781–791.

Kopp, B., Rist, F., & Mattler, U. (1996). N200 in the flanker task as a neurobehavioral tool for investigating executive control. *Psychophysiology, 33*, 282–294.

MacDonald, A. W., Cohen, J. D., Stenger, V. A., & Carter, C. S. (2000). Dissociating the role of the dorsolateral prefrontal and anterior cingulate cortex in cognitive control. *Science, 288*, 1835–1838.

Ochsner, K. N., Bunge, S. A., Gross, J. J., & Gabrieli, J. D. E. (2002). Rethinking feelings: An fMRI study of the cognitive regulation of emotion. *Journal of Cognitive Neuroscience, 14*, 1215–1229.

Ochsner, K. N., Kossyln, S. M., Cosgrove, G. R., Cassem, E. H., Price, B. H., Nierenberg, A. A., et al. (2001). Deficits in visual cognition and attention following bilateral anterior cingulotomy. *Neuropsychologia, 39*, 219–230.

Posner, M. I., & Fan, J. (2008). Attention as an organ system. In J. Pomerantz (Ed.), *Neurobiology of perception and communication: From synapse to society: The 4th De Lange Conference* (pp. 31–61). Cambridge, UK: Cambridge University Press.

Posner, M. I., & Raichle, M. E. (1994). *Images of mind.* New York: Scientific American Books.

Posner, M. I., & Raichle, M. E. (Eds.). (1998). Overview: The neuroimaging of human brain function. *Proceedings of the National Academy of Sciences USA, 95*, 763–764.

Posner, M. I., & Rothbart, M. K. (1998). Attention, self-regulation and consciousness. *Philosophical Transactions of the Royal Society of London B, 353*, 1915–1927.

Posner, M. I., & Rothbart, M. K. (2000). Developing mechanisms of self-regulation. *Development and Psychopathology, 12*, 427–441.

Posner, M. I., & Rothbart, M. K. (2007). Research on attention networks as a model for the integration of psychological science. *Annual Review of Psychology, 58*, 1–23.

Posner, M. I., Rothbart, M. K., & Sheese, B. E. (2007). Attention genes. *Developmental Science, 10*, 24–29.

Posner, M. I., Sheese, B., Odludas, Y., & Tang, Y. (2006). Analyzing and shaping neural networks of attention. *Neural Networks, 19*, 1422–1429.

Rainville, P., Duncan, G. H., Price, D. D., Carrier, B., & Bushnell, M. C. (1997). Pain affect encoded in human anterior cingulated but not somatosensory cortex. *Science, 277*, 968–970.

Ridderinkhof, K. R., van der Molen, M. W., Band, P. H., & Bashore, T. R. (1997). Sources of interference from irrelevant information: A developmental study. *Journal of Experimental Child Psychology, 65*, 315–341.

Rothbart, M. K., & Bates, J. E. (1998). Temperament. In W. Damon (Series Ed.) & N. Eisenberg (Vol. Ed.), *Handbook of child psychology: Vol. 3. Social, emotional and personality development* (5th ed., pp. 105–176). New York: Wiley.

Rothbart, M. K., Ellis, L. K., Rueda, M. R., & Posner, M. I. (2003). Developing mechanisms of conflict resolution. *Journal of Personality, 71*, 1113–1143.

Rueda, M. R., Checa, P., & Santonja, M. (2008, April). *Training executive attention in preschoolers: Lasting effects and transfer to affective self-regulation.* Paper presented at the annual meeting of the Cognitive Neuroscience Society, San Francisco.

Rueda, M. R., Fan, J., McCandliss, B., Halparin, J. D., Gruber, D. B., Pappert, L., et al. (2004). Development of attentional networks in childhood. *Neuropsychologia, 42*, 1029–1040.

Rueda, M. R., Posner, M. I., Rothbart, M. K., & Davis-Stober, C. P. (2004). Development of the time course for processing conflict: An event-related potentials study with 4 year olds and adults. *BMC Neuroscience, 5*(39), 1–13.

Rueda, M. R., Rothbart, M. K., McCandliss, B. D., Saccomanno, L., & Posner, M. I. (2005). Training, maturation and genetic influences on the development of executive attention. *Proceedings of the National Academy of Sciences USA, 102*, 14931–14936.

Ruff, H. A., & Rothbart, M. K. (1996). *Attention in early development: Themes and variations.* New York: Oxford University Press.

Rumbaugh, D. M., & Washburn, D. A. (1995). Attention and memory in relation to learning: A comparative adaptation perspective. In G. R. Lyon & N. A. Krasenor (Eds.), *Attention, memory and executive function* (pp. 199–219). Baltimore: Brookes.

Sheese, B. E., Voelker, P. M., Rothbart, M. K., & Posner, M. I. (2007). Parenting quality interacts with genetic variation in dopamine receptor DRD4 to influence temperament in early childhood. *Development and Psychopathology, 19*, 1039–1046.

Simon, H. A. (1969). *The sciences of the artificial.* Cambridge, MA: MIT Press.

Sridharan, D., Levitin, D. J., & Menon, V. (2008). A critical role for the right fronto-insular cortex in switching between central-executive and default-mode networks. *Proceedings of the National Academy of Sciences USA, 105*(34), 12569–12574.

Thorndike, E. L. (1903). *Educational psychology.* New York: Teachers College Press.

Titchener, E. B. (1909). *Experimental psychology of the thought processes.* New York: Macmillan.

Turken, A. U., & Swick, D. (1999). Response selection in the human anterior cingulate cortex. *Nature Neuroscience, 2*(10), 920–924.

van Veen, V., & Carter, C. S. (2002). The timing of action-monitoring processes in the anterior cingulate cortex. *Journal of Cognitive Neuroscience, 14*(4), 593–602.

Venter, J. C., Adams, M. D., Myers, E. W., Li, P. W., Mural, R. J., Sutton, G. G., et al. (2001). The sequence of the human genome. *Science, 291*, 1304–1335.

Voelker, P., Sheese, B. E., Rothbart, M. K., & Posner, M. I. (2009). Variations in *COMT* gene interact with parenting to influence attention in early development. *Neuroscience, 164*, 121–130.

Welch, M. C. (2001). The prefrontal cortex and the development of executive function in childhood. In A. F. Kalverboer & A. Gramsbergen (Eds.), *Handbook of brain and behavior in human development* (pp. 767–790). Dordrecht, The Netherlands: Kluwer Academic.

Wright, R. D., & Ward, L. E. (2008). *Orienting of attention.* New York: Oxford University Press.

CHAPTER 16

A Bidirectional Model of Executive Functions and Self-Regulation

CLANCY BLAIR
ALEXANDRA URSACHE

E xecutive functions are cognitive abilities that are important for organizing informa- tion, for planning and problem solving, and for orchestrating thought and action in goal-directed behavior. As such they are aspects of psychological ability that assist the individual in self-regulation and self-control. As aspects of cognition that are important for rational thinking and planful behavior, however, executive functions are not synony- mous with self-regulation and self-control; that is, people do not always act rationally or purposefully when regulating behavior, and they may act rationally and with deliberation when experiencing a failure of self-regulation and a loss of self-control (Stanovich, 2009). Executive thinking skills can and often do facilitate self-regulation and self-control, but the relation of higher order, more effortful or deliberative aspects of self-regulation, such as executive functions, to lower order, more automatic aspects of self-regulation, such as the regulation of emotion, attention, and stress physiology, is somewhat unclear. Execu- tive functions can serve a critical higher-level or top-down role in behavior regulation and act as a primary mechanism of effortful self-regulation but are to some extent as much a consequence as a cause of reactivity and regulation in lower-order, more automatic emotion, attention, and stress response systems. Accordingly, this chapter describes a bidirectional developmental model in which brain areas that underlie executive functions reciprocally interact with brain areas associated with the control of attention, emotion, and stress physiology. Because relations among executive functions, emotion, attention, and stress physiology are bidirectional, or *cybernetic* (Luu & Tucker, 2004), meaning that they interact in an adaptive feedback loop in response to environmental cues, execu- tive function and self-regulation development are highly influenced by experience. In this, self-regulation development is understood as a process through which experience directs or canalizes development in ways that maximize the individual's potential to act advantageously in various contexts and circumstances.

DEFINING AND MEASURING EXECUTIVE FUNCTIONS

Stated simply, *executive functions* refer to aspects of cognition that are called on in situations when brain and behavior cannot run on automatic. More specifically, executive functions describe interrelated cognitive abilities that are required when one must intentionally or deliberately hold information in mind, manage and integrate information, and resolve conflict or competition between stimulus representations and response options. In this process of integration and control, it is generally agreed that executive functions include *working memory*, defined as the active maintenance or updating of information over a relatively short time period; *inhibitory control*, defined as the activation of specific information and inhibition of automatic but nonoptimal or incorrect responses; and cognitive flexibility or *attentional set–shifting* ability, defined as the ability to shift flexibly the focus of attention or cognitive set and to adjust behavior accordingly. In general, these aspects of cognition are important for planning, future-directed thinking, and monitoring of behavior; all of which are aspects of cognitive experience encompassed by definitions of executive functions.

The nature of executive functioning as integrated working memory, inhibitory control, and attentional set–shifting processes is seen in classic measures of the construct. For example, in the well-known Stroop color–word task, participants are presented with a word that names a color such as *red*. The word *red*, however, is written in a text color, such as green, that is incongruent with the color word. Participants first complete a series of trials in which they are asked to read the color name rather than name the color in which the word is written. This is relatively easy because reading simple color words is for fluent readers a highly automatic process. However, when the task is switched in a subsequent block of trials and participants must respond by naming the color of the text (in this example *green*) rather than reading the color word, the task becomes more difficult and requires executive functions because reading is a highly automatic process and the natural tendency to read the color word must be inhibited, and interference from the presence of the incongruent written word must be overcome when naming the color of text in which the color word is printed.

Another classic measure of executive function is the Wisconsin Card Sorting Task, in which participants are asked to sort cards by one of three possible dimensions—color, shape, or quantity, each of which is simultaneously represented on the cards. Having sorted by one dimension, say color, the participant is required to follow subtle cues from the examiner and to switch the relevant dimension being attended to and sort by one of the other two dimensions. For example, if first sorting by color, the participant is required to inhibit this previously relevant dimension and do what is referred to as *shift cognitive set* and no longer view the cards in terms of color but in terms of shape or quantity.

Yet another widely used measure of executive function is what is referred to as an *n*-back updating task, in which the individual is presented with a series of stimuli and asked to respond when the presented stimulus matches a stimulus presented either one, two, or three stimuli previously. For example, on a 2-back version of the task, the participant should respond when the present stimulus matches the stimulus presented two stimuli previously.

UNITY AND DIVERSITY OF EXECUTIVE FUNCTION

Given the presence of distinct working memory, inhibitory control, and attentional set–shifting components of executive function, researchers have been interested in the extent to which executive function is really a single integrated, unitary construct or whether it is better represented by its distinct component processes. Results from a number of experiments, including behavioral (Friedman et al., 2006; Miyake et al., 2000), neural imaging (Wager, Jonides, & Reading, 2004), and clinical neuropsychological research (Stuss et al., 2002), indicate that the components of executive function can be clearly differentiated. For example, the analysis of young adults completing simple tasks thought to capture the tripartite division of executive functions into attention-shifting, inhibitory control, and working memory components has indicated the presence of distinct yet correlated latent factors for each aspect of executive function. As well, tasks commonly used in the literature to measure executive functions, for example, the Wisconsin Card Sorting Task described earlier, or the Tower of Hanoi, a planning and sequencing task that requires participants to rearrange disks or balls among a set of pegs with a minimum number of moves, have been shown to involve one or more of the components of executive function (Miyake et al., 2000). Furthermore, from the standpoint of localization of function in the brain, clinical (Robbins, 1996; Stuss et al., 2002) and neural imaging research (Wager et al., 2004; Wager, Jonides, Smith, & Nichols, 2005) indicate common and unique regions of cerebral activity associated with the various component processes of executive function. Overwhelmingly, however, this research has indicated that brain regions associated with executive functions are centered in prefrontal cortex (PFC) and in associated posterior and subcortical limbic and brain stem regions highly interconnected with PFC.

EXECUTIVE FUNCTIONS AND HUMAN DEVELOPMENT

Generally speaking, the relation of executive function to self-regulation is seen in the idea that executive function abilities work as an integrated whole to organize complex information and regulate thought and action in goal-directed ways (Fuster, 2002). Such a role for executive functions is seen in the types of problems individuals have in regulating emotion and behavior in the instance of damage to PFC and related networks, and also in pathologies affecting the chemical and neural functions of PFC and related brain systems (Mayberg, 2002; Robbins & Arnsten, 2009). Deficits in executive functions are a primary aspect of cognitive impairment in a number of disorders and psychopathologies (Pennington & Ozonoff, 1996; Zelazo & Müller, 2002), and performance on executive function tasks is positively associated with various aspects of cognitive and social competence throughout the lifespan (Blair & Razza, 2007; Hughes & Ensor, 2007; West, 1996; Zelazo, Craik, & Booth, 2004).

Influential theories of PFC function and cognitive control emphasize the ways in which executive functions represent the integration and selective maintenance and coordination of information and actions (Mesulam, 2002; Miller & Cohen, 2001). For example, clinical studies indicate that individuals with damage to PFC have little difficulty representing specific information but are noticeably impaired on goal-directed tasks and on tasks in which an automatic or prepotent response must be inhibited, ambiguity resolved and salient distracters ignored, and in which contextual cues must be used to guide correct responding (Duncan, Burgess, & Emslie, 1995). This broad integrating and organizing role for executive functions in directing behavior is embodied in a number of theories addressing the neural basis for cognitive control, such as Miller and Cohen's (2001) integrative theory and Duncan's (2001) adaptive coding model. In both of these theories, PFC is understood to maintain goal representations and to orchestrate activity in multiple neural systems, particularly when well-established or habitual responding must be overridden to achieve the goal. In their broad form, however, research and theory on executive functions raise fundamental questions concerning the source of control and regulation of cognitive processes and the origin of intentionality or goal directedness. In the PFC's organizing role, there seems to be a need to postulate an organizing agent or homunculus that prioritizes information and directs cognitive control processes. Solving this homunculus problem requires determining how the brain selectively attends to and prioritizes information among multiple diverse sources of potentially conflicting information. Doing so also necessitates conclusions concerning the extent of free will and intentionality in human behavior.

More concretely, cognitive psychologists have focused their efforts on specific pieces of the executive function puzzle and have developed programs of research that emphasize one or more of the component processes of executive function. For example, the well-known working memory model of Alan Baddeley (2003) and collaborators (see Hofmann, Friese, Schmeichel, & Baddeley, Chapter 11, this volume) emphasizes the integrated nature of executive functions but has tended to focus more on the information maintenance aspect of working memory than on the executive control aspect of executive function. In contrast, Randal Engle, Michael Kane, and collaborators have tended to focus more on the control aspect and on the ability to maintain information in the focus of attention in tasks in which interference from competing information is high (e.g., Kane & Engle, 2002).

In the study of the development of executive function in early childhood, Adele Diamond has focused primarily on the inhibitory control aspect of executive function. She suggests that a first step in executive function development is the ability to inhibit responding to overcome what is termed *attentional inertia* (Kirkham, Cruess, & Diamond, 2003). In Diamond's theoretical approach, an inhibitory deficit is indicated when children at approximately age 3 years fail to shift cognitive set in the prototypical measure of executive function for children, the dimensional change card sorting task (Zelazo, 2006), an appropriate task for young children, modeled on the Wisconsin Card Sorting Task. Instead of three dimensions of the stimuli represented with multiple values per dimension and multiple shifts, the dimensional change card sorting task presents only two dimensions, two values per dimension and one shift. In the dimensional change card sorting task children are presented cards with pictures of a shape, for example, either a rabbit or a boat, and the rabbits and boats can be either red or blue. Children are instructed to attend to one of the dimensions and to sort the cards by that dimension ("We are going to play the shape game. In the shape game, rabbits go here and boats go here"). After correctly sorting by this dimension, children are then asked to switch and sort the cards by the second dimension ("Now we are going to play the color game. In the color game, blue ones go here and red ones go here"). Support for Diamond's inhibitory account of the failure to shift cognitive set in the task is found in data indicating that when the inhibitory demand of the task is reduced, as in versions of the task in which color and shape dimensions on the cards to be sorted are separated rather than integrated, the average age at which children are able to switch dimensions is reduced (A. Diamond, Carlson, & Beck, 2005; Kirkham et al., 2003; Kloo & Perner, 2005).

In contrast, Zelazo proposes that the primary cause of age-related change in executive function both early and late in the lifespan is the development and decline of the ability to reason or reflect on rules, and to generate and apply higher-order knowledge of conditional relations among sets of rules (Zelazo et al., 2004). As outlined in the revised version of the cognitive complexity and control theory (CCC-R), Zelazo, Müller, Frye, and Marcovitch (2003), emphasize an integrative approach that identifies a shift in the individual's ability to maintain a representation and to guide behavior based on that representation as essential to the emergence of executive functions. Young children lack the ability to reflect on lower-order rules, such as simple if–then statements, and this prevents them from embedding lower-order rules in higher-order rules that specify which lower-order rule to follow in a given context. The CCC-R theory suggests that reflection and higher-order rule formation enable processes of inhibition and redirection of attention; that is, once the child has a schema of higher-order rules, he or she is then able to inhibit responding and redirect attention to the context-appropriate rule. Conversely, in older age, as basic cognitive abilities that support hierarchical representation or rules and reflection on rule pairs declines, deficits in executive functions are increasingly apparent (Zelazo et al., 2004).

In the study of executive function in later adulthood, researchers have also emphasized both inhibitory control and working memory as sources of general decline in mental ability. For example, similar to Diamond's account, Dempster (1992) proposed that inhibitory deficits, primarily decreasing ability to resist interference from competing information and distraction, are central aspects of cognitive decline. In contrast, similar to Zelazo's account, West (1996) suggested that a more inclusive definition of executive functions, one that combines inhibition and resistance to distraction with information maintenance, provides a better description of the type of cognitive deficits experienced with aging that lead to executive function deficits. A number of studies have supported an executive function explanation of cognitive aging. For example, executive function is more strongly related to measures of fluid intelligence in the very old and the very young (Zook, Davalos, Delosh, & Davis, 2004). However, a number of studies have also demonstrated that changes in other underlying abilities, namely, speed of processing (Salthouse, 1996), are perhaps best able to explain changes in mental abilities with age.

EXECUTIVE FUNCTIONS AND SELF-REGULATION: A BIDIRECTIONAL THEORY

From the foregoing it is evident that research and theory support the idea that executive functions are aspects of cognition that can be key contributors to the self-regulation of behavior. As aspects of cognition that enable the organization of information, resistance to distraction, and planning and problem solving, executive functions are in one sense synonymous with self-regulation. When examining executive function abilities, however, it is clear that they are highly interrelated with and also dependent on activity in emotion, attention, and stress response systems. Accordingly, this chapter proceeds from a definition of *self-regulation* as the primarily, but not necessarily, volitional management of attention and arousal, including stress physiology and emotional arousal, for the purposes of goal-directed action. Within this definition of self-regulation, executive functions have been described in a number of theories as playing a top-down role in directing attention and organizing cognitive resources (Miller & Cohen, 2001), and in regulating emotion (Ochsner & Gross, 2005; see McRae, Ochsner, & Gross, Chapter 10, this volume). It is important to recognize, however, that from a bottom-up perspective, executive functions are also dependent on attention, emotion, and stress arousal (Blair & Dennis, 2009; Gray, 2004; Luu & Tucker, 2004); that is, in contexts that lead to particularly high or low levels of attentional focus and emotion and stress arousal, executive functions are impaired (Alexander, Hillier, Smith, Tivarus, & Beversdorf, 2007; Arnsten & Goldman-Rakic, 1998; Lupien, Gillin, & Hauger, 1999; Ramos & Arnsten, 2007). Although executive functions are primary mechanisms of self-regulation in a top-down framework, they are themselves dependent on the regulation of attention and emotion through bottom-up, nonexecutive processes. In other words, the relation between executive functions and the control of attention and emotion is bidirectional and operates in an interactive feedback loop.

The nature of executive function from both top-down and bottom-up perspectives is best seen within the framework of research on temperament (Derryberry & Rothbart, 1997; see Rothbart, Ellis, & Posner, Chapter 24, this volume). In this theory, *temperament* is defined by early emerging biologically based tendencies or predispositions to a given level of emotionality in infancy, both positive and negative, followed by development in infancy of alerting and orienting aspects of attention and somewhat later, during the toddler period, of the ability volitionally to control attention, referred to as *executive attention*. Executive attention, the aspect of attention that registers conflict between stimuli or between stimulus and response options, and is activated in response to error (Colombo, 2001; Posner & Rothbart, 2000). The developmental relation between level of emotionality and the effortful regulation of emotional reactivity, primarily through attention control, referred to as *effortful control*, defines temperament. Relations between emotionality and developing control of emotionality through attention have been demonstrated in a number of studies with young children (Gerardi-Caulton, 2000; Rothbart, Ellis, Rueda, & Posner, 2003; see Rueda, Posner, & Rothbart, Chapter 15, this volume). A child characterized by a high level of positive emotionality and approach behavior, and relatively low levels of effortful control is considered to have a temperament characterized by extraversion and surgency. In contrast, a child with a high level of fear emotionality and low approach and poor effortful control is said to have a temperament type characterized by high negative affectivity.

This theoretical model of temperament is based on the neurobiological interaction between cognition and emotion, and as such has some fairly direct implications for understanding executive functions. Specifically, the neural systems that underlie emotionality are primarily located in limbic and brain stem structures that rapidly register experience and nonconsciously or automatically activate stress physiology and motor, emotion, and attention response systems to deal with contingencies in the environment. These response systems are understood to vary between individuals in their resting level of activity and in the arousal threshold at which they are activated. A temperamentally anxious individual is thought to have a relatively high resting state and a relatively low threshold for activation in interrelated stress physiology, attention, emotion, and motor response systems (Kagan, 1994). The opposite is considered to be the case for a temperamentally calm individual. Components of stress physiology that are active in response to arousal include the sympathetic–adrenal–medullary system, which rapidly mobilizes visceral functions such as heart rate to deal with acute stress, and the limbic hypothalamic–pituitary–adrenal (HPA) axis component of the stress response, which controls levels of the glucocorticoid hormone cortisol that are important for longer term reactivity to threat or uncertainty (Gunnar & Quevedo, 2007).

In terms of attention, all three aspects of attention—alerting, orienting, and executive attention (Posner & Rothbart, 2007)—are activated automatically in response to environmental contingencies. Alerting and orienting responses are seen in the way attention is captured in emotionally arousing contexts, and in the narrowing and focusing of attention that occurs in response to highly arousing stimuli. Alerting and orienting away from an emotional stimulus are, of course, also important for regulating emotion. In highly emotionally arousing situations, however, it is very difficult to redirect attention, and any redirection of attention for the purpose of self-regulation in these contexts is primarily *exogenous*, which means that it is prompted by persons or events external to the individual rather than self-directed. In infancy and early childhood this is seen in the fact that distraction and reorienting are primary ways in which caregivers attempt to regulate emotion in infants and young children (Harman, Rothbart, & Posner, 1997; Stifter & Braungart, 1995).

Similar to alerting and orienting aspects of attention, executive attention can be engaged automatically by contingencies in the environment, namely, conflicting information and error. Like these first two aspects of attention, it can be directed intentionally to regulate emotion and behavior in response to conflicting information, primarily by calling on and engaging executive functions (Botvinick, Cohen, & Carter, 2004; Carter & van Veen, 2007). As such, executive attention ability is an important precursor for the development of executive functions and can first be measured effectively in the preschool period using tasks that induce cognitive conflict between stimuli and on which errors are more likely, such as flanker or Simon tasks. For example, in a flanker task, the participant is asked to indicate the direction in which a central stimulus, an arrow, or, for children, a smiling fish, is pointing. On certain trials for the task this central stimulus is congruent (facing the same direction) with the flanking stimuli, that is, those on either side of it, and on other trials the direction of the central stimulus is incongruent (facing the opposite direction) with the flanking stimuli. In a Simon-type task, stimulus and response locations are either congruent or incongruent, and responding on incongruent trials is slowed relative to responding on congruent trials; as with the Stroop color–word task, responding on flanker and Simon tasks is delayed and less accurate on incongruent than on congruent trials.

Brain imaging research has indicated that the registration of conflict associated with flanker and Simon tasks is associated with increased activity in the anterior segment of an area of the brain known as *cingulate cortex* (Bush, Lu, & Posner, 2000; Ridderinkhof, Ullsperger, Crone, & Nieuwenhuis, 2004). Furthermore, neural imaging has indicated that, having registered conflict, the anterior cingulate signals the PFC to activate executive functions (Kerns et al., 2004; MacDonald, Cohen, Stenger, & Carter, 2000). These relations between brain and behavior are of particular interest because the anterior cingulate cortex (ACC) links limbic areas of emotion processing with areas of PFC important for executive functions (Allman, Hakeem, Erwin, Nimchinsky, & Hof, 2001). The neuroanatomical association of executive attention with the ACC is consistent with the understanding of the role of attention in self-regulation. With the recognition of conflict, the ACC signals the PFC to initiate activity in dorsal and ventrolateral regions associated with executive functions. As such, the ACC and related regions of PFC form what is considered to be the primary neural substrate for executive functions (Miller & Cohen, 2001). When cognitive conflict cannot be resolved, however, or the information to be managed overwhelms the ability and resources of the individual, PFC activity is reduced (Callicott et al., 1999; Rypma, Prabhakaran, Desmond, Glover, & Gabrieli, 1999), and activity in regions of ACC and limbic structures can trigger a stress response and increase neuroendocrine hormone activity (Critchley, 2005), leading to increased emotional and stress arousal and to difficulty controlling attention and using executive functions.

Differentiating Executive Functions from Executive Attention

Relations among PFC, ACC, limbic structures, and stress physiology in the interaction of top-down and bottom-up processes of regulation form the basis for the bidirectional model of executive functions. Of particular interest in this model is the distinction between executive attention and executive functions. Although these are overlapping constructs, the bidirectional model considers executive attention, as with orienting and alerting aspects of attention, to be a relatively fast psychophysical phenomenon, and executive functions to be somewhat slower and more consciously effortful or deliberate; that is, executive attention is the attentional component of executive functions and as such is important for directing cognitive resources in situations that require the engagement of PFC to resolve conflict by holding information in working memory, inhibiting automatic responses, and shifting perspective or cognitive set as needed.

As a set of cognitive abilities that are important for resolving conflicting information and maintaining task focus and goal-directedness, executive function provides the mechanism whereby the individual's cognitive and motivational resources are directed to new and potentially confusing and disruptive information, and behavior is directed in ways that allow for purposeful engagement with the environment. Goal-directedness is a hallmark of theoretical models of executive functions, and in this respect executive functions are central aspects of a volitional, free will–based definition of self-regulation and self-control through which the autonomous individual directs thinking, feeling, and will as a purposeful agent in the world. Executive functions interact with the knowledge base and prior experience to guide behavior. Here executive functions are important contributors to reasoning ability and to the aspect of intelligence associated with reasoning ability, referred to as *fluid* as opposed to crystallized or knowledge-based intelligence (Blair, 2006). A number of studies have demonstrated that working memory, inhibitory control, and attentional set shifting factors that comprise executive function are uniquely related to measures of general intelligence (Friedman et al., 2006) and indicate that executive functions, working memory in particular, may serve as the basis for individual differences in intelligence (Carpenter, Just, & Shell, 1990; Gustafsson, 1984).

The Inverted U

From a bottom-up perspective, however, one in keeping with a developmental systems approach that emphasizes bidirectional relations among influences on behavior (Cairns, Elder, & Costello, 1996), executive functions, although essential to self-regulation, are just as appropriately characterized as dependent on rather than as determinants of self-regulation. This characterization of executive functions is based on the neurobiology of the cognition–emotion interaction described earlier, and on behavioral and neuroscience research demonstrating the ways in which emotional arousal affects attention and cognitive ability. It is well established that a high level of emotional arousal reduces the ability flexibly to control attention and impairs executive functions (Arnsten & Goldman-Rakic, 1998; Dennis & Chen, 2007; Lupien, Gillin, & Hauger, 1999). This relation, however, is only one instance of a general relation between emotion and cognition (Blair & Dennis, 2009). Just as emotional processes at very high levels can disrupt executive functions, emotion at moderate levels facilitates attention and executive functions. In this, the relation between emotion and cognition follows an inverted U-shape first described by Robert Yerkes and John Dodson (1908). The *Yerkes–Dodson principle* states that performance on a given cognitive task increases with arousal up to a given threshold, then decreases as arousal rises beyond the threshold level. This principle, however, applies specifically to complex aspects of cognition, such as executive functions. In their original and subsequent experiments, Yerkes and Dodson demonstrated that the inverted U-shape relation between arousal and performance is specific to complex learning tasks, such as those involving executive functions. For relatively simple and reactive forms of cognition and behavior, such as fear conditioning, attention narrowing, and traumatic or emotional memory formation, the relation between arousal and performance is linear and positive (D. M. Diamond, Campbell, Park, Halonen, & Zoladz, 2007).

The specific relation of the Yerkes–Dodson principle to complex cognition is seen in the neurobiology of emotion–cognition interactions that underlie executive functions. Experiments with animal models demonstrate that neural activity in PFC in the neural substrate for executive functions is dependent to some extent on relative levels of stress hormones and related neuromodulators that originate in limbic and brain stem areas. For example, at a very low level of arousal, levels of neuromodulators, including norepinephrine, dopamine, and glucocorticoids, are low and synaptic activity in PFC is limited. As levels of these neurochemicals rise, however, activity in the neural substrate for PFC increases as specific neural receptors become occupied (Arnsten & Li, 2005; Robbins & Arnsten, 2009). With increase beyond a moderate level, however, receptors become saturated, and neural activity in PFC begins to decrease. Conversely, as levels of neuromodulators continue to rise and activity in PFC decreases, activity in posterior brain areas associated with reactive responses to stimulation and long-term memory formation of emotionally arousing events increases (Arnsten, 2000; D. M. Diamond et al., 2007). In this way the inverted U-shaped relation between arousal and performance first describe by Yerkes and Dodson (1908) at the behavioral level is mirrored in neural activity at the biological level.

THE DEVELOPMENT OF EXECUTIVE FUNCTIONS

Characterization of executive functions as an aspect of self-regulation important for but also dependent on the regulation of emotion and attention provides a framework for understanding influences on the development of executive function abilities. Couched in the neurobiology of emotion–cognition interaction, executive function ability is a manifestation of a cooperative relation between bottom-up and top-down influences. From a developmental standpoint, it has been known for some time that the single best predictor in infancy of later cognitive competence is a measure of attention that is dependent on alerting and orienting responses known as habituation–dishabituation. *Habituation* is defined as a decrement in attention to a repeatedly or continuously presented stimulus, while *dishabituation* is defined as the reactivation of attention to a novel stimulus following habituation. The relative efficiency with which infants habituate to a repeatedly presented stimulus and then dishabituate to a novel stimulus has been demonstrated in a number of studies to be a robust correlate of later IQ. Examinations of habituation–dishabituation between the ages of 6 and 12 months to IQ measured between 2 and 8 years later have yielded correlations ranging from .25 to .61 (Kavsek, 2004). Remarkably, one study examining relations between habituation and dishabituation in infancy, and receptive verbal ability and academic achievement 21 years later obtained correlations of .34 and .32 that, when corrected for unreliability in the outcome measures, increased to .59 and .53.

Given a close relation between executive functions and attention and between executive functions, particularly working memory, and general mental ability (Kane, Hambrick, & Conway, 2005) it is likely that executive functions are an important mediator of the relation between attention in infancy and later general cognitive competence. No studies have as yet examined this possibility directly. Available studies of temperament linking the early development of alerting and orienting aspects of attention with emotionality and the development of executive attention (Rothbart et al., 2003) suggest that individual differences in habituation–dishabituation would be a significant indicator of executive function development. The few studies using neural imaging methods appropriate for infants and children have demonstrated that habituation–dishabituation behavior is associated with neural activity in PFC. Although PFC is relatively slow to develop, it is, of course, active in novelty detection in infancy as seen in the use of using near infrared spectroscopy to measure a relative increase in the ratio of oxygenated to deoxygenated hemoglobin in frontal cortex in 3-month-old infants in response to a habituation–dishabituation procedure (Nakano, Watanabe, Homae, & Taga, 2009). Functional neuroimaging of attention to unattended novel events in adults has also indicated activation in specific regions of PFC and hippocampus, demonstrating the role of prefrontal–limbic neural circuitry in novelty detection (Yamaguchi, Hale, D'Esposito, & Knight, 2004).

In theory, given ongoing development of PFC throughout childhood into the young adult years (Toga, Thompson, & Sowell, 2006), the variety of influences on infant attention, emotion, and stress physiology, primarily those associated with early rearing experience and the conditions of the home environment, are likely to influence the development of neural networks that underlie executive function development and thereby the development of self-regulation (Blair, in press). In particular, available evidence indicates that adverse rearing environments, such as those overrepresented in poverty, detrimentally affect cognitive development through processes involving attention, emotion, and stress physiology. For example, in a longitudinal study that my colleagues and I are conducting with children and families living in predominantly low-income and nonurban communities in two geographically distinct regions of the United States, we demonstrated that the conditions of poverty, including low income and low maternal education, and most importantly, low levels of prototypically sensitive and responsive maternal caregiving behavior are associated with elevated stress physiology in infancy, as indicated by infants' stress hormone cortisol at 7, 15, and 24 months of age (Blair et al., 2008, in press). Furthermore, we found that environmental effects of poverty on stress physiology, as measured by cortisol levels, represents a mediating path through which the environment affects executive function ability at age 3 years (Blair et al., in press). Remarkably, in this study, which contained African American as well as white participants, cortisol was elevated in African American children even when we controlled for family characteristics and parenting behavior, and elevated cortisol, along with maternal caregiving and conditions of poverty, fully explained observed associations between African American ethnicity and low executive function and IQ. Given that African American participants in this sample, as in the United States generally, are considerably worse off than whites due to conditions of poverty (true for every variable we examined, including income, maternal education, household crowding, and neighborhood safety), it is likely that African American ethnicity in this sample represents a marker of deep and persistent poverty. As such, results suggest that noted racial gaps in cognitive ability and school achievement in the United States reflect, in addition to well-documented inequalities in educational opportunity, the adverse effects of poverty on stress physiology, with cascading effects on self-regulation and executive functions.

Although this is the first study of its kind to examine associations among the conditions of poverty, stress physiology, and executive functions in early childhood, our findings are consistent with prior studies examining relations among poverty and stress physiology (Evans, 2003) and poverty and executive functions (Noble, McCandliss, & Farah, 2007). For example, in a longitudinal sample of children seen at ages 9 and 13 years, increased cumulative risk in the home, including both physical and psychosocial characteristics of the home environment, were associated with elevated stress physiology. However, the association between cumulative risk and elevated stress physiology was observed only among children whose mothers were observed to have low levels of responsive involvement with children, suggesting that a close and caring relationship can buffer the effects of environmental risk on stress physiology (Evans, Kim, Ting, Tesher, & Shannis, 2007). As well, in a further follow-up of the sample at age 17 years, the working memory aspect of executive function was significantly lower for participants with both a greater number of childhood years in poverty and elevated stress physiology. Furthermore, when covaried, stress physiology was shown to account for the relation between years spent in poverty and working memory deficits (Evans & Schamberg, 2009); that is, as with our findings relating stress physiology to executive function development in early childhood, the effect of poverty on executive function in adolescence in the study by Evans and Schamberg was found to a considerable extent to be attributable to the effect of poverty on stress physiology.

Data demonstrating relations among early experience, activity in stress response systems, and the development of executive functions are of strong interest given evidence of neurobiological mechanisms through which these relations occur. As noted earlier, activity in the neural substrate for executive functions is influenced by levels of stress hormones. Furthermore, the role of early experience in the development of stress physiology that is important for executive functions is consistent with a well-described model in rats, demonstrating that the behavior of the rat mother essentially programs the development of the HPA component of the stress response (Meaney, 2001). In rat mothers, high levels of licking and grooming, and a style referred to as arched back nursing during the first postnatal week, have been shown to affect the expression of a gene that codes for the density of glucocorticoid receptors in the hippocampus. Rats born to mothers with high levels of licking and grooming and arched back nursing have a greater density of glucocorticoid receptors in the hippocampus, a major structure in the regulation of glucocorticoid levels, and are therefore better able to regulate stress physiology. In contrast, offspring of mothers with lower levels of licking and grooming and arched back nursing have lower levels of glucocorticoid receptors in the hippocampus, are more reactive and less well-regulated physiologically, and more anxious and fearful behaviorally (Caldji et al., 1998; Liu et al., 1997). Furthermore, offspring of low licking and grooming and arched back nursing mothers perform less well on cognitive tasks, such as complex learning and memory tasks (Liu, Diorio, Day, Frances, & Meaney, 2000). However, consistent with the Yerkes–Dodson principle outlined earlier, offspring of low licking and grooming and arched back nursing mothers are more reactive to stimulation in the environment and exhibit faster fear conditioning (Champagne et al., 2008).

The extent to which the model of development in rats generalizes to humans or to nonhuman primates (Parker, Buckmaster, Justus, Schatzberg, & Lyons, 2005) is not currently known. It is likely, however, that this research reflects a general model describing the way in which early experience shapes or programs the developing organism to meet an expected environment. In such a biological sensitivity to context model (Boyce & Ellis, 2005), stress reactivity is understood to shape processes of self-regulation to optimize the functioning of the individual within that environment. Specifically, physiological reactivity to stress is thought to be increased in both advantaged and disadvantaged environments. In advantaged environments, in which resources and support are high and predictable, this increase is conducive to the development of effortful self-regulation, such as that associated with executive functions, because stress physiology tends to be well regulated in advantaged environments. Physiologically speaking, in response to stimulation provided through sensitive and responsive caregiving, levels of stress hormones increase to ranges that are conducive to synaptic activity in PFC associated with executive functions. As well, increases in stress hormone levels in supportive environments are sufficiently well regulated so as not to rise above a threshold range and lead to decreased activity in PFC and increased activity in posterior regions and subcortical regions associated with reactive responses to stimulation. In contrast, disadvantaged environments, primarily in the context of poverty, as described earlier, are more likely to be over- or understimulating (McLoyd, 1998). Environments that are excessively or unpredictably over- or understimulating are likely to lead to particularly high or low and not well-regulated levels of stress hormones and are therefore associated with reduced neural activity in PFC and poor executive function. Furthermore, in the higher-risk environment, caregiver support for the regulation of physiological reactivity is frequently low due to stress on caregivers and general conditions of the home environment that interfere with sensitive and responsive caregiving.

Although speculative to some extent, the biological sensitivity model is based upon clear evidence concerning the relation of experience to the development of stress physiology and that of stress physiology to emotion and cognition. It is known that the stress response is under strong social control in early childhood (Gunnar & Donzella, 2002), and that social relationships and the controllability of events are primary influences on reactivity and regulation in stress response systems (Dickerson & Kemeny, 2004). To this end, the theoretical model linking early attention, emotion, and stress physiology as precursors of executive functions and the development of the effective self-regulation of behavior suggests a plausible mechanism of effects through which poverty "gets under the skin" to affect development at multiple levels of influence. To this end, the biological sensitivity to context model provides a comprehensive explanation for the efficacy of early intervention programs for children from high-risk backgrounds. Longitudinal follow-up of several programs modeled on responsive educational caregiving for infants and children from high-risk backgrounds has demonstrated sustained effects on cognitive ability and positive life outcomes. For example, several longitudinal intervention projects, providing early educational care to high-risk samples of infants and preschoolers, such as the Abecedarian Experiment (Ramey & Campbell, 1991) and the Perry Preschool Study (Schweinhart et al., 2005), have produced long-term effects into adulthood on a number outcomes associated with self-regulation and self-control, such as greater job and marital stability, and reduced rates of arrest and incarceration (Reynolds & Temple, 2006). Longer-term results from these programs may be attributable to program effects on self-regulation given that program effects on IQ, an outcome of early interest, tended to fade shortly after the intervention phase of the programs ended in early childhood (Campbell, Pungello, Miller-Johnson, Burchinal, & Ramey, 2001; Heckman, Malofeeva, Pinto, & Savelyev, 2009). A self-regulation hypothesis for long-term effects of early intervention is consistent with the model of self-regulation development outlined here and with current thinking about best approaches to maximizing human development potential (Heckman, 2006, 2007).

CONCLUSION AND FUTURE DIRECTIONS

In this chapter we have presented a model in which executive functions are seen to be both top-down mechanisms of self-regulation and aspects of cognitive ability that themselves are dependent on bottom-up processes associated with the regulation of emotion, attention, and stress physiology. In applying the bidirectional developmental science approach to executive functions, we have described these cognitive abilities as emerging from early developing processes of emotionality and attention that are the primary constituents of temperament. From this model of temperament, the chapter has examined executive functions from the perspective of biological sensitivity to context. The biological sensitivity theory is based upon studies demonstrating that early experience essentially primes or programs the physiological response to stress in order to promote the expression of behaviors that are likely to be adaptive and advantageous within the expected environment. In environments that are high in social and economic resources, and appropriately stimulating and supportive, attention, emotion, and stress physiology develop in ways that promote executive function abilities and higher-order self-regulation. In contrast, in low-resource, less predictable environments, attention, emotion, and stress physiology are more reactive and less conducive to executive function abilities. The application of the biological sensitivity model to executive functions is based in the neurobiology of PFC circuitry and considers how stress physiology may promote or limit the development of executive functions in the service of self-regulation in specific contexts (Blair, 2010).

Given the applicability of a biological sensitivity to context model to self-regulation and the development of executive functions, at least three directions for future research are indicated. The first concerns the application of the model to education and to the promotion of human development potential. Self-regulation, including the regulation of attention, emotion, and stress physiology, is a primary influence on educational achievement. Numerous studies with preschool and early school-age children have indicated that executive functions are robust predictors of academic achievement above and beyond measured intelligence (Blair & Razza, 2007; McClelland et al., 2007; Normandeau & Guay, 1998; Palisin, 1986) and provide support for the general theoretical model in which self-regulation is understood to be the basis for school readiness (Blair, 2002). Similarly, in older children, investigators have employed a social cognitive approach (Dweck & Leggett, 1988) to examine aspects of self-regulation relating to self-perceptions (Skinner, Zimmer-Gembeck, & Connell, 1998), self-attributions (Eccles & Wigfield, 2002), self-discipline (Duckworth & Seligman, 2005), and motivational orientations (Elliott & Dweck, 1988) that are conducive to engagement and persistence in academic learning tasks (Dweck, 1999). Future work on self-regulation and academic achievement could profitably examine bidirectional relations among executive functions and attention, emotion, and stress physiology, and consider the extent to which particular types of experiences and educational curricula, from the perspective of the Yerkes–Dodson principle, lead to optimal levels of arousal and engagement.

In the process of promoting self-regulation to improve educational outcomes, however, it appears that it is important to start early, in the preschool and early elementary grades. As noted earlier, longitudinal follow-ups of well-known early intervention programs have demonstrated long-term effects of preschool intervention on educational achievement and on numerous life outcomes that appear to be due to program benefits to self-regulation. An important future direction for evaluations of similar types of readiness programs, such as the Tools of the Mind program (Bodrova & Leong, 2007), an early educational curriculum that focuses specifically on self-regulation development, is to include measures of attention, emotion, and stress physiology, as well as executive functions, in randomized designs and to link these measures to specific program activities and to measures of neural activity that underlie executive functions and self-regulation. Such research can help to confirm and clearly establish the efficacy of these programs in fostering self-regulation and promoting positive outcomes.

A second direction for future research concerns the applicability of the bidirectional model of executive functions to research and theory indicating that self-regulation is a limited resource (Baumeister, Vohs, & Tice, 2007; Schmeichel & Baumeister, 2004). The limited resource model suggests that failures of self-regulation result from a depletion of as yet unspecified self-regulatory resources (see Bauer & Baumeister, Chapter 4, this volume). As well, the limited resource model identifies executive functions as central to self-regulation ability and as being particularly vulnerable to resource depletion. Data in support of the limited resource model are consistent with the bidirectional model of executive functions. The bidirectional model suggests that the depletion of regulatory ability is a function of the relation of stress physiology to neural activity in PFC circuits that support executive functions. With repeated regulatory challenges, the activation of attention, emotion, and stress physiology in response to those challenges rise to levels that are not conducive to executive functions. In terms of the Yerkes–Dodson principle, self-regulation in the limited resource model is a complex cognitive ability and, as such, is most easily accomplished when arousal is in an optimal range. When arousal is outside of this optimal range, whether at the low or high end of the inverted U-shaped curve, self-regulatory attempts are more likely to meet with failure. Although the limited resource model generally refers to self-regulatory strength and to self-regulation capacity as muscle, it may be that an analogy to an engine in which stress hormones are more or less literally the fuel that powers the engine may be equally apt.

A third, somewhat more mundane but essential direction for future research concerns ongoing advances in the measurement of executive functions. Research and theory have been increasingly clear in the definition and measurement of executive functions (Garon, Bryson, & Smith, 2008; Miyake et al., 2000; Zelazo et al., 2003), and the differentiation of executive functions from other aspects of cognitive ability, particularly general intelligence (Blair, 2006). The measures available to researchers interested in executive functions, however, have for the most part been adapted from clinical neuropsychology and were originally designed to identify failures of executive functions in the instance of damage to specific brain areas. Although this tradition has been invaluable in identifying the types of tasks that elicit executive functions, the focus in neuropsychological research on the presence or absence of executive ability, rather than the demarcation of a continuum of ability, renders these tasks less suitable for developmental use, particularly the study of intraindividual change. Currently, a number of available tasks are effective in measuring executive function ability in early childhood (A. Diamond & Taylor, 1996; Zelazo, 2006). Until recently, however, none have been available that are suitable for longitudinal use. Accordingly, we developed a task battery for use with children in the 3- to 6-year-old age range and are evaluating its psychometric properties (Willoughby, Blair, Wirth, Greenberg, and the Family Life Project Investigators, in press) and change over time in ability. Similarly, an adaptation of the dimensional card sorting task by Carlson, Beck, and Pang (2009) that decreases difficulty for young children (2.5 to 3 years) by separating the dimensions on the cards to be sorted, and increases difficulty for older children (6 to 7 years) by adding an indicator on the cards that determines the relevant sorting dimension, is being developed for longitudinal use.

In conclusion, ongoing examination of executive function development longitudinally in relation to measures of attention, emotion, and stress physiology will help to validate the construct and begin to provide data on the normative developmental course of executive functions and their role in self-regulation development in childhood. Further research, including improved measures, will help to clarify the relation of developmental trajectories of executive function abilities to the self-regulation of behavior and attention, and to salient indicators of success in life, such as school achievement, prosocial behavior, and relative stability in friendships, jobs, and romantic relationships. Although there remains a great deal to be learned, this chapter has outlined ways in which biology and experience are intertwined in executive function development, and how executive functions both regulate and are regulated by responses to the environment. While top-down processes of executive function are a mechanism of self-regulation, bottom-up processes of emotion, attention, and the stress response affect executive function ability, such that the relation of executive functions to self-regulation generally is best characterized as bidirectional.

ACKNOWLEDGMENTS

This work was supported by the National Institute of Child Health and Human Development (Grant No. P01 HD39667), with cofunding from the National Institute on Drug Abuse (Grant No. R01 HD51502).

REFERENCES

Alexander, J. K., Hillier, A., Smith, R. M., Tivarus, M. E., & Beversdorf, D. Q. (2007). Beta-adrenergic modulation of cognitive flexibility during stress. *Journal of Cognitive Neuroscience, 19*, 468–478.

Allman, J. M., Hakeem, A., Erwin, J. M., Nimchinsky, E., & Hof, P. (2001). The anterior cingulate cortex: The evolution of an interface between emotion and cognition. *Annals of the New York Academy of Sciences, 935*, 107–117.

Arnsten, A. F. (2000). Through the looking glass: Differential noradenergic modulation of prefrontal cortical function. *Neural Plasticity, 7*, 133–146.

Arnsten, A. F., & Goldman-Rakic, P. S. (1998). Noise stress impairs prefrontal cortical cognitive function in monkeys: Evidence for a hyperdopaminergic mechanism. *Archives of General Psychiatry, 55*(4), 362–368.

Arnsten, A. F., & Li, B. M. (2005). Neurobiology of executive functions: Catecholamine influences on prefrontal cortical functions. *Biological Psychiatry, 57*(11), 1377–1384.

Baddeley, A. (2003). Working memory: Looking back and looking forward. *Nature Reviews Neuroscience, 4*(10), 829–839.

Baumeister, R. F., Vohs, K. D., & Tice, D. M. (2007). The strength model of self-control. *Current Directions in Psychological Science, 16*, 351–355.

Blair, C. (2002). School readiness: Integrating cognition and emotion in a neurobiological conceptualization of children's functioning at school entry. *American Psychologist, 57*(2), 111–127.

Blair, C. (2006). How similar are fluid cognition and general intelligence?: A developmental neuroscience perspective on fluid cognition as an aspect of human cognitive ability. *Behavioral and Brain Sciences, 29*(2), 109–160.

Blair, C. (in press). Stress and the development of self-regulation in context. *Child Development Perspectives.*

Blair, C., & Dennis, T. (2009). An optimal balance: Emotion–cognition integration in context. In S. Calkins & M. Bell (Eds.), *Child development at the intersection of cognition and emotion* (pp. 17–36). Washington DC: American Psychological Association.

Blair, C., Granger, D. A., Kivlighan, K. T., Mills-Koonce, R., Willoughby, M., Greenberg, M. T., et al. (2008). Maternal and child contributions to cortisol response to emotional arousal in young children from low-income, rural communities. *Developmental Psychology, 44*, 1095–1109.

Blair, C., Granger, D., Willoughby, M., Mills-Koonce, R., Cox, M., Greenberg, M. T., et al. (in press). Salivary cortisol mediates effects of poverty and parenting on executive functions in early childhood. *Child Development.*

Blair, C., & Razza, R. P. (2007). Relating effortful control, executive function, and false belief understanding to emerging math and literacy ability in kindergarten. *Child Development, 78*(2), 647–663.

Bodrova, E., & Leong, D. J. (2007). *Tools of the Mind: The Vygotskian approach to early childhood education* (2nd ed.). Upper Saddle River, NJ: Pearson.

Botvinick, M. M., Cohen, J. D., & Carter, C. S. (2004). Conflict monitoring and anterior cingulate cortex: An update. *Trends in Cognitive Sciences, 8*(12), 539–546.

Boyce, W. T., & Ellis, B. J. (2005). Biological sensitivity to context: I. An evolutionary-developmental theory of the origins and functions of stress reactivity. *Development and Psychopathology, 17*(2), 271–301.

Bush, G., Luu, P., & Posner, M. I. (2000). Cognitive and emotional influences in anterior cingulate cortex. *Trends in Cognitive Sciences, 4*(6), 215–222.

Cairns, R. B., Elder, G. H., & Costello, E. J. (Eds.). (1996). *Developmental science.* New York: Cambridge University Press.

Caldji, C., Tannenbaum, B., Sharma, S., Francis, D., Plotsky, P. M., & Meaney, M. J. (1998). Maternal care during infancy regulates the development of neural systems mediating the expression of fearfulness in the rat. *Proceedings of the National Academy of Sciences USA, 95*(9), 5335–5340.

Callicott, J. H., Mattay, V. S., Bertolino, A., Finn, K., Coppola, R., Frank, J. A., et al. (1999). Physiological characteristics of capacity constraints in working memory as revealed by functional MRI. *Cerebral Cortex, 9*(1), 20–26.

Campbell, F. A., Pungello, E. P., Miller-Johnson, S., Burchinal, M., & Ramey, C. T. (2001). The development of cognitive and academic abilities: Growth curves from an early childhood educational experiment. *Developmental Psychology, 37*, 231–242.

Carlson, S. M., Beck, D. M., & Pang, K. C. (2009, April). *Measurement of executive function in preschoolers: Component processes.* Poster presented at the biennial meeting of the Society for Research in Child Development, Denver, CO.

Carpenter, P. A., Just, M. A., & Shell, P. (1990). What one intelligence test measures: A theoretical account of the processing in the raven progressive matrices test. *Psychological Review, 97*(3), 404–431.

Carter, C. S., & van Veen, V. (2007). Anterior cingulate cortex and conflict detection: An update of theory and data. *Cognitive, Affective, and Behavioral Neuroscience, 7*(4), 367–379.

Champagne, D. L., Bagot, R. C., van Hasselt, F., Ramakers, G., Meaney, M. J., de Kloet, E. R., et al. (2008). Maternal care and hippocampal plasticity: Evidence for experience-dependent structural plasticity, altered synaptic functioning, and differential responsiveness to glucocorticoids and stress. *Journal of Neuroscience, 28*(23), 6037–6045.

Colombo, J. (2001). The development of visual attention in infancy. *Annual Review of Psychology, 52*, 337–367.

Critchley, H. D. (2005). Neural mechanisms of autonomic, affective, and cognitive integration. *Journal of Comparative Neurology, 493*(1), 154–166.

Dempster, F. N. (1992). The rise and fall of the inhibitory mechanism: Toward a unified theory of cognitive development and aging. *Developmental Review, 12*(1), 45–75.

Dennis, T. A., & Chen, C. C. (2007). Neurophysiological mechanisms in the emotional modulation of attention: The interplay between threat sensitivity and attentional control. *Biological Psychology, 76*(1–2), 1–10.

Derryberry, D., & Rothbart, M. (1997). Reactive and effortful processes in the organization of temperament. *Development and Psychopathology, 9*, 633–652.

Diamond, A., Carlson, S. M., & Beck, D. M. (2005). Preschool children's performance in task switching on the dimensional change card sort task: Separating the dimensions aids the ability to switch. *Developmental Neuropsychology, 28*(2), 689–729.

Diamond, A., & Taylor, C. (1996). Development of an aspect of executive control: Development of the abilities to remember what I said and to "do as I say, not as I do." *Developmental Psychobiology, 29*, 315–334.

Diamond, D. M., Campbell, A. M., Park, C. R., Halonen, J., & Zoladz, P. R. (2007). The temporal dynamics model of emotional memory processing: A synthesis on the neurobiological basis of stress-induced amnesia, flashbulb and traumatic memories, and the Yerkes–Dodson law. *Neural Plasticity, 2007*, 60803.

Dickerson, S. S., & Kemeny, M. E. (2004). Acute stressors and cortisol responses: A theoretical integration and synthesis of laboratory research. *Psychological Bulletin, 130*(3), 355–391.

Duckworth, A. L., & Seligman, M. E. (2005). Self-discipline outdoes IQ in predicting academic performance of adolescents. *Psychological Science, 16*(12), 939–944.

Duncan, J. (2001). An adaptive coding model of neural function in prefrontal cortex. *Nature Reviews Neuroscience, 2*(11), 820–829.

Duncan, J., Burgess, P., & Emslie, H. (1995). Fluid intelligence after frontal lobe lesions. *Neuropsychologia, 33*(3), 261–268.

Dweck, C. S. (1999). *Self-theories: Their role in motivation, personality, and development.* Ann Arbor, MI: Psychology Press/Taylor & Francis Group.

Dweck, C. S., & Leggett, E. L. (1988). A social-cognitive approach to motivation and personality. *Psychological Review, 95*(2), 256–273.

Eccles, J. S., & Wigfield, A. (2002). Motivational beliexecutive functions, values, and goals. *Annual Review of Psychology, 53*, 109–132.

Elliott, E. S., & Dweck, C. S. (1988). Goals: An approach to motivation and achievement. *Journal of Personality and Social Psychology, 54*(1), 5–12.

Evans, G. W. (2003). A multimethodological analysis of cumulative risk and allostatic load among rural children. *Developmental Psychology, 39*(5), 924–933.

Evans, G.W., Kim, P., Ting, A., Tesher, H., & Shannis, D. (2007). Cumulative risk, maternal responsiveness, and allostatic load among young adolescents. *Developmental Psychology, 43*, 341–351.

Evans, G. W., & Schamberg, M. A. (2009). Childhood poverty, chronic stress, and adult working memory. *Proceedings of the National Academy of Sciences USA, 106*(16), 6545–6549.

Friedman, N. P., Miyake, A., Corley, R. P., Young, S. E., DeFries, J. C., & Hewitt, J. K. (2006). Not all executive functions are related to intelligence. *Psychological Science, 17*(2), 172–179.

Fuster, J. M. (2002). Physiology of executive functions: The perception–action cycle. In D. T. Stuss & R. T. Knight (Eds.), *Principles of frontal lobe function* (pp. 96–108). Oxford, UK: Oxford University Press.

Garon, N., Bryson, S. E., & Smith, I. M. (2008). Executive function in preschoolers: A review using an integrative framework. *Psychological Bulletin, 134*, 31–60.

Gerardi-Caulton, G. (2000). Sensitivity to spatial conflict and the development of self-regulation in children 24–36 months of age. *Developmental Science, 3*(4), 397–404.

Gray, J. R. (2004). Integration of emotion and cognitive control. *Current Directions in Psychological Science, 13*, 46–48.

Gunnar, M., & Quevedo, K. (2007). The neurobiology of stress and development. *Annual Review of Psychology, 58*, 145–173.

Gunnar, M. R., & Donzella, B. (2002). Social regulation of the cortisol levels in early human development. *Psychoneuroendocrinology, 27*(1–2), 199–220.

Gustafsson, J. (1984). A unifying model for the structure of intellectual abilities. *Intelligence, 8*(3), 179–203.

Harman, C., Rothbart, M. K., & & Posner, M. I. (1997). Distress and attention interactions in early infancy. *Motivation and Emotion, 21*, 27–43.

Heckman, J. (2006). Skill formation and the economics of investing in disadvantaged children. *Science, 312*, 1900–1902.

Heckman, J. (2007). The economics, technology, and neuroscience of human capability formation. *Proceedings of the National Academy of Sciences USA, 104*, 13250–13255.

Heckman, J., Malofeeva, L., Pinto, R., & Savelyev, P. (2009, April). *The powerful role of noncognitive skills in explaining the effects of the Perry Preschool Program.* Paper presented at the biennial meeting of the Society for Research in Child Development, Denver, CO.

Hughes, C., & Ensor, R. (2007). Executive function and theory of mind: Predictive relations from ages 2 to 4. *Developmental Psychology, 43*(6), 1447–1459.

Kagan, J. (1994). On the nature of emotion. *Monographs of the Society for Research in Child Development, 59*(2–3), 7–24.

Kane, M. J., & Engle, R. W. (2002). The role of prefrontal cortex in working-memory capacity, executive attention, and general fluid intelligence: An individual-differences perspective. *Psychonomic Bulletin and Review, 9*(4), 637–671.

Kane, M. J., Hambrick, D. Z., & Conway, A. R. A. (2005). Working memory capacity and fluid intelligence are strongly related constructs: Comment on Ackerman, Beier, and Boyle (2005). *Psychological Bulletin, 131*(1), 66–71.

Kavsek, M. (2004). Predicting later IQ from infant visual habituation and dishabituation: A meta-analysis. *Journal of Applied Developmental Psychology, 25*(3), 369–393.

Kerns, J. G., Cohen, J. D., MacDonald, A. W., III, Cho, R. Y., Stenger, V. A., & Carter, C. S. (2004). Anterior cingulate conflict monitoring and adjustments in control. *Science, 303*, 1023–1026.

Kirkham, N. Z., Cruess, L., & Diamond, A. (2003). Helping children apply their knowledge to their behavior on a dimension-switching task. *Developmental Science, 6*(5), 449–467.

Kloo, D., & Perner, J. (2005). Disentangling dimensions in the dimensional change card-sorting task. *Developmental Science, 8*(1), 44–56.

Liu, D., Diorio, J., Day, J. C., Francis, D. D., & Meaney, M. J. (2000). Maternal care, hippocampal neurogenesis, and cognitive development in rats. *Nature Neuroscience, 3*, 799–806.

Liu, D., Diorio, J., Tannenbaum, B., Caldji, C., Francis, D., Freedman, A., et al. (1997). Maternal care, hippocampal glucocorticoid receptors, and hypothalamic–pituitary–adrenal responses to stress. *Science, 277*, 1659–1662.

Lupien, S. J., Gillin, C. J., & Hauger, R. L. (1999). Working memory is more sensitive than declarative memory to the acute effects of corticosteroids: A dose–response study in humans. *Behavioral Neuroscience, 113*(3), 420–430.

Luu, P., & Tucker, D. M. (2004). Self-regulation by the medial frontal cortex: Limbic representation of motive set-points. In M. Beauregard (Ed.), *Consciousness, emotional self-regulation and the brain* (pp. 123–161). Amsterdam: Benjamins.

MacDonald, A. W., III, Cohen, J. D., Stenger, V. A., & Carter, C. S. (2000). Dissociating the role of the dorsolateral prefrontal and anterior cingulate cortex in cognitive control. *Science, 288*, 1835–1838.

Mayberg, H. S. (2002). Mapping mood: An evolving emphasis on frontal–limbic interactions. In D. T. Stuss & R. T. Knight (Eds.), *Principles of frontal lobe function* (pp. 376–391). Oxford, UK: Oxford University Press.

McClelland, M. M., Cameron, C. E., Connor, C. M., Farris, C. L., Jewkes, A. M., & Morrison, F. J. (2007). Links between behavioral regulation and preschoolers' literacy, vocabulary, and math skills. *Developmental Psychology, 43*(4), 947–959.

McLoyd, V. C. (1998). Socioeconomic disadvantage and child development. *American Psychologist, 53*(2), 185–204.

Meaney, M. J. (2001). Maternal care, gene expression, and the transmission of individual differences in stress reactivity across generations. *Annual Review of Neuroscience, 24*, 1161–1192.

Mesulam, M. M. (2002). The human frontal lobes: Transcending the default mode through contingent encoding. In D. T. Stuss & R. T. Knight (Eds.), *Principles of frontal lobe function* (pp. 8–30). Oxford, UK: Oxford University Press.

Miller, E. K., & Cohen, J. D. (2001). An integrative theory of prefrontal cortex function. *Annual Review of Neuroscience, 24*, 167–202.

Miyake, A., Friedman, N. P., Emerson, M. J., Witzki, A. H., Howerter, A., & Wager, T. D. (2000). The unity and diversity of executive functions and their contributions to complex "frontal lobe" tasks: A latent variable analysis. *Cognitive Psychology, 41*(1), 49–100.

Nakano, T., Watanabe, H., Homae, F., & Taga, G. (2009). Prefrontal cortical involvement in young infants' analysis of novelty. *Cerebral Cortex, 19*, 455–463.

Noble, K. G., McCandliss, B. D., & Farah, M. J. (2007). Socioeconomic gradients predict individual differences in neurocognitive abilities. *Developmental Science, 10*(4), 464–480.

Normandeau, S., & Guay, F. (1998). Preschool behavior and first-grade school achievement: The mediational role of cognitive self-control. *Journal of Educational Psychology, 90*(1), 111–121.

Ochsner, K. N., & Gross, J. J. (2005). The cognitive control of emotion. *Trends in Cognitive Sciences, 9*(5), 242–249.

Palisin, H. (1986). Preschool temperament and performance on achievement tests. *Developmental Psychology, 22*(6), 766–770.

Parker, K. J., Buckmaster, C. L., Justus, K. R., Schatzberg, A. F., & Lyons, D. M. (2005). Mild early life stress enhances prefrontal-dependent response inhibition in monkeys. *Biological Psychiatry, 57*, 848–855.

Pennington, B. F., & Ozonoff, S. (1996). Executive functions and developmental psychopathology. *Journal of Child Psychology and Psychiatry and Allied Disciplines, 37*(1), 51–87.

Posner, M. I., & Rothbart, M. K. (2000). Developing mechanisms of self-regulation. *Development and Psychopathology, 12*(03), 427–441.

Posner, M. I., & Rothbart, M. K. (2007). Research on attention networks as a model for the integration of psychological science. *Annual Review of Psychology, 58*, 1–23.

Ramey, C. T., & Campbell, A. F. (1991). Poverty, early childhood education, and academic competence: The Abecedarian Experiment. In A. C. Huston (Ed.), *Children in poverty: Child development and public policy* (pp. 190–221). Cambridge, UK: Cambridge University Press.

Ramos, B. P., & Arnsten, A. F. (2007). Adrenergic pharmacology and cognition: Focus on the prefrontal cortex. *Pharmacology and Therapeutics, 113*, 523–536.

Reynolds, A. J., & Temple, J. (2006). Cost-effective early childhood development programs from preschool to third grade. *Annual Review of Clinical Psychology, 4*, 109–139.

Ridderinkhof, K. R., Ullsperger, M., Crone, E. A., & Nieuwenhuis, S. (2004). The role of the medial frontal cortex in cognitive control. *Science, 306*, 443–447.

Robbins, T. W. (1996). Dissociating executive functions of the prefrontal cortex. *Philosophical Transactions of the Royal Society of London B: Biological Sciences, 351*, 1463–1470.

Robbins, T. W., & Arnsten, A. F. (2009). The neuropsychopharmacology of fronto-executive function: Monoaminergic modulation. *Annual Review of Neuroscience, 32*, 267–287.

Rothbart, M. K., Ellis, L. K., Rueda, M. R., & Posner, M. I. (2003). Developing mechanisms of temperamental effortful control. *Journal of Personality, 71*(6), 1113–1143.

Rypma, B., Prabhakaran, V., Desmond, J. E., Glover, G. H., & Gabrieli, J. D. (1999). Load-dependent roles of frontal brain regions in the maintenance of working memory. *NeuroImage, 9*(2), 216–226.

Salthouse, T. A. (1996). The processing-speed theory of adult age differences in cognition. *Psychological Review, 103*(3), 403–428.

Schmeichel, B. J., & Baumeister, R. F. (2004). Self-regulatory strength. In R. F. Baumeister & K. D. Vohs (Eds.), *Handbook of self-regulation: Research, theory, and applications* (pp. 84–98). New York: Guilford Press.

Schweinhart, L. J., Montie, J., Xiang, Z., Barnett, W. S., Belfield, C. R., & Nores, M. (2005). *Lifetime effects: The High/Scope Perry Preschool study through age 40* (Monographs of the High/Scope Educational Research Foundation, No. 14). Ypsilanti, MI: High/Scope Press.

Skinner, E. A., Zimmer-Gembeck, M. J., & Connell, J. P. (1998). Individual differences and the development of perceived control. *Monographs of the Society for Research in Child Development, 63*(2–3).

Stanovich, K. (2009). *What intelligence tests miss: The psychology of rationale thought.* New Haven, CT: Yale University Press.

Stifter, C. A., & Braungart, J. M. (1995). The regulation of negative reactivity in infancy: Function and development. *Developmental Psychology, 31*(3), 448–455.

Stuss, D. T., Alexander, M. P., Floden, D., Binns, M. A., Levine, B., McIntosh, A. R., et al. (2002). Fractionation and localization of distinct frontal lobe processes. In D. Stuss & R. Knight

(Eds.), *Principles of frontal lobe function* (pp. 392–407). Oxford, UK: Oxford University Press.

Toga, A. W., Thompson, P. M., & Sowell, E. R. (2006). Mapping brain maturation. *Trends in Neurosciences, 29*(3), 148–159.

Wager, T. D., Jonides, J., & Reading, S. (2004). Neuroimaging studies of shifting attention: A meta-analysis. *NeuroImage, 22*(4), 1679–1693.

Wager, T. D., Jonides, J., Smith, E. E., & Nichols, T. E. (2005). Toward a taxonomy of attention shifting: Individual differences in fMRI during multiple shift types. *Cognitive, Affective, and Behavioral Neuroscience, 5*(2), 127–143.

West, R. L. (1996). An application of prefrontal cortex function theory to cognitive aging. *Psychological Bulletin, 120*(2), 272–292.

Willoughby, M., Blair, C., Wirth, R. J., Greenberg, M., & the Family Life Project Investigators (in press). The measurement of executive function at age 3: Psychometric properties and criterion validity of a new battery of tasks. *Psychological Assessment.*

Yamaguchi, S., Hale, L. A., D'Esposito, M., & Knight, R. T. (2004). Rapid prefrontal–hippocampal habituation to novel events. *Journal of Neuroscience, 24*(23), 5356–5363.

Yerkes, R. M., & Dodson, J. D. (1908). The relation of strength of stimulus to rapidity of habit formation. *Journal of Comparative Neurology and Psychology, 18*, 459–482.

Zelazo, P. D. (2006). The dimensional change card sort (DCCS): A method of assessing executive function in children. *Nature Protocols, 1*(1), 297–301.

Zelazo, P. D., Craik, F., & Booth, L. (2004). Executive function across the lifespan. *Acta Psychologica, 115*, 167–183.

Zelazo, P. D., & Müller, U. (2002). Executive function in typical and atypical development. In U. Goswami (Ed.), *Handbook of childhood cognitive development* (pp. 445–469). Oxford, UK: Blackwell.

Zelazo, P. D., Müller, U., Frye, D., & Marcovitch, S. (2003). The development of executive function in early childhood. *Monographs of the Society for Research in Child Development, 68*(3).

Zook, N. A., Davalos, D. B., Delosh, E. L., & Davis, H. P. (2004). Working memory, inhibition, and fluid intelligence as predictors of performance on Tower of Hanoi and London tasks. *Brain and Cognition, 56*(3), 286–292.

CHAPTER 17

Aging and Self-Regulation

WILLIAM VON HIPPEL
JULIE D. HENRY

A trophy of the brain is a normal part of aging. Just as muscle and bone mass decline in late adulthood, so too does the brain gradually shrink in total volume and weight. The frontal and temporal lobes, in particular, often show substantial atrophy with age (Dempster, 1992; Scahill et al., 2003; West, 1996). The frontal and temporal lobes support a number of important mental processes, but for our purposes in this chapter we focus on executive functions and emotions. Age-related atrophy of the frontal and temporal lobes can lead to changes in both of these areas, with important consequences for self-regulation later in life. Our goal in this chapter is to review research that concerns the consequences of age-related losses in emotion and executive processes for self-regulation and social functioning. We turn first to a consideration of the consequences of deficits in executive functions.

AGING, EXECUTIVE FUNCTIONS, AND SELF-CONTROL

Like executives in a complex organization, the mental processes known as *executive functions* are responsible for initiating, planning, and coordinating the basic cognitive processes with which we navigate our everyday lives. Executive functions include planning, task switching, and inhibition of thought and behavior. Thus, rather than being considered a unitary ability, executive functions refer to the ensemble of higher-order processes that permit contextually sensitive, flexible behavior. Because executive functions impose particular demands on frontal neural substrates, and because these structures are subject to age-related deterioration, aging has been linked to diminished executive control (Dempster, 1992; Hasher, Zacks, & May, 1999; West, 1996).

Because failures at thought control lead to contamination of ongoing mental activities with unwanted information, age-related deficits in inhibitory ability have been implicated in a variety of cognitive deficits (Hasher et al., 1999). Executive functions are not only important for regulating cognitive activity but they also play a central role in social functioning. Indeed, many theorists believe that it was the demands of social living that led to the development of such large frontal lobes in humans (Dunbar & Shultz, 2007), and there is considerable evidence for social abnormalities in populations with executive impairment (Stuss & Levine, 2002). Thus, despite the fact that aging is associated with improvement in some aspects of socioemotional functioning (Blanchard-Fields, 2007; Carstensen, Gottman, & Levenson, 1995), age-related executive deficits have the potential to disrupt social behavior in a variety of domains. In the first part of this chapter we review the evidence for this possibility.

Aging, Inhibition, and Prejudice

It is common knowledge that older Americans tend to be more prejudiced than their younger counterparts. It is also widely assumed that the root cause of this age difference lies in the historical periods in which different generations were socialized. Consistent with these lay beliefs, research supports the notion that people were more prejudiced 60 years ago than they are today (Schuman, Steeh, Bobo, & Krysan, 1997). Nevertheless, this "generational" explanation for age differences in prejudice may be only part of the story.

In an influential model of prejudice, Devine (1989) proposed that because American culture is suffused with stereotypes concerning African Americans, these stereotypes become overlearned and are automatically activated upon encounters with individual African Americans. What differentiates nonprejudiced from prejudiced people is not whether prejudiced thoughts are activated, but whether people inhibit those thoughts and replace them with more egalitarian beliefs. Prejudiced people endorse the stereotypic thoughts that are automatically activated, and nonprejudiced people reject and subsequently inhibit the stereotypic thoughts. This model suggests that older adults might be more prejudiced than younger adults because they can no longer inhibit their unintentionally activated stereotypes. There are now several lines of research that support this possibility.

In a study of explicit stereotyping and prejudice, von Hippel, Silver, and Lynch (2000) found that older white adults show greater stereotyping and prejudice toward blacks than do younger white adults. This age difference emerged despite the fact that the older adults were more concerned about impression management and more motivated than the younger adults to control their prejudices. Older adults also performed more poorly than younger adults on a measure of inhibitory ability, in which they read paragraphs aloud, some of which contained distracting text that they were not to vocalize. Perhaps most importantly, this age difference in inhibition fully mediated the age differences in stereotyping and prejudice; that is, older adults only showed greater stereotyping and prejudice to the degree that they also showed greater difficulty inhibiting their responses in general. Additionally, individual differences in inhibition were associated with individual differences in prejudice among both older and younger adults. This finding suggests that the link between inhibition and prejudice in older adults is not simply a by-product of their shared relationship with general cognitive decline or early stages of dementia. Rather, because younger adults also show a correlation between inhibitory ability and prejudice, there appears to be something unique about inhibition that plays a critical role in the prevention of prejudice.

There are, of course, interpretive problems associated with the findings of von Hippel and colleagues (2000), and subsequent research has addressed these issues in a variety of ways. First, it is possible that older adults are no more prejudiced than younger adults, but they are simply more willing to express their prejudices in the politically correct confines of the university laboratory. To address this possibility, Henry, von Hippel, and Baynes (2009) asked a close friend or family member of the participants to report on the participants' prejudice level. Participants then completed two measures of executive control—a Trail Making Test (which requires participants to trace a pathway among randomly scattered letters and numbers, alternating between letters and numbers, and thus to inhibit the natural tendency to follow alphabetic or numeric sequences) and a phonemic fluency test (which requires self-initiated retrieval of words that begin with a particular letter, thereby eventually requiring participants to inhibit words that have previously been retrieved). Henry and colleagues found that older adults were more prejudiced than younger adults (according to their peers), and that this age difference in peer-reported prejudice was mediated by participants' own performance on measures of executive control.

This finding addresses the problems associated with political correctness and social desirability, but it does not circumvent the fact that prejudice is still measured as public expression. To address this issue, Radvansky, Copeland, and von Hippel (2010) conducted an experiment in which older and younger adults were presented with stories that contained stereotype-suggestive sentences that were not explicitly stereotypic. After these suggestive sentences, participants were occasionally interrupted to complete a lexical decision task assessing activation of a word highly related to the stereotypic inference (e.g., after the sentence, "Susan saw that Jamal didn't help," participants were tested with the word *lazy*). Participants were also presented with lexical decisions after inference-inviting sentences that were stereotype neutral (e.g., the sentence "Jamal watched with anticipation," followed by the word *hungry*) and after sentences in which no inference was likely (which were used as control sentences). Results revealed that compared to the lexical decisions in the control sentences, younger adults were faster to identify the inference-relevant neutral words but slower to identify the inference-relevant stereotypic words. Older adults were also faster to identify the neutral words, but nonsignificantly faster rather than slower to identify the stereotypic words.

These findings suggest that younger adults inhibit their stereotypic inferences as they encode new information, but older adults fail to do so. Two different types of modeling data reveal results that are consistent with this possibility. First, Gonsalkorale, Sherman, and Klauer (2009) used the quadruple process model (Conrey, Sherman, Gawronski, Hugenberg, & Groom, 2005) to examine the source of age differences in implicit prejudice that emerged in a large national data set with the Implicit Association Test (IAT; Greenwald, McGhee, & Schwarz, 1998). Their modeling results indicated that older adults are less successful than younger adults in regulating automatic bias toward African Americans, but show no differences in degree of bias itself. Second, Stewart, von Hippel, and Radvansky (2009) conceptually replicated this result using the process dissociation procedure (Jacoby, 1991). Stewart and colleagues (2009) found that age differences in implicit prejudice toward African Americans emerged only in the control component of implicit prejudice, with older participants showing decreased control over their automatic biases. Furthermore, this age difference in prejudice control was mediated by age differences in the reading with distraction task used in von Hippel and colleagues (2000). Finally, Stewart and colleagues also found that self-reported motivation to be non-prejudiced only translated into low prejudice responses on the IAT when participants also had good control over their automatic biases. The results of Gonsalkorale and colleagues and Stewart and colleagues suggest that age differences in prejudice are the result of poor inhibitory control of prejudicial associations and are not just evidence of a greater willingness among older adults to express their prejudices.

Aging, Inhibition, and Social Inappropriateness

Age-related inhibitory losses have also been implicated in two types of social inappropriateness. First, older adults are more likely than younger adults to talk excessively and about topics that are irrelevant to the stream of conversation (Pushkar et al., 2000). This "off-target verbosity" is associated with diminished inhibitory ability (as indexed via the Trail Making Test, the Stroop test, and verbal fluency), which leaves older adults less capable of stopping their conversation and remaining on topic.

Inhibition also appears to be necessary to restrain oneself from verbalizing thoughts that are better left unsaid (von Hippel & Gonsalkorale, 2005); thus, inhibitory deficits can lead older adults to make socially inappropriate remarks. Consistent with this possibility, von Hippel and Dunlop (2005) found that older adults are more likely than younger adults (according to their peers) to inquire about private issues in public settings, and that this age difference in peer-reported social inappropriateness is mediated by their own inhibitory deficits (measured with a trivia test [Yoon, May, & Hasher, 2000] that includes misleading items that require respondents to inhibit their initial response; e.g., answering "black" to the question "What color are a tiger's spots?"). Furthermore, these age differences emerged despite the fact that older and younger adults agree that it is inappropriate to inquire about such issues in public settings. Indeed, older adults in particular felt less close to those who inquired about private issues in public. These findings suggest the presence of a dissociation between knowledge of social rules and the ability to follow them that is consistent with frontal lobe damage.

This finding of increased social inappropriateness with age has been conceptually replicated by Henry and colleagues (2009), who found that older adults' peers were more likely than younger adults' peers to report that they engaged in a variety of socially inappropriate behaviors. Furthermore, this peer-reported increase in social inappropriateness was again mediated by participants' own performance on the Trail Making Test and verbal fluency. Importantly, the effect of executive decline was found to be independent of the effect of general cognitive decline, suggesting that increased social inappropriateness in late life is not just a sign of early stages of dementia.

If these effects of executive decline are indeed distinct from the effects of incipient dementia, then it should also be the case that younger adults who have relatively poor inhibitory functioning are more likely to make socially inappropriate comments. To test this possibility, von Hippel and Gonsalkorale (2005) told young adult white subjects that they were participating in a study on the effects of food chemicals on memory. Half of the participants were then told by a Chinese experimenter that they were going to eat her favorite food, which was also the national dish of China. The other participants were simply told by a white experimenter that they would be eating Chinese food. Independent of this social pressure manipulation, half of the participants were then asked to remember an eight-digit number, whereas half were not given this task.

In close proximity to the participant's face, the experimenter then opened a dish containing an intact chicken foot, including the claws, cooked in a Chinese style. A hidden video camera revealed that participants were least likely to make a negative expression or comment if they were not cognitively busy, and if the Chinese experimenter had placed social pressure on them with her claims about the food's cultural and personal significance. Additionally, only in this condition did participants show a negative relationship between inhibitory ability (measured via the Stroop task) and the likelihood of making a negative expression or comment. These results suggest that younger adults also rely on their inhibitory ability to restrain socially inappropriate comments because only when they were motivated to pretend to like the chicken foot and had all of their mental faculties available did a difference in responses to the foot emerge between good and poor inhibitors. These results suggest that increased social inappropriateness with age is not just a sign of early stages of dementia because younger adults also appear to rely on inhibition to keep socially inappropriate thoughts in check. Thus, as with prejudice, there appears to be something unique about the role played by inhibition in the relationship between age and social inappropriateness.

Aging, Inhibition, and Depression

Poor inhibitory ability is not only associated with cognitive and social problems, but it is also related to depression (Hertel, 1997). Although depression might cause inhibitory deficits, age-related inhibitory deficits might also contribute to late-onset depression by impairing control of excessive rumination. Note, however, that inhibitory deficits should not lead all, or even most, older adults to excessive rumination. Rather, only those older adults who rely on inhibitory control to stop themselves from ruminating (either chronically or when confronted by negative life events) are likely to develop problems with rumination if they have poor executive control. Older adults who are disinclined to ruminate and those who ruminate but do not try to suppress their ruminative thoughts should not show a relationship between inhibition and rumination.

Deficits in executive control are particularly apparent in depression that has its initial onset in older adulthood (typically defined as at or after 60 years of age; for a review, see Alexopoulos, 2003). This suggests that inhibitory deficits may contribute to depressive symptoms because they bring decreased capacity for self-regulation in the face of negative life events. Additionally, age-related deficits in executive control may increase vulnerability to depression among older adults who may have been prone to depressive patterns of thinking throughout their lives. According to these possibilities, late-onset depression is more likely than early-onset depression to be associated with deficits in executive control. As such, among depressed older adults, late onset of symptoms should be associated with poor inhibitory ability, whereas early onset of symptoms may or may not be associated with inhibitory ability (because poor inhibition is only one of many possible causal factors in early-onset depression). Moreover, the relation between inhibitory deficits and late-onset depression should be mediated by rumination.

Consistent with this reasoning, von Hippel, Vasey, Gonda, and Stern (2008) found that inhibitory deficits (measured via the Stroop task, the reading with distraction task described earlier, and a working memory task) predicted greater depression among late-onset but not early-onset depressed older adults, and that inhibitory deficits had their impact via their role in rumination; that is, among older adults with late-onset depression, poorer inhibition predicted increased rumination, which in turn predicted increased depression. In contrast, among older adults with early-onset depression, inhibitory deficits were not associated with ruminative tendencies, suggesting that these individuals were not relying on inhibition to control their rumination and had in all likelihood developed depression for other reasons.

Aging, Inhibition, and Problem Gambling

Analogous to the case with late-onset depression, poor inhibitory ability is unlikely to lead to gambling problems in all or even most older adults. Rather, inhibitory deficits might lead to gambling problems only among those who enjoy gambling and have ready access to gambling sites. To test this possibility, von Hippel and colleagues (2009) recruited older adults from various gambling establishments, and measured their executive control and self-reported level of gambling problems. They found that older adults who gamble have greater gambling problems to the degree that they also have poor executive control (measured via the Trail Making Test). In a follow-up study, von Hippel and colleagues replicated this relationship and also found that self-reported gambling problems predicted greater depression via their impact on financial stress. Furthermore, these relationships emerged independent of general cognitive decline. These findings suggest that older adults who enjoy gambling are likely to develop greater gambling problems if they suffer losses in inhibitory control, and furthermore, that these gambling problems are important in that they appear to cause significant financial distress and consequent depression.

The problem with these studies, however, is that they rely exclusively on self-report measures of gambling problems. If deficits in inhibitory functioning cause gambling problems because they make it difficult for older adults to restrain their urge to gamble, then they should also lead to greater perseverance at gambling in the face of losses. To test this possibility, von Hippel and Hucker (2006; reported in von Hippel, 2007) conducted an experiment in which older adults recruited from gambling venues played a computerized gambling game with real winnings. Because people show reliable circadian rhythms in their inhibitory control—with most older adults showing better inhibitory control in the morning than in the afternoon (May & Hasher, 1998)—participants were randomly assigned to play the gambling game either in the morning or the afternoon. The game was preprogrammed to appear random but initially to provide more wins than losses. After participants had accumulated some winnings, they were told that they could continue to play for as long as they liked, or until they lost all their winnings. Unbeknownst to them, at that point the program shifted, so that the game no longer provided any wins, thereby enabling the assessment of perseverance in the absence of reward. Consistent with predictions, older adults responded more readily to the absence of reward and stopped playing more quickly in the morning than in the afternoon, and this effect was most pronounced among older adults whose circadian rhythms identified them most clearly as "morning types." These findings implicate inhibitory deficits in gambling perseverance, but because circadian rhythms influence general cognitive functioning in addition to inhibitory control (May & Hasher, 1998), it remains for further research to establish that inhibition is the mechanism underlying this effect.

AGING, EMOTIONAL EXPERIENCE, AND SELF-CONTROL

Age-related losses in emotional recognition, experience, and expression also have the potential to lead to difficulties regulating social behavior in late adulthood. The next section of this chapter reviews evidence on how age-related changes in emotion processing can lead to self-regulation difficulties in late adulthood.

Emotion Recognition

The face is a particularly important source of nonverbal emotional information and from a very early age basic emotions are represented clearly on the human face. Deficits in normal facial affect recognition are therefore a critical factor in poor communication, and are associated with interpersonal problems and the development and maintenance of psychopathology (Mogg, Millar, & Bradley, 2000; Pollak & Tolley-Schell, 2003).

Although emotion recognition relies on multiple cognitive processes that are subserved by a large array of neural structures, difficulty recognizing specific emotions has been observed in normal aging and linked to age-related brain changes (e.g., Calder et al., 2003; Sullivan & Ruffman, 2004). The predominant pattern across all emotions and modalities is of age-related decline, with recognition of anger and sadness particularly impaired, but older adults are potentially *better* than young adults at recognizing disgust (Ruffman, Henry, Livingstone, & Phillips, 2008). These age-related deficits appear to emerge due to the demands that the decoding of emotions imposes on specific frontal, temporal, and limbic neural substrates (Calder et al., 2003; Sullivan & Ruffman, 2004).

Difficulties understanding emotional signals have implications for social interactions in old age. Indeed, emotion misrecognition is associated with reduced social competence and interest, poor interpersonal functioning and communication, reduced quality of life, and inappropriate social behavior (Carton, Kessler, & Pape, 1999; Phillips, Scott, Henry, Mowat, & Bell, in press; Shimokawa et al., 2001). While no study to date has assessed the relationship between emotion recognition and self-regulation in the context of normal adult aging, several clinical studies support the importance of emotion recognition in self-regulation. For instance, emotion misrecognition plays a significant role in the behavioral problems and social skills difficulties that characterize attention-deficit/hyperactivity disorder (ADHD) (Kats-Gold, Besser, & Priel, 2007), a disorder widely regarded as involving impaired self-regulation (Barkley, 1997). Deficits in emotion recognition are also related to self-regulation problems in individuals with substance use dependencies (Verdejo-García, Rivas-Pérez, Vilar-López, & Pérez-García, 2007). Thus, despite the need for direct evidence of the role of emotion recognition problems in self-regulatory failure in late adulthood, the extant research strongly supports the likely relationship between the two.

Cognitive and Affective Empathy

Empathy can be divided into cognitive and affective components. While the affective component concerns emotional *responses* to the cognitive or affective state of another, the cognitive component focuses on *understanding* another's internal mental state. Cognitive empathy, theory of mind (ToM), and perspective taking are therefore regarded as overlapping constructs. In the literature on aging, empathy research has focused almost exclusively on assessment of the cognitive component, typically identifying age-related deficits in this capacity (Bailey & Henry, 2008). In addition, because the self-perspective is the cognitive default (Decety et al., 1997), to see the world from another's perspective requires active inhibition of the prepotent self-perspective. In part because of inhibitory deficits (Hasher et al., 1999), as we enter late adulthood it becomes more difficult to see things from someone else's point of view.

Deficits in empathy are likely to incur social costs because empathetic skills are considered an essential prerequisite for social functioning (Baron-Cohen & Wheelwright, 2004). In the only study to date that tested whether age-related changes in empathy relate to social outcomes, older adults reported reduced capacity for cognitive but not affective empathy compared to younger adults (Bailey, Henry, & von Hippel, 2008). Older adults also reported participating in fewer social activities. Furthermore, this age-related decline in social functioning was partially mediated by reductions in the ability to understand others' mental states. This mediational finding implies that older adults might be unintentionally driving away some social partners due to a reduced capacity for empathy.

As with emotion recognition, one of the ways by which empathetic difficulties may incur social costs is via reduced capacity for self-regulation. The management of conflict between selfish and prosocial motivations depends on self-regulatory energy (DeWall, Baumeister, Gailliot, & Maner, 2009), and feelings of empathy for others promote the desire for self-control that permits one to override the default selfish response. Consistent with this possibility, Braaten and Rosén (2000) found that although boys with ADHD did not differ from controls on emotional intensity or responses, they exhibited less empathy. Braaten and Rosén suggested that reduced empathy may lead to fewer prosocial behaviors, which may in turn lead to the social rejection often experienced by those with ADHD. Age-related reductions in empathy may similarly compromise self-regulatory efforts to behave prosocially in late adulthood, thereby incurring social costs.

Self-Conscious Emotions

Self-conscious emotions have been closely linked to self-regulation. For example, Beer, Heerey, Keltner, Scabini, and Knight (2003) found that deficient behavioral regulation following orbitofrontal damage is related to inappropriate self-conscious emotions, as well as deficits in interpreting the self-conscious emotions of others. Furthermore, simply *anticipating* self-conscious emotions is sufficient to promote greater self-control efforts (Giner-Sorolla, 2001). These data suggest that the adaptive regulation of social behavior is dependent on self-conscious emotions and their underlying appraisal processes.

Different literatures generate different predictions about how age may be related to self-conscious emotions. On the one hand, age-related losses may be anticipated because self-conscious emotions are more cognitively complex than the basic emotions, requiring the ability to self-reflect and to be aware of how our actions might be perceived by others. Consequently, cognitive empathy plays an important role in self-conscious emotions. In conjunction with atrophy of the orbitofrontal area, age-related losses in cognitive empathy therefore have the potential to lead to reduced self-conscious emotional responding.

In contrast to these predictions, evidence for age-related gains in some aspects of emotion regulation predict that only the experience and expression of *negative* self-conscious emotion may be reduced; the experience of positive self-conscious emotion may be enhanced. For example, socioemotional selectivity theory suggests that older adults may be more effective than younger adults at engaging in the emotion regulation strategy of situation selection—planning contact with people they already know and love rather than pursuing interactions with more peripheral social contacts (Carstensen, Fung, & Charles, 2003).

To provide a preliminary assessment of whether there are age differences in the experience of self-conscious emotion, Henry, Waters, von Hippel, and Ruffman (2009) had younger, middle-aged, and older adults complete self-report, interview-based, and behavioral measures focused on their experiences of embarrassment, pride, shame, and guilt. The results indicated that although experiences of the negative self-conscious emotions were less likely to be reported by the older adult group, when these emotions were experienced, their perceived emotional intensity did not differ between the age groups. In addition, when older adults were asked to *imagine* themselves in situations that might elicit negative self-conscious emotion, there were no age differences in perceived reactions to those situations. These data imply that age per se may not affect the ability to experience negative self-conscious emotion, but enhanced emotion regulation skills may lead to greater avoidance of situations likely to elicit such emotions (Birditt, Fingerman, & Almeida, 2005; Carstensen et al., 2003). However, this is but a single study, and no research to date has assessed whether the expression of self-conscious emotion is altered in late adulthood. As noted previously, not only the experience but also the appropriate outward display of self-conscious emotion has been linked to various positive social outcomes.

POSITIVE VERSUS NEGATIVE SOCIAL CONSEQUENCES OF AGING

Our focus in this chapter has been on the negative social consequences that emerge from age-related atrophy of the frontal and temporal lobes. It should be noted, however, that some of these negative effects might be offset by other changes in social and cognitive functioning that emerge in late adulthood. For example, it is well known that older adults attend more to positive emotions than do younger adults, and older adults indeed show decreased responding in the amygdala (a brain region involved in emotional experience) to negative but not to positive events (Mather et al., 2004). This increased positivity and decreased negativity with age has a number of important social consequences, such as a more affectionate style of conflict resolution (Carstensen et al., 1995). Older adults are also more effective than younger adults at solving some types of social problems, in part because they are more likely to integrate their long-term emotional goals with their immediate instrumental intentions (Blanchard-Fields, 2007).

These studies suggest that there are likely to be circumstances in which the social behavior of older adults is facilitated by increases in wisdom, positivity, and priority of relationship motives, and other circumstances in which social behavior is disrupted by deficits in executive control and emotion processing. Indeed, the same circumstances might involve both countervailing forces. Evidence for such a possibility can be seen in the research of von Hippel, Henry, and Matovic (2008), who found that older adults show levels of social satisfaction similar to those of younger adults, despite spending more time alone and engaging in fewer social activities. Additionally, older adults reported neither more nor fewer uplifts from the experiences that they shared with younger adults. Yet this apparent stability in social experience masked underlying countercurrents whereby age-related losses were suppressing the effect of age-related gains. On the loss side of the ledger, in addition to spending more time alone and engaging in fewer social activities, older adults also had poorer working memory than younger adults. All three of these factors played a mediating role in decreasing social satisfaction among older adults, and when they were included as mediators, a suppression effect emerged, whereby aging was now associated with residual *increases* in social satisfaction and uplifts from social experiences. Thus, at the aggregate level, the losses offset the gains, but in the case of any single individual, there is clearly the potential for age-related losses, gains, or stasis in social functioning and satisfaction.

FUTURE DIRECTIONS

The findings reviewed here on aging and self-regulatory deficits suggest a variety of directions for future research. Perhaps most notably, this review highlights the need to combine cognitive and affective approaches to the study of aging and self-regulation because changes in cognitive and affective processes have the potential to augment or attenuate each other's effects. For example, declines in executive functioning have the potential to exacerbate age-related declines in perspective taking and empathy, but enhanced emotion regulation and prioritization in late life have the potential to offset some of the social consequences of executive decline (von Hippel, Henry, et al., 2008). Thus, future research on aging and self-regulation would benefit from integrating cognitive and affective approaches. With this goal in mind, we briefly outline a few possible themes for future research on aging and self-regulation.

Social Functioning

Loneliness and social isolation have broad negative implications for physical health and mental well-being, with the strongest effects in late adulthood (House, Landis, & Umberson, 1988). Although there are many causes of loneliness in this age group, deficits in executive functioning and increased social inappropriateness are possible sources of reduced social satisfaction (von Hippel & Dunlop, 2005; von Hippel, Henry, et al., 2008). Additionally increased difficulty taking the perspective of another (Bailey & Henry, 2008) might also contribute to poorer social functioning and subsequent loneliness (Bailey et al., 2008). Taken together, these possibilities suggest that some social problems are increased in older adulthood because of self-regulatory failures arising from executive dysfunction.

Age-related changes in emotional responding also have the potential to disrupt self-control efforts in social domains and, as noted earlier, one possible route is through the altered experience of self-conscious emotion. Self-conscious emotions, such as pride, guilt, shame, and embarrassment, are critical determinants of self-control behaviors in social contexts that motivate interpersonal etiquette and personal hygiene, and inhibit transgression of social standards. Such emotions also promote reparative actions to mend social relations following transgressions (Tracy & Robins, 2007). Furthermore, any decrease in felt arousal to negative outcomes should also reduce experience of self-conscious emotions that arise in relation to negative cues (e.g., guilt). Future research might profitably explore whether, when, and how altered emotional experience interacts with diminished executive control to influence self-regulation of social behavior and consequent social outcomes.

Finances

The percentage of adults over the age of 65 who gamble has risen dramatically over the past 30 years, as have rates of problem gambling in this age group (Petry, 2005). It is unclear from these trends, however, why gambling problems are increasing among older adults. It could be that the increased accessibility of gambling, in combination with the availability of leisure time and expendable income, leads some older adults to develop gambling problems. Alternatively, as suggested earlier, it is possible that gambling problems in older adults are at least partially the result of age-related reductions in the capacity for self-regulation. Problems with executive control might be compounded by changes in emotional experience because reduced arousal in reaction to losses (but not wins) may increase the weighting placed on positive relative to negative feedback, making it more difficult to inhibit the urge to gamble. These notions raise the possibility that gambling establishments might be taking advantage of older adults who have problems with self-control and limited opportunities to earn back their losses. At the same time, the current findings also suggest new avenues for treatment of gambling problems among older adults. For example, older adults might gamble more wisely if they adhere to their circadian rhythms and avoid gambling in the afternoon or evening. As with social functioning, future research might profitably examine the conjoint effects of executive losses and increased positivity on levels of gambling problems in older adults.

Health

Like many other demographic groups in industrialized nations, older adults are increasingly struggling with obesity (e.g., Australian Institute of Health and Welfare, 2004). These obesity trends have important health, economic, and social consequences, with a recent longitudinal study of nearly 4,000 older adults identifying a relationship between increasing body mass index and functional impairment (Lang, Llewellyn, Alexander, & Melzer, 2008). The increased prevalence of obesity in late adulthood may be partially attributable to reduced capacity for self-regulation. Excess body weight has been strongly linked to lifestyle factors, such as reduced exercise and increased food consumption. Because exercising can be onerous, maintaining a healthy routine can depend on the ability to resist the temptation to relax and to induce oneself to exercise. Furthermore, because fattening foods are readily available, maintenance of a healthy body weight also depends on the ability to resist frequent dietary temptations. Self-regulatory failures in late adulthood may therefore manifest themselves in increased body weight. Indeed, in a sample of otherwise healthy adults, those who were overweight exhibited reduced executive control relative to their normal-weight counterparts (Gunstad et al., 2007). Furthermore, any diminution of felt arousal to negative (but not positive) outcomes may increase the emphasis placed on the immediate positive feelings derived from eating a tempting food relative to the negative long-term consequences of weight gain. At this point there are no empirical tests of these possibilities, but changes in emotional responding and losses in executive functioning could easily be precursors of weight gain and other health problems in late adulthood.

Forewarning

Although the data reviewed in this chapter suggest a variety of self-regulation problems experienced by older adults due to deficits in executive functioning and changes in emotional experiences, older adults are likely to be able to compensate for many of these changes. For example, older adults typically manage their poorer memory for details by relying on higher-level representations that contain the primary points of the information they learned (Radvansky & Dijkstra, 2007). In a similar manner, older adults might also develop strategies that minimize their difficulties with self-regulation brought about by executive decline or emotional changes.

In support of such a possibility, recent evidence suggests that older adults can inhibit stereotypes just as effectively as younger adults when they know the stereotype is irrelevant at encoding (Radvansky, Lynchard, & von Hippel, 2009). In their study, Radvansky and colleagues (2009) presented younger and older adults with stories about a person with a stereotypically male or female occupation (e.g., plumber vs. babysitter). Half of the time, participants were explicitly given a gender label when first learning about the protagonist (e.g., "The babysitter was a young boy who . . . "), and half the time they were not (e.g., "The babysitter was a young teenager who . . . "). Additionally, half of the time the gender of the protagonist was occupation-stereotypic and half the time it was counterstereotypic. Later in the story, participants encountered a pronoun that communicated the gender of the protagonist, and the critical measure was whether they read the sentence containing the counterstereotypic pronoun more slowly than the sentence containing the stereotypic pronoun. Results indicated that both younger and older adults read the sentence containing the counterstereotypic pronoun more slowly when they had not initially been provided an explicit gender label, but both younger and older adults read the counterstereotypic pronoun just as quickly as the stereotypic pronoun when they had already been provided a gender label.

These findings suggest that older adults are just as capable as young adults of putting aside their stereotypes when they know at the moment they encounter the person that their stereotypes are irrelevant to the situation at hand. These findings are also consistent with informal observations from our laboratory that older adults are often just as capable as younger adults of suppressing a socially inappropriate response when they know in advance that the need to suppress a response is likely to be imminent. Older adults seem to get themselves into trouble primarily when they cannot anticipate the self-regulatory demands in advance and prepare themselves for it. This possibility suggests that interventions might be designed around the idea of forewarning older adults who are having self-regulatory difficulties. The mechanisms and boundary conditions involved in the effectiveness of forewarning, and indeed the search for and development of other compensatory strategies, would seem to be a worthwhile direction for future research.

REFERENCES

Alexopoulos, G. S. (2003). Role of executive function in late-life depression. *Journal of Clinical Psychiatry, 64*(Suppl. 14), 18–23.

Australian Institute of Health and Welfare (2004). *Obesity trends in older Australians* [Bulletin No. 12]. Canberra, Australia: Author.

Bailey, P. E., & Henry, J. D. (2008). Growing less empathic with age: Disinhibition of the self-perspective. *Journals of Gerontology B: Psychological Sciences and Social Sciences, 63*, P219–P226.

Bailey, P. E., Henry, J. D., & von Hippel, W. (2008). Empathy and social functioning in late adulthood. *Aging and Mental Health, 12*, 499–503.

Barkley, R. A. (1997). Behavioral inhibition, sustained attention, and executive functions: Constructing a unified theory of ADHD. *Psychological Bulletin, 121*, 65–94.

Baron-Cohen, S., & Wheelwright, S. (2004). The Empathy Quotient: An investigation of adults with Asperger syndrome or high functioning autism and normal sex differences. *Journal of Autism and Developmental Disorders, 34*, 163–175.

Beer, J. S., Heerey, E. A., Keltner, D., Scabini, D., & Knight, R. T. (2003). The regulatory function of self-conscious emotion: Insight from patients with orbitofrontal damage. *Journal of Personality and social Psychology, 85*, 594–604.

Birditt, K. S., Fingerman, K. L., & Almeida, D. M. (2005). Age differences in exposure and reactions to interpersonal tensions: A daily diary study. *Psychology and Aging, 20*(2), 330–340.

Blanchard-Fields, F. (2007). Everyday problem solving and emotion: An adult developmental perspective. *Current Directions in Psychological Science, 16*, 26–31.

Braaten, E. B., & Rosén, L. A. (2000). Self-regulation of affect in attention deficit-hyperactivity disorder (ADHD) and non-ADHD boys: Differences in empathic responding. *Journal of Consulting and Clinical Psychology, 68*, 313–321.

Calder, A. J., Keane, J., Manly, T., Sprengelmeyer, R., Scott, S., Nimmo-Smith, I., et al. (2003). Facial expression recognition across the adult life span. *Neuropsychologia, 41*, 195–292.

Carstensen, L. L., Fung, H. H., & Charles, S. T. (2003). Socioemotional selectivity theory and the regulation of emotion in the second half of life. *Motivation and Emotion, 27*, 103–123.

Carstensen, L. L., Gottman, J. M., & Levenson, R. W. (1995). Emotional behavior in long-term marriage. *Psychology and Aging, 10*, 140–149.

Carton, J. S., Kessler, E. A., & Pape, C. L. (1999). Nonverbal decoding skills and relationship well-being in adults. *Journal of Nonverbal Behavior, 23*, 91–100.

Conrey, F. R., Sherman, J. W., Gawronski, B., Hugenberg, K., & Groom, C. J. (2005). Separating multiple processes in implicit social cognition: The quad model of implicit task performance. *Journal of Personality and Social Psychology, 89*, 469–487.

Decety, J., Grezes, J., Costes, N., Perani, D., Jeannerod, M., Procyk, E., et al. (1997). Brain activity during observation of actions: Influence of action content and subject's strategy. *Brain, 120*, 1763–1777.

Dempster, F. N. (1992). The rise and fall of the inhibitory mechanism: Toward a unified theory of cognitive development and aging. *Developmental Review, 12*, 45–75.

Devine, P. G. (1989). Stereotypes and prejudice: Their automatic and controlled components. *Journal of Personality and Social Psychology, 56*, 5–18.

DeWall, C. N., Baumeister, R. F., Gailliot, M. T., & Maner, J. K. (2009). Depletion makes the heart grow less helpful: Helping as a function of self-regulatory energy and genetic relatedness. *Personality and Social Psychology Bulletin, 34*, 1653–1662.

Dunbar, R., & Shultz, S. (2007). Evolution in the social brain. *Science, 317*, 1344–1347.

Giner-Sorolla, R. (2001). Guilty pleasures and grim necessities: Affective attitudes in dilemmas of self-control. *Journal of Personality and Social Psychology, 80*, 206–221.

Gonsalkorale, K., Sherman, J. W., & Klauer, K. C. (2009). Aging and prejudice: Diminished regulation of automatic race bias among older adults. *Journal of Experimental Social Psychology, 45*, 1081–1087.

Greenwald, A. G., McGhee, D. E., & Schwartz, J. K. L. (1998). Measuring individual differences in implicit cognition: The Implicit Association Test. *Journal of Personality and Social Psychology, 74*, 1464–1480.

Gunstad, J., Paul, R. H., Cohen, R. A., Tate, D. F., Spitznagel, M. B., & Gordon, E. (2007). Elevated body mass index is associated with executive dysfunction in otherwise healthy adults. *Comprehensive Psychiatry, 48*, 57–61.

Hasher, L., Zacks, R. T., & May, C. P. (1999). Inhibitory control, circadian arousal, and age. In D. Gopher & A. Koriat (Eds.), *Attention and performance XVII: Cognitive regulation of performance: Interaction of theory and application* (pp. 653–675). Cambridge, MA: MIT Press.

Henry, J. D., von Hippel, W., & Baynes, K. (2009). Social inappropriateness, executive control, and aging. *Psychology and Aging, 24*, 239–244.

Henry, J. D., Waters, M., von Hippel, W., & Ruffman, T. (2009). *Aging and self-conscious emotions.* Unpublished manuscript, University of New South Wales.

Hertel, P. T. (1997). On the contribution of deficient cognitive control to memory impairment in depression. *Cognition and Emotion, 11*, 569–583.

House, J. S., Landis, K. R., & Umberson, D. (1988). Social relationships and health. *Science, 241*, 540–545.

Jacoby, L. L. (1991). A process dissociation framework: Separating automatic from intentional uses of memory. *Journal of Memory and Language, 30*, 513–541.

Kats-Gold, I., Besser, A., & Priel, B. (2007). The role of simple emotion recognition skills among school aged boys at risk of ADHD. *Journal of Abnormal Child Psychology, 35*, 363–378.

Lang, I. A., Llewellyn, D. J., Alexander, K., & Melzer, D. (2008). Obesity, physical function, and mortality in older adults. *Journal of the American Geriatrics Society, 56*, 1474–1478.

Mather, M., Canli, T., English, T., Whitfield, S., Wais, P., Ochsner, K., et al. (2004). Amygdala responses to emotionally valenced stimuli in older and younger adults. *Psychological Science, 15*, 259–263.

May, C. P., & Hasher, L. (1998). Synchrony effects in inhibitory control over thought and action. *Journal of Experimental Psychology: Human Perception and Performance, 24*, 363–379.

Mogg, K., Millar, N., & Bradley, B. P. (2000). Biases in EMs to threatening facial expressions in generalized anxiety disorder and depressive disorder. *Journal of Abnormal Psychology, 109*, 695–704.

Petry, N. M. (2005). *Pathological gambling: Etiology, comorbidity, and treatment.* Washington, DC: American Psychological Association.

Phillips, L. H., Scott, C., Henry, J. D., Mowat, D., & Bell, S. (in press). Emotion perception in Alzheimer's disease and mood disorders in old age. *Psychology and Aging.*

Pollak, S. D., & Tolley-Schell, S. A. (2003). Selective attention to facial emotion in physically abused children. *Journal of Abnormal Psychology, 112*, 323–338.

Pushkar, D., Basevitz, P., Arbuckle, T., Nohara-LeClair, M., Lapidus, S., & Peled, M. (2000). Social behavior and off-target verbosity in elderly people. *Psychology and Aging, 15*, 361–374.

Radvansky, G. A., Copeland, D. E., & von Hippel, W. (2010). Stereotype activation, inhibition, and aging. *Journal of Experimental Social Psychology, 46*, 51–60.

Radvansky, G. A., & Dijkstra, K. (2007). Aging and situation model processing. *Psychonomic Bulletin and Review, 14*, 1027–1042.

Radvansky, G. A., Lynchard, N. A., & von Hippel, W. (2009). Aging and stereotype suppression. *Aging, Neuropsychology, and Cognition, 16*, 22–32.

Ruffman, T., Henry, J. D., Livingstone, V., & Phillips, L. H. (2008). A meta-analytic review of emotion recognition and aging: Implications for neuropsychological models of aging. *Neuroscience and Biobehavioral Reviews, 32*, 863–881.

Scahill, R. I., Frost, C., Jenkins, R., Whitewell, J. L., Rossor, M. N., & Fox, N. C. (2003). A longitudinal study of brain volume changes in normal aging using serial registered magnetic resonance imaging. *Archives of Neurology, 60*, 989–994.

Schuman, H., Steeh, C., Bobo, L., & Krysan, M. (1997). *Racial attitudes in America: Trends and interpretations*. Cambridge, MA: Harvard University Press.

Shimokawa, A., Yatomi, N., Anamizu, S., Torii, S., Isono, H., Sugai, Y., et al. (2001). Influence of deteriorating ability of emotional comprehension on interpersonal behaviour in Alzheimer-type dementia. *Brain and Cognition, 47*, 423–433.

Stewart, B. D., von Hippel, W., & Radvansky, G. A. (2009). Age, race, and implicit prejudice: Using process dissociation to separate the underlying components. *Psychological Science, 20*, 164–168.

Stuss, D. T., & Levine, B. (2002). Adult clinical neuropsychology: Lessons from studies of the frontal lobes. *Annual Review of Psychology, 53*, 401–433.

Sullivan, S., & Ruffman, T. (2004). Emotion recognition deficits in the elderly. *International Journal of Neuroscience, 114*, 94–102.

Tracy, J. L., & Robins, R. W. (2007). Emerging insights into the nature and function of pride. *Current Directions in Psychological Science, 16*, 147–150.

Verdejo-García, A., Rivas-Pérez, C., Vilar-López, R., & Pérez-García, M. (2007). Strategic self-regulation, decision-making and emotion processing in poly-substance abusers in their first year of abstinence. *Drug and Alcohol Dependence, 86*, 139–146.

von Hippel, W. (2007). Aging, executive functioning and social control. *Current Directions in Psychological Science, 16*, 240–244.

von Hippel, W., & Dunlop, S. M. (2005). Aging, inhibition, and social inappropriateness. *Psychology and Aging, 20*, 519–523.

von Hippel, W., & Gonsalkorale, K. (2005). "That is bloody revolting!": Inhibitory control of thoughts better left unsaid. *Psychological Science, 16*, 497–500.

von Hippel, W., Henry, J. D., & Matovic, D. (2008). Aging and social satisfaction: Offsetting positive and negative effects. *Psychology and Aging, 23*, 435–439.

von Hippel, W., Ng, L., Abbott, L., Caldwell, S., Gill, G., & Powell, K. (2009). Executive functioning and gambling: Performance on the Trail Making Test is associated with gambling problems in older adult gamblers. *Aging, Neuropsychology, and Cognition, 16*, 654–670.

von Hippel, W., Silver, L. A., & Lynch, M. E. (2000). Stereotyping against your will: The role of inhibitory ability in stereotyping and prejudice among the elderly. *Personality and Social Psychology Bulletin, 26*, 523–532.

von Hippel, W., Vasey, M. W., Gonda, T., & Stern, T. (2008). Executive function deficits, rumination and late-onset depressive symptoms in older adults. *Cognitive Therapy and Research, 32*, 474–487.

West, R. L. (1996). An application of prefrontal cortex function theory to cognitive ageing. *Psychological Bulletin, 120*, 272–292.

Yoon, C., May, C. P., & Hasher, L. (2000). Aging, circadian arousal patterns, and cognition. In D. C. Park & N. Schwarz (Eds.), *Cognitive aging: A primer* (pp. 151–171). Philadelphia: Psychology Press.

PART IV

SOCIAL DIMENSION OF SELF-REGULATION

CHAPTER 18

The Sociometer, Self-Esteem, and the Regulation of Interpersonal Behavior

MARK R. LEARY
JENNIFER GUADAGNO

Most discussions of self-regulation have focused on the generic psychological processes that allow people to control their thoughts, emotions, and behaviors—processes that are nonspecific with regard to the action being regulated (Baumeister, Heatherton, & Tice, 1994; Carver & Scheier, 1981; Mischel, 1996). For example, TOTE (test–operate–test–exit) and other cybernetic models of self-control (Carver & Scheier, 1981) can be applied to many domains, and the same basic processes are involved regardless of the nature of the self-control task at hand.

In addition to these general-purpose self-regulatory systems, people also possess mechanisms that are dedicated to particular functions. Such mechanisms operate in a circumscribed range of situations and handle only one kind of regulatory problem. This chapter examines one such mechanism—the *sociometer*—that appears to be involved in the control of interpersonal behavior. Most previous writing and research regarding the sociometer have emphasized its connection to self-esteem, but, as we will see, its functions go far beyond simply affecting how people feel about themselves (Leary & Baumeister, 2000).

According to evolutionary psychologists, the human mind is composed of distinct, domain-specific modules that evolved because they solved recurrent problems involving survival and reproduction in the past (Samuels, 2000). Recurrent challenges in the ancestral environment led to the evolution of systems designed to meet those challenges. So, for example, theorists have posited regulatory modules that help people to avoid toxic substances, identify potential mates, detect group members who cheat, and ostracize those who may be infected with parasites.

Many of these systems—such as those involving fear and disgust—protect people from physical threats directly. Other systems, however, evolved to serve interpersonal functions by helping people behave toward others in ways that facilitated their own survival and reproduction. Such systems have clear adaptive benefits, but their effects on well-being are mediated by the responses of other people.

THE SOCIOMETER

The fundamental prerequisite of interpersonal life is that a person be minimally accepted by other people and avoid wholesale rejection. Virtually all social affordances—such as friendship, social support, group memberships, social influence, and pair-bonds—require the individual to be accepted by others. Furthermore, only those who have established supportive relationships can count on others' assistance in terms of food sharing, protection, and care when ill, injured, or old. Because of the adaptive advantages of being accepted by other people, human beings possess a strong need for acceptance and belonging (Baumeister & Leary, 1995; Leary & Allen, in press). Furthermore, given the vital importance of social acceptance and the disastrous consequences of rejection throughout evolution, human beings have developed a psychological system that monitors and responds to events that are relevant to interpersonal acceptance and rejection.

Regulatory systems generally possess three features. They monitor the internal or external environments for cues that signal advantageous or disadvantageous circumstances, evoke positive or negative feelings when such cues are detected, and motivate behaviors that help the individual to capitalize on opportunity or avert threat. Thus, a module that evolved to facilitate acceptance and avoid rejection would be expected to respond to cues indicating real or potential rejection, evoke feelings that alert the individual to the threat, and motivate the person to behave in ways that minimize the probability of rejection and promote acceptance.

Detecting Threats to Relational Value

According to sociometer theory, people possess a sociometer that monitors the interpersonal environment for cues that are relevant to a person's *relational value* in the eyes of other people—the degree to which other people regard their relationships with the individual as valuable or important (Leary, 2002). What we colloquially call *rejection* and *acceptance* are the end points on a continuum of relational value.

People are exceptionally sensitive to events that have implications for their relational value and readily pick up on subtle cues related to their social standing (Weisbuch, Sinclair, Skorinko, & Eccleston, 2009). In fact, people monitor the environment for cues relevant to their relational value on a preattentive level. For example, the *cocktail party effect*, in which a person orients toward his or her name in the noisy hubbub of a party (Cherry, 1953), demonstrates nonconscious vigilance for indications of how one is regarded by others. In addition, people think a good deal about other people's perceptions and evaluations of them and try to anticipate how others will react to them in future situations. Some of these are idle imaginings, but others evoke deep concern when they suggest that one's past, present, or future relational value is lower than desired.

The Warning System

At least since Darwin, theorists have agreed that emotions serve to alert us to events with potential implications for our well-being. Emotions shift attention to critical features of the environment, motivate behaviors that respond to these events, and reinforce actions that deal effectively with them. So, for example, threatening stimuli evoke subjective fear and an action tendency to avoid or escape the feared stimulus, and such actions are reinforced by a decline in the aversive feelings. Of course, a functional analysis does not imply that all emotions are adaptive. People may react dysfunctionally when they misappraise a situation or misjudge the most effective response to it. Even so, emotions evolved because they help people regulate their behavior, and emotions are fundamentally involved in self-regulation (Carver & Scheier, 1981, Chapter 1, this volume).

The affective output of the sociometer serves precisely these functions. Indications that one is approved of or accepted—that one's relational value is high—lead to positive affect. Indications that one is disapproved of or rejected—that one's relational value is low (or declining)—lead to negative affect. Studies have shown that perceived rejection (i.e., low relational value) is associated with negative emotions such as hurt feelings, jealousy, and sadness, and with increased attention to the problematic interpersonal situation (Leary, Koch, & Hechenbleikner, 2001).

Typically, whenever people experience acceptance and rejection, they also feel good or bad *about themselves*. Sociometer theory suggests that these self-relevant feelings—state self-esteem—are part of this regulatory system (Leary, 2006). When the sociometer detects cues that connote unacceptably low relational value, it not only triggers negative affect but also instigates a process to assess whether one's low relational value is due to some personal action, shortcoming, or deficiency. In most cases, people entertain the possibility that their low relational value is at least partly their own fault, which leads them to feel bad about themselves, that is, to experience lowered state self-esteem. However, when people are certain that their exclusion by other people does not reflect on them personally, their state self-esteem is unaffected (Leary, Tambor, Terdal, & Downs, 1995). These effects on self-esteem have even been demonstrated on an international level. Countries in which people have frequent interactions with friends have higher nationwide self-esteem than countries without strong social practices, even when researchers control for happiness, individualism, neuroticism, and economic factors (Denissen, Penke, Schmitt, & van Aken, 2008).

Some critics have correctly observed that a regulatory system with the properties of a sociometer need not involve any connection to the self. After all, other species of animals possess systems that regulate interactions with conspecifics, but we would not invoke the concept of self-esteem in accounting for their reactions. This objection is partially correct. An animal does not need self-esteem to regulate its social behavior. Prior to the evolution of self-awareness, our hominid ancestors presumably interacted effectively even though they lacked the capacity for conscious self-reflection. In the absence of self-awareness, however, this system could respond only to social cues in the immediate environment. The detection of certain "rejection" cues (e.g., frowns, disinterest, or angry gestures) would likely have elicited negative affect and motivated efforts to appease, ingratiate, or withdraw, all of which could have happened without a self.

With the appearance of self-awareness, however, people's reactions to rejection-relevant cues became more complex. Although early human beings would still have responded to immediate cues relevant to acceptance, changes in the self would have added a new layer of cognitive processing. Improvements in the extended self, which processes information about the individual over time, would have allowed people to ponder past rejections and anticipate possible rejections in the future (Leary & Buttermore, 2003). The ability to feel good or bad about future events would have been an important development in self-regulation, allowing people to anticipate others' reactions and thereby detering actions that might result in rejection.

In brief, prior to the time that human beings became fully capable of self-related thought, people would have had a sociometer of sorts, but it would have responded only to concrete social cues in the immediate situation and its operation would have been based exclusively on affect. Once people could think about themselves over time, adopt others' perspectives of them, and conceptualize themselves symbolically, they would have had a modern sociometer that led them to feel good and bad *about themselves* as a result of the real or imagined evaluations of other people. Furthermore, with a modern conceptual self, they could consciously think about and evaluate themselves, use other people's reactions to them to assess their abilities and worth, and judge themselves according to other people's standards. As a result, merely thinking about other people's evaluations of them could evoke feelings about symbolic aspects of the self.

The (So-Called) Self-Esteem Motive

Most conceptualizations of self-esteem have not explained precisely what self-esteem does or why it is important (Leary, 1999). The assumption has been that people's feelings about themselves are related to important outcomes such as achievement, positive interpersonal relations, and psychological well-being (Mecca, Smelser, & Vasconcellos, 1989), but few efforts have been made to explain what functions people's feelings about themselves might serve. To complicate matters, most psychologists have assumed that people have a *need* for self-esteem, without asking why people should need to feel good about themselves.

Sociometer theory answers this question by proposing that, contrary to how it may appear, people do not have a need for self-esteem (Leary, 2006; Leary & Downs, 1995). Rather, people only appear to seek self-esteem because they often behave in ways that maintain or increase their relational value. The behaviors that have been attributed to efforts to maintain self-esteem reflect people's efforts to maintain relational value in other people's eyes. They appear to be seeking self-esteem because self-esteem is an output of the gauge that monitors their success in promoting relational value (Leary, 2006). This is not to say that people do not occasionally cognitively override the sociometer to avoid negative feelings, but these intrapsychic, self-serving reactions reflect a hedonistic effort to avoid negative affect rather than a need for self-esteem per se.

Do All Changes in Self-Esteem Involve Acceptance and Rejection?

The traditional conceptualization views *self-esteem* as an individual's personal self-evaluation—an assessment of whether one has achieved one's personal goals or lived up to personal standards. Conceptualizing self-esteem as a person's private self-evaluation has had important, and perhaps unfortunate, consequences for understanding self-esteem. If we start with the assumption that self-esteem is a person's private self-evaluation, it is but a short step to conclude that healthy self-esteem ought not to be affected by other people's evaluations. Several theorists have taken this step by suggesting self-esteem that is affected by other people is not "true" or "healthy" self-esteem (Deci & Ryan, 1995). Furthermore, many people insist that how they feel about themselves is not affected by other people's reactions to them.

The data tell a different story, however, suggesting that events with implications for acceptance and rejection affect self-esteem in most individuals. In two studies (Leary et al., 2003), we selected groups of participants who either believed that their self-esteem was affected by acceptance and approval or strongly denied that acceptance and approval had any effect whatsoever on how they felt about themselves. Then, we gave both groups feedback indicating a low or high degree of approval/acceptance from other participants and measured their state self-esteem. The results of both studies unequivocally showed that the two groups did not respond differently to the social acceptance and rejection manipulation. Similar results from Lemay and Ashmore (2006) showed that trait self-esteem was related to perceived regard from others, even for people who believed that their self-esteem was not contingent on others' beliefs about them. The fact that the sociometer responds to rejection even among people who deny it (and may be unaware of it) suggests that contingent self-esteem is an inherent and normal feature of human nature that often works outside of people's conscious awareness.

However, even if we accept the claim that self-esteem naturally responds to cues regarding one's relational value, we may ask whether self-esteem is ever affected by events that have no implications for acceptance and rejection. One possibility involves situations in which people feel good about themselves when they achieve or do good deeds even though no one else is privy to their behavior or, conversely, feel bad about themselves when they do (or even contemplate) some reprehensible thing that no one else will ever know. Where are the implications for acceptance and rejection of private behaviors such as these? The answer is that, as a regulatory mechanism, the sociometer cannot afford to wait until one is already rejected to respond. Just as the mechanism that elicits fear and avoidance cannot wait until a threat is immediately present, the sociometer must warn people *in advance* about the possibility of low relational value. Thus, the sociometer should warn us that our relational value is in potential jeopardy even when we contemplate performing some dark act or receive feedback that only we know about (Guay, Delisle, Fernet, Julien, & Senécal, 2008). Only then can it deter us from engaging in behaviors that might jeopardize our relational value. Furthermore, people may experience lowered self-esteem when they think that their actions may lead them to be rejected in the near future, and those who believe that they are more likely to be devalued, such as people who are low in trait self-esteem, are more likely to show this effect (Haupt & Leary, 1997).

In brief, people appear to possess a sociometer that monitors their interpersonal worlds for information relevant to relational value, alerts them through unpleasant emotions and lowered state self-esteem when their relational value is lower than desired or declining, and motivates behavior that helps to enhance relational value. This system is essential for helping people to regulate their interpersonal behavior in ways that minimize the potential for rejection.

THE CALIBRATION OF THE SOCIOMETER
AND INTERPERSONAL SELF-REGULATION

Self-regulatory systems function optimally when they accurately monitor relevant aspects of the world, thus reflecting the true state of the environment in which the organism is operating. Unfortunately, like many meters and gauges, the sociometer may be miscalibrated such that it does not accurately reflect the person's relational value to others. Miscalibration undermines the sociometer's ability to regulate behavior in ways that maintain an acceptable level of interpersonal acceptance, and as we will see, many interpersonal and psychological difficulties can be conceptualized as miscalibrations of the sociometer.

One might expect that a properly calibrated sociometer would respond to relational evaluation in a linear fashion, with equal increments or decrements in relational value resulting in equal changes in emotion and state self-esteem. However, Leary, Haupt, Strausser, and Chokel (1998) showed that this is not the case. In four experiments, participants imagined or received one of several levels of feedback, ranging from extreme rejection to extreme acceptance. Although state self-esteem increased with relational value, the function was curvilinear. Figure 18.1 shows the general form of the relationship between relational value (i.e., acceptance–rejection) and state self-esteem. As can be seen, the sociometer is more sensitive to small changes in relational value in the neutral to moderately positive range of relational value than in the rejecting and highly accepting ranges. With declining relational value, state self-esteem hits its lowest point long before feedback is maximally rejecting, so that people's response to feedback that reflects slightly negative relational value is similar to that reflecting maximally negative value. One explanation for this pattern is that once relational value drops just below neutral, further decrements have few, if any, tangible consequences. Generally, people simply ignore or ostracize individuals whose relationships they do not value, no matter how strongly they devalue those individuals. As a result, being greatly devalued is not much

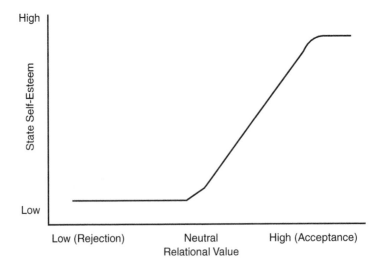

FIGURE 18.1. The relationship between relational value and state self-esteem.

more troubling than being moderately devalued. Similarly, once relational value reaches a moderately high level, further increases in relational value do not affect state self-esteem, probably for the same reason. Once people value and accept us moderately, increases in our relational value rarely have additional benefits. Thus, beyond a certain point, there is little reason for the system to respond to increasing acceptance.

Between neutral and high relational value, however, small changes in relational value have notable consequences. Being relationally valued just a little is certainly more advantageous than being viewed neutrally, and being valued moderately is better than being valued just a little. As a result, people are sensitive to gradations in relational value in this range.

Trait Self-Esteem

Trait self-esteem—a person's typical or average level of self-esteem—is also relevant to interpersonal self-regulation. If we view the sociometer as a gauge that assesses relational value, then trait self-esteem is the resting position of the sociometer in the absence of incoming interpersonal feedback. It is where the indicator on the gauge rests when explicit cues relevant to one's relational value are not present.

The sociometer of a person with high trait self-esteem rests at a relatively high position, indicating a high degree of relational value when it is in "standby mode" (Figure 18.2A). Because of past experiences, such individuals implicitly assume that they are generally acceptable people with whom others value having relationships. Trait self-esteem correlates highly with the degree to which people believe that they are acceptable individuals who possess attributes that other people value (see Denissen et al., 2008; Leary & MacDonald, 2003; Leary, Tambor, et al., 1995; Lemay & Ashmore, 2006; MacDonald, Saltzman, & Leary, 2003).

In contrast, the sociometer of a person with low trait self-esteem rests at a point indicating a low to moderate degree of relational value (Figure 18.2B). Theorists have noted that people who score "low" on measures of trait self-esteem rarely possess truly low self-esteem. Rather, their feelings about themselves are neutral or mixed, often with some combination of positive and negative judgments (Baumeister, Tice, & Hutton, 1989).

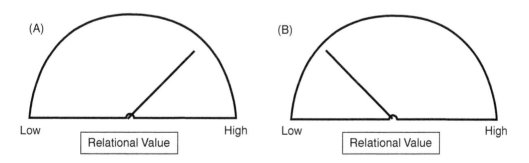

FIGURE 18.2. (A) The sociometer of a person with high trait self-esteem rests in a position that indicates relatively high relational value in the absence of incoming interpersonal feedback. (B) The sociometer of a person with low trait self-esteem rests in a relatively low position in the absence of incoming interpersonal feedback.

This suggests that few people's sociometers chronically register no relational value, probably because most people have a least a few people who value relationships with them.

Viewed from the sociometer perspective, what are typically regarded as effects of trait self-esteem are more accurately conceptualized as the effects of a sociometer that tends to operate in a particular range of relational value. Because of the set points of their sociometers, people with low versus high self-esteem react to acceptance and rejection differently (Nezlek, Kowalski, Leary, Blevins, & Holgate, 1997). For example, people with low trait self-esteem are not anxious, depressed, jealous, lonely, or rejection-sensitive *because* they have low self-esteem (as others have suggested) but because they go through life detecting a relatively low degree of relational value. Likewise, people with low self-esteem do not engage in the array of dysfunctional behaviors attributed to them *because* they have low self-esteem (Heaven, 1986; Kaplan, 1980; Rosenberg, Schooler, & Schoenbach, 1989) but because they regularly detect inadequate acceptance in their interpersonal environments and, thus, resort to extreme measures to boost their relational value (Leary, 1999; Leary, Schreindorfer, & Haupt, 1995).

It may be tempting to conclude that people who score low in trait self-esteem suffer from poorly calibrated sociometers, but that is not necessarily the case. Many people with low trait self-esteem have well-calibrated sociometers that accurately detect their relatively low degree of relational value. However, some people with low self-esteem probably detect lower relational evaluation from others than actually exists, and their sociometers can be viewed as miscalibrated. In the following sections, we examine ways in which a miscalibrated sociometer may lead to emotional distress and problems with self-regulation.

When the Sociometer Is Set Too Low

One type of miscalibration occurs when the sociometer is set "too low"—that is, when it detects less relational value in the interpersonal environment than actually exists. This situation, which is shown in Figure 18.3, is comparable to a fuel gauge that indicates less gas in the tank than there really is (causing the driver to be more anxious about running out of gas than is warranted).

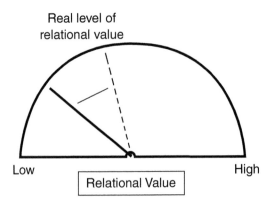

FIGURE 18.3. A person with a sociometer that is calibrated low chronically experiences less relational value (and, thus, lower self-esteem) than is warranted by the situation.

One consequence of this kind of miscalibration is an oversensitivity to cues that connote relational devaluation. The system will register a high proportion of false positives, interpreting benign (or even mildly favorable) interpersonal events as potential threats to acceptance. Because this miscalibrated sociometer responds as if relational value is unacceptably low, the person experiences frequent episodes of low state self-esteem, along with rejection-related emotions, such as social anxiety, jealousy, guilt, and embarrassment (Leary et al., 2001; Leary & MacDonald, 2003) and interpersonal defensiveness (Wood, Heimpel, Manwell, & Whittington, 2009).

Of course, people who have low trait self-esteem do not necessarily have miscalibrated sociometers; many people with low self-esteem accurately perceive that they have low relational value to others; thus, their sociometers are working properly. However, some people who have low trait self-esteem may be biased to perceive less acceptance than actually exists. Koch (2002) found that people who scored low in trait self-esteem tend to respond to evaluatively ambiguous primes as though they were negative. Similarly, people who feel less valued by their spouses are more likely to perceive benign or ambiguous spousal behavior (e.g., partner being in a bad mood) as rejecting and consequently feel worse about themselves the next day (Murray, Griffin, Rose, & Bellavia, 2003).

Having such an improperly calibrated sociometer compromises the person's ability to self-regulate optimally. By responding to interpersonal events as though they connote lower relational value than is the case, people overreact, both emotionally and behaviorally. Such reactions can become self-fulfilling prophecy because people who often feel devalued often pull back from or attack relational partners, leading those individuals to withdraw (DeHart, Pelham, & Murray, 2004; Downey, Freitas, Michealis, & Khouri, 1998; Murray, Holmes, MacDonald, & Ellsworth, 1998). Not surprisingly, then, the degree to which people's self-esteem was influenced by their partners' actions on a day-to-day basis predicted relationship decline over the course of a year for both partners (Murray, Bellavia, Rose, & Griffin, 2003). People with low self-esteem are also more likely to base their social decisions on the likelihood of being accepted by their peers (Anthony, Wood, & Holmes, 2007), and their unwillingness to take social risks limits the number of new people and groups with which they become acquainted, lowering their opportunities of being accepted, thus maintaining their level of low self-esteem.

When the Sociometer Is Set Too High

The sociometer may also be set "too high"—like a fuel gauge that indicates more gas than is actually in the tank (see Figure 18.4). In this case, people chronically detect that others value them more as social interactants and relational partners than they actually do. Subjectively, such an optimistic miscalibration may seem beneficial because the person has high self-esteem and rarely experiences the aversive emotions associated with feeling devalued or rejected. Indeed, the prevailing view has been that positive illusions regarding one's acceptability and worth are psychologically beneficial (Murray, Holmes, & Griffin, 1996; Taylor & Brown, 1988).

However, if we think of self-esteem and affect as the output of a sociometer designed for interpersonal self-regulation, the fallacy of this view becomes apparent. A sociometer that is calibrated too high (as in Figure 18.4) leads people to overestimate their relational value and, thus, show inadequate concern for how others perceive and evaluate them. Such a miscalibrated sociometer will fail to warn them when their acceptance by other people

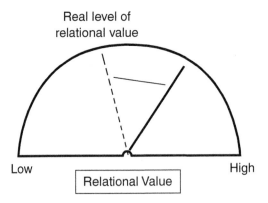

FIGURE 18.4. A person with a sociometer that is calibrated high chronically experiences greater relational value (thus, higher self-esteem) than is warranted by the situation.

is in jeopardy. Although a driver on a lonely stretch of highway may take great comfort in seeing that the fuel gauge is well above "Empty," this consolation is badly misplaced if the gas tank is actually running dry. Social life requires that people understand how they are perceived, evaluated, and accepted by others. Although it is sometimes wise to disregard others' evaluations, effective behavior cannot be predicated on erroneous perceptions of other people's reactions. Believing that one's relational value is higher than it is results in negative consequences for both the individual and those with whom he or she interacts.

At minimum, the person whose sociometer is calibrated too high will be disliked, if not rejected, for being haughty, conceited, or snobbish (Leary, Bednarski, Hammon, & Duncan, 1997). Worse, people who overestimate their relational value (and have undeservedly high self-esteem) tend to influence, dominate, and exploit other people (Emmons, 1984). They also tend to respond defensively and aggressively to suggestions that they are not as wonderful as their sociometers suggest (Baumeister, Smart, & Boden, 1996; Emmons, 1984). Furthermore, people who believe they have generally high relational value may be insufficiently restrained in mistreating or hurting other people because they assume they are so highly valued. In part, a well-placed concern for potential rejection helps to keep behavior within socially acceptable bounds.

The extreme case of this miscalibration is narcissism, in which people feel more special, important, and self-satisfied than objective feedback warrants (Raskin, Novacek, & Hogan, 1991). Conceptualizing narcissism as arising from a sociometer that is calibrated too high helps to explain the paradox of why narcissists have grandiose self-views yet react strongly to criticism. With a sociometer that is set too high, narcissists feel better about themselves than they objectively ought to feel. Thus, when they receive clear-cut feedback indicating that other people do not value and accept them, a discrepancy arises between how they feel about themselves and how other people feel about them. Because the powerful, subjective reality of their miscalibrated sociometer convinces them that they are important or valuable, they conclude that other people's negative evaluations are biased and unfair, and this sense of being devalued unfairly produces their defensiveness and anger. On occasion, unable to discount negative feedback and rejection, a narcissist may realize that his or her relational value is not as high as assumed, resulting in a devastating crash in self-esteem.

The problems that arise for people whose sociometers are calibrated too high highlight the risks of raising people's self-esteem artificially. Although psychologists, educators, and politicians have advocated raising self-esteem as a way to improve mental health, decrease maladaptive behavior, and eliminate social problems (Mecca et al., 1989), raising self-esteem in a manner that is not commensurate with people's true relational value is a recipe for disaster. Convincing people that they are acceptable, worthy, and lovable individuals despite the fact that they regularly treat others in unacceptable ways is analogous to adjusting one's fuel gauge so that it shows more gas in the tank than there is. The person may feel temporarily good about circumstances but suffer negative consequences in the long run (Robins & Beer, 2001).

When the Sociometer Is Excessively or Insufficiently Sensitive

Some people's sociometers underreact or overreact to cues that are relevant to relational value. Having a sociometer that is either excessively or insufficiently sensitive to interpersonal appraisals creates yet other problems with interpersonal self-regulation.

Hypersensitivity

An overactive sociometer leads people to experience extreme swings in affect and state self-esteem on the basis of minor changes in the interpersonal environment. Mild signs of acceptance may evoke high self-esteem and euphoria, and mild signs of disinterest or disapproval may crush self-esteem and elicit despair (see Figure 18.5).

This seems to be the case for people with unstable self-esteem. Kernis and Goldman (2003) suggested that unstable self-esteem reflects "fragile, vulnerable feelings of immediate self-worth that are influenced by potentially self-relevant events" (p. 114). This view is undoubtedly correct, and sociometer theory helps to explain the source of highly variable self-esteem. When the sociometer overresponds to events that are relevant to relational value, people display swings in self-esteem that are out of proportion to the evaluative implications of those events. Indeed, the personality factors associated with unstable self-esteem are those that characterize a person with an unstable sociometer. For example, high dependence on other people makes their reactions particularly important, an impov-

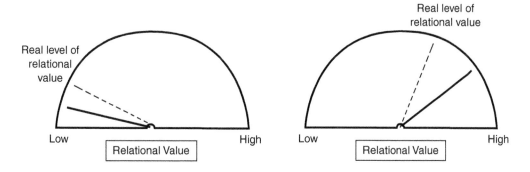

FIGURE 18.5. A person with a hypersensitive sociometer experiences greater swings in perceived relational value (thus, self-esteem) than are warranted by the situation.

erished self-concept fails to provide an anchor from which one can assess one's relational value independently of immediate feedback, and overreliance on social approval renders one's value in other people's eyes more important than it needs to be (see Butler, Hokanson, & Flynn, 1994; Kernis, Paradise, Whitaker, Wheatman, & Goldman, 2000). The literature on self-esteem instability (see Kernis & Goldman, 2003) can be integrated, if we assume that people with unstable self-esteem have hyperactive sociometers.

A person's attachment style is also related to self-regulation, and the sociometer may be involved. Srivastava and Beer (2005) suggested that anxiously attached individuals have a reactive sociometer because they employ hyperactive strategies to monitor others' reactions to them and are more vigilant to signs of possible acceptance and rejection. Additionally, Pietromonaco and Barrett (2006) found that nonsecurely attached individuals are more likely than securely attached individuals to seek acceptance and liking from others. In particular, people with a preoccupied attachment style are more likely to rely on others for help in regulating what they think and feel about themselves, and their evaluations of themselves are associated with the degree to which they feel cared for and understood by another person.

Hyposensitivity

A hypoactive sociometer is relatively insensitive to changes in relational value (see Figure 18.6). Large changes in one's relational value to other people result in only slight movement in the sociometer and negligible changes in state self-esteem. A sociometer that does not react to interpersonal feedback cannot adequately assess the person's relational value. Although instances arise in which a person ought to disregard other people's reactions, chronically doing so leads the person to be ostracized by everyone because he or she fails to react intelligently to situations that ought to convey low or declining relational value.

In extreme cases, people's sociometers are essentially out of service. If being valued and adored has the same subjective effect as being devalued and detested, then the person is incapable of interpersonal self-regulation. The person who rarely experiences anxiety, hurt feelings, or guilt in situations in which others dislike, detest, or ostracize him or her may have a broken sociometer. Although no direct evidence bears on this point, one exemplar of an insensitive or "stuck" sociometer would seem to be the antisocial (or

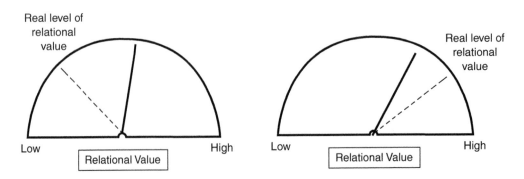

FIGURE 18.6. A person with a hyposensitive sociometer experiences smaller changes in perceived relational value (thus, self-esteem) than are warranted by the situation.

sociopathic) personality, which is characterized by impaired empathy and a weak conscience. The selfish, manipulative, and hurtful behaviors of the person with antisocial personality disorder seem to stem from indifference to how his or her actions are perceived and evaluated by other people, and to the ostracism that often results. A person with an antisocial personality is deceitful, egocentric, irresponsible, and manipulative (Lykken, 1995)—characteristics that most people try to avoid because they likely lead to rejection. This is not to say that an out-of-order sociometer lies at the heart of sociopathy (although it might), but it does suggest that sociopaths have broken sociometers.

SECONDARY SATISFACTION OF SELF-ESTEEM

As noted, sociometer theory suggests that people's apparent efforts to protect their self-esteem stem from an interest in maintaining their relational value to other people. Although it is easy to see how public behaviors may enhance one's image and value to other people, one can ask whether people sometimes try to maintain self-esteem in their own heads.

The ability to self-reflect allows people to override their natural and immediate reactions by reconstruing the personal meaning of events. As a result, people sometimes interpret events that objectively ought to make them feel bad about themselves in ways that allow them to maintain self-esteem. In essence, people can cognitively override the sociometer. One such example involves implicit self-esteem compensation, whereby people experience a boost in self-esteem after their belongingness is threatened (Rudman, Dohn, & Fairchild, 2007). Compensatory cognitive strategies help to buffer against threats, but there has been considerable debate regarding whether these self-serving biases or positive illusions are beneficial to people's well-being (Colvin & Block, 1994; Robins & Beer, 2001; Taylor & Brown, 1988).

Viewing self-esteem as a sociometer involved in self-regulation suggests that these biases and illusions are probably detrimental. The sociometer effectively regulates interpersonal relations only to the extent that it provides a reasonably accurate picture of other people's reactions to the individual vis-à-vis acceptance and rejection. In overriding and fooling the system, positive illusions increase the likelihood of misregulation. Positive illusions about the self undoubtedly make people feel better and, occasionally, allow them to maintain a positive attitude and motivation in the face of adversity. But, over the long haul, positive illusions circumvent the sociometer's function. Convincing oneself that one is more acceptable than one actually is makes no more sense than convincing oneself that the car's gas tank contains more gasoline than it really does. It may make one feel better temporarily but, to the extent that it deters appropriate or remediative action, the ultimate outcome will often be negative.

CONCLUSIONS

Conceptualizing the sociometer as a psychological mechanism that monitors people's social environments and helps them minimize the likelihood of rejection is helpful in thinking about the self-regulation of interpersonal behavior. Research supports the idea that people possess a regulatory mechanism that responds to changes in relational value, and the concept of a sociometer provides an overarching framework for conceptualizing a variety of phenomena, such as self-esteem, interpersonal emotions, reactions to rejection, individual differences in rejection sensitivity, and personality disorders (particularly the narcissistic and antisocial disorders). Importantly, the metaphor of the sociometer as a psychological gauge of relational value may also provide insights into what goes wrong when people self-regulate in dysfunctional ways that damage their relationships with other people.

REFERENCES

Anthony, D., Wood, J., & Holmes, J. (2007). Testing sociometer theory: Self-esteem and the importance of acceptance for social decision making. *Journal of Experimental Social Psychology, 43,* 425–432.

Baumeister, R. F., Heatherton, T. F., & Tice, D. M. (1994). *Losing control: How and why people fail at self-regulation.* San Diego, CA: Academic Press.

Baumeister, R. F., & Leary, M. R. (1995). The need to belong: Desire for interpersonal attachments as a fundamental human motivation. *Psychological Bulletin, 117,* 497–529.

Baumeister, B. F., Smart, L., & Boden, J. M. (1996). Relation of threatened egotism to violence and aggression: The dark side of high self-esteem. *Psychological Review, 103,* 5–33.

Baumeister, R. F., Tice, D. M., & Hutton, D. G. (1989). Self-presentational motivations and personality differences in self-esteem. *Journal of Personality, 57,* 547–579.

Butler, A. C., Hokanson, J. E., & Flynn, H. A. (1994). A comparison of self-esteem lability and low self-esteem as vulnerability factors for depression. *Journal of Personality and Social Psychology, 66,* 166–177.

Carver, C. S., & Scheier, M. F. (1981). *Attention and self-regulation: A control theory approach to human behavior.* New York: Springer-Verlag.

Cherry, E. C. (1953). Some experiments on the recognition of speech, with one and with two ears. *Journal of Acoustical Society of America, 25,* 975–979.

Colvin, C. R., & Block, J. (1994). Do positive illusions foster mental health?: An examination of the Taylor and Brown formulation. *Psychological Bulletin, 116,* 3–20.

Deci, E. L., & Ryan, R. M. (1995). Human agency: The basis for true self-esteem. In M. H. Kernis (Ed.), *Efficacy, agency, and self-esteem* (pp. 31–50). New York: Plenum Press.

DeHart, T., Pelham, B., & Murray, S. (2004). Implicit dependency regulation: Self-esteem, relationship closeness, and implicit evaluations of close others. *Social Cognition, 22,* 126–146.

Denissen, J. J. A., Penke, L., Schmitt, D. P., & van Aken, M. A. G. (2008). Self-esteem reactions to social interactions: Evidence for sociometer mechanisms across days, people, and nations. *Journal of Personality and Social Psychology, 95,* 181–196.

Downey, G., Freitas, A. L., Michealis, B., & Khouri, H. (1998). The self-fulfilling prophecy in close relationships: Do rejection sensitive women get rejected by romantic partners? *Journal of Personality and Social Psychology, 75,* 545–560.

Emmons, R. A. (1984). Factor analysis and construct validity of the Narcissistic Personality Inventory. *Journal of Personality Assessment, 48,* 291–300.

Guay, F., Delisle, M., Fernet, C., Julien, É., & Senécal, C. (2008). Does task-related identified regulation moderate the sociometer effect?: A study of performance feedback, perceived inclusion, and state self-esteem. *Social Behavior and Personality, 36,* 239–254.

Haupt, A. L., & Leary, M. R. (1997). The appeal of worthless groups: Moderating effects of trait self-esteem. *Group Dynamics: Theory, Research, and Practice, 1,* 124–132.

Heaven, P. C. (1986). Correlates of conformity in three cultures. *Journal of Personality and Social Psychology, 54,* 883–887.

Kaplan, H. B. (1980). *Deviant behavior in defense of self.* New York: Academic Press.

Kernis, M. H., & Goldman, B. M. (2003). Stability and variability in self-concept and self-esteem. In M. R. Leary & J. P. Tangney (Eds.), *Handbook of self and identity* (pp. 106–127). New York: Guilford Press.

Kernis, M. H., Paradise, A. W., Whitaker, D., Wheatman, S., & Goldman, B. (2000). Master of one's psychological domain?: Not likely if one's self-esteem is unstable. *Personality and Social Psychology Bulletin, 26,* 1297–1305.

Koch, E. J. (2002). Relational schemas, self-esteem, and the processing of social stimuli. *Self and Identity, 1,* 271–279.

Leary, M. R. (2001). Toward a conceptualization of interpersonal rejection. In M. R. Leary (Ed.), *Interpersonal rejection* (pp. 3–20). New York: Oxford University Press.

Leary, M. R. (2002). The interpersonal basis of self-esteem: Death, devaluation, or deference? In J. Forgas & K. D. Williams (Eds.), *The social self: Cognitive, interpersonal, and intergroup perspectives* (pp. 143–159). New York: Psychology Press.

Leary, M. R. (2006). Sociometer theory and the pursuit of relational value: Getting to the root of self-esteem. *European Review of Social Psychology, 16,* 75–111.

Leary, M. R., & Allen, A. B. (in press). Belonging motivation: Establishing, maintaining, and repairing relational value. In D. Dunning (Ed.), *Social motivation.* New York: Psychology Press.

Leary, M. R., & Baumeister, R. F. (2000). The nature and function of self-esteem: Sociometer theory. In M. P. Zanna (Ed.), *Advances in experimental social psychology* (Vol. 32, pp. 1–62). San Diego, CA: Academic Press.

Leary, M. R., Bednarski, R., Hammon, D., & Duncan, T. (1997). Blowhards, snobs, and narcissists: Interpersonal reactions to excessive egotism. In R. M. Kowalski (Ed.), *Aversive interpersonal behaviors* (pp. 111–131). New York: Plenum Press.

Leary, M. R., & Buttermore, N. (2003). The evolution of the human self: Tracing the natural history of self-reflection. *Journal for the Theory of Social Behaviour, 33,* 365–404.

Leary, M. R., & Downs, D. L. (1995). Interpersonal functions of the self-esteem motive: The self-esteem system as a sociometer. In M. Kernis (Ed.), *Efficacy, agency, and self-esteem* (pp. 123–144). New York: Plenum Press.

Leary, M. R., Gallagher, B., Fors, E. H., Buttermore, N., Baldwin, E., Lane, K. K., et al. (2003). The invalidity of personal claims about self-esteem. *Personality and Social Psychology Bulletin, 29,* 623–636.

Leary, M. R., Haupt, A. L., Strausser, K. S., & Chokel, J. T. (1998). Calibrating the sociometer: The relationship between interpersonal appraisals and state self-esteem. *Journal of Personality and Social Psychology, 74,* 1290–1299.

Leary, M. R., Koch, E., & Hechenbleikner, N. (2001). Emotional responses to interpersonal rejection. In M. R. Leary (Ed.), *Interpersonal rejection* (pp. 145–166). New York: Oxford University Press.

Leary, M. R., & MacDonald, G. (2003). Individual differences in self-esteem: A review and theoretical integration. In M. R. Leary & J. P. Tangney (Eds.), *Handbook of self and identity* (pp. 401–418). New York: Guilford Press.

Leary, M. R., Schreindorfer, L. S., & Haupt, A. L. (1995). The role of low self-esteem in emotional and behavioral problems: Why is low self-esteem dysfunctional? *Journal of Social and Clinical Psychology, 14,* 297–314.

Leary, M. R., Tambor, E., Terdal, S., & Downs, D. L. (1995). Self-esteem as an interpersonal monitor: The sociometer hypothesis. *Journal of Personality and Social Psychology, 68,* 518–530.

Lemay, E., & Ashmore, R. (2006). The relationship of social approval contingency to trait self-esteem: Cause, consequence, or moderator? *Journal of Research in Personality, 40,* 121–139.

Lykken, D. T. (1995). *The antisocial personalities.* Hillsdale, NJ: Erlbaum.

MacDonald, G., Saltzman, J. L., & Leary, M. R. (2003). Social approval and trait self-esteem. *Journal of Research in Personality, 37,* 23–40.

Mecca, A. M., Smelser, N. J., & Vasconcellos, J. (1989). *The social importance of self-esteem.* Berkeley: University of California Press.

Mischel, W. (1996). From good intentions to willpower. In P. M. Gollwitzer & J. A. Bargh (Eds.), *The psychology of action: Linking cognition and motivation to behavior* (pp. 197–218). New York: Guilford Press.

Murray, S. L., Bellavia, G., Rose, P., & Griffin, D. W. (2003). Once hurt, twice hurtful: How perceived regard regulates daily marital interaction. *Journal of Personality and Social Psychology, 84,* 126–147.

Murray, S. L., Griffin, D. W., Rose, P., & Bellavia, G. M. (2003). Calibrating the sociometer: The relational contingencies of self-esteem. *Journal of Personality and Social Psychology, 85,* 63–84.

Murray, S. L., Holmes, J. G., & Griffin, D. W. (1996). The benefits of positive illusions: Idealization and the construction of satisfaction in close relationships. *Journal of Personality and Social Psychology, 70,* 79–98.

Murray, S. L., Holmes, J. G., MacDonald, G., & Ellsworth, P. C. (1998). Through the looking glass darkly?: When self-doubts turn into relationship insecurities. *Journal of Personality and Social Psychology, 75,* 1459–1480.

Nezlek, J. B., Kowalski, R. M., Leary, M. R., Blevins, T., & Holgate, S. (1997). Personality moderators of reactions to interpersonal rejection: Depression and trait self-esteem. *Personality and Social Psychology Bulletin, 23,* 1235–1244.

Pietromonaco, P., & Barrett, L. (2006). What can you do for me?: Attachment style and motives underlying esteem for partners. *Journal of Research in Personality, 40,* 313–338.

Raskin, R., Novacek, J., & Hogan, R. (1991). Narcissism, self-esteem, and defensive self-enhancement. *Journal of Personality, 59,* 19–38.

Robins, R. W., & Beer, J. S. (2001). Positive illusions about the self: Short-term benefits and long-term costs. *Journal of Personality and Social Psychology, 80,* 340–352.

Rosenberg, M., Schooler, C., & Schoenbach, C. (1989). Self-esteem and adolescent problems: Modeling reciprocal effects. *American Sociological Review, 54,* 1004–1018.

Rudman, L., Dohn, M., & Fairchild, K. (2007). Implicit self-esteem compensation: Automatic threat defense. *Journal of Personality and Social Psychology, 93,* 798–813.

Samuels, R. (2000). Massively modular minds: Evolutionary psychology and cognitive architecture. In P. Carruthers & A. Chamberlain (Eds.), *Evolution and the human mind* (pp. 13–46). Cambridge, UK: Cambridge University Press.

Srivastava, S., & Beer, J. (2005). How self-evaluations relate to being liked by others: Integrating sociometer and attachment perspectives. *Journal of Personality and Social Psychology, 89,* 966–977.

Taylor, S. E., & Brown, J. D. (1988). Illusion and well-being: A social psychological perspective on mental health. *Psychological Bulletin, 116,* 193–210.

Weisbuch, M., Sinclair, S. A., Skorinko, J. L., & Eccleston, C. P. (2009). Self-esteem depends on the beholder: Effects of subtle value cue. *Journal of Experimental Social Psychology, 45,* 143–148.

Wood, J. V., Heimpel, S. A., Manwell, L. A., & Whittington, E. J. (2009). This mood is familiar and I don't deserve to feel better anyway: Mechanisms underlying self-esteem differences in motivation to repair sad moods. *Journal of Personality and Social Psychology, 96,* 363–380.

CHAPTER 19

Early Attachment Processes and the Development of Emotional Self-Regulation

SUSAN D. CALKINS
ESTHER M. LEERKES

The construct of emotional self-regulation and its role in successful adaptation has been examined quite extensively, particularly in the early childhood period. Drawing from theoretical and empirical work in the developmental (Cole, Martin, & Dennis, 2004) and clinical fields (Keenan, 2000; Sroufe, 2000), we define *emotional self-regulation* as those behaviors, skills, and strategies, whether conscious or unconscious, automatic or effortful, that serve to modulate, inhibit, and enhance emotional experiences and expressions. The capacity to exercise self-control over the expression of emotion, particularly negative emotions, develops over the first years of life and has particular importance for the unfolding of appropriate and adaptive social behavior during the preschool (i.e., 3 to 5 years) and early school years (i.e., 6 to 12 years) (Eisenberg & Fabes, 2006; Eisenberg, Smith, & Spinrad, Chapter 14, this volume). Furthermore, the lack of adequate development of control over emotion (as well as, in some instances, overcontrol of emotion) may be a precursor to the development of psychopathology (Calkins & Dedmon, 2000; Calkins & Fox, 2002; Cicchetti, Ackerman, & Izard, 1995; Keenan, 2000).

The broad construct of emotional self-regulation has been studied in many ways, including the examination of specific strategies and their effects on affective experience and expression. For example, research reveals that specific emotion regulation strategies, such as self-comforting, help seeking, and distraction, may assist the young child in managing early temperament-driven frustration and fear responses in situations where the control of negative emotions may be necessary (Stifter & Braungart, 1995). Moreover, emotion regulation skills may be useful in situations that elicit positive affective arousal, in that they allow the child to keep such arousal within a manageable and pleasurable range (Grolnick, Cosgrove, & Bridges, 1996). Failure to acquire adaptive emotional regulation skills leads to difficulties in areas such as social competence and school adjustment (Eisenberg & Fabes, 2006; Graziano, Reavis, Keane, & Calkins, 2007). Thus, the acquisition of emotion regulation skills and strategies is considered a critical achievement of early childhood (Bronson, 2000; Sroufe, 1996).

One important assumption of much of the research on the acquisition of emotional self-regulation is that parental caregiving practices may support or undermine such development, thus contributing to observed individual differences among young children's emotional skills (Morris, Silk, Steinberg, Myers, & Robinson, 2007; Thompson, 1994). In infancy, there is an almost exclusive reliance on parents for the regulation of emotion. Over time, interactions with parents in emotion-laden contexts teach children that the use of particular strategies may be more useful than other strategies for the reduction of emotional arousal (Sroufe, 1996). Although caregiving practices are often attributed a role in the development of emotion regulation, the specific processes by which these practices affect children's development are often left unspecified (Fox & Calkins, 2003).

One hypothesis about the way in which caregiving practices affect developing emotion regulation is through the emerging attachment relationship and the experience, over the course of infancy, of attachment-related processes. Attachment processes are often activated in emotionally evocative contexts and serve specific emotion regulatory functions. Thus, it is likely that they contribute to the acquisition of the repertoire of self-regulated emotional skills that develops in the child over the course of infancy and toddlerhood.

In this chapter, we examine the early development of emotional self-regulation processes across the first 2 years of life. First, we briefly review the emergence of these processes as a function of normative development in the affective, motor, and cognitive domains. Next, we address the role of specific types of attachment experiences within the family context, and examine both short-term and long-term emotional consequences of attachment processes. We conclude with recommendations for future research, including an examination of the integration of different levels of self-regulation and a focus on mechanisms that explain the effects of attachment processes on these multiple levels.

EMOTIONAL REGULATION IN EARLY CHILDHOOD: NORMATIVE DEVELOPMENT

Dramatic developments are observed during the infancy and toddler periods of development in terms of emotional self-regulation skills and abilities. The process may be broadly described as one in which the relatively passive and reactive neonate becomes a child capable of self-initiated behaviors that serve a regulatory function (Calkins, 1994; Kopp, 1982; Sroufe, 1996). This process has also been described as one in which the infant progresses from near complete reliance on caregivers for regulation to independent self-regulation. As the infant makes this transition, specific strategies and behaviors become organized into the infant's repertoire of emotional self-regulation that may be used in a variety of contexts.

Kopp (1982) provides an excellent overview of the early developments in emotional self-regulation. This description has been verified by studies of both normative development (Buss & Goldsmith, 1998; Rothbart, Ziaie, & O'Boyle, 1992) and individual differences (Stifter & Braungart, 1995). These descriptions provide an explanation of how infants develop and utilize a rich behavioral repertoire of strategies in the service of reducing, inhibiting, amplifying, and balancing different affective responses. It is also clear from these descriptions that functioning in a variety of nonemotional domains, including motor, language and cognition, and social development, is implicated in these changes (Kopp, 1989, 1992).

Early efforts at emotional self-regulation, those occurring prior to about 3 months of age, are thought to be controlled largely by physiological mechanisms that are innate (Kopp, 1982). By 3 months of age, primitive mechanisms of self-soothing, such as sucking, simple motor movements (e.g., turning away), and reflexive signaling in response to discomfort, often in the form of crying, are the primary processes operating, independent of caregiver intervention (Kopp, 1982; Rothbart et al., 1992).

The period between 3 and 6 months of age marks a major transition in infant development. First, sleep–wake cycles and eating and elimination processes have become more predictable, signaling an important biological transition. Second, the ability of the infant to control arousal levels voluntarily begins to emerge. This control depends largely on attentional control mechanisms and simple motor skills (Rothbart, Ellis, & Posner, Chapter 24, this volume; Rothbart et al., 1992; Ruff & Rothbart, 1996), and leads to coordinated use of attention engagement and disengagement, particularly in contexts that evoke negative affect. Infants are now capable of engaging in self-initiated distraction, moving attention away from the source of negative arousal to more neutral, nonsocial stimuli. For example, the ability to shift attention away from a negative event (e.g., something frightening) to a positive distracter leads to decreases in the experience of negative affect (Crockenberg & Leerkes, 2004). Importantly, though, there are clear individual differences in the ability to utilize attention successfully to control emotion and behavior. Rothbart (1986) found increases in positive affect and decreases in infants' distress from 3 to 6 months during episodes of focused attention, suggesting that attentional control is tied to affective experience. Moreover, the experience of negative affect is believed to interfere with the child's ability to explore and learn about the environment (Ruff & Rothbart, 1996). Consequently, there are clear implications of early emotional self-regulation for development in a range of domains.

By the end of first year of life, infants become much more active and purposeful in their attempts to control affective arousal (Kopp, 1982). First, they begin to employ organized sequences of motor behavior that enable them to reach, retreat, redirect, and self-soothe in a flexible manner that suggests they are responsive to environmental cues. Second, their signaling and redirection become explicitly social as they recognize that caregivers and others may behave in a way that will assist them in the regulation of affective states (Rothbart et al., 1992).

During the second year of life, the transition from passive to active methods of emotional self-regulation is complete (Rothbart et al., 1992). Although infants are not entirely capable of controlling their own affective states by this age, they are capable of using specific strategies to attempt to manage different affective states, albeit sometimes unsuccessfully (Calkins & Dedmon, 2000; Calkins, Gill, Johnson, & Smith, 1999). Moreover, during this period, infants begin to respond to caregiver directives and, as a consequence of this responsivity, compliance and behavioral self-control begin to emerge (Kopp, 1989). This shift is supported by developments in the motor domain, as well as changes in representational ability and the development of language skills. Brain maturation contributes as well, and by the end of toddlerhood, children have executive control abilities that allow control of arousal, regulation of affective expression, and inhibition and activation of behavior (Bronson, 2000).

Empirical evidence supports the notion that both biological and innate dispositions, such as the temperamental disposition of the child, certain cognitive skills, and the underlying neural and physiological systems that support and are engaged in the processes of control, and environmental experiences, such as the manner in which caregivers socialize emotional responses in the child, contribute to emerging emotional self-regulation (Fox & Calkins, 2003; Raikes, Robinson, Bradley, Raikes, & Ayoub, 2007). Clearly, though, emotional self-regulatory processes begin to develop in the context of dyadic interactions (Sroufe, 1996). Such interactions contribute to both normative developments and individual variability in emotional self-regulation (Cassidy, 1994). Although multiple dimensions of caregiving may contribute to the development of self-regulation (Eisenberg, Cumberland, & Spinrad, 1998; Morris et al., 2007), one important dimension of the dyadic relationship is the attachment relationship that develops between caregivers and infants over the first year of life. In the next section, attachment theory is reviewed briefly, with an emphasis on the way in which attachment processes affect developing emotional self-regulation.

ATTACHMENT PROCESSES IN EARLY EMOTIONAL DEVELOPMENT

Current theorizing about childhood attachment and its role in emotional functioning and behavioral adjustment has its roots in the work of John Bowlby (1969/1982), whose evolutionary theory of attachment emphasizes the biological adaptiveness of specific attachment behaviors displayed during the infancy period. Such behaviors permit the infant to initiate and maintain contact with the primary caregiver, which serves a survival purpose (Bowlby, 1988). In typical development, infants exhibit a repertoire of behaviors, including looking, crying, and clinging, that allow them to signal and elicit support from the primary caregiver in times of external threat. Bowlby argued that, by the end of the first year of life, the interactive history between the infant and caregiver, including times of stress or external threat, produces an attachment relationship that provides a sense of security for the infant and significantly influences the child's subsequent adaptation to a variety of challenges (Bowlby, 1988).

Bowlby hypothesized that the mechanism through which early parent–child attachment affects later functioning is via the *internal working model*, a cognitive representation of the self and the caregiver that is constructed out of repeated early interactions. Such representations provide the infant and/or young child with a guide to expectations about his or her own emotional responding, and the likelihood and success of caregiver intervention in managing this affective responding. Thus, the experience of sensitive caregiving was hypothesized to lead to a secure attachment and expectations that emotional needs would either be met by the caregiver or be managed with skills developed through interactions with the caregiver.

Numerous developmental scientists have conducted tests of Bowlby's theory, though Mary Ainsworth, the most noted, conducted pioneering naturalistic and observational studies that focused on individual differences in mother–infant attachment relationships (Ainsworth, Blehar, Waters, & Wall, 1978). Ainsworth theorized that while all infants become attached to primary caregivers, the quality of this attachment varies as a function of the relationship history. She developed an empirical paradigm, the Strange Situation, to assess individual variation in infants' exploratory and security-seeking behaviors during a series of brief, but increasingly stressful episodes that comprised interactions with a stranger, and separations from and reunions with the caregiver. On the basis of infant behavior displayed in the Strange Situation, particularly those behaviors that reflected the dyad's ability to manage stress, she characterized infants as securely or insecurely attached, with either resistant or avoidant profiles. Secure infants engaged in exploration and positive affect sharing during the low-stress context, and proximity seeking in the high stress context of separation, and were comforted upon the mother's return. In contrast, insecurity was indexed by either heightened distress and difficulty calming (referred to as *resistance* or *ambivalence*), or active avoidance of the caregiver during the high-stress context of separation. More recent research with high-risk samples led to the identification of a fourth group. Disorganized infants engage in contradictory and odd behaviors during the Strange Situation that appear to reflect the lack of a single coherent attachment strategy (e.g., freezing, stereotypies) (Main & Solomon, 1990). Importantly, Ainsworth and numerous others (see De Wolff & Van IJzendoorn, 1997, for a review) reported that the quality of different types of attachment relationships could be predicted by the quality of maternal caregiving observed during the first year of life. Ainsworth argued that experience of consistent sensitive and responsive caregiving teaches the infant about appropriate expectations regarding others and allows the infant to experience a reduction in arousal level as a consequence of caregiver behaviors (Ainsworth et al., 1978). Over time, the infant's supported and independent use of regulatory strategies is reinforced by the accompanying reduction in arousal and positive reinforcement from the mother. As a consequence, the infant is able to develop a sense of efficacy in the ability to self-regulate (Bell & Ainsworth, 1972).

More recently, Sroufe (1996) has argued that emotional development is inextricably linked with social development, with the course of emotional development described as the transition from dyadic regulation of affect to self-regulation of affect. He argues that the ability to self-regulate arousal levels is embedded in affective interactions between infant and caregiver. These interactions provide infants with the experience of arousal escalation and reduction as a function of caregiver interventions, distress reactions that are relieved through caregiver actions, and positive interactions with the caregiver (Sroufe, 1996). Such experiences contribute to the working model of affect-related expectations that transfer from the immediate caregiving environment to the larger social world of peers and others.

Cassidy (1994) has also addressed the role of attachment processes in the development of emotional self-regulation. She argues that patterns of affective responding in the context of the attachment relationship are actually strategies that infants use to allow their attachment needs to be met. The open and flexible emotional communication that is characteristic of a secure attachment allows the infant to express comfortably and safely both positive and negative affect, ensuring proximity and comfort from the responsive caregiver. Moreover, the different strategies of insecure infants provide these infants with a means of meeting their own needs within the context of a less-than-optimal caregiving environment. The heightened distress characterizing resistant infants serves as a clear signal to gain the attention of the inconsistent or unresponsive caregiver. In a similar manner, avoidant behavior serves the adaptive purpose of minimizing the attachment relationship and has the effect of allowing the infant to maintain needed proximity without threatening the relationship with the caregiver through displays of overt sadness or anger. Importantly, though, these short-term adaptations of the different patterns displayed by insecure infants may lead to long-term difficulties in other contexts. For example, heightened emotion expression, in the context of peer relationships, may lead to problematic peer interactions and have implications for the development of social competence (Cassidy, 1994).

Other recent theoretical perspectives focus on the biological processes involved in the regulation of attachment and emotion processes (Field, 1994; Fox & Hane, 2008). For example, Hofer (1994; Polan & Hofer, 1999) addresses the multiple psychobiological roles that the caregiver plays in regulating infant behavior and physiology early in life. Based on his research with infant rat pups, he describes these "hidden regulators" as operating at multiple sensory levels (e.g., olfactory, tactile, and oral) and influencing multiple levels of behavioral and physiological functioning in the infant. So, for example, maternal tactile stimulation may have the effect of lowering the infant's heart rate during a stressful situation, which may in turn support a more adaptive behavioral response. Moreover, removal of these regulators, during separation, for example, disrupts the infant's functioning at multiple levels as well. Clearly, then, opportunities for individual differences in the development of emotional self-regulation may emerge from differential rearing conditions providing more or less psychobiological regulation. Consistent with this view, maternal holding and rocking are particularly effective at reducing infant distress (Jahromi, Putnam, & Stifter, 2004), and mother–infant skin-to-skin contact has been linked with greater physiological and emotional regulation in premature infants (Feldman, Weller, Sirota, & Eidelman, 2002).

The psychobiological interpretation of attachment theory also offers insight into the mechanism by which interactive experiences across the first year of life become integrated into the internal working model that Bowlby articulated. For example, Hofer (1994) describes how the biological experience of infant–caregiver interactions becomes a representational structure that guides affective functioning. He argues that these early interactions are, in fact, regulatory experiences that contribute to an inner affective experience composed of sensory, physiological, and behavioral responses. Over time, these affective experiences lead to organized representations, the integration of which is the internal working model. These organized mental representations are ultimately what guide the child's behavior, rather than the individual sensory and physiological components to which the infant responded earlier in infancy (Hofer, 1994).

Schore (2000) extends these psychobiological ideas even further in arguing that interactive experiences between caregiver and child that are the essential elements of the emerging attachment relationship also affect the development of the prefrontal cortex. The right hemisphere in particular, he notes, is especially influenced by experiences in the social world, and, in turn, determines the regulation and coping skills that young children develop. Support for the role of the right frontal cortex in human behavioral and emotional regulation has emerged (Fox, 1994; Fox & Hane, 2008). For example, chronic exposures to stress and/or high cortisol levels may result in impaired functioning in the regions of the brain associated with inhibition and regulation, such as the prefrontal cortex (Goldsmith & Davidson, 2004). Thus, there appears to be a compelling conceptual rationale for investigating whether and how caregivers affect infants' emerging self-regulatory system at multiple levels.

From this brief review of current theorizing in the area of attachment and emotional self-regulation, it is clear that multiple possible pathways to the development of emotional self-regulation in infancy and early childhood likely involve attachment processes. Moreover, these theoretical perspectives suggest that empirical evidence for the role of attachment processes in the development of emotional self-regulation may come from a number of different directions. First, attachment processes may be predictive of specific emotional responses in the context of the relationship dyad itself, and may be observed empirically in behavioral end emotional responses to the Strange Situation or in other interactions between the caregiver and the infant. Second, attachment processes may be implicated in the development and use of specific strategies outside the context of the attachment relationship, for example, during tasks requiring more independent self-regulation of emotion. Third, attachment processes may affect the development and functioning of physiological processes that support emotional self-regulation. Fourth, attachment processes may be implicated in the patterns of behavioral and social adaptation children display as they move from the social world of the family to that of school and peers, patterns that are often considered to be proxies for self-regulatory skills. In the next section, we examine evidence for each of these propositions.

ATTACHMENT PROCESSES
AND THE DEVELOPMENT OF EMOTIONAL SELF-REGULATION

Attachment and Emotional Regulation in Dyadic Contexts

The research examining attachment and emotion regulation processes in contexts that activate the attachment system is consistent in its findings. In multiple studies in different laboratories, researchers have demonstrated that infants with secure attachment relationships utilize strategies that include social referencing and express a need for social intervention (Braungart & Stifter, 1991; Nachmias, Gunnar, Manglesdorf, Parritz, & Buss, 1996). These same researchers report that insecure–avoidant children are more likely to use self-soothing and solitary exploration with toys (Braungart & Stifter, 1991; Nachmias et al., 1996). The strategies of both secure and insecure infants seem to reflect a history of experiences and expectations regarding the availability of the caregiver as an external source of emotional self-regulation, expectations that are clearly important when the attachment system becomes activated during the stressful context of the strange situation. Thus, the research examining direct links between attachment and emotional self-regulation in situations that activate the attachment system reveals clear behavioral differences between secure and insecure infants.

Attachment and Emerging Autonomous Emotional Self-Regulation

The pattern of findings linking attachment and specific emotion regulation behaviors in contexts less likely to activate the attachment system are somewhat consistent with findings observed in the Strange Situation. First, Diener, Manglesdorf, McHale, and Frosch (2002) observed that attachment classification predicted infants' regulatory strategies during a mildly stressful task in which infants were left with nothing to do while their parents completed a questionnaire. Infants in secure attachment relationships with both parents used strategies emphasizing social orientation. Likewise, in a challenging problem-solving task, during which the mother was present, toddlers classified as secure a year earlier engaged in more maternal help seeking than did avoidant and disorganized toddlers (Schieche & Spangler, 2005). In contrast, mother-reported attachment security was unrelated to the use of mother-oriented regulation strategies during laboratory tasks designed to elicit fear and frustration, but it was linked with more positive and less negative affect, suggesting more adaptive emotion regulation among secure children (Smith, Calkins, & Keane, 2006). Similarly, infants classified as secure at 15 months of age were less likely than avoidant infants to be classified as dyregulated on the basis of high negative affect and defiance during a compliance task at 24 months (National Institute of Child Health and Human Development (NICHD) Early Child Care Research Network, 2004). Importantly, this effect was significant, independent of a variety of demographic characteristics, infant temperament, and maternal sensitivity, indicating that the link was robust and not merely an artifact of maternal sensitivity.

Few scholars have examined links between attachment security and emotional regulation processes beyond the infancy period. In a study of preschoolers' use of specific anger control strategies during a waiting paradigm, a secure attachment in infancy predicted greater use of attentional distraction linked to successful waiting (Gilliom, Shaw, Beck, Schonberg, & Lukon, 2002). Likewise, 7-year-olds classified as securely attached in infancy reported greater expectations that others would help them emotionally and instrumentally during peer provocations (Ziv, Oppenheim, & Sagi-Schwartz, 2004). This supports the view that children with a secure attachment history have positive expectations of others that may contribute to the use of other-oriented regulation strategies beyond infancy.

Attachment processes have also been implicated in the development of fear, anger, and joy across the first 3 years of life (Kochanska, 2001). Consistent with other research (Calkins & Fox, 1992), Kochanska (2001) found that insecure–resistant infants were more fearful than other infants. In addition, across the second and third year of life, insecure infants displayed a different pattern with respect to the display of both positive and negative affect. Secure infants showed a predictable decline in the display of negative affect, while insecure infants displayed an increase, as well as a decrease, in positive affect. Presumably, by age 3, decreases in the expression of negative affect observed among securely attached children are, at least in part, a function of emerging control of such expression. A notable finding of this study was that, over time, avoidant infants display an increase in fear reactions, a finding that supports Cassidy's notion that emotion minimization, while effective in the short term, may lead to difficulties later in development. Clearly, the strategy of minimization is either ineffective over time, or leads to repeated experiences of internal arousal that eventually become difficult to contain. These data provide support for the notion that early attachment processes are implicated in the development of affective functioning, an important component of which is self-regulation.

Studies examining the relations between aspects of parenting thought to be linked to attachment and emotional self-regulation are also of interest. These studies are worth noting because they are conducted with toddlers, children for whom there are clear expectations of emerging autonomous emotional control. In one study of mothers and toddlers, for example, we examined the relations between maternal behavior across a variety of different situations and child emotional self-control in frustrating situations (Calkins, Smith, Gill, & Johnson, 1998). Our analyses indicated that maternal negative and controlling behavior (thought to be reflective of intrusive behavior characteristic of insecure attachment relationships) was related to the use of orienting to or manipulating the object of frustration (a barrier box containing an attractive toy) and negatively related to the use of distraction techniques. Likewise, maternal nonresponsiveness and disengagement following toddler distress cues were linked with children's use of ineffective attentional control strategies during a delay of gratification task (Mischel & Ayduk, Chapter 5, this volume; Rodriguez et al., 2005). These data are important in light of findings that the ability to control attention and engage in distraction has been related to the experience of less emotional arousal and reactivity (Calkins, 1997; Crockenberg & Leerkes, 2004; Grolnick et al., 1996) and to the display of early externalizing (Calkins & Dedmon, 2000; Crockenberg, Leerkes, & Barrig Jó, 2008) and internalizing (Crockenberg & Leerkes, 2006) behavior problems. Finally, maternal sensitivity to infant distress cues, but not nondistress cues, at 6 months was linked with less affect dysregulation at age 2 among temperamentally reactive infants (Leerkes, Blankson, & O'Brien, 2009). That sensitivity to distress was a particularly salient predictor of attachment security in the same sample (McElwain & Booth-LaForce, 2005), suggests that attachment-related processes may account for this effect.

Attachment and Physiological Self-Regulation

Researchers have examined whether attachment processes also affect physiological indices of emotional self-regulation. Much of this early work is reviewed by Fox and Hane (2008), who note that multiple physiological indices have been examined, including measures of heart rate, cortisol, and brain electrical activity during the Strange Situation. More recent work in this area has included the assessment of additional indices of self-regulation during the Strange Situation, examination of attachment-based differences in physiological regulation outside of the Strange Situation, attention to the coupling between physiological and behavioral indices of regulation across attachment groups, and attention to gene × environment interactions.

Cortisol findings indicate that insecurely attached and disorganized infants are more stressed during the Strange Situation, as demonstrated by elevated cortisol levels (Fox & Hane, 2008). One study demonstrated that infants who were securely attached to their mothers had lower cortisol levels than did insecurely attached infants during the adaptation to child care (i.e., the 2 days that their mothers introduced them to the child care setting by remaining present) (Ahnert, Gunnar, Lamb, & Barthel, 2004). Several studies suggest that attachment security may be especially beneficial to stress responses among temperamentally reactive infants; that is, attachment security buffered temperamentally fearful or inhibited infants from elevated cortisol levels during the Strange Situation (Nachmias et al., 1996; Spangler & Schieche, 1998), inoculations (Gunnar, Broderson, Nachmias, Buss, & Rigatuso, 1996), and difficult problem-solving tasks during which the mother was present (Schieche & Spangler, 2005).

In a recent investigation, infants' vagal withdrawal, a measure of physiological regulation (Porges, 2007), and salivary alpha-amylase, a measure of autonomic reactivity (Granger et al., 2006) were assessed simultaneously across episodes of the Strange Situation (Hill-Soderlund et al., 2008). Avoidant infants demonstrated greater increases in vagal withdrawal across the Strange Situation and consistently high salivary alpha-amylase in comparison to the secure infants indicating greater sympathetic arousal and greater internal efforts to self-regulate. The authors speculated that this pattern represents hyperactivation of the coping system, which may contribute to burnout and lead to the underarousal of physiological coping systems and less well-controlled behavior over time. That avoidant attachment has been consistently linked with externalizing behaviors, as reviewed below, is consistent with this perspective.

A number of researchers have also examined the extent to which physiological and behavioral indices of emotion regulation are coupled differently for infants with varying attachment classifications. On average, results suggest less coupling among avoidant infants, in that they do not appear distressed behaviorally, but their elevated cortisol levels suggest otherwise in the Strange Situation (Spangler & Grossman, 1993; Zelenko et al., 2005) and other contexts (Ahnert et al., 2004). This mismatch is consistent with Cassidy's (1994) view that avoidant infants learn to minimize the expression of negative affect.

Recent advances in genetics have led to the identification of two dopamine receptor genes (*DRD2* and *DRD4 long*) that are linked with problems reflecting emotional and behavioral undercontrol (see Propper et al., 2008, for a review), and each has been demonstrated to interact with attachment-related processes in predicting children's physiological emotional control. For example, maternal sensitivity during the first year buffered infants with the *DRD2* risk allele from negative effects on vagal withdrawal during a distressing task (Propper et al., 2008). Likewise, an attachment-based intervention was primarily effective in reducing daily cortisol levels and externalizing behaviors among infants with the *DRD4* long allele (Bakermans-Kranenburg, Van IJzendoorn, Mesman, Alink, & Juffer, 2008; Bakermans-Kranenburg, Van IJzendoorn, Pijlman, Mesman, & Juffer, 2008). These data suggest that a secure attachment may be particularly beneficial to the development of emotional self-regulation in children who are predisposed to emotion regulation difficulties. Additional work in this area is needed to determine whether these effects are robust across studies, whether other emotion-linked genes demonstrate a comparable effect, and whether such effects are in fact explained by attachment security.

One difficulty with this work, in general, is that the extent to which the measures reflect emotional tone or reactivity versus emotional self-regulation is not often clear. For example, elevated cortisol level could reflect heightened distress, an indicator of reactivity, or poor regulatory abilities, or a combination of both. Clearly, though, the measures support the notion that specific components of the attachment process are physiological in nature, as evidenced by normative changes in physiology across episodes of the Strange Situation. Moreover, there is emerging evidence of individual differences in emotion-related physiology as a function of attachment status.

Attachment and Behavioral Self-Regulation

In examining the relation between attachment processes and emotional regulation that is less proximal to the dyadic caregiver–child relation, it is important to examine the behavior problem literature. Within this literature, problems of both an internalizing and externalizing nature are often defined by self-regulatory difficulties (Barkley, 1997; Keenan, 2000). For example, in characterizing children with early externalizing behavior problems, there is often reference to a lack of control, undercontrol, or poor regulation

(Lewis & Miller, 1990). In characterizing the behavior of children with internalizing disorders, there is often a discussion of overcontrol (Calkins & Fox, 2002). Rarely do these investigations examine specific emotion regulation strategies or processes (but for exceptions see Calkins & Dedmon, 2000; Gilliom et al., 2002). Rather, it is often assumed that the behavioral symptoms themselves (e.g., aggression, in the case of externalizing, or withdrawal, in the case of internalizing) either are strategies for regulation (Calkins, 1994) or they reflect a lack of adaptive strategies (Keenan, 2000). Thus, the child behavior problem literature is an appropriate place to examine the relation between attachment and emerging emotional self-regulation.

There is a large empirical literature examining the relations between attachment and child behavior problems, particularly the more salient and disruptive externalizing behavior problems such as aggression or oppositional defiant disorder (ODD). Several studies have shown that insecure infant attachment, particularly avoidant attachment, is predictive of later externalizing behavior problems in children (Burgess, Marshall, Rubin, & Fox, 2003; McElwain, Cox, Burchinal, & Macfie, 2003; Shaw, Owens, Giovanelli, & Winslow, 2001; Shaw, Owens, Vondra, Keenan, & Winslow, 1996). Attachment disorganization has also been linked to externalizing in research (Lyons-Ruth, Easterbrooks, & Cibelli, 1997; Madigan, Moran, Schuengel, Pederson, & Otten, 2007; Munson, McMahon, & Spieker, 2001; Smeekens, Riksen-Walraven, & van Bakel, 2007). In contrast, though, Bates and colleagues (Bates & Bayles, 1988; Bates, Maslin, & Frankel, 1985) failed to show that attachment security at 13 months predicted later behavior problems at 3, 5, or 6 years of age. These researchers concluded that the link between externalizing behavior and attachment could not be supported. However, it is important to note that attachment classifications may not consistently predict later behavior problems because attachment status can change as children move beyond infancy, particularly if parenting quality and environmental risk change (Cicchetti, Cummings, Greenberg, & Marvin, 1990). Consistent with this view, data from the NICHD study of early child care demonstrated that an insecure attachment during infancy was linked with behavior problems at age 3 only if maternal sensitivity at 24 months was low (Belsky & Fearon, 2002) and with behavior problems in kindergarten and first grade if parenting quality did not improve over time (NICHD Early Child Care Research Network, 2006).

An examination of concurrent relations between attachment status and child behavior problems, as opposed to early attachment security as a predictor of later behavior problems, may be more useful to understanding the processes underlying the display and maintenance of problematic behavior. For example, in an extensive study of the concurrent factors that distinguish preschool boys with and without a clinical diagnosis of ODD, Greenberg and colleagues (DeKlyen, Speltz, & Greenberg, 1998; Greenberg, Speltz, DeKlyen, & Endriga, 1991; Speltz, Greenberg, & DeKlyen, 1990) found that the preschool boys with a clinical diagnosis of ODD were more likely than the boys in the control group to be insecurely attached.

In examining attachment processes as predictors of internalizing spectrum problems, results have been even less consistent. Several studies have found relations, but the types of insecurity that predict outcomes differ, as does the developmental lag between attachment predictors and outcomes. For example, Shaw and colleagues found that toddler insecurity predicted both internalizing and externalizing problems at preschool age (Vondra, Shaw, Swearingen, Cohen, & Owens, 2001), but disorganized attachment in infancy predicted toddlers' internalizing problems (Shaw, Keenan, Vondra, Delliquadri, & Giovanelli, 1997). Among school-age children, ambivalent–resistant attachment in infancy predicted internalizing symptoms in three studies (Lewis, Feiring, McGuffog, & Jaskir, 1984; NICHD Early Child Care Research Network, 2006; Renken, Egeland, Marvinney, Mangelsdorf, & Sroufe, 1989), whereas avoidant attachment (Lyons-Ruth et al., 1997) and disorganized attachment (NICHD Early Child Care Research Network, 2006) each predicted internalizing in one study. Finally, resistant attachment in infancy predicted adolescent anxiety disorders even after researchers controlled for infant temperament and maternal anxiety symptoms (Warren, Huston, Egeland, & Sroufe, 1997). Thus, across studies, there is fairly consistent evidence that attachment security is linked with better behavioral self-regulation.

Summary

This review of research examining the effects of early relationships on the development of emotional self-regulation seems to demonstrate that the proximal effects of this relationship are quite evident. Infants in secure attachment relationships utilize effective and appropriate caregiver-directed behaviors to elicit supportive caregiving in times of stress. In addition, there is evidence from the psychophysiological literature that predictable biological responses can be expected from infants in contexts that activate the attachment system, as well as evidence for the effects of attachment security on this responding. Beyond this immediate dyadic context, though, there are also effects of the attachment relationship on emotional self-regulation. Secure infants and children use effective strategies when engaged in tasks that require more autonomous emotional control than the anticipated external control provided in dyadic regulation. More distal effects of attachment on behavioral and emotional self-regulation that underlie adaptive functioning in preschool and early childhood have also been observed. However, clear interpretation of these data may require a more systematic evaluation of both the timing of the effects of attachment and the influence of other environmental factors, and the role of mediating and moderating variables.

FUTURE DIRECTIONS IN THE STUDY OF ATTACHMENT PROCESSES AND EMOTIONAL SELF-REGULATION

The theoretical and empirical work reviewed to this point suggest that that there are clear implications of attachment processes in the development of emotional self-regulation. Nevertheless, there is reason to think that future studies of these phenomena could clarify the nature and extent of these relations.

First, empirical work that is more focused on process than on simple associations might be more informative in elucidating the complex ways that attachment and emotion regulation influence development. For example, it might be useful to examine the role of emotion regulation as a mediator of the relations between early attachment and other, more complex kinds of self-regulation. In one of the few studies that have examined such a hypothesis, Contreras, Kerns, Weimer, Gentzler, and Tomich (2000) observed that specific dimensions of emotion regulation, including arousal and attention deployment, mediated the relation between attachment and peer social behavior. A movement toward a focus on specific styles or strategies of emotional control might provide greater specificity with respect to the role of attachment in behavioral adjustment.

A second step that might help to illuminate these processes would be to continue to address the issue of moderators of the relation between attachment and regulation. Evidence to date suggests that the nature of the association between attachment and emotional self-regulation varies based on temperament, a genetic predisposition toward emotional problems, and change in the caregiving environment over time. Identification of other factors, such as subsequent positive peer relations or positive relationships with alternative caregivers that may ameliorate the negative effects of an insecure attachment on emotional regulation, is needed. It may also be useful to examine parent gender as a moderator of links between attachment processes and emotional regulation because young children may learn different lessons about emotions within the context of the father–child relationship given stylistic parenting differences between mothers and fathers (Parke, 2002). A focus on moderated effects will provide greater specificity in prediction, while preserving the important role of attachment processes in emotional functioning.

Third, it is clear that the direction of effects in development is not always from parent to child. Transactional influences from the environment to the child and back again are clearly responsible for some pathways in development. Moreover, it must be acknowledged that the child plays an important role in the dyadic interactions with caregivers that lead to the development of attachment relationships (Calkins, 1994). For example, infant affect regulation and parental sensitivity at 4 months were interrelated, and both predicted subsequent attachment classifications (Braungart-Rieker, Garwood, Powers, & Wang, 2001). Transactional influences may obscure the identification of longer-term effects of attachment on emotional processes but clearly are important to understanding developmental pathways (Cicchetti, 1993).

Finally, it may be more useful to adopt an approach that considers multiple levels of analysis of self-regulation. Bowlby's original theory of attachment, and subsequent elaboration of the theory, place emotional development at the center of attachment processes. For this reason, the theory has clear implications for the emergence of early emotional self-regulation. However, self-regulation occurs on a number of different, and likely interrelated, levels, including physiological, attentional, emotional, behavioral, cognitive, and interpersonal or social processes (Calkins & Fox, 2002; Eisenberg et al., Chapter 14, this volume; Eisenberg et al., 2000; Posner & Rothbart, 2000; Rueda, Posner, & Rothbart, Chapter 15, this volume). We advocate an approach that integrates biological and cognitive phenomena into both theoretical and empirical explications about the development of emotional and behavioral self-regulation. Embedding emotional self-regulation in a larger self-regulatory framework has the advantage of allowing researchers to understand the multiple levels of infant and child functioning that may be influenced by the emerging attachment relationship.

ACKNOWLEDGMENT

The writing of this chapter was supported by a National Institutes of Health grant to Susan D. Calkins (No. MH 74077).

REFERENCES

Ahnert, L., Gunnar, M., Lamb, M., & Barthel, M. (2004). Transition to child care: Associations with infant–mother attachment, infant negative emotion, and cortisol elevations. *Child Development, 75,* 639–650.

Ainsworth, M., Blehar, M., Waters, E., & Wall, S. (1978). *Patterns of attachment.* Hillsdale, NJ: Erlbaum.

Bakermans-Kranenburg, M., Van IJzendoorn, M., Mesman, J., Alink, L., & Juffer, F. (2008). Effects of an attachment-based intervention on daily cortisol moderated by dopamine receptor D4: A randomized control trial on 1- to 3-year-olds screened for externalizing behavior. *Development and Psychopathology, 20,* 805–820.

Bakermans-Kranenburg, M., Van IJzendoorn, M., Pijlman, F., Mesman, J., & Juffer, F. (2008). Experimental evidence for differential susceptibility: Dopamine D4 receptor polymorphism (DRD4 VNTR) moderates intervention effects on toddlers' externalizing behavior in a randomized controlled trial. *Developmental Psychology, 44,* 293–300.

Barkley, R. A. (1997). *ADHD and the nature of self-control.* New York: Guilford Press.

Bates, J. E., & Bayles, K. (1988). Attachment and the development of behavior problems. In J. Belsky & T. Nezworski (Eds.), *Clinical implications of attachment* (pp. 253–299). Hillsdale, NJ: Erlbaum.

Bates, J. E., Maslin, C. A., & Frankel, K. A. (1985). Attachment security, mother–child interaction and temperament as predictors of behavior-problem ratings at age three years. In I. Bretherton & E. Waters (Eds.), Growing points in attachment theory and research. *Monographs of the Society for Research in Child Development, 50*(1–2, Serial No. 209), 167–193.

Bell, S., & Ainsworth, M. (1972). Infant crying and maternal responsiveness. *Child Development, 43,* 1171–1190.

Belsky, J., & Fearon, R. M. P. (2002). Early attachment security, subsequent maternal sensitivity, and later child development: Does continuity in development depend upon continuity of caregiving? *Attachment and Human Development, 3,* 361–387.

Bowlby, J. (1969/1982). *Attachment and loss: Vol. 1. Attachment.* New York: Basic Books.

Bowlby, J. (1988). *A secure vase.* New York: Basic Books.

Braungart, J. M., & Stifter, C. A. (1991). Regulation of negative reactivity during the Strange Situation: Temperament and attachment in 12-month-old infants. *Infant Behavior and Development, 14,* 349–367.

Braungart-Rieker, J., Garwood, M., Powers, B., & Wang, X. (2001). Parental sensitivity, infant affect, and affect regulation: Predictors of later attachment. *Child Development, 72,* 252–270.

Bronson, M. B. (2000). *Self-regulation in early childhood: Nature and nurture.* New York: Guilford Press.

Burgess, K. B., Marshall, P. J., Rubin, K. H., & Fox, N. A. (2003). Infant attachment and temperament as predictors of subsequent externalizing problems and cardiac physiology. *Journal of Child Psychology and Psychiatry, 44,* 819–831.

Buss, K. A., & Goldsmith, H. H. (1998). Fear and anger regulation in infancy: Effects on the temporal dynamics of affective expression. *Child Development, 69,* 359–374.

Calkins, S. D. (1994). Origins and outcomes of individual differences in emotional regulation. In N. A. Fox (Ed.), Emotion regulation: Behavioral and biological considerations. *Monographs of the Society for Research in Child Development, 59*(2–3, Serial No. 240), 53–72.

Calkins, S. D. (1997). Cardiac vagal tone indices of temperamental reactivity and behavioral regulation in young children. *Developmental Psychobiology, 31,* 125–135.

Calkins, S. D., & Dedmon, S. A. (2000). Physiological and behavioral regulation in two-year-old children with aggressive/destructive behavior problems. *Journal of Abnormal Child Psychology, 2,* 103–118.

Calkins, S. D., & Fox, N. A. (1992). The relations among infant temperament, security of attachment and behavioral inhibition at 24 months. *Child Development, 63,* 1456–1472.

Calkins, S. D., & Fox, N. A. (2002). Self-regulatory processes in early personality development: A multilevel approach to the study of childhood social withdrawal and aggression. *Development and Psychopathology, 14,* 477–498.

Calkins, S. D., Gill, K. A., Johnson, M. C., & Smith, C. (1999). Emotional reactivity and emotion regulation strategies and predictors of social behavior with peers during toddlerhood. *Social Development, 8,* 310–341.

Calkins, S. D., Smith, C. L., Gill, K. L., & Johnson, M. C. (1998). Maternal interactive style across contexts: Relations to emotional, behavioral and physiological regulation during toddlerhood. *Social Development, 7,* 350–369.

Cassidy, J. (1994). Emotion regulation: Influences of attachment relationships. In N. A. Fox (Ed.), Emotion regulation: Behavioral and biological considerations. *Monographs of the Society for Research in Child Development, 59*(2–3, Serial No. 240), 228–283.

Cicchetti, D. (1993). Developmental psychopathology: Reactions, reflections, projections. *Developmental Review, 13,* 471–502.

Cicchetti, D., Ackerman, B., & Izard, C. (1995). Emotions and emotion regulation in developmental psychopathology. *Development and Psychopathology, 7,* 1–10.

Cicchetti, D., Cummings, E. M., Greenberg, M. T., & Marvin, R. S. (1990). An organizational perspective on attachment beyond infancy: Implications for theory, measurement, and research. In M. T. Greenberg, D. Cicchetti, & E. M. Cummings (Eds.), *Attachment in the preschool years* (pp. 3–50). Chicago: University of Chicago Press.

Cole, P., Martin, S., & Dennis, T. (2004, March). Emotion regulation as a scientific construct: Methodological challenges and directions for child development research. *Child Development, 75,* 317–333.

Contreras, J., Kerns, K. A., Weimer, B., Gentzler, A., & Tomich, P. (2000). Emotion regulation as a mediator of associations between mother–child attachment and peer relationships in middle childhood. *Journal of Family Psychology, 14,* 111–124.

Crockenberg, S. C., & Leerkes, E. M. (2004). Infant and maternal behaviors regulate infant reactivity to novelty at 6 months. *Developmental Psychology, 40,* 1123–1132.

Crockenberg, S. C., & Leerkes, E. M. (2006). Infant and maternal behavior moderate reactivity to novelty to predict anxious behavior at 2.5 years. *Development and Psychopathology, 18,* 17–34.

Crockenberg, S., Leerkes, E., & Barrig Jó, P. (2008). Predicting aggressive behavior in the third year from infant reactivity and regulation as moderated by maternal behavior. *Development and Psychopathology, 20,* 37–54.

DeKlyen, M., Speltz, M. L., & Greenberg, M. T. (1998). Fathering and early onset conduct problems: Positive and negative parenting, father–son attachment, and the marital context. *Clinical Child and Family Psychology Review, 1,* 3–21.

De Wolff, M., & Van IJzendoorn, M. (1997). Sensitivity and attachment: A meta-analysis on parental antecedents of infant attachment. *Child Development, 68,* 571–591.

Diener, M., Mangelsdorf, S., McHale, J., & Frosch, C. (2002). Infants' behavioral strategies for emotion regulation with fathers and mothers: Associations with emotional expressions and attachment quality. *Infancy, 3,* 153–174.

Eisenberg, N., Cumberland, A., & Spinrad, T. L. (1998). Parental socialization of emotion. *Psychological Inquiry, 9,* 241–273.

Eisenberg, N., & Fabes, R. (2006). Emotion regulation and children's socioemotional competence. *Child psychology: A handbook of contemporary issues* (2nd ed., pp. 357–381). New York: Psychology Press.

Eisenberg, N., Guthrie, I. K., Fabes, R. A., Shepard, S., Losoya, S., Murphy, B. C., et al. (2000). Prediction of elementary school children's externalizing problem behaviors from attention and behavioral regulation and negative emotionality. *Child Development, 71,* 1367–1382.

Feldman, R., Weller, A., Sirota, L., & Eidelman, A. (2002). Skin-to-skin contact (kangaroo care) promotes self-regulation in premature infants: Sleep–wake cyclicity, arousal modulation, and sustained exploration. *Developmental Psychology, 38,* 194–207.

Field, T. (1994). The effects of mother's physical and emotional unavailability on emotion regulation. In N. A. Fox (Ed.), Emotion regulation: Behavioral and biological considerations. *Monographs of the Society for Research in Child Development, 59*(2–3, Serial No. 240), 208–227.

Fox, N., & Calkins, S. D. (2003). The development of self-control of emotion: Intrinsic and extrinsic influences. *Motivation and Emotion, 27,* 7–26.

Fox, N. A. (1994). Dynamic cerebral process underlying emotion regulation. In N. A. Fox (Ed.), Emotion regulation: Behavioral and biological considerations. *Monographs of the Society for Research in Child Development, 59*(2–3, Serial No. 240), 152–166.

Fox, N. A., & Hane, A. A. (2008). Studying the biology of human attachment. In J. Cassidy & P. R. Shaver (Eds.), *Handbook of attachment: Theory, research, and clinical applications* (2nd ed., pp. 217–240). New York: Guilford Press.

Gilliom, M., Shaw, D., Beck, J., Schonberg, M., & Lukon, J. (2002). Anger regulation in disadvantaged preschool boys: Strategies, antecedents, and the development of self-control. *Developmental Psychology, 38,* 222–235.

Goldsmith, H., & Davidson, R. (2004). Disambiguating the components of emotion regulation. *Child Development, 75,* 361–365.

Granger, D., Kivlighan, K., Blair, C., El-Sheikh, M., Mize, J., Lisonbee, J., et al. (2006). Integrating the measurement of salivary *a*-amylase into studies of child health, development, and social relationships. *Journal of Personal and Social Relationships, 23,* 267–290.

Graziano, P., Reavis, R., Keane, S., & Calkins, S. (2007). The role of emotion regulation in children's early academic success. *Journal of School Psychology, 45,* 3–19.

Greenberg, M. T., Speltz, M. L., DeKlyen, M., & Endriga, M. C. (1991). Attachment security in preschoolers with and without externalizing behavior problems: A replication. *Development and Psychopathology, 3,* 413–430.

Grolnick, W., Cosgrove, T., & Bridges, L. (1996). Age-graded change in the initiation of positive affect. *Infant Behavior and Development, 19,* 153–157.

Gunnar, M. R., Broderson, L., Nachmias, M., Buss, K., & Rigatuso, J. (1996). Stress reactivity and attachment security. *Developmental Psychobiology, 29,* 191–204.

Hill-Soderlund, A., Mills-Koonce, W., Propper, C., Calkins, S., Granger, D., Moore, G., et al. (2008). Parasympathetic and sympathetic responses to the strange situation in infants and mothers from avoidant and securely attached dyads. *Developmental Psychobiology, 50,* 361–376.

Hofer, M. A. (1994). Hidden regulators in attachment, separation, and loss. In N. A. Fox (Ed.), Emotion regulation: Behavioral and biological considerations. *Monographs of the Society for Research in Child Development, 59*(2–3, Serial No. 240), 192–207.

Jahromi, L., Putnam, S., & Stifter, C. (2004). Maternal regulation of infant reactivity from 2 to 6 months. *Developmental Psychology, 40,* 477–487.

Keenan, K. (2000). Emotion dysregulation as a risk factor for child psychopathology. *Clinical Psychology: Science and Practice, 7,* 418–434.

Kochanska, G. (2001). Emotional development in children with different attachment histories: The first three years. *Child Development, 72,* 474–490.

Kopp, C. (1982). Antecedents of self-regulation: A developmental perspective. *Developmental Psychology, 18,* 199–214.

Kopp, C. (1989). Regulation of distress and negative emotions: A developmental view. *Developmental Psychology, 25,* 243–254.

Kopp, C. (1992). Emotional distress and control in young children. In N. Eisenberg & R. Fabes (Eds.), *Emotion and its regulation in early development: New directions for child development* (pp. 7–23). San Francisco: Jossey-Bass/Pfeiffer.

Leerkes, E. M., Blankson, A. N., & O'Brien, M. (2009). Differential effects of maternal sensitivity to infant distress and nondistress on social–emotional functioning. *Child Development, 80*, 762–775.

Lewis, M., Feiring, C., McGuffog, C., & Jaskir, J. (1984). Predicting psychopathology in six-year-olds from early social relations. *Child Development, 55*, 123–136.

Lewis, M. G., & Miller, S. (1990). *Handbook of developmental psychopathology.* New York: Plenum Press.

Lyons-Ruth, K., Easterbrooks, M., & Cibelli, C. (1997). Infant attachment strategies, infant mental lag, and maternal depressive symptoms: Predictors of internalizing and externalizing problems at age 7. *Developmental Psychology, 33*, 681–692.

Madigan, S., Moran, G., Schuengel, C., Pederson, D., & Otten, R. (2007). Unresolved maternal attachment representations, disrupted maternal behavior and disorganized attachment in infancy: Links to toddler behavior problems. *Journal of Child Psychology and Psychiatry, 48*, 1042–1050.

Main, M., & Solomon, J. (1990). Procedures for identifying infants as disorganized/disoriented during the Ainsworth Strange Situation. In M. T. Greenberg (Ed.), *Attachment in the preschool years: Theory, research, and intervention* (pp. 121–160). Chicago: University of Chicago Press.

McElwain, N., & Booth-LaForce, C. (2006). Maternal sensitivity to infant distress and nondistress as predictors of infant–mother attachment security. *Journal of Family Psychology, 20*, 247–255.

McElwain, N., Cox, M., Burchinal, M., & Macfie, J. (2003). Differentiating among insecure mother–infant attachment classifications: A focus on child–friend interaction and exploration during solitary play at 36 months. *Attachment and Human Development, 5*, 136–164.

Morris, A., Silk, J., Steinberg, L., Myers, S., & Robinson, L. (2007). The role of the family context in the development of emotion regulation. *Social Development, 16*, 361–388.

Munson, J. A., McMahon, R. J., & Spieker, S. J. (2001). Structure and variability in the developmental trajectory of children's externalizing problems: Impact of infant attachment, maternal depressive symptomatology, and child sex. *Development and Psychopathology, 13*, 277–296.

Nachmias, M., Gunnar, M., Mangelsdorf, S., Parritz, R. H., & Buss, K. (1996). Behavioral inhibition and stress reactivity: The moderating role of attachment security. *Child Development, 67*, 508–522.

NICHD Early Child Care Research Network. (2004). Affect dysregulation in the mother–child relationship in the toddler years: Antecedents and consequences. *Development and Psychopathology, 16*, 43–68.

NICHD Early Child Care Research Network. (2006). Infant–mother attachment classification: Risk and protection in relation to changing maternal caregiving quality. *Developmental Psychology, 42*, 38–58.

Parke, R. (2002). Fathers and families. In M. H. Bornstein (Ed.) *Handbook of parenting: Vol. 3. Being and becoming a parent* (2nd ed., pp. 27–73). Mahwah, NJ: Erlbaum.

Polan, H. J., & Hofer, M. A. (2008). Psychobiological origins of infants attachment and its role in development. In J. Cassidy & P. R. Shaver (Eds.), *Handbook of attachment: Theory, research, and clinical applications* (2nd ed., pp. 158–172). New York: Guilford Press.

Porges, S. (2007). The polyvagal perspective. *Biological Psychology, 74*, 116–143.

Posner, M. I., & Rothbart, M. K. (2000). Developing mechanisms of self-regulation. *Development and Psychopathology, 12*, 427–441.

Propper, C., Moore, G., Mills-Koonce, W., Halpern, C., Hill-Soderlund, A., Calkins, S., et al.

(2008). Gene–environment contributions to the development of infant vagal reactivity: The interaction of dopamine and maternal sensitivity. *Child Development, 79,* 1377–1394.

Raikes, H., Robinson, J., Bradley, R., Raikes, H., & Ayoub, C. (2007). Developmental trends in self-regulation among low-income toddlers. *Social Development, 16,* 128–149.

Renken, B., Egeland, B., Marvinney, D., Mangelsdorf, S., & Sroufe, L. A. (1989). Early childhood antecedents of aggressive and passive withdrawal in early elementary school. *Journal of Personality, 57,* 257–282.

Rodriguez, M., Ayduk, O., Aber, J., Mischel, W., Sethi, A., & Shoda, Y. (2005). A contextual approach to the development of self-regulatory competencies: The role of maternal unresponsivity and toddlers' negative affect in stressful situations. *Social Development, 14,* 136–157.

Rothbart, M., Ziaie, H., & O'Boyle, C. (1992). Self-regulation and emotion in infancy. In N. Eisenberg & R. Fabes (Eds.), *Emotion and its regulation in early development: New directions for child development* (pp. 7–23). San Francisco: Jossey-Bass/Pfeiffer.

Rothbart, M. K. (1986). Longitudinal observation of infant temperament. *Developmental Psychology, 22,* 356–365.

Ruff, H., & Rothbart, M. K. (1996). *Attention in early development.* New York: Oxford University Press.

Schieche, M., & Spangler, G. (2005). Individual differences in biobehavioral organization during problem-solving in toddlers: The influence of maternal behavior, infant–mother attachment, and behavioral inhibition on the attachment–exploration balance. *Developmental Psychobiology, 46,* 293–306.

Schore, A. (2000). Attachment and the regulation of the right brain. *Attachment and Human Development, 2,* 23–47.

Shaw, D., Owens, E., Giovanelli, J., & Winslow, E. (2001). Infant and toddler pathways leading to early externalizing disorders. *Journal of the American Academy of Child and Adolescent Psychiatry, 40,* 36–43.

Shaw, D. S., Keenan, K., Vondra, J., Delliquadri, E., & Giovanelli, J. (1997). Antecedents of preschool children's internalizing problems: A longitudinal study of low-income families. *Journal of the American Academy of Child and Adolescent Psychiatry, 36,* 1760–1767.

Shaw, D. S., Owens, E. B., Vondra, J. I., Keenan, K., & Winslow, E. B. (1996). Early risk factors and pathways in the development of early disruptive behavior problems. *Development and Psychopathology, 8,* 679–699.

Smeekens, S., Riksen-Walraven, J., & van Bakel, H. (2007). Multiple determinants of externalizing behavior in 5-year-olds: A longitudinal model. *Journal of Abnormal Child Psychology, 35,* 347–361.

Smith, C. L., Calkins, S. D., & Keane, S. P. (2006). The relation of maternal behaviour and attachment security to toddlers' emotions and emotion regulation. *Research in Human Development, 3,* 21–31.

Spangler, G., & Grossman, K. E. (1993). Biobehavioral organization in securely and insecurely attached infants. *Child Development, 64,* 1439–1450.

Spangler, G., & Schieche, M. (1998). Emotional and adrenocortical responses of infants to the Strange Situation: The differential function of emotional expression. *International Journal of Behavioral Development, 22,* 681–706.

Speltz, M. L., Greenberg, M. T., & DeKlyen, M. (1990). Attachment in preschoolers with disruptive behavior: A comparison of clinic-referred and nonproblem children. *Development and Psychopathology, 2,* 31–46.

Sroufe, A. L. (1996). *Emotional development: The organization of emotional life in the early years.* New York: Cambridge University Press.

Sroufe, L. A. (2000). Early relationships and the development of children. *Infant Mental Health Journal, 21,* 67–74.

Stifter, C. A., & Braungart, J. M. (1995). The regulation of negative reactivity in infancy: Function and development. *Developmental Psychology, 31,* 448–455.

Thompson, R. A. (1994). Emotion regulation: A theme in search of definition. In N. A. Fox (Ed.), The development of emotion regulation: Biological and behavioral considerations. *Monographs of the Society for Research in Child Development, 59*(2–3, Serial No. 240), 25–52.

Vondra, J. I., Shaw, D. S., Swearingen, L., Cohen, M., & Owens, E. B. (2001). Attachment stability and emotional and behavioral regulation from infancy to preschool age. *Development and Psychopathology, 13,* 13–33.

Warren, S., Huston, L., Egeland, B., & Sroufe, L. (1997). Child and adolescent anxiety disorders and early attachment. *Journal of the American Academy of Child and Adolescent Psychiatry, 36,* 637–644.

Zelenko, M., Kraemer, H., Huffman, L., Gschwendt, M., Pageler, N., & Steiner, H. (2005). Heart rate correlates of attachment status in young mothers and their infants. *Journal of the American Academy of Child and Adolescent Psychiatry, 44,* 470–476.

Ziv, Y., Oppenheim, D., & Sagi-Schwartz, A. (2004). Social information processing in middle childhood: Relations to infant–mother attachment. *Attachment and Human Development, 6,* 327–348.

CHAPTER 20

When People Strive
for Self-Harming Goals
Sacrificing Personal Health for Interpersonal Success

CATHERINE D. RAWN
KATHLEEN D. VOHS

Nineteen-year-old Sam Spady was in many ways the typical college sophomore. She had pledged a sorority but struggled to juggle her coursework with Greek events. Living on campus, she missed her family and was sometimes overheard saying how she wished she could sleep in her own bed at her family's house. Sam did not have the opportunity to sleep in her own bed after September 5, 2004, because she died that night by overdosing on alcohol. Sam attended party after party and became so drunk that she could not stand on her own. According to reports, she drank for 11 hours straight—long past the point of pleasure even for the most experienced drinkers ("Frat suspended," 2004; "Samantha Spady," n.d.). An autopsy revealed that Sam's blood alcohol content was 0.43 (0.07 or 0.10 is the legal limit for driving in most U.S. states).

Teenagers' automobile safety records likewise show patterns of undue riskiness in the presence of peers (Simons-Morton, Lerner, & Singer, 2005). It is not that teens are simply novice drivers and that is why they get into accidents: When there are two other teens in the car, the probability of an accident quintuples relative to when a teenager drives alone ("How many teens," n.d.). When asked, teens report a change in their driving behavior with friends, in that almost half (44%) admit they drive recklessly when friends accompany them.

Yet adolescents are not alone in following their friends to leap from metaphorical bridges. Social psychology abounds with demonstrations of conformity across the lifespan (Asch, 1955, 1956; Cialdini, 2009; Sherif, 1935). People who seek to persuade others know full well the power of social proof and tailor their messages to create the impression that "everyone" is using their product, frequenting their service, or behaving in a certain way (e.g., Goldstein, Cialdini, & Griskevicius, 2008). The hope of social inclusion strongly motivates behavior (Baumeister & Leary, 1995). Moreover, social isolation, or even the mere threat of it, changes thoughts, feelings, and behavior, mostly not for the better (Baumeister, DeWall, Ciarocco, & Twenge, 2005; Twenge, Baumeister, DeWall, Ciarocco, & Bartels, 2007; Twenge, Baumeister, Tice, & Stucke, 2001). Yet could a desire for interpersonal rewards, such as attaining acceptance and avoiding exclusion, motivate people to override basic desires for self-protection?

We argue that the answer is "yes": People can and do deliberately engage in self-harming actions to gain interpersonal acceptance. Moreover, these personally risky actions require self-control exertion to enact if people feel repelled by those actions in the first place. They often feel repelled by risky acts—after all, protecting the self is paramount (death only has to win once; life has to win every day; Baumeister, Bratslavsky, Finkenauer, & Vohs, 2001). Yet people may be willing to override aversion to distasteful or risky behavior when they think it will bring social acceptance. Sam Spady might have thought she was fitting into the wild party scene ("Samantha Spady," n.d.) at the fraternity house where she did much of her drinking that night. To be sure, a lonely college woman might seek social inclusion by going along with the perceived norms of the group. Hence, people might risk harm to the self if they believe there is a prize for overcoming personal aversions, including self-protective impulses. Such self-control for personal harm, we argue, is often aimed at the valuable prize of social inclusion.

The key implication of the self-control for personal harm model for self-control theory is that some behaviors that may appear disinhibited are actually performed using self-control strength. Going on a nonlethal alcohol binge might represent self-control exertion or self-control failure. If a prospective drinker has a strong attraction to alcohol and wants to get intoxicated, then bingeing would mean that our drinker is acquiescing to urges. Similarly, if the driver of a car likes to drive faster than is safe for most cars on the roadway, going well over the speed limit is a failure to self-regulate.

However, if a prospective drinker or driver has an impulse to avoid these dangerous activities, then binge drinking or fast driving would require overriding an impulse not to perform such an act, which means self-control exertion. Thus, self-control can be used to enact behaviors that have a high degree of probable self-harm. Taken in the abstract, the only way to know whether an action could have resulted from self-control failure or exertion is to know the nature of the actor's impulse toward that action. This is one of the main take-away points of this chapter: Canonical self-regulation acts or self-regulation failures cannot generically be judged as one or the other (successful or failed self-regulation) if the judge does not know the incipient feelings of the actor. An underage drinker swallowing beer at a sorority party, contrary to the stereotypic view, might be exerting a lot of self-control to choke down each bitter gulp.

SELF-CONTROL OFTEN IS USED FOR GOOD OUTCOMES, BUT NOT ALWAYS

Self-control is exerted when people force themselves to deny an impulse to do something (e.g., stopping oneself from eating another piece of warm pecan pie) or to do something they would prefer to avoid (e.g., jogging) (Baumeister, Schmeichel, & Vohs, 2007; Vohs & Baumeister, 2004). It is indisputable that self-control can lead to positive outcomes. Dispositionally high self-control predicts greater personal and interpersonal well-being, including academic achievement, high self-esteem, skillful perspective-taking ability, low aggression, effective coping strategies, and the ability to stop interpersonal conflict from escalating (Finkel & Campbell, 2001; Mischel, Shoda, & Peake, 1988; Tangney, Baumeister, & Boone, 2004). At the state level, people who have been depleted of their self-control resources tend to engage in actions that have negative personal consequences that include truncating study time, eating unhealthy foods, mismanaging their public impressions, and making irrational decisions (Baumeister, Bratslavsky, Muraven, & Tice, 1998; Pocheptsova, Amir, Dhar, & Baumeister, 2009; Schmeichel, Vohs, & Baumeister, 2003; Vohs, Baumeister, & Ciarocco, 2005; Vohs & Heatherton, 2000).

There is a clear link between high self-control and outcomes that carry positive consequences for the self and relationships, and we take no issue with this robust finding. Yet in the literature, processes of self-control failure and exertion sometimes have been conflated with behavioral outcomes. For example, self-control has been dubbed "the moral muscle" (Baumeister & Exline, 1999), suggesting that chiefly virtuous acts result from self-control exertion. This moniker conceals the possibility that self-control can be used to engage in immoral, unhealthy, risky, and otherwise ill-advised actions. A parallel might be made with intelligence. Although being intelligent is clearly associated with good outcomes in life, intelligence in itself is neither good nor bad. Highly intelligent people with dastardly intentions, after all, can form extremely devious plans.

Making matters muddier, some actions have been equated with self-control failure based on normative assumptions about what is considered tempting in Western culture. Overconsumption of alcohol, overspending, smoking, unsafe sex, gambling, overeating, and criminal behaviors have been identified as domains that invite self-control failure (Baumeister, Heatherton, & Tice, 1994; Baumeister et al., 2007; Gottfredson & Hirschi, 1990).

Furthermore, recent theories have begun defining the urges involved in self-control dilemmas as necessarily appetitive. Hofmann, Friese, and Wiers (2009) state that impulses have "strong incentive value" that is hedonic and prepares the person to go toward the arousing stimulus (p. 114; see also Hoffman, Friese, & Strack, 2009). The current perspective offered in this chapter firmly disagrees with this notion that de facto urges are aimed at consuming an alluring temptation, and considers it to conflate unnecessarily the notion of an urge with the approach–avoidance nature of the urge. In short, we do not take issue with research indicating that behaviors that risk self-harm often result from self-control failure, or that self-control is often used to achieve normatively good outcomes. Yet necessarily inferring a process of self-control exertion or failure by viewing a behavior demonstrates faulty logic.

The process of self-control is conceptually independent of the particular action that it avoids or to which it leads. People vary in the extent to which they are attracted to any behavior; risky, self-harming behaviors are no different. Logically it follows that actions normatively understood as resulting from self-control failures can result from self-control exertion, at least some of the time. Actions that may appear to be self-control failures because of their obvious costs to the self can result from self-control exertion, in the same manner as actions resulting in self-improvement. It is imperative to know the nature of someone's impulse toward any action before inferring whether it resulted from self-control exertion or failure.

The distinction between the process of self-control and its behavioral outcomes is rarely emphasized, yet such a conflation obscures the fact that people can engage in self-control for personal harm. People engage in risky behaviors for many reasons. Some people enjoy the thrill of risk taking. Others enjoy the physical sensations. Still others simply do not perceive the risk involved. Others, we argue, are in fact repelled by the thought of putting themselves in harm's way. Yet they sometimes engage in those risky behaviors because they think they will be rewarded for doing so. Theoretically, the process of overcoming an aversion to a risky behavior to gain expected rewards requires self-control.

This process begs the question: What kinds of rewards would lead people to force themselves to engage in a risky behavior they do not want to do, such as an 11-hour drinking binge or driving recklessly? In other words, when is self-control for personal harm likely to occur? Many rewards can motivate people to overcome an aversion to a risky behavior. For example, some people enjoy the personal challenge of overcoming a fear. Other people expect the action to be rewarding eventually, after repeated attempts, despite its aversive qualities at present. In many cases, however, we propose that the expectation of social rewards is a key motivator. People may self-harm—and exert self-control to do so—in order to reap anticipated social benefits.

We have focused on social rewards as motivator for a number of reasons. First, a substantial literature documents their importance (Baumeister & Leary, 1995; Eisenberger, Lieberman, & Williams, 2003; Leary, Tambor, Terdal, & Downs, 1995; see Leary & Guadagno, Chapter 18, this volume). Second, in everyday life, there is often tension between what is good for the self and what is good for one's standing in valued groups (Heine & Ruby, 2010). From an evolutionary perspective, navigating a tension between interpersonal goals and intrapersonal goals, desires, and preferences may have been a key benefit in the development of self-control (Vohs & Heatherton, 2000).

Sometimes interpersonal and intrapersonal goals align, which theoretically reduces the amount of self-control required to engage in or avoid a particular action. When an action serves neither personal preferences or goals nor interpersonal goals, the action should be unlikely to occur, and avoiding the action should take no self-control. When an action serves both intrapersonal and interpersonal goals, engaging in the act should take self-control only to the extent that the action is unappealing initially. For example, if Fred has an important goal to lose weight to improve both his personal health and his ability to attract a romantic partner, then hopping in the pool may still require some self-control if he dislikes swimming. If Sally has those same goals but intrinsically enjoys swimming, then to start swimming will not require self-control. From this perspective, actions tend to take less self-control when interpersonal goals align with intrapersonal goals and preferences.

Conflicts between intrapersonal and interpersonal goals—like those highlighted in this chapter—present people with self-control dilemmas. Choosing to forego a close friend's birthday party to study for a midterm exam may take substantial self-control because interpersonal harmony is sacrificed at the expense of an intrapersonal goal to succeed academically. This kind of self-control exertion (i.e., sacrificing interpersonal for intrapersonal gain) is sometimes heralded as a good use of self-control, at least in North America, in that it aligns with the Protestant Work Ethic (see Sanchez-Burks, 2002, for discussion of prioritization of personal over relational concerns).

By the same token, sacrificing personal health for interpersonal success should also require self-control. For example, consider Barney, who recently took an embarrassing pay cut and is very concerned that he now has no spare money after his bills are paid. His closest friends get together to play poker every Friday, and Barney views playing as a crucial way to connect with them. He may force himself to play and to spend money he knows he cannot afford, thereby causing great anxiety. This kind of situation may be interpreted as self-control failure because of normative beliefs that self-harming actions such as gambling are intrinsically appealing (Baumeister et al., 1994). But for Barney, sitting down at that poker table takes a great deal of self-control. His financial health—and, hence, his personal well-being—conflict with his interpersonal relationships and his incipient impulse is to conserve his money and not play. In this case, acting in a relationship-enhancing way would require self-control (Finkel & Campbell, 2001), despite what it might look like to outsiders.

THREE CONDITIONS UNDER WHICH PEOPLE ARE LIKELY TO EXERT SELF-CONTROL FOR PERSONAL HARM IN THE SERVICE OF INTERPERSONAL GAIN

This chapter highlights circumstances in which people exert self-control to overcome an aversion to a risky behavior to gain social rewards for doing so. We propose that these events, which have been ignored or miscategorized in the literature, are most likely to occur when three conditions are met: (1) when people are averse to a particular risky behavior, but (2) they have a strong desire to be accepted by a specific group, and (3) when they perceive the self-harming behavior as a central means of being accepted by that group. When these three conditions are in place, people are likeliest to exert the requisite self-control to engage in that risky action.

Aversion to a Self-Harming Action

There is variation in the extent to which people are initially attracted to self-harming behaviors such as drinking alcohol, smoking, promiscuous sex, gambling, overspending, and overeating. The notion of Type 1 and Type 2 alcoholism is one such demonstration (Irwin, Schuckit, & Smith, 1990). Type 1 alcoholics feel distress in combination with their excessive drinking, are more responsive to treatment, and develop alcoholism in adulthood. Type 2 alcoholics have problems (fighting, etc.) associated with drinking, feel little remorse about drinking, and develop the problem before adulthood. It is probably fair to say that Type 2 alcoholics have, at baseline, a stronger urge to drink than do Type 1 alcoholics.

Alcohol consumption and other kinds of "ephemeral, low-priority enticements" (Fishbach, Friedman, & Kruglanski, 2003) are often presumed to be inherently attractive. However, we do not assume that this is always the case. For example, when people first try self-harming actions such as smoking or drinking alcohol, many recoil at the physical sensations and taste. Some people go on to acquire appetites for self-harming behaviors, but the point is that it is common to feel aversion toward them, at least initially (Fallon & Rozin, 1983).

Strong Desire to Be Accepted by Someone or a Group

The promise of rewards must be sufficiently important to motivate one to overcome a loathed behavior. Much research has shown that, in general, social rewards (including gaining acceptance and avoiding rejection) are highly motivating (Baumeister & Leary,

1995). We propose that perceiving the acceptance, or continued acceptance, by a specific person or a group as vital may provide the motivation to overcome a strong aversion to self-harm. People with strong motivation can overcome strong urges and self-control deficits (Baumeister & Vohs, 2007; Muraven & Slessareva, 2003), suggesting that people with an intense desire to be socially accepted may be particularly willing to exert self-control and, consequently, self-harm despite their aversion to the self-harming act. The expectation of important social rewards can spur the self-control exertion process to override aversion to a self-harming behavior.

Perceive the (Self-Harming) Action as the Central Means to Acceptance

When people feel a strong aversion toward a self-harming action but perceive it as the route to gaining highly valued social acceptance (or avoiding rejection), it should require self-control despite appearances of self-control failure. In terms of goals, when interpersonal goals conflict with intrapersonal goals and preferences in this way, it takes self-control to do the requisite action.

Empirical evidence for the self-control for personal harm model is considered next. The three criteria presented here have provided a broad conceptual frame for searching the literature. As expected, a variety of literature suggests that people sometimes feel averse to actions commonly coded as self-control failures, yet they engage in them for social rewards.

DO PEOPLE EXERT SELF-CONTROL FOR PERSONAL HARM TO GAIN SOCIALLY?

Empirical evidence shows that people engage in self-harming actions for social gain. Moreover, there is evidence that domains normatively viewed as tempting are not always so. When considered in tandem, the literature presents the possibility that sometimes people use self-control to do self-harming acts that are normatively encoded as resulting from self-control failures.

Alcohol Consumption

Alcohol consumption, particularly overconsumption, often is linked to self-control failures (Hull & Slone, 2004; Sayette & Griffin, Chapter 27, this volume). However, surveys have shown that the initial taste of alcohol is unpleasant to many people (Fallon & Rozin, 1983; Moore & Weiss, 1995). Countless manufacturers offer sweetened and diluted versions of alcoholic beverages to entice those who dislike the taste of alcohol, particularly "entry-level drinkers" (McCreanor, Greenaway, Barnes, Borell, & Gregory, 2005; Mosher & Johnsson, 2005). Ample survey data, coupled with the existence of these sweetened products, show that the taste of alcohol is often unpleasant, particularly for early consumption experiences. Yet many people go on to consume alcohol regularly, suggesting that at some point they had to overcome an initial taste aversion.

Despite the unpleasant taste, a key predictor of alcohol consumption frequency is the expectation of social benefits, including acceptance from others and having confidence in conversations (Brown, Goldman, & Christiansen, 1985; Roehling & Goldman, 1987). Results of a 2-year longitudinal study showed that the degree to which young adolescents (ages 11–14) expected alcohol to ease social interactions positively predicted their alcohol consumption habits by the end of the study (Smith, Goldman, Greenbaum, & Christiansen, 1995). It is plausible that the hope of social rewards led some of these adolescents to overcome a preexisting aversion to the taste of alcohol that was likely present for many of them (Fallon & Rozin, 1983; Moore & Weiss, 1995).

When people no longer anticipate social rewards from consuming alcohol, they stop drinking so much of it. Research on pluralistic ignorance regarding alcohol consumption norms has shown that alcohol consumption is affected by people's beliefs about how valued others feel about drinking it (Schroeder & Prentice, 1998). People who have been taught that their peers do not enjoy consuming alcohol as much as it appears they do (based on their consumption) subsequently drink less alcohol than those who maintain that their peers heartily enjoy consuming alcohol. This pattern suggests that people intrinsically desire to consume much less alcohol than they actually do in contexts where alcohol consumption is quite prevalent. The desire to fit in with the peer group seems to motivate some people to drink more alcohol than they would like, suggesting that at least some self-control is being used to consume alcohol.

Recent research has examined the drinking habits over time of people who explicitly reported a dislike of consuming alcohol (Rawn & Vohs, 2011). People who believed concurrently that their friends enjoyed drinking alcohol but that they themselves did not enjoy it went on to consume alcohol at least weekly 2 months later. In contrast, people who reported concurrently disliking alcohol and believing their friends also disliked it did not drink any alcohol 2 months later. These new data suggest that fitting in with desirable others can motivate people to force themselves to overcome their intrinsic distaste for alcohol, but only if those desirable others enjoy drinking it.

Tobacco Use

Starting to smoke is a physically unpleasant experience, and even tobacco companies acknowledge this reality (DiFranza et al., 2004; Teague, 1973). About three-fourths of people who have tried smoking report that their first experience was distasteful and did not make them want to try another cigarette (DiFranza et al., 2004). In response to this strong aversion most people have to their first experiences with smoking, tobacco companies have tried to mask the taste by flavoring products with menthol (Hersey et al., 2006) and fruit (e.g., cherry, peach; Montana Department of Revenue, 2007). In Indonesia, companies such as Marlboro have added cloves to appeal to the local palate and to numb the throat, thereby making it easier for new smokers to inhale smoke (Brummit, 2007). Indeed, in September 2009, a ban on flavored tobacco went into effect in the United States, in an effort by the Federal Drug Administration to curb smoking. The U.S. Congress concluded that flavors such as spice, cinnamon, vanilla, chocolate, clove, strawberry, grape, or cherry were too appealing to children. Hence, the idea is to remove the enticing flavors that otherwise enable young smokers to perform the behavior of smoking without having to (in our words) exert the self-control needed to prevail over the ill-taste of unflavored tobacco.

Clearly, the initial taste of cigarettes is aversive to many. Yet some people endure their first horrid experiences and acquire a taste for (and addiction to) tobacco. Research shows that the expectation of social rewards, including presenting an attractive public self-image and gaining friendship with desirable others, impels people to overcome their initial aversion to smoking. To this point, only a tiny proportion of people smoke their first cigarette by themselves (Friedman, Lichtenstein, & Biglan, 1985; Hahn et al., 1990). The fact that the vast majority of people first try smoking among friends suggests that the social context is a key component of starting smoking.

Longitudinal evidence supports the role of anticipated social rewards in overcoming an initial distaste for smoking. For instance, one study examined the impact of *trait self-monitoring* (Snyder, 1974), which describes the degree to which people stick with one consistent set of behaviors and preferences (i.e., low in self-monitoring) or are "social chameleons" who change with the interpersonal context (i.e., high in self-monitoring). This study focused on 11-year-olds who believed that smoking was common among their peers (Perrine & Aloise-Young, 2004). Results showed that those children who scored highest in self-monitoring (i.e., who were most concerned with presenting a public self-image that matched that of the crowd) were three times more likely than children who scored low in self-monitoring to begin smoking within a year. A desire to portray the self in sync with one's peers, coupled with the perception that smoking is a common activity among those peers, seems to lead young adolescents to overcome the unpleasant taste of starting to smoke.

More convincingly, another study showed that smoking commencement was influenced by the smoking habits of a desired friend (Aloise-Young, Graham, & Hansen, 1994). In this study, adolescents who were outsiders (i.e., those who were not identified as a friend by any peers) tended to begin smoking over the course of a year if they desired friendship from a smoker. Outsiders who desired friendship from a nonsmoker were half as likely as those who desired friendship from a smoker to begin smoking during that same year. Moreover, outsiders who desired friendship from a smoker adjusted their frequency of smoking to match that of their would-be friend. This study suggests that people will overcome an aversion to smoking cigarettes if they think it will lead to social acceptance.

Binge Eating

Satiation from food is accompanied by a variety of signals, including gastric distension, intestinal peptide release, and oral sensations (French & Cecil, 2001). Eating past the point of physical satiety signals requires overriding their input, and results in uncomfortable and even painful side effects. Long-term binge eating, which is clinically considered a self-control failure (American Psychiatric Association, 1994), heightens risks of obesity, depression, and anxiety (Reichborn-Kjennerud, Bulik, Sullivan, Tambs, & Harris, 2004). Binge eating is a physically aversive activity.

Despite the plethora of immediate and longer-term negative consequences for the self, research shows that people will binge-eat in order to fit in with others. Such research suggests that self-control exertion may sometimes lead people to overcome the physically aversive consequences and binge-eat for social rewards. For example, sorority members binge-eat only to the extent that binge-eating is socially rewarded in their particular sorority (Crandall, 1988). In a sorority in which the norm was to binge-eat a moderate amount, members became more popular over time to the extent that they binge-ate a moderate amount, and less popular to the extent that they binge-ate much more or much less than the norm. In a second sorority, the norm was to binge-eat as much as possible; over the course of a year, women in this sorority became more popular if they binged a large amount, and less popular if they did not binge-eat enough. When friendship subgroups, rather than individuals, were considered the unit of analysis, the same pattern was found, such that subgroups became more popular within the sororities to the extent that their members typically binge-ate in line with the sorority norm.

This study was recently replicated and extended, showing more clearly that people binge-eat in order to fit in. In the summer, when the sorority disbanded, the frequency of members' binge-eating episodes (and in this study purging, too), dropped precipitously (Zalta & Keel, 2006). In this case, people do not seem to enjoy engaging in bulimic behaviors, but instead cease when those actions are no longer immediately socially rewarded by peers. These studies show that people binge-eat in order to be liked by others, they are rewarded for doing so, and they suggest that such actions may take self-control to overcome their aversive properties.

Drugs and Delinquency

Illicit drug use and delinquent behaviors, including vandalism, theft, and other criminal acts, have the potential to result in severe costs to the self in both the short and the long term. It is well known that delinquent acts may result in a criminal record, financial penalties, or incarceration. Drug use has the potential to cause addiction, financial expense, physical damage to the body, and legal trouble. Despite a dearth of research, there is some support for the possibility that at least some people have an aversive impulse toward trying drugs. The perception that drugs are used commonly by valued peers is a stronger predictor of drug use than is the expectation that drugs will result in a desirable effect (Eisenthal & Udin, 1972), suggesting that attraction to drugs for their own sake is not the key motivating factor in drug use. Moreover, despite the fact that non-drug-users tend to expect more negative effects as a result of drug use than do users (Linkovich-Kyle & Dunn, 2001; O'Connor, Fite, Nowlin, & Colder, 2007), some nonusers go on to try drugs. The expectation of social rewards may provide adequate incentive for nonusers to try these drugs they know can cause serious consequences. From a different perspective, people are often wary about trying or continuing to use their prescription medications, which again suggests that some people have an aversive impulse toward drug use (Britten, Stevenson, Gafaranga, Barry, & Bradley, 2004; Givens et al., 2006). Together with anecdotal evidence from many discussion boards for people who are scared to try drugs, we conclude that at least some people feel an aversive impulse toward drug use. Desire to be liked by peers (or to follow orders from an authority, as in the case of prescription medicines), may lead people to overcome their aversion to drug use.

Peer pressure has emerged as a key predictor of engagement in a variety of delinquent acts and drug use (Kung & Farrell, 2000; Wolfe, Lennox, & Cutler, 1986), sometimes in addition to desire for popularity (Santor, Messervey, & Kusumakar, 2000). Moreover, in one study, incoming freshmen who were especially concerned with fitting in used more recreational drugs during their first year than did their less socially concerned counterparts in their first and third years, but only if those eager freshmen perceived drug use as instrumental to being liked (Wolfe et al., 1986). This result suggests that some people use harmful drugs in strategic ways to gain acceptance.

More recently, experimental evidence revealed that people will engage in aggressive acts toward the self (i.e., giving oneself a painful electric shock) in order to fit in with an established group norm (Sloan, Berman, Zeigler-Hill, Greer, & Mae, 2006), especially when everyone in the group is self-harming in this way (as opposed to only some group members; Sloan, Berman, Zeigler-Hill, & Bullock, 2009). Desire to fit in with others seems to provide ample incentive for people to accept the negative personal consequences for a variety of delinquent acts, including immediately painful self-shocks. We argue that illicit drug use and many delinquent behaviors (and perhaps self-shocking, although we doubt it) are often viewed as resulting from self-control failure. What this literature suggests is that sometimes people overcome aversions to a variety of potentially dangerous actions in order to gain interpersonal success, which suggests self-control exertion.

Sexual Behaviors

Some sexual practices, such as promiscuous sex and sex without adequate protection, carry personal risks of unwanted pregnancy and sexually transmitted infections that range in consequences from unpleasant to lethal. Moreover, people clearly differ in the kinds of sexual behaviors they find appealing (Scorolli, Ghirlanda, Enquist, Zattoni, & Jannini, 2007). One reason that people engage in sexual practices they perceive to be risky or unappealing is to be liked by other people, including their sexual partners. For example, adolescent girls report a willingness to engage in sexual acts they perceive to be risky, immoral, or unpleasant, if they perceive that those acts will strengthen their romantic relationships (Cornell & Halpern-Felsher, 2006; Halpern-Felsher, Cornell, Kropp, & Tschann, 2005; Purdie & Downey, 2000).

Many people report having participated in consensual unwanted sex; that is, engaging in sexual acts to please a partner, despite their lack of personal desire to do so (Impett & Peplau, 2003). Although it is typically women who report having consensual unwanted sex (O'Sullivan & Allgeier, 1998; Sprecher, Hatfield, Cortese, Potapova, & Levitskaya, 1994), men report it, too, as do people in both short- and long-term relationships, regardless of gender (Impett & Peplau, 2003). This research clearly supports the self-control for personal harm model, showing that people sometimes have sex when they do not want to do so in order to gain social rewards (in this case, harmony with one's partner).

Some people desire interpersonal acceptance to such a degree that they are willing to risk their lives for it. In a small, understudied subculture of gay men, testing positive to the human immunodeficiency virus (HIV) is perceived to be a desirable social status that is accompanied by a community of support (Grov & Parsons, 2006; Tewksbury, 2006). This community is called the Poz Brotherhood, and some men actively seek to become infected with HIV in order to join it. This outrageous example highlights the contextual elements that we proposed would most likely lead people to subjugate their personal well-being for social rewards. First, these men, arguably, are averse to dying (after all, if they wanted to die immediately, there are more efficient routes). They strongly desire membership in a specific group and expect valuable social support that accompanies entrance into that brotherhood. Crucially, there is only one way to join this group, which is to become infected with HIV. These men have overcome an aversion to death in order to join a social group they perceive to be desirable.

Summary

People will consume alcohol, smoke cigarettes, use illicit drugs, shock themselves, engage in criminal acts, have sex, and seek HIV-positive status in order to gain social rewards. When considered together, substantial research and theory support our view that people sometimes risk their personal well-being in order to be liked by others. Furthermore, data suggest that people exert self-control to overcome intrinsic aversions to these acts.

THEORETICAL IMPLICATIONS AND EXTENSIONS

Two theories relate closely to the view that people engage in potentially self-harming behaviors in order to fit in with others. The theory of planned behavior and deviance regulation theory hold social inclusion as a driving force in determining whether and how people decide to enact behaviors that may lead to short-term damage for the actor. Yet neither specifies the mechanism by which such risky behaviors might be enacted.

The theory of planned behavior (TPB; Ajzen, 1985, 1991) is a well-supported and commonly used model for predicting behavior (Ajzen & Cote, 2008). According to the theory of planned behavior, behavior emerges from behavioral intentions, which are derived from social pressure to perform a behavior (i.e., subjective norms), personal attitudes toward the behavior, and a belief that one can enact the behavior (i.e., self-efficacy). This model has been profitably applied to explain numerous behaviors, including condom use (Albarracín, Johnson, Fishbein, & Muellerleile, 2001) and alcohol consumption (e.g., Collins & Carey, 2007; Huchting, Lac, & LaBrie, 2008). In TPB models, the three predictors of behavioral intention are considered simultaneously and without interaction.

The self-control for personal harm model suggests that this first-order model may miss cases in which people's personal attitudes toward a behavior are negative but they feel social pressure to enact it. In theoretical discussions of the TPB, there is an awareness that the relative power of the three predictors likely varies as a function of the particular behavior and population (e.g., Ajzen & Cote, 2008), but interactions among predictors typically are not modeled in empirical studies (cf. Wallace, Paulson, Lord, & Bond, 2005).

Deviance regulation theory (DRT; Blanton & Christie, 2003) posits that people desire to be distinguished from others, yet do so in socially accepted ways lest they be rejected for extreme deviance. In this model, behaviors that distinguish people from others in their group are viewed as being tied to one's identity. People must walk the line between adopting behaviors that become distinguishing characteristics and conforming to restrictions their social groups impose to avoid rejection. The notion of social rejection from extreme deviation is echoed in our model as well. Yet our model places at the center the process of self-control, which is absent from DRT. Marrying the self-control for personal harm model with deviance regulation, though, leads to the notion that self-control is the process through which some deviant behavior is enacted. In other words, we predict that the people who are most successful at managing their deviance (not too much, and not too little) are those with high self-control; those who are least successful at managing their deviance (i.e., by engaging in no acts or acts that are too extreme for the group) are either chronically or temporarily low in self-control.

Our theory suggests that the predictive power of the TPB and DRT may be improved to the extent that interactions among predictors are modeled in addition to the first-order effects. Also, we propose that those models need to specify the psychological mechanism through which people come to enact behavior. It is possible that behaviors may arise through self-control in different ways (i.e., through self-control failure or exertion), depending on the degree of conflict among attitudes, subjective norms, and self-efficacy. Future research could merge the ideas proposed in the self-control for personal harm model with these related models for a comprehensive understanding of *why* (e.g., to regulate one's social standing or to conform to peer pressure) and *how* (i.e., self-control processes) people enact risky behaviors.

CONCLUSIONS

This chapter has presented a new self-control for personal harm model. Some caveats are in order, though, before we draw our conclusions. First, it is not necessary that the reward toward which people are orienting be interpersonal but, like many scholars (e.g., Baumeister & Leary, 1995; Leary et al., 1995), we assume that much of what people do is aimed at securing and maintaining social inclusion. Second, it is not necessary for an act of self-control to lead to self-injurious outcomes.

Rather, our model underscores that the process of self-control is separate from the outcome. This means that people can engage in self-control to achieve ill-aims or that people can achieve normatively good outcomes through no use of self-control. Notably, the current theory also does not preordain that urges be aimed at consuming attractive temptations (cf. Hofmann, Friese, & Wiers, 2009); urges can and often are aimed at avoiding loathsome stimuli, such as that involved in new and unwanted encounters.

In summary, the self-control for personal harm model we have presented here states that people who want to belong to a group and are unsure of how otherwise to become included may turn to behaviors that they do not desire to perform, but that they think will lead to acceptance. To perform these behaviors, the individual needs self-control. This means that self-control can be used for behaviors that are not only good or moral but also harmful to the self, and these behaviors still fit squarely in the definition of self-control, in that they require overriding an incipient impulse with a goal in mind. By viewing these behaviors as self-control endeavors, researchers will have a firmer grasp on how they come about and what can be done to alter them.

REFERENCES

Ajzen, I. (1985). From intentions to actions: A theory of planned behavior. In J. Kuhl & J. Beck-mann (Eds.), *Action control: From cognition to behavior* (pp. 11–39). Heidelberg: Springer.

Ajzen, I. (1991). The theory of planned behavior. *Organizational Behavior and Human Decision Processes, 50*, 179–211.

Ajzen, I., & Cote, N. G. (2008). Attitudes and the prediction of behavior. In W. D. Crano & R. Prislin (Eds.), *Attitudes and attitude change* (pp. 289–311). New York: Psychology Press.

Albarracín, D., Johnson, B. T., Fishbein, M., & Muellerleile, P. A. (2001). Theories of reasoned action and planned behavior as models of condom use: A meta-analysis. *Psychological Bulletin, 127*, 142–161.

Aloise-Young, P. A., Graham, J. W., & Hansen, W. B. (1994). Peer influence of smoking initiation during early adolescence: A comparison of group members and group outsiders. *Journal of Applied Psychology, 79*, 281–287.

American Psychiatric Association. (1994). *Diagnostic and statistical manual of mental disorders* (4th ed.). Washington, DC: Author.

Asch, S. E. (1955). Opinions and social pressure. *Scientific American, 193*, 31–35.

Asch, S. E. (1956). Studies of independence and conformity: A minority of one against a unanimous majority. *Psychological Monographs, 70*(9, Whole No. 416).

Baumeister, R. F., Bratslavsky, E., Finkenauer, C., & Vohs, K. D. (2001). Bad is stronger than good. *Review of General Psychology, 5*, 323–370.

Baumeister, R. F., Bratslavsky, E., Muraven, M., & Tice, D. M. (1998). Ego depletion: Is the active self a limited resource? *Journal of Personality and Social Psychology, 74*, 1252–1265.

Baumeister, R. F., DeWall, C. N., Ciarocco, N. J., & Twenge, J. M. (2005). Social exclusion impairs self-regulation. *Journal of Personality and Social Psychology, 88*, 589–604.

Baumeister, R. F., & Exline, J. J. (1999). Virtue, personality, and social relations: Self-control as the moral muscle. *Journal of Personality, 67*, 1165–1194.

Baumeister, R. F., Heatherton, T. F., & Tice, D. M. (1994). *Losing control: How and why people fail at self-regulation*. San Diego, CA: Academic Press.

Baumeister, R. F., & Leary, M. R. (1995). The need to belong: Desire for interpersonal attachments as a fundamental human motivation. *Psychological Bulletin, 117*, 497–529.

Baumeister, R. F., Schmeichel, B. J., & Vohs, K. D. (2007). Self-regulation and the executive function: The self as controlling agent. In A. W. Kruglanski & E. T. Higgins (Eds.), *Social psychology: Handbook of basic principles* (2nd ed., pp. 516–539). New York: Guilford Press.

Baumeister, R. F., & Vohs, K. D. (2007). Self-regulation, ego depletion, and motivation. *Social and Personality Psychology Compass, 1*, 115–128.

Blanton, H., & Christie, C. (2003). Deviance regulation: A theory of action and identity. *Review of General Psychology, 7*, 115–149.

Britten, N., Stevenson, F., Gafaranga, J., Barry, C., & Bradley, C. (2004). The expression of aversion to medicines in general practice consultations. *Social Science and Medicine, 59*, 1495–1503.t

Brown, S. A., Goldman, M. S., & Christiansen, B. A. (1985). Do alcohol expectancies mediate drinking patterns of adults? *Journal of Consulting and Clinical Psychology, 53*, 512–519.

Brummit, C. (2007, July 3). Clove Marlboro launched in Indonesia. *USA Today*. Retrieved March 6, 2009, from *www.usatoday.com/money/economy/2007-07-03-3435618843_x.htm*.

Cialdini, R. B. (2009). *Influence: Science and practice* (5th ed.). Boston: Allyn & Bacon.

Collins, S. E., & Carey, K. B. (2007). The theory of planned behavior as a model of heavy episodic drinking among college students. *Psychology of Addictive Behaviors, 21*, 498–507.

Cornell, J. L., & Halpern-Felsher, B. L. (2006). Adolescents tell us why teens have oral sex. *Journal of Adolescent Health, 38*, 299–301.

Crandall, C. S. (1988). Social contagion of binge eating. *Journal of Personality and Social Psychology, 55*, 588–598.

DiFranza, J. R., Savageau, J. A., Fletcher, K., Ockene, J. K., Rigotti, N. A., McNeill, A. D., et al. (2004). Recollections and repercussions of the first inhaled cigarette. *Addictive Behaviors, 29*, 261–272.

Eisenberger, N. I., Lieberman, M. D., & Williams, K. D. (2003). Does rejection hurt?: An fMRI study of social exclusion. *Science, 302*, 290–292.

Eisenthal, S., & Udin, H. (1972). Psychological factors associated with drug and alcohol usage among Neighborhood Youth Corps enrollees. *Developmental Psychology, 7*, 119–123.

Fallon, A. E., & Rozin, P. (1983). The psychological bases of food rejections by humans. *Ecology of Food and Nutrition, 13*, 15–26.

Finkel, E. J., & Campbell, W. K. (2001). Self-control and accommodation in close relationships: An interdependence analysis. *Journal of Personality and Social Psychology, 81*, 263–277.

Fishbach, A., Friedman, R. S., & Kruglanski, A. W. (2003). Leading us not into temptation: Momentary allurements elicit overriding goal activation. *Journal of Personality and Social Psychology, 84*, 296–309.

Frat suspended after student's body found inside lounge. (2004). Retrieved December 4, 2009, from *www.thedenverchannel.com/news/3713302/detail.html*.

French, S. J., & Cecil, J. E. (2001). Oral, gastric and intestinal influences on human feeding. *Physiology and Behavior, 74*, 729–734.

Friedman, L. S., Lichtenstein, E., & Biglan, A. (1985). Smoking onset among teens: An empirical analysis of initial situations. *Addictive Behaviors, 10*, 1–13.

Givens, L. L., Datto, C. J., Ruckdeschel, K., Knott, K., Zubritsky, C., Oslin, D. W., et al. (2006). Older patients' aversion to antidepressants: A qualitative study. *Journal of General Internal Medicine, 21*, 146–151.

Goldstein, N. J., Cialdini, R. B., & Griskevicius, V. (2008). A room with a viewpoint: Using normative appeals to motivate environmental conservation in a hotel setting. *Journal of Consumer Research, 35*, 472–482.

Gottfredson, M. R., & Hirschi, T. (1990). *A general theory of crime*. Stanford, CA: Stanford University Press.

Grov, C., & Parsons, J. T. (2006). Bug Chasing and Gift Giving: The potential for HIV transmission among barebackers on the Internet. *AIDS Education and Prevention, 18*, 490–503.

Hahn, G., Charlin, V. L., Sussman, S., Dent, C. W., Manzi, J., Stacy, A. W., et al. (1990). Adolescents' first and most recent use situations of smokeless tobacco and cigarettes: Similarities and differences. *Addictive Behaviors, 15*, 439–448.

Halpern-Felsher, B. L., Cornell, J. L., Kropp, R. Y., & Tschann, J. M. (2005). Oral versus vaginal sex among adolescents: Perceptions, attitudes, and behavior. *Pediatrics, 115*, 845–851.

Heine, S. J., & Ruby, M. B. (2010). Cultural psychology. *Wiley Interdisciplinary Reviews: Cognitive Science, 1*, 254–266.

Hersey, J. C., Ng, S. W., Nonnemaker, J. M., Mowery, P., Thomas, K. Y., Vilsaint, M.-C., et al. (2006). Are menthol cigarettes a starter product for youth? *Nicotine and Tobacco Research, 8*, 403–413.

Hofmann, W., Friese, M., & Strack, F. (2009). Impulse and self-control from a dual-systems perspective. *Perspectives in Psychological Science, 4*, 162–176.

Hofmann, W., Friese, M., & Wiers, R. W. (2008). Impulsive versus reflective influences on health behavior: A theoretical framework and empirical review. *Health Psychology Review, 2*, 11–137.

How many teens die in car wrecks? (n.d.). Retrieved December 9, 2009, from *www.keepthedrive.com/statistics.aspx*.

Huchting, K., Lac, A., & LaBrie, J. W. (2008). An application of the theory of planned behavior to sorority alcohol consumption. *Addictive Behaviors, 33*, 538–551.

Hull, J. G., & Slone, L. B. (2004). Alcohol and self-regulation. In R. F. Baumeister & K. D. Vohs (Eds.), *Handbook of self-regulation: Research, theory, and applications* (pp. 466–491). New York: Guilford Press.

Impett, E. A., & Peplau, L. A. (2003). Sexual compliance: Gender, motivational, and relationship perspectives. *Journal of Sex Research, 40*, 87–100.

Irwin, M., Schuckit, M. A., & Smith, T. L. (1990). Clinical importance of age at onset in Type 1 and Type 2 primary alcoholics. *Archives of General Psychiatry, 47*, 320–324.

Kung, E. M., & Farrell, A. D. (2000). The role of parents and peers in early adolescent substance use: An examination of mediating and moderating effects. *Journal of Child and Family Studies, 9*, 509–528.

Leary, M. R., Tambor, E. S., Terdal, S. K., & Downs, D. L. (1995). Self-esteem as an interpersonal monitor: The sociometer hypothesis. *Journal of Personality and Social Psychology, 68*, 518–530.

Linkovich-Kyle, T. L., & Dunn, M. E. (2001). Consumption-related differences in the organization and activation of marijuana expectancies in memory. *Experimental and Clinical Psychopharmacology, 9*, 334–342.

McCreanor, T., Greenaway, A., Barnes, H. M., Borell, S., & Gregory, A. (2005). Youth identity formation and contemporary alcohol marketing. *Critical Public Health, 15*, 251–262.

Mischel, W., Shoda, Y., & Peake, P. K. (1988). The nature of adolescent competencies predicted by preschool delay of gratification. *Journal of Personality and Social Psychology, 54*, 687–696.

Montana Department of Revenue. (June 26, 2007). Listed product of little cigars classified as cigarettes for taxation purposes and youth access laws. Retrieved March 6, 2009, from *mt.gov/revenue/forbusinesses/littlecigars/little_cigar_classification_list_of_little_cigars.pdf.*

Moore, M., & Weiss, S. (1995). Reasons for non-drinking among Israeli adolescents of four religions. *Drug and Alcohol Dependence, 38*, 45–50.

Mosher, J. F., & Johnsson, D. (2005). Flavored alcoholic beverages: An international marketing campaign that targets youth. *Journal of Public Health Policy, 26*, 326–342.

Muraven, M., & Slessareva, E. (2003). Mechanisms of self-control failure: Motivation and limited resources. *Personality and Social Psychology Bulletin, 29*, 894–906.

O'Connor, R. M., Fite, P. J., Nowlin, P. R., & Colder, C. R. (2007). Children's beliefs about substance use: An examination of age differences in implicit and explicit cognitive precursors of substance use initiation. *Psychology of Addictive Behaviors, 21*, 525–533.

O'Sullivan, L. F., & Allgeier, E. R. (1998). Feigning sexual desire: Consenting to unwanted sexual activity in heterosexual dating relationships. *Journal of Sex Research, 35*, 234–243.

Perrine, N. E., & Aloise-Young, P. A. (2004). The role of self-monitoring in adolescents' susceptibility to passive peer pressure. *Personality and Individual Differences, 37*, 1701–1716.

Pocheptsova, A., Amir, O., Dhar, R., & Baumeister, R. F. (2009). Deciding without resources: Resource depletion and choice in context. *Journal of Marketing Research, 46*, 344–355.

Purdie, V., & Downey, G. (2000). Rejection sensitivity and adolescent girls' vulnerability to relationship-centered difficulties. *Child Maltreatment, 5*, 338–349.

Rawn, C. D., & Vohs, K. D. (2011). *Longitudinal study of potentially risky behaviors.* Manuscript in preparation.

Reichborn-Kjennerud, T., Bulik, C., Sullivan, P. F., Tambs, K., & Harris, J. R. (2004). Psychiatric and medical symptoms in binge eating in the absence of compensatory behaviors. *Obesity Research, 12*, 1445–1454.

Roehling, P. V., & Goldman, M. S. (1987). Alcohol expectancies and their relationship to actual drinking experiences. *Psychology of Addictive Behaviors, 1*, 108–113.

Samantha Spady. (n.d.). Retrieved December 4, 2009, from *compelledtoact.com/tragic_listing/spady.htm.*

Sanchez-Burks, J. (2002). Protestant relational ideology and (in)attention to relational cues in work settings. *Journal of Personality and Social Psychology, 83*, 919–929.

Santor, D. A., Messervey, D., & Kusumakar, V. (2000). Measuring peer pressure, popularity, and conformity in adolescent boys and girls: Predicting school performance, sexual attitudes, and substance abuse. *Journal of Youth and Adolescence, 29*, 163–182.

Schmeichel, B. J., Vohs, K. D., & Baumeister, R. F. (2003). Ego depletion and intelligent performance: Role of the self in logical reasoning and other information processing. *Journal of Personality and Social Psychology, 85*, 33–46.

Schroeder, C. M., & Prentice, D. A. (1998). Exposing pluralistic ignorance to reduce alcohol use among college students. *Journal of Applied Social Psychology, 28*, 2150–2180.

Scorolli, C., Ghirlanda, S., Enquist, M., Zattoni, S., & Jannini, E. A. (2007). Relative prevalence of different fetishes. *International Journal of Impotence Research, 19*, 432–437.

Sherif, M. (1935). A study of some social factors in perception. *Archives of Psychology, 27*, 23–46.

Simons-Morton, B., Lerner, N., & Singer, J. (2005). The observed effects of teenage passengers on the risky driving behavior of teenage drivers. *Accident Analysis and Prevention, 37*, 973–982.

Sloan, P. A., Berman, M. E., Zeigler-Hill, V., & Bullock, J. S. (2009). Group influences on self-aggression: Conformity and dissenter effects. *Journal of Social and Clinical Psychology, 28*, 535–553.

Sloan, P. A., Berman, M. E., Zeigler-Hill, V., Greer, T. F., & Mae, L. L. (2006). Group norms and self-aggressive behavior. *Journal of Social and Clinical Psychology, 25*, 1107–1121.

Smith, G. T., Goldman, M. S., Greenbaum, P. E., & Christiansen, B. A. (1995). Expectancy for social facilitation from drinking: The divergent paths of high-expectancy and low-expectancy adolescents. *Journal of Abnormal Psychology, 104*, 32–40.

Snyder, M. (1974). Self-monitoring of expressive behaviour. *Journal of Personality and Social Psychology, 30*, 526–537.

Sprecher, S., Hatfield, E., Cortese, A., Potapova, E., & Levitskaya, A. (1994). Token resistance to sexual intercourse and consent to unwanted intercourse: College students' dating experiences in three countries. *Journal of Sex Research, 31*, 125–132.

Tangney, J. P., Baumeister, R. F., & Boone, A. L. (2004). High self-control predicts good adjustment, less pathology, better grades, and interpersonal success. *Journal of Personality, 72*, 271–322.

Teague, C. E. (1973, February 2). *Research planning memorandum on some thoughts about new brands of cigarettes for the youth market.* Winston-Salem, NC: R. J. Reynolds Tobacco Co. Retrieved March 6, 2009, from *ltdlimages.library.ucsf.edu/imagese/e/d/y/edy62d00.*

Tewksbury, R. (2006). "Click here for HIV": An analysis of Internet-based Bug Chasers and Bug Givers. *Deviant Behavior, 27*, 379–395.

Twenge, J. M., Baumeister, R. F., DeWall, C. N., Ciarocco, N. J., & Bartels, J. M. (2007). Social exclusion decreases prosocial behavior. *Journal of Personality and Social Psychology, 92*, 56–66.

Twenge, J. M., Baumeister, R. F., Tice, D. M., & Stucke, T. S. (2001). If you can't join them, beat them: Effects of social exclusion on aggressive behavior. *Journal of Personality and Social Psychology, 81*, 1058–1069.

Vohs, K. D., & Baumeister, R. F. (2004). Understanding self-regulation: An introduction. In R. F. Baumeister & K. D. Vohs (Eds.), *Handbook of self-regulation* (pp. 1–9). New York: Guilford Press.

Vohs, K. D., Baumeister, R. F., & Ciarocco, N. (2005). Self-regulation and self-presentation: Regulatory resource depletion impairs impression management and effortful self-presentation depletes regulatory resources. *Journal of Personality and Social Psychology, 88*, 632–657.

Vohs, K. D., & Heatherton, T.F. (2000). Self-regulatory failure: A resource-depletion approach. *Psychological Science, 11*, 249–254.

Wallace, D. S., Paulson, R. M., Lord, C. G., & Bond, C. F., Jr. (2005). Which behaviors do attitudes predict?: Meta-analyzing the effects of social pressure and perceived difficulty. *Review of General Psychology, 9*, 214–227.

Wolfe, R. N., Lennox, R. D., & Cutler, B. L. (1986). Getting along and getting ahead: Empirical support for a theory of protective and acquisitive self-presentation. *Journal of Personality and Social Psychology, 50*, 356–361.

Zalta, A. K., & Keel, P. K. (2006). Peer influence on bulimic symptoms in college students. *Journal of Abnormal Psychology, 115*, 185–189.

CHAPTER 21

The Effects of Social Relationships on Self-Regulation

ELI J. FINKEL
GRÁINNE M. FITZSIMONS

The last few decades of the 20th century were fat times for self-regulation research. Scholars introduced exciting new theories and research methods that reverberated throughout psychology and beyond. Most of this research examined individuals who set goals, sought to achieve them, and monitored their progress, all largely by themselves (for a review, see Baumeister, Heatherton, & Tice, 1994). The research largely neglected the role of social relationships in influencing self-regulatory processes.

This intrapersonal emphasis contrasted sharply with major approaches to self-regulation outside of the ivory tower. For example, Alcoholics Anonymous, which is one of the most famous and influential approaches to understanding self-regulation, accepts as a core tenet that individuals cannot conquer their destructive drinking behavior without help from other people. According to the opening sentence the organization's website, "Alcoholics Anonymous is a fellowship of men and women who share their experience, strength and hope with each other that they may solve their common problem and help others to recover from alcoholism." In short, self-regulation, at least insofar as destructive drinking is concerned, requires help from others.

Over the past decade, a growing body of research has emerged to support the idea that social relationships have strong and wide-ranging effects on people's self-regulatory success (see Vohs & Finkel, 2006), and one goal of this chapter is to review this research. Our second goal is to incorporate into our review of this topic disparate findings (from various subdisciplines of psychology) that have not typically been conceptualized in terms of the effects of social relationships on self-regulation. Our third and final goal is to identify largely neglected research topics linking social relationships to self-regulation.

Toward these goals, we adopt Carver and Scheier's (1982) model of self-regulation as an organizing framework (also see Baumeister, Schmeichel, & Vohs, 2007). In particular, our review focuses on three key components of self-regulation: (1) *goal setting and initiation*, or the processes by which individuals decide which goals to pursue; (2) *goal operation*, or the processes by which individuals alter their thoughts, feelings, or behaviors to make progress toward achieving their goals; and (3) *goal monitoring*, or the processes by which individuals evaluate the degree to which they are making progress toward achieving their goals and are likely to make progress in these efforts in the future.

We begin by defining terms and addressing issues of scope. The term *self-regulation* refers to the processes by which the self alters its own responses or inner states in a goal-directed manner (see Baumeister et al., 2007). We use the terms *self-regulation* and *goal pursuit* interchangeably. Our primary focus is on the influence that *close* relationship partners, also called *significant others* (romantic partners, parents, etc.), have on people's self-regulation. However, we also review research involving nonclose relationship partners (even strangers) when the available research involving close relationship partners is sparse and the processes at play are likely to be relevant to close relationships. Such topics often suggest promising directions for future research.

INTERPERSONAL INFLUENCES ON GOAL INITIATION

We begin by discussing interpersonal influences on the first component of goal pursuit—the preliminary processes people employ to set or initiate goals (Carver & Scheier, 1982). In this broad category of *goal initiation*, we include both fully deliberate processes, such as explicit goal setting, and nondeliberate processes, such as automatic goal activation. Research over the past decade has established that although goal activation frequently emerges via internal and independent processes, it can also emerge via interpersonal processes. Relationship partners can influence goal initiation by assigning goals, inspiring goals, or triggering goals.

Assigning Goals

A quick review of experimental research on self-regulation makes clear that other people can initiate one's goals: Although many self-regulation studies examine participants' ongoing real-life goal pursuits (e.g., Fishbach, Friedman, & Kruglanski, 2003; Fitzsimons & Shah, 2008), many others examine goals initiated in response to experimental manipulations. As an example, consider the classic delay of gratification experiments (Mischel, 1974; Mischel, Shoda, & Rodriguez, 1989). The experimenter assigned children the goal of resisting the impulse to consume an inferior reward in the moment (e.g., one marshmallow) to earn a superior reward later in the session (e.g., two marshmallows). Similarly, studies of implementation intentions sometimes involve the experimenter assigning goals to participants (e.g., assigning students the goal of writing a report during a busy holiday; Gollwitzer & Brandstätter, 1997).

Organizational and developmental psychologists have explored this process of explicit goal assignment outside of the laboratory. According to an extensive review of goal setting in organizations (Locke & Latham, 1990, 2002), when goals are externally assigned (i.e., the manager sets the goal for the employee), they shape performance just as strongly as when goals are "participatively set" (i.e., the employee takes part in the goal setting), as long as the goal's purpose is explained (Latham, Erez, & Locke, 1988).

Externally assigned goals influence performance by changing the employee's goal setting and sense of self-efficacy. For example, when a supervisor assigns a particularly challenging goal, this improves performance because it increases both the ambitiousness of the employee's goal and the employee's self-efficacy (see Locke & Latham, 2002); after all, employees whose supervisor assigns them a challenging goal can typically conclude that the supervisor believes they can accomplish it. Similarly, parentally assigned goals can shape children's goal setting and subsequent performance (Caulkins, Smith, Gill, & Johnson, 1998; Marjoribanks, 1979; Zimmerman, Bandura, & Martinez-Pons, 1992), although the mechanisms through which parents' achievement-relevant goal setting impacts children's own goal initiation are not well understood (Martinez-Pons, 2002; Zimmerman et al., 1992).

Inspiring Goals

In addition to assigning explicit goals, relationship partners can also affect one's goal initiation by serving as models of behavior that can inspire the adoption of new standards. According to social learning theory (Bandura, 1986), one can adopt new goals by observing and imitating the actions of a model. Modeled goal pursuits that lead to positive outcomes for the model are especially likely to motivate one to adopt the new action (Bandura, 1986; Zimmerman & Koussa, 1979), presumably because one also seeks the positive end states associated with performing that action. A number of studies have demonstrated that close relationship partners can inspire one's goals via modeling. For example, parents who modeled good self-regulation had children with stronger academic self-regulation and academic achievement than parents who did not (Martinez-Pons, 2002), and parents who modeled good exercise behavior had children with better fitness habits than parents who did not (Davison, Cutting, & Birch, 2003).

Triggering Goals

The preceding discussion notwithstanding, people frequently initiate goals on their own. Indeed, people are often alone, absorbed in their own thoughts, when goals come to mind and motivate goal pursuit. Are these situations outside the influence of social relationships? Over the past decade, scholars have employed social cognitive procedures to demonstrate empirically that goal-relevant actions, even when they are initiated and pursued in isolation, are often socially triggered.

In particular, research on automatic goal pursuit has suggested one route through which relationship partners can shape goal initiation. Individuals repeatedly initiate and pursue specific goals in the company of the same significant others, such as romantic partners, colleagues, and family members. Over time, due to this repetition, individuals develop strong associations between these goals and these significant others (Miller & Read, 1991; Moretti & Higgins, 1999). Based on these strong associations, exposure to those significant others can be sufficient to activate the linked goal, which, once activated, can subsequently shape perception and behavior. Thus, the presence of significant others can trigger goal-directed action, even in the absence of any awareness on the part of goal pursuers, who likely perceive their actions as unaffected by external influence (Wegner & Wheatley, 1999).

Importantly, research has shown that this process can be triggered without the physical presence of significant others; their mere psychological presence has been shown to be sufficient to trigger goals and initiate goal-directed behavior (Andersen, Reznik, & Manzella, 1996; Fitzsimons & Bargh, 2003; Shah, 2003a). This idea was first explored in the context of studies on transference, which found that when a new person resembled a significant other, motivation toward the significant other was transferred to the new person (Andersen et al., 1996). For example, in one study, participants reported stronger approach goals toward a stranger who resembled a positive significant other and stronger avoidance goals toward a stranger who resembled a negative significant other.

Building on those findings, research has demonstrated that simply reminding people of their significant others produces goal-directed behavior—from helping behavior to achievement-oriented behavior—in line with goals associated with those others (Fitzsimons & Bargh, 2003; Shah, 2003a). When participants were primed with close relationship partners, the goals they commonly pursued within those relationships became active and guided behavior. For example, one study examined how significant-other priming affected college students' motivation to perform well on an academic achievement task (Fitzsimons & Bargh, 2003). In a mass testing session, participants reported the goals they commonly pursued with each of a number of important relationship partners, including their mothers. Researchers grouped participants into two categories: those who spontaneously reported a goal to achieve academically to please their mothers, and those who did not mention such a goal with their mothers. In a laboratory session later in the term, participants completed a supraliminal priming procedure, in which they described either their mothers' physical appearance or their path to school, then performed an academic achievement task. Participants primed with their mothers significantly outperformed control participants, but only if they had reported a goal to achieve academically to please their mothers. The impact of significant others on individuals' goal-directed action was further shown to depend on features of the relationship. For example, in one study, only participants who believed their fathers cared about their academic performance and reported a close relationship with him responded to subliminal primes *father* and *dad* by working harder on an academic achievement task (Shah, 2003a).

Of course, not everyone hopes to please every relationship partner, or seeks to fulfill every relationship partner's goals. As such, thinking about others will not always lead individuals to behave in line with the others' goals. For example, when individuals perceive significant others as controlling, they can react against the goals of those others (Chartrand, Dalton, & Fitzsimons, 2007). In one study, participants primed with a controlling significant other who wanted them to work hard subsequently solved fewer anagrams than participants primed with a controlling other who wanted them to have fun. Similarly, participants who scored high in the individual-difference tendency toward psychological reactance (Brehm, 1966) also responded to significant-other priming by pursuing goals counter to the desires of their loved ones (Chartrand et al., 2007).

Complementing this research demonstrating that activating representations of relationship partners can influence goal pursuit in a specific goal context is research demonstrating that activating relationship insecurities can alter individuals' general motivational orientation (Cavallo, Fitzsimons, & Holmes, 2009, 2010). Several studies showed that worries about a romantic partner's dedication can temporarily prompt individuals to initiate and pursue safety-oriented goals in general, outside of the relationship. For example, when participants were led to doubt their romantic partners' commitment, they chose more cautious financial investments and showed greater accessibility of safety-related constructs.

Just thinking about close relationships, then, can initiate goal pursuit and shape behavior outside of the relationship context. In addition, simply watching another person pursue a goal can trigger goal-directed action on the part of the observer. In *goal contagion*, individuals automatically infer goals underlying others' actions and subsequently pursue those goals themselves (Aarts, Gollwitzer, & Hassin, 2004; see Papies & Aarts, Chapter 7, this volume). In one study, half of the heterosexual male participants read a story in which the main character's actions implied he was pursuing a goal to have casual sex, while another half read a story with similar content that did not imply such a goal. Participants then had the opportunity to ingratiate themselves to another student by working to improve a task allegedly designed by that student. Participants who read a story implying the goal of seeking casual sex were more helpful, but only when they believed the other student was female, suggesting that their actions might have been guided by an underlying goal to seek sex themselves. Although these experiments involved fictional characters, we believe they have implications for close relationships. Given their high interdependence, close relationship partners are frequently and repeatedly exposed to each other's goal pursuits. As such, over time, such partners may be particularly likely to adopt each other's goals without conscious intention.

In summary, these programs of research suggest that the goals that people initiate and choose to pursue are shaped by the presence—physical or psychological—of others. Of course, people are not passive copycats who mimic every action pursued by others, nor are they mindless automatons who pursue every goal activated by others. To date, little research has examined the limiting or boundary conditions of these phenomena, or of priming effects more broadly. Future research could fruitfully explore the psychological and social situations most and least likely to imbue people with the ability to trigger goals in others.

INTERPERSONAL INFLUENCES ON GOAL OPERATION

Once individuals have set and initiated a goal, they must pursue some goal-relevant course of action to make progress toward achieving it. In this section, we discuss interpersonal influences on the second component of goal pursuit—the mechanisms by which individuals seek to reduce discrepancies between their current and their desired states (Carver & Scheier, 1982). In this broad category of *goal operation*, we review evidence that relationship partners can influence individuals' success at achieving such discrepancy reduction. A relationship partner can have such an effect by providing social support, influencing one's psychological resources, influencing one's motivation, or altering one's goal-pursuit strategies. Our review focuses more on the former two processes (social support and resources) than on the latter two (motivation and strategies) because they have garnered considerably more attention in the scholarly literature. (A fifth process, in which a relationship partner fosters appropriate disengagement from one's goals, has been largely neglected.)

Providing Social Support

A general means by which interpersonal processes affect the operation stage of self-regulation is via *social support*, which we define broadly as a suite of interpersonal processes whereby another person helps an individual engage in effective self-regulation. Social support has been particularly well-studied in the domain of health behaviors (see Reblin & Uchino, 2008). Because virtually all of us seek to be healthy and fit rather than unhealthy and flabby, and because self-regulatory failures in health-related domains (e.g., overeating, lack of exercise, smoking) are rampant (see Baumeister, Heatherton, & Tice, 1994), the effects of social processes on health behaviors are prototypical examples of how such processes can promote effective self-regulation. For example, individuals with strong social support adhere better to medical regimens than do individuals with weak social support (for a meta-analytic review, see DiMatteo, 2004). Such individuals also exercise more, engage in more physical activity in general, sleep more regular hours, are more likely to use seat belts when driving, consume more fruits and vegetables, and are more likely to quit smoking (Allgöwer, Wardle, & Steptoe, 2001; Cohen & Lichtenstein, 1990; Davison et al., 2003; Eyler et al., 1999; Novak & Webster, 2009; Reblin & Uchino, 2008). People with poorer social support die younger, and this association appears to be mediated in part through such health behaviors (Uchino, 2004). However, because much of this research is correlational, it remains unclear to what extent positive relationships promote good self-regulation in the health domain, and to what extent good self-regulation promotes positive relationships (for a review of researching examining the link between self-regulation and relationship functioning, see Fitzsimons & Finkel, Chapter 22, this volume).

Several lines of research suggest that the effects of social support on self-regulation are not limited to the domain of health behaviors. For example, individuals whose romantic partners strongly (vs. weakly) support and encourage their goals in domains such as academics, career, friendships, and fitness, have significantly greater confidence that these goals are achievable and are ultimately more likely to achieve them (Brunstein, Dangelmayer, & Schultheiss, 1996; Feeney, 2004). Research on the *dependency paradox* demonstrates that individuals who are willing to be dependent upon a romantic partner pursue their goals with greater autonomy than do individuals who are less willing to be dependent (Feeney, 2007). Thus, close others can positively impact goal progress.

Indeed, individuals who respond to an activated goal by selectively drawing closer to goal-supportive others are more successful in their goal pursuits over time than are individuals whose feelings of closeness to others' are unaffected by the others' goal support (Fitzsimons & Shah, 2008). In a study combining social cognitive and longitudinal procedures, first-year university students rated their closeness to achievement-instrumental and -noninstrumental friends one time when achievement goals were primed and another time when they were not. Students who drew closer to their goal-instrumental friends when achievement goals were primed (relative to when such goals were not primed) adhered better to their studying goals and ultimately earned higher grades than their counterparts who did not.

An extended program of research on the Michelangelo phenomenon investigates one social support process through which relationship partners positively predict one's goal achievement. The *Michelangelo phenomenon* describes a process whereby a relationship partner "sculpts" one toward achieving on one's ideal-self goals—those goals that are essential to helping an individual become the person he or she aspires to become (Drigotas, Rusbult, Wieselquist, & Whitton, 1999; for a review, see Rusbult, Finkel, & Kumashiro, 2009). The metaphor underlying this phenomenon comes from Michelangelo Buonarroti's sculpting process. Michelangelo "conceived his figures as lying hidden in the block of marble. . . . The task he set himself as a sculptor was merely to extract the ideal form" (Gombrich, 1995, p. 313). The sculptor hammers, chisels, and polishes the raw material to reveal the beautiful figure slumbering within.

Humans, too, have ideal forms (Higgins, 1987; Markus & Nurius, 1986), and although humans are better equipped than blocks of marble to grow toward their ideal self without external intervention, research on the Michelangelo phenomenon suggests that close relationship partners can facilitate such growth. To the degree that such a partner views one as already approximating one's ideal self and behaves in accord with this view, one grows over time toward this ideal. Such personal growth positively predicts individuals' personal and relational well-being (Drigotas, 2002; Drigotas et al., 1999).

Scholars interested in the circumstances under which the sculpting process is most successful have examined aspects of (1) the sculptor (the relationship partner), (2) the raw material/sculpture (the self), or (3) the fit between the sculptor and the raw material/sculpture (the interaction between the relationship partner and the self). For example, one study of committed relationship partners demonstrated that dispositional tendencies in either the sculptor or the sculpture to move with sustained dedication from one goal state or strategy to another (*locomotion* tendencies; see Kruglanski et al., 2000) facilitated both growth toward the ideal self and relationship well-being, presumably because high locomotion tendencies promote action and change (Kumashiro, Rusbult, Finkenauer, & Stocker, 2007). This study also demonstrated that dispositional tendencies in either the sculptor or the sculpture, both to evaluate which goals and goal pursuit strategies are optimal and to appraise goal performance (*assessment* tendencies), inhibited growth toward the ideal self and relationship well-being, presumably because high assessment tendencies promote extensive evaluation and stasis.

Other research has explored characteristics of the relationship between the sculptor and the sculpture that influence Michelangelo processes. For example, one recent series of studies tested the hypothesis that the Michelangelo phenomenon works especially smoothly to the extent that the sculptor approximates the sculpture's ideal self (Rusbult, Kumashiro, Kubacka, & Finkel, 2009). When the sculptor does so, he or she tends to be successful at affirming the sculpture, which in turn predicts both the sculpture's growth toward the ideal self and relationship well-being, including a reduced likelihood of breakup.

Influencing Resources

A second means by which interpersonal processes affect the operation stage of self-regulation is by influencing individuals' psychological resources. An influential theory suggests that self-regulation functions like a muscle (Baumeister, Vohs, & Tice, 2007; Muraven & Baumeister, 2000). According to this "strength model" of self-regulation, all acts of deliberate self-regulation require that individuals tap into a limited and depletable resource called *self-regulatory strength*. Just as physical exertion can deplete muscular strength, self-regulatory exertion can deplete self-regulatory strength, which can impair one's self-regulatory efforts.

A large body of evidence demonstrates that various interpersonal processes influence the degree to which the interactants subsequently possess limited versus plentiful self-regulatory strength. Research on *high-maintenance interaction*, which refers to the degree to which social interaction requires energy exertions beyond those required to perform the task itself, demonstrates that effortful social interaction can deplete self-regulatory resources (Finkel et al., 2006). In one study, research participants performed a 3-minute, collaborative maze task with a research confederate. The experimenter gave the participant a computer joystick and assigned her the task of navigating the maze. To make the maze task collaborative, the experimenter placed a visual occlusion between the participant and the computer screen, explaining that the other participant—actually the research confederate—would talk the participant through the maze task (e.g., "Up, left, left, right, down"). By random assignment, half of the participants experienced a low-maintenance interaction in which the confederate's instructions made the interaction efficient, whereas the other half experienced a high-maintenance interaction in which the confederate's instructions made the interaction inefficient (e.g., "Wait, hold on, go back, I meant left"). Relative to participants who had experienced the low-maintenance interaction, participants who had experienced the high-maintenance interaction subsequently were both lazier (they were more likely to prefer a simple, unrewarding activity to a challenging, potentially rewarding one) and more mentally unfocused (they solved fewer anagrams).

Dozens of additional studies have demonstrated this high-maintenance interaction effect across diverse forms of interpersonal interaction. For example, relative to participants engaging in easy, well-practiced forms of self-presentation, participants engaging in challenging, novel forms were more depleted, persisting for less time on an arithmetic task (Vohs, Baumeister, & Ciarocco, 2005). Relative to either nonbiased white participants or white participants engaging in a same-race interaction, racially biased white participants engaging in a interracial interaction were more depleted, exhibiting greater cognitive interference on the Stroop (1935) color-naming task (Richeson & Shelton, 2003; Richeson & Trawalter, 2005). Relative to participants who were subtly and nonverbally mimicked (an affiliation cue) by an interaction partner from whom they expected warm treatment (an employee or a same-race interaction partner), participants who were mimicked by an interaction partner from whom they did not expect such treatment (a supervisor or a cross-race interaction partner) were more depleted, exhibiting greater Stroop interference (Dalton, Chartrand, & Finkel, in press). Relative to male participants who had just interacted with another male, male participants who had just interacted with a female were more depleted, exhibiting impaired performance on concentration-intensive tasks, especially to the degree that participants perceived the female as attractive or were trying to make a good impression on her (Karremans, Verwijmeren, Pronk, & Reitsma, 2009); female participants did not show a parallel effect.

A related line of research demonstrates that being socially excluded impairs one's self-regulation (Baumeister, DeWall, Ciarocco, & Twenge, 2005). For example, relative to participants who had just been socially included, participants who had been socially excluded were more depleted, eating more than twice as many fattening cookies.

An intriguing new program of research demonstrates that merely empathizing with another person who is exerting self-control can be sufficient to deplete one's self-regulatory resources (Ackerman, Goldstein, Shapiro, & Bargh, 2009). In one study, participants read a first-person account of a waiter or waitress who arrived to work hungry, worked at a high-quality restaurant, and was not allowed to eat on the job. Participants then indicated how much money they would be willing to spend on a series of luxury goods. Half of the participants simply read the story (low perspective-taking condition), whereas the other half immersed themselves in the story as if they actually were the hungry waiter or waitress (high perspective-taking condition). Building upon previous work demonstrating that depleted individuals are willing to pay more than nondepleted individuals for luxury goods (Vohs & Faber, 2007), participants in the high perspective-taking condition subsequently reported a willingness to spend more money on these luxury goods than did participants in the low perspective-taking condition (Ackerman et al., 2009).

Fortunately, the effect of social processes on people's self-regulatory resources is not always negative. Recent research suggests that other people can sometimes bolster people's self-regulatory strength. For example, participants assigned to act out target terms such as *Olympics* and *helicopter* while playing charades (a game where the performer acts out the target terms, trying to get the guesser to identify them correctly) experienced bolstered strength, exhibiting a significant increase in handgrip persistence from before to after the game if the guesser was well-synchronized with them, but not if the guesser was not (Knowles, Finkel, & Williams, 2007). In another series of studies, relative to participants who were primed with thoughts about nonfamilial topics, participants who were primed with thoughts about a close family member appeared to be less depleted, as demonstrated by superior performance on language and math tasks, and by greater restraint when tempted by unhealthy cookies (Stillman, Tice, Fincham, & Lambert, 2009).

Influencing Motivation

A third means by which interpersonal processes affect the operation stage of self-regulation is by influencing individuals' motivation to achieve a given goal. Research has shown that relationship partners can sometimes increase motivation. For example, other people can serve as an inspiration or a role model for one's goal pursuits, especially insofar as (1) those people are successful in a domain that is important to the self, (2) their achievement does not seem unattainable, and (3) they encourage strategies that match the self's general motivational orientation to pursue desirable outcomes rather than avoid undesirable outcomes (Lockwood, Jordan, & Kunda, 2002; Lockwood & Kunda, 1997; cf. Tesser, Millar, & Moore, 1988). In these circumstances, role models can motivate individuals to expend more effort and to persist longer toward goal achievement than they otherwise would.

In addition to increasing individuals' motivation, relationship partners can (unintentionally) decrease it. They can exacerbate the gap between individuals' goal-relevant intentions (e.g., intending to read law periodicals regularly to reach the goal of becoming a lawyer) and behavior (e.g., actually reading the periodicals) (Gollwitzer, Sheeran, Michalski, & Seifert, 2009). In several experiments, people were less likely to follow through on their goal-relevant intentions when others were made aware of these intentions. It seems that having other people recognize one's intentions can be satisfying in and of itself, diminishing the need to work hard toward goal achievement.

Altering Strategies

A fourth means by which interpersonal processes affect the operation stage of self-regulation is by influencing the goal pursuit strategies people employ. For example, a romantic partner might help one improve one's study habits in advance of a major exam. To date, this topic has been largely neglected. However, some of psychology's classic findings provide compelling illustrations of how other people can promote or impair one's self-regulation by fostering one strategy over another. For example, the research on delay of gratification discussed earlier demonstrates that an experimenter not only can set goals for children but also that his or her strategic advice influences how successful children are at resisting the temptation to indulge immediately in the inferior reward to earn a superior reward a little while later (Mischel, 1974; Mischel et al., 1989). Whereas children who were instructed to think about the rewards (e.g., the taste and texture of the marshmallows) while waiting exhibited poor delay performance, children who were instructed to think fun, distracting thoughts exhibited impressive delay performance.

This delay of gratification research provides compelling evidence that relationship partners can promote or impair individuals' self-regulatory success by altering the strategies those individuals employ. Investigating such strategic processes in close relationships, and perhaps individuals' reactance to receiving strategic advice from significant others (Brehm, 1966), is a promising direction for future research.

INTERPERSONAL INFLUENCES ON GOAL MONITORING

Once individuals have operated on the environment in an attempt to make progress toward their goals, they frequently benefit from discerning the degree to which their efforts have been successful thus far and evaluating their likelihood of future success. In this section, we discuss interpersonal influences on the third component of goal pursuit—the evaluative processes people employ to ascertain whether their operating processes are actually helping them progress toward achieving their goals, and the degree to which they feel confident that their goal pursuit efforts will be effective in the future (Carver & Scheier, 1982). *Goal monitoring* involves individuals' thoughts, feelings, and perceptions about goals and their progress thus far, as well as their expectations about the likelihood of future progress. The goal-monitoring process helps goal pursuers decide how much effort to devote to the goal and what goal pursuit strategies might be most effective. Relationship partners can influence goal monitoring (either by doing the monitoring themselves or by influencing individuals' monitoring tendencies) by helping to evaluate both goal progress to date and the likelihood of goal progress in the future.

Evaluating Goal Progress

Some of the best research on the role of relationship partners in monitoring one's goal progress has taken place in the health domain. For example, research has examined the impact of parental monitoring of their child's adherence to the prescribed medical regimen for managing the child's diabetes (Anderson, Ho, Brackett, Finkelstein, & Laffel, 1997; La Greca et al., 1995). Relative to children whose parents were less involved in blood glucose monitoring and insulin administration, children with more involved parents exhibited better metabolic control. These effects of parental involvement in blood glucose monitoring appear to be mediated by their effects on the child's monitoring of his or her own blood glucose (Anderson et al., 1997).

In the achievement domain, research has tested the influence of relationship partners on people's interest in accurate (vs. defensively biased or incomplete) goal monitoring. In a recent pair of studies, students at a prestigious university took a challenging (and bogus) intelligence test and received feedback that their performance was "poor" (Kumashiro & Sedikides, 2005). Participants then indicated the degree to which they wanted to learn more about their poor performance. This information would allegedly improve their ability to monitor their performance and perhaps help them develop strategies for reducing the discrepancy between their goal to exhibit intelligence and their ostensibly weak performance on this intelligence test. Students who brought to mind a close, positive relationship partner were subsequently more willing to learn about the nature of their poor performance than were students who brought to mind either a close, negative relationship partner or a nonclose relationship partner. Given that most (and likely all) of these students possessed the goals both to be intelligent and to perform tasks in a way that demonstrates this intelligence, this bolstered willingness to learn more about their poor performance suggests that close, positive relationship partners make people willing to attend to information that is valuable for monitoring their goal progress, even when such monitoring is likely to portray important aspects of the self in a harsh light.

In addition to research on health and intelligence, scholars interested in caregiving have also examined relationship partners' progress monitoring tendencies. For example, research on adult attachment theory suggests that monitoring of partners' progress toward important goals is an inherent part of responsive caregiving (Feeney & Collins, 2001). A responsive caregiver provides the right amount and type of support for the current needs of the partner; failure to do so—for example, by providing a small amount of support when the partner's needs are high, or a large amount when the partner's needs are low—can produce negative relationship outcomes (Dakoff & Taylor, 1990; Feeney & Collins, 2001). Indeed, accurate monitoring of the partner's needs for support when pursuing a stressful or difficult goal may be essential for the successful provision of responsive support. In one experiment, participants who believed their partners were highly nervous about an upcoming speech provided stronger levels of emotional support than participants who believed their partners were less nervous (Feeney & Collins, 2001). This modulation suggests that participants were aware of and responsive to their partners' expectations and worries about their performance, an awareness that required monitoring of his or her goal progress.

Finally, close relationship partners often share information with each other about their goal performance, which provides an opportunity for partners to affect each other's goal monitoring. For example, when partners respond enthusiastically (vs. neutrally) to news of individuals' good performance, those individuals tend to regard the event more positively (Reis et al., 2009).

Evaluating the Likelihood of Future Success

An important part of the goal monitoring process is assessing whether one is likely to make substantial goal progress in the future. Several lines of research investigate the role of other people in helping individuals make such assessments. For example, in a recent study in the social cognitive tradition, relative to individuals who had been subliminally primed with the names of significant others who had low expectations for their self-regulatory success, individuals who had been subliminally primed with the names of significant others who had high expectations for their self-regulatory success believed that they were more likely to attain their goals. Consequently, they persisted longer in their goal pursuit behavior and were more likely to experience goal success (Shah, 2003b).

Other research also examines the role of relationship partners in altering assessments of one's ability to achieve successful goal-pursuit in the future, even though this research typically is not couched in such terms. For example, research on social comparison processes has revealed that people often compare their goal-directed performance to the performance of romantic partners, friends, family members, and colleagues (Pinkus, Lockwood, Schimmack, & Fournier, 2008). Social comparison is essentially a monitoring process: By looking at others' performance, people gain information about not only their own relative performance but also their likelihood of future relative success or failure. Typically, after comparing their own performance to the performance of more successful others (upward comparisons) in self-relevant domains, individuals report lower self-efficacy and show decreased motivation; after comparing their own performance to the performance of less successful others (downward comparisons) in self-relevant domains, individuals report higher self-efficacy and show increased motivation (Festinger, 1954; Suls, Martin, & Wheeler, 2002; Tesser, 1988; Wood, 1989). In close romantic relationships, however, these tendencies are diminished or even reversed (Beach et al., 1998; Pinkus et al., 2008). For example, in several studies, people responded more positively when comparing their own performance upward (vs. downward) to the performance of close romantic partners in self-relevant domains (Lockwood, Dolderman, Sadler, & Gerchak, 2004; Pinkus et al., 2008). Within close relationships then, upward comparisons may not consistently lower self-efficacy and motivation because the other can be seen as an extension of the self, with shared fate.

According to social comparison theory, then, people look to others' actions to assess their own relative progress (Festinger, 1954). According to another classic theory—social learning theory—people also look to the *consequences* of others' actions to determine expectations of their own success (Schunk, 1987; Schunk & Zimmerman, 1997): When similar others succeed, observers infer that their own success is likelier; thus, they have higher self-efficacy and motivation. When similar others struggle, observers infer that that their own success is less likely; thus, they have lower self-efficacy and motivation. Modeled goal pursuit can thus provide valuable goal-monitoring information.

CONCLUSION

In this chapter, we have reviewed the burgeoning literature on the effects of social relationships on self-regulation. This review has demonstrated that relationships affect all three components of self-regulation—goal setting and initiation, goal operation, and goal monitoring—in powerful and diverse ways. It has also identified several areas where no research yet links close relationships to self-regulation. Indeed, it is best to conceptualize this review as a snapshot of a research area at about 10 years of age. The good news is that this area is maturing quickly. Given the rapidly expanding rate of research linking social relationships to self-regulation, we look forward to seeing the updated coverage of this topic in the third edition of this *Handbook.* because that version will surely fill many of the empirical gaps in the present version and incorporate exciting and heretofore unimagined new developments.

ACKNOWLEDGMENTS

The writing of this chapter was supported by a National Science Foundation grant (No. 719780) awarded to Eli J. Finkel and a Social Sciences and Humanities Research Council of Canada grant awarded to Gráinne M. Fitzsimons. Any opinions, findings, and conclusions or recommendations expressed in this material are those of the authors and do not necessarily reflect the views of the funding agencies. Authorship ordering was determined by flipping a Loonie.

REFERENCES

Aarts, H., Gollwitzer, P. M., & Hassin, R. (2004). Goal contagion: Perceiving is for pursuing. *Journal of Personality and Social Psychology, 87,* 23–37.

Ackerman, J. M., Goldstein, N. J., Shapiro, J. R., & Bargh, J. A. (2009). You wear me out: The vicarious depletion of self-control. *Psychological Science, 20,* 326–332.

Allgöwer, A., Wardle, J., & Steptoe, A. (2001). Depressive symptoms, social support, and personal health behaviors in young men and women. *Health Psychology, 20,* 223–227.

Andersen, S. M., Reznik, I., & Manzella, L. M. (1996). Eliciting facial affect, motivation, and expectancies in transference: Significant-other representations in social relations. *Journal of Personality and Social Psychology,* 71, 1108–1129.

Anderson, B., Ho, J., Brackett, J., Finkelstein, D., & Laffel, L. (1997). Parental involvement in diabetes management tasks: relationships to blood glucose monitoring adherence and metabolic control in young adolescents with insulin-dependent diabetes mellitus. *Journal of Pediatrics, 130,* 257–265.

Bandura, A. (1986). *Social foundations of thought and action: A social cognitive theory.* Englewood Cliffs, NJ: Prentice-Hall.

Baumeister, R. F., DeWall, C. N., Ciarocco, N. J., & Twenge, J. M. (2005). Social exclusion impairs self-regulation. *Journal of Personality and Social Psychology, 88,* 589–604.

Baumeister, R. F., Heatherton, T. F., & Tice, D. M. (1994). *Losing control: How and why people fail at self-regulation.* New York: Academic Press.

Baumeister, R. F., Schmeichel, B. J., & Vohs, K. D. (2007). Self-regulation and the executive function: The self as controlling agent. In A. W. Kruglanski & E. T. Higgins (Eds.), *Social psychology: Handbook of basic principles* (2nd ed., pp. 516–539). New York: Guilford Press.

Baumeister, R. F., Vohs, K. D., & Tice, D. M. (2007). The strength model of self-control. *Current Directions in Psychological Science, 16,* 351–355.

Beach, S. R. H., Tesser, A., Fincham, F. D., Jones, D. J., Johnson, D., & Whitaker, D. J. (1998). Pleasure and pain in doing well, together: An investigation of performance-related affect in close relationships. *Journal of Personality and Social Psychology, 74,* 923–938.

Brehm, J. W. (1966). *A theory of psychological reactance.* New York: Academic Press.

Brunstein, J. C., Dangelmayer, G., & Schultheiss, O. C. (1996). Personal goals and social support in close relationships: Effects on relationship mood and marital satisfaction. *Journal of Personality and Social Psychology, 71,* 1006–1019.

Carver, C. S., & Scheier, M. F. (1982). Control theory: A useful conceptual framework for personality–social, clinical, and health psychology. *Psychological Bulletin, 92,* 111–135.

Caulkins, S. D., Smith, C. L., Gill, K. L., & Johnson, M. C. (1998). Maternal interactive style across contexts: Relations to emotional, behavioral and physiological regulation during toddlerhood. *Social Development, 7,* 350–369.

Cavallo, J. C., Fitzsimons, G. M., & Holmes, J. G. (2009.) Taking chances in the face of threat: Romantic risk regulation and approach motivation. *Personality and Social Psychology Bulletin, 35,* 737–751.

Cavallo, J. C., Fitzsimons, G. M., & Holmes, J. G. (2010). When self-protection overreaches: Relationship specific threat activates domain-general avoidance motivation. *Journal of Experimental Social Psychology, 48,* 1–8.

Chartrand, T. L., Dalton, A., & Fitzsimons, G. J. (2007). Relationship reactance: When priming significant others triggers opposing goals. *Journal of Experimental Social Psychology, 43,* 719–726.

Cohen, S., & Lichtenstein, E. (1990). Partner behaviors that support quitting smoking. *Journal of Consulting and Clinical Psychology, 58,* 304–309.

Dakoff, G. A., & Taylor, S. E. (1990). Victims' perceptions of social support: What is helpful from whom? *Journal of Personality and Social Psychology, 58,* 80–89.

Dalton, A. N., Chartrand, T. L., & Finkel, E. J. (in press). The schema-driven chameleon: How mimicry affects executive and self-regulatory resources. *Journal of Personality and Social Psychology.*

Davison, K. K., Cutting, T. M., & Birch, L. L. (2003). Parents' activity-related parenting practices predict girls' physical activity. *Medicine and Science in Sports and Exercise, 35,* 1589–1905.

DiMatteo, R. M. (2004). Social support and patient adherence to medical treatment: A meta-analysis. *Health Psychology, 23,* 207–218.

Drigotas, S. M. (2002). The Michelangelo phenomenon and personal well-being. *Journal of Personality, 70,* 59–77.

Drigotas, S. M., Rusbult, C. E., Wieselquist, J., & Whitton, S. (1999). Close partner as sculptor of the ideal self: Behavioral affirmation and the Michelangelo phenomenon. *Journal of Personality and Social Psychology, 77,* 293–323.

Eyler, A. A., Brownson, R. C., Donatelle, R. J., King, A. C., Brown, D., & Sallis, J. F. (1999). Physical activity social support and middle- and older-aged minority women: Results from a U.S. survey. *Social Science and Medicine, 49,* 781–789.

Feeney, B. C. (2004). A secure base: Responsive support of goal strivings and exploration in adult intimate relationships. *Journal of Personality and Social Psychology, 87,* 631–648.

Feeney, B. C. (2007). The dependency paradox in close relationships: Accepting dependence promotes independence. *Journal of Personality and Social Psychology, 92,* 268–285.

Feeney, B. C., & Collins, N. L. (2001). Predictors of caregiving in adult intimate relationships: An attachment theoretical perspective. *Journal of Personality and Social Psychology, 80,* 972–994.

Festinger, L. (1954). A theory of social comparison processes. *Human Relations, 7,* 117–140.

Finkel, E. J., Campbell, W. K., Brunell, A. B., Dalton, A. N., Chartrand, T. L., & Scarbeck, S. J. (2006). High-maintenance interaction: Inefficient social coordination impairs self-regulation. *Journal of Personality and Social Psychology, 91,* 456–475.

Fishbach, A., Friedman, R. S., & Kruglanski, A. W. (2003). Leading us not unto temptation: Momentary allurements elicit overriding goal activation. *Journal of Personality and Social Psychology, 84,* 296–309.

Fitzsimons, G. M., & Bargh, J. A. (2003). Thinking of you: Nonconscious pursuit of interpersonal goals associated with relationship partners. *Journal of Personality and Social Psychology, 84,* 148–164.

Fitzsimons, G. M., & Shah, J. Y. (2008). How goal instrumentality shapes relationship evaluations. *Journal of Personality and Social Psychology, 95,* 319–337.

Gollwitzer, P. M., & Brandstätter, V. (1997). Implementation intentions and effective goal pursuit. *Journal of Personality and Social Psychology, 73*, 186–199.

Gollwitzer, P. M., Sheeran, P., Michalski, V., & Seifert, A. E. (2009). When intentions go public: Does social reality widen the intention-behavior gap? *Psychological Science, 20*, 612–618.

Gombrich, E. H. (1995). *The story of art* (16th ed.). London: Phaidon Press.

Higgins, E. T. (1987). Self-discrepancy: A theory relating self and affect. *Psychological Review, 94*, 319–340.

Karremans, J. C., Verwijmeren, T., Pronk, T. M., & Reitsma, M., (2009). Interacting with women can impair men's cognitive functioning. *Journal of Experimental Social Psychology, 45*, 1041–1044.

Knowles, M. L., Finkel, E. J., & Williams, K. (2007). *Bolstering self-regulation through social lubrication*. Unpublished manuscript, Northwestern University.

Kruglanski, A. W., Thompson, E. P., Higgins, E. T., Atash, M. N., Pierro, A., Shah, J. Y., et al. (2000). To "do the right thing" or "just do it": Locomotion and assessment as distinct self-regulatory imperatives. *Journal of Personality and Social Psychology, 79*, 793–815.

Kumashiro, M., Rusbult, C. E., Finkenauer, C., & Stocker, S. L. (2007). To think or to do: The impact of assessment and locomotion orientation on the Michelangelo phenomenon. *Journal of Social and Personal Relationships, 24*, 591–611.

Kumashiro, M., & Sedikides, C. (2005). Taking on board liability-focused information: Close positive relationships as a self-bolstering resource. *Psychological Science, 16*, 732–739.

La Greca, A. M., Auslander, W. F., Greco, P., Spetter, D., Fisher, E. B., & Santiago, J. V. (1995). I get by with a little help from my family and friends: Adolescents' support for diabetes care. *Journal of Pediatric Psychology, 20*, 449–476.

Latham, G. P., Erez, M., & Locke, E. (1988). Resolving scientific disputes by the joint design of crucial experiments by the antagonists: Application to the Erez–Latham dispute regarding participation in goal setting. *Journal of Applied Psychology, 73*, 753–772.

Locke, E. A., & Latham, G. P. (1990). *A theory of goal setting and task performance*. Englewood Cliffs, NJ: Prentice-Hall.

Locke, E. A., & Latham, G. P. (2002). Building a practically useful theory of goal setting and task motivation: A 35-year odyssey. *American Psychologist, 57*, 705–717.

Lockwood, P., Dolderman, D., Sadler, P., & Gerchak, L. (2004). Feeling better about doing worse: Social comparisons in romantic relationships. *Journal of Personality and Social Psychology, 87*, 80–95.

Lockwood, P., Jordan, C. H., & Kunda, Z. (2002). Motivation by positive or negative role models: Regulatory focus determines who will best inspire us. *Journal of Personality and Social Psychology, 83*, 854–864.

Lockwood, P., & Kunda, Z. (1997). Superstars and me: Predicting the impact of role models on the self. *Journal of Personality and Social Psychology, 73*, 93–103.

Marjoribanks, K. (1979). *Families and their learning environments: An empirical analysis*. London: Routledge & Kegan Paul.

Markus, H., & Nurius, P. (1986). Possible selves. *American Psychologist, 41*, 954–969.

Martinez-Pons, M. (2002). Parental influences on children's academic self-regulatory development. *Theory Into Practice, 41*, 126–131.

Miller, L. C., & Read, S. J. (1991). On the coherence of mental models of persons and relationships: A knowledge structure approach. In G. J. O. Fletcher & F. Fincham (Eds.), *Cognition in close relationships* (pp. 69–99). Hillsdale, NJ: Erlbaum.

Mischel, W. (1974). Processes in delay of gratification. In L. Berkowitz (Ed.), *Advances in experimental social psychology* (Vol. 7, pp. 249–292). New York: Academic Press.

Mischel, W., Shoda, Y., & Rodriguez, M. L. (1989). Delay of gratification in children. *Science, 244*, 933–938.

Moretti, M. M., & Higgins, E. T. (1999). Own versus other standpoints in self-regulation: Developmental antecedents and functional consequences. *Review of General Psychology, 3*, 188–223.

Muraven, M., & Baumeister, R. F. (2000). Self-regulation and depletion of limited resources: Does self-control resemble a muscle? *Psychological Bulletin, 126*, 247–259.

Novak, S. A., & Webster, G. D. (2009). *Honey, you don't want fries with that: A daily diary study of spousal social control during the partner's weight loss attempt.* Unpublished manuscript, Hofstra University.

Pinkus, R. T., Lockwood, P., Schimmack, U., & Fournier, M. (2008). For better and for worse: Everyday social comparisons between romantic partners. *Journal of Personality and Social Psychology, 95*, 1180–1201.

Reblin, M., & Uchino, B. N. (2008). Social and emotional support and its implication for health. *Current Opinion in Psychiatry, 21*, 201–205.

Reis, H. T., Smith, S. M., Carmichael, C. L., Caprariello, P. A., Tsai, F., Rodrigues, A., et al. (2009). *Are you happy for me?: How sharing positive events with others provides personal and interpersonal benefits.* Unpublished manuscript, University of Rochester, Rochester, NY.

Richeson, J. A., & Shelton, J. N. (2003). When prejudice does not pay: Effects of interracial contact on executive function. *Psychological Science, 14*, 287–290.

Richeson, J. A., & Trawalter, S. (2005). Why do interracial interactions impair executive function?: A resource depletion account. *Journal of Personality and Social Psychology, 88*, 934–947.

Rusbult, C. E., Finkel, E. J., & Kumashiro, M. (2009). The Michelangelo phenomenon. *Current Directions in Psychological Science, 18*, 305–309.

Rusbult, C. E., Kumashiro, M., Kubacka, K. E., & Finkel, E. J. (2009). "The part of me that you bring out": Ideal similarity and the Michelangelo phenomenon. *Journal of Personality and Social Psychology, 96*, 61–82.

Schunk, D. H. (1987). Peer models and children's behavioral change. *Review of Educational Research, 57*, 140–174.

Schunk, D. H., & Zimmerman, B. J. (1997). Social origins of self-regulatory competence. *Educational Psychologist, 32*, 195–208.

Shah, J. Y. (2003a). Automatic for the people: How representations of significant others implicitly affect goal pursuit. *Journal of Personality and Social Psychology, 84*, 661–681.

Shah, J. Y. (2003b). The motivational looking glass: How significant others implicitly affect goal appraisals. *Journal of Personality and Social Psychology, 85*, 424–439.

Stillman, T. F., Tice, D. M., Fincham, F. D., & Lambert, N. M. (2009). The psychological presence of family improves self-control. *Journal of Social and Clinical Psychology, 28*, 498–529.

Stroop, J. R. (1935). Studies of interference in serial verbal reactions. *Journal of Experimental Psychology, 18*, 643–662.

Suls, J., Martin, R., & Wheeler, L. (2002). Social comparison: Why, with whom and with what effect? *Current Directions in Psychological Science, 11*, 159–163.

Tesser, A. (1988). Toward a self-evaluation maintenance model of social behavior. In L. Berkowitz (Ed.), *Advances in experimental social psychology* (Vol. 21, pp. 181–227). New York: Academic Press.

Tesser, A., Millar, M., & Moore, J. (1988). Some affective consequences of social comparison and reflection processes: the pain and pleasure of being close. *Journal of Personality and Social Psychology, 54*, 49–61.

Uchino, B. N. (2004). *Social support and physical health: Understanding the health consequences of our relationships.* New Haven, CT: Yale University Press.

Vohs, K. D., Baumeister, R. F., & Ciarocco, N. (2005). Self-regulation and self-presentation: Regulatory resource depletion impairs impression management and effortful self-presentation depletes regulatory resources. *Journal of Personality and Social Psychology, 88*, 632–657.

Vohs, K. D., & Faber, R. J. (2007). Spent resources: Self-regulatory resource availability affects impulse buying. *Journal of Consumer Research, 33,* 537–547.

Vohs, K. D., & Finkel, E. J. (Eds.). (2006). *Self and relationships: Connecting intrapersonal and interpersonal processes.* New York: Guilford Press.

Wegner, D. M., & Wheatley, T. P. (1999). Apparent mental causation: Sources of the experience of will. *American Psychologist, 54,* 480–492.

Wood, J. V. (1989). Theory and research concerning social comparisons of personal attributes. *Psychological Bulletin, 106,* 231–248.

Zimmerman, B. J., Bandura, A., & Martinez-Pons, M. (1992). Self-motivation for academic attainment: The role of self-efficacy beliefs and personal goal setting. *American Educational Research Journal, 29,* 663–676.

Zimmerman, B. J., & Koussa, R. (1979). Social influences on children's toy preferences: Effects of model rewardingness and affect. *Contemporary Educational Psychology, 4,* 55–66.

CHAPTER 22

The Effects of Self-Regulation on Social Relationships

GRÁINNE M. FITZSIMONS
ELI J. FINKEL

Why does it matter if someone can push himself to run another mile on a dreary February morning or stop himself from reading online sports news at work? In other words, what are the downstream consequences of self-regulation? A large body of research within personality, organizational, and social psychology has demonstrated that self-regulation has significant consequences for the individual. Good self-regulators—those who can withstand temptations, persist through obstacles, and delay gratification, for example—are likelier to be physically healthier, more successful in their careers, and experience more life satisfaction and well-being (Bandura, 1982; Baumeister, Heatherton, & Tice, 1994; Emmons, 1986; Locke & Latham, 2002; Mischel, Shoda, & Rodriguez, 1989).

Given the ubiquity of self-regulation efforts in everyday life, and the fact that many acts of self-regulation occur within social contexts, the consequences of self-regulation likely extend beyond self-directed accomplishments to social and interpersonal relationships as well. However, until recently, most empirical research on self-regulation has neglected its consequences for relationships with others. This neglect of interpersonal consequences is surprising given that self-regulation is crucial for social success even in informal social settings. Imagine a day care playgroup or a tailgate party: No one likes the kid who wails when she can't get her way, and no one likes the drunk who throws up on the lawn. Indeed, so crucial is self-regulation to humans' social well-being that researchers have theorized that it may have evolved primarily to serve this function (Baumeister, 2005; Heatherton & Vohs, 1998; Rawn & Vohs, 2006).

In this chapter, we discuss support for the importance of self-regulation in social contexts by examining its role within one particular—and important—social context: that of close relationships. (Although we focus on close relationships, we also review research involving broader social contexts when the research has immediate relevance for close relationships.) We present research from a number of different programs of study that highlight the direct relationship consequences of *self-regulation*, defined broadly as the processes by which the self alters its own responses or inner states in a goal-directed manner (see Baumeister, Schmeichel, & Vohs, 2007; Rawn & Vohs, 2006). We discuss the relationship consequences of *self-regulatory strength* (how much self-regulation people have), *self-regulatory content* (what people are regulating toward), and *self-regulatory strategies* (how people self-regulate).

PART 1: SELF-REGULATORY STRENGTH

Given the high everyday interdependence of most close relationship partners, the self-regulation abilities of one partner have unavoidable fallout for the other partner (Kelley, 1979). If one partner struggles with self-control, the other partner suffers. If one partner takes on a challenging goal pursuit, his or her resources for relationship goals are depleted. Low levels of self-regulatory strength are likely a major vulnerability in a close relationship partner, while high levels are likely a major asset. In this section, we discuss how close relationships are affected by the strength of the self's regulatory abilities.

Individual Differences in Self-Regulatory Strength

Individuals vary in the degree to which they can self-regulate successfully in everyday life. According to one prominent model, exertions of self-regulation depend upon a limited, unitary resource, *self-regulatory strength* (Baumeister, Vohs, & Tice, 2007; Muraven & Baumeister, 2000). Just as some individuals have more physical strength than others, so too do some individuals have more self-regulatory strength—more reserves of this limited capacity to engage in self-control efforts—than others.

Several lines of research have demonstrated that individual differences in self-regulatory strength have important implications for interpersonal relationships. Scholars have measured these individual differences—which assess the degree to which individuals are successful at regulating their thoughts, feelings, or behaviors in a goal-directed manner—with self-reports, cognitive tasks, and behavioral tasks. In typical research employing self-reports, participants indicate their agreement with items assessing general self-regulatory success (e.g., "I am able to work effectively toward long-term goals"). Such research demonstrates that individuals who report greater (vs. lesser) self-regulatory success in general also report superior relationship functioning: They respond to partner offenses more constructively and less violently, experience less family conflict and less anger, and have better communication skills (Finkel & Campbell, 2001; Finkel, DeWall, Slotter, Oaten, & Foshee, 2009; Tangney, Baumeister, & Boone, 2004).

In typical research assessing individual differences in self-regulatory strength with cognitive tasks, participants perform a computer-based task assessing their facility at overriding automatic cognitive responses. For example, the Stroop (1935) task, perhaps the most famous of these cognitive self-regulation tasks (also called *executive control tasks* or *executive functioning tasks*), requires that participants override their automatic tendency to read the name of a certain color (e.g., *red*), instead reporting the color of the font in which that name is printed (e.g., *blue*). Individuals vary in their ability to override their automatic tendency to read the word, and this variability functions as a cognitive measure of self-regulation. Research demonstrates that individuals who exhibit strong (vs. weak) self-regulatory ability on these cognitive tasks tend to be more polite and less interpersonally offensive (von Hippel & Gonsalkorale, 2005). In addition, they tend to be more forgiving of a close relationship partner's transgressions, apparently because they are more effective at controlling their ruminations about the transgressions (Pronk, Karremans, Overbeek, Vermulst, & Wigboldus, in press).

In typical research assessing individual differences in self-regulatory strength with behavioral tasks, participants perform a laboratory-based task assessing their success at resisting the urge to enact a tempting behavior that is counterproductive to their longer-term self-interest. The most famous example of such research poses young children with a dilemma (Mischel, 1974): They can have a relatively small treat right away (e.g., a marshmallow), or they can wait for an unknown period of time for a more desirable treat (e.g., two marshmallows). In one study, the number of seconds children delayed gratification (i.e., waited for the more desirable treat) predicted their parents' assessments of their ability to maintain friendships and get along with peers 10 years later (Mischel, Shoda, & Peake, 1988). In subsequent research, the length of time the children delayed gratification predicted their teacher's positive assessments of their interpersonal functioning (less aggressive behavior and greater peer acceptance), at least for socially insecure children (Ayduk et al., 2000). Whereas the ability to delay gratification did not predict interpersonal functioning among socially secure children, it appeared to be crucial in helping rejection-sensitive children manage their social anxieties in socially acceptable ways.

Situational Fluctuations in Self-Regulatory Strength

Many recent studies have looked beyond individual differences in self-regulatory ability to examine how situational factors can influence self-control and, consequently, alter relationship processes. According to the strength model of self-regulation (Baumeister, Vohs, et al., 2007; Muraven & Baumeister, 2000), just as physical exertion can exhaust a muscle, self-regulatory exertion can exhaust self-regulatory strength, thereby impairing performance on subsequent tasks requiring self-control. A number of studies have now found evidence that depleted self-regulatory resources impair interpersonal functioning. For example, depletion produces ineffective self-presentation (Vohs, Baumeister, & Ciarocco, 2005): Relative to nondepleted individuals, depleted individuals tend to talk too much, to be arrogant, or to self-disclose inappropriately. Depletion also negatively affects individuals' behavior during relationship conflicts (Finkel & Campbell, 2001). Relative to nondepleted individuals, depleted individuals tend to respond in a less constructive, more retaliatory fashion to relationship offenses. Recent research has applied these ideas to the domains of interpersonal aggression and intimate partner violence (DeWall, Baumeister, Stillman, & Gailliot, 2007; Finkel et al., 2009). In one study, participants either engaged or did not engage in a depleting attention-regulation task prior to experiencing or not experiencing a provocation by their romantic partner (Finkel et al., 2009). The experimenter then informed participants that they had been randomly assigned to the role of director, and their partner to the role of actor, for a yoga pose task. Participants determined how long their partner had to maintain body poses; they were told that maintaining the body poses would be painful for their partner, but would not cause any long-term physical damage. Depleted participants forced their partner to maintain these body poses 68% longer than did nondepleted participants, but only if their partner had provoked them. In the absence of provocation, depletion had no effect on assigned pose duration, presumably because nonprovoked participants had no aggressive impulses to inhibit in the first place.

A follow-up study examined how bolstering self-regulatory strength may generate positive relationship consequences over time. The strength model not only predicts that exerting self-regulation depletes self-regulatory strength in the short run but also that people can bolster their self-regulatory strength over time with training (Baumeister, Gailliot, DeWall, & Oaten, 2006). In one study (Finkel et al., 2009), participants attended two laboratory sessions, 2 weeks apart, at which they were depleted before they completed a self-report measure of intimate partner violence. This measure asked participants to indicate how "physically aggressive" they would be in response to a series of partner transgressions (e.g., "I walk in and catch my partner having sex with someone"). In the 2-week period between the laboratory sessions, participants were assigned either to one of two self-regulation systematic bolstering regimens (controlling either their verbal or physical behavior during everyday tasks) or to a no-intervention control condition. Participants in both bolstering regimens exhibited a significant reduction in their self-reported aggressive tendencies from the first to the second session, whereas participants in the control condition exhibited no change. These findings suggest that strengthening general self-regulatory ability leads to improved relationship functioning.

PART 2: SELF-REGULATORY CONTENT

In addition to the *amount* or *strength* of self-regulatory ability, another important aspect of self-regulation that impacts social relationships is the *content* of the self-regulatory pursuit. By definition, self-regulation is directed toward some kind of outcome or end state, and the content of that end state has implications for relationships. Again, given the high interdependence of many close relationships, the content of one partner's personal goals has fallout for the other partner: If one partner aims to lose weight before the holidays, then this has consequences for the other partner (e.g., to eat more healthfully whether he or she wants to or not). This is perhaps even more true for interpersonal goals. If one partner aims to build a closer relationship, this has consequences for the other partner (e.g., to spend less time with friends and more time with the partner).

Beyond these obvious practical effects of one partner's goal content on the other partner's everyday life, the content of each partner's goals has important consequences for the well-being of the relationship. In this section, we discuss two illustrations of how goal content affects relationships. First, we describe a program of research that outlines a goal content model of relationship phenomena, outlining how the pursuit of different interpersonal goals influences relationship well-being. Second, we describe several programs of research that examine the impact of personal goals on individuals' feelings about partners who make those goal contents more versus less likely to be realized.

Interpersonal Goal Content

One of the most well-documented self-regulatory challenges within close relationships is to balance the content of two competing goals—to promote the health and well-being of the relationship, and to protect the self from rejection and pain (Murray, Holmes, & Collins, 2006). These goals are often incompatible: First, to promote the goal of maintaining a happy, healthy romantic relationship, people must engage in actions oriented toward the relationship, not the self. To be responsive and committed partners, people need to "put themselves out there," to become dependent on their partners, to rely on them for help, to express love and caring—essentially, to behave in ways that would make any subsequent rejection even more painful. Unfortunately, then, the very actions that encourage satisfaction of a relationship-promoting goal are the same actions that threaten satisfaction of a basic self-protection goal: to minimize vulnerability to rejection and hurt. Similarly, the actions that help to satisfy the self-protection goal (behaving dismissively toward the partner, distancing, etc.) are damaging to relationship well-being (Murray, Bellavia, Rose, & Griffin, 2000). Murray and her colleagues (2006) refer to the process by which individuals cope with these two conflicting goals as *risk regulation*: If close relationship partners hope to maintain satisfying relationships, then they must regulate their thoughts, feelings, and actions to overcome self-protective motivations in favor of relationship-promoting ones.

According to the *risk regulation model* (Murray et al., 2006), people regulate their dependency (their willingness to make themselves vulnerable to the pain of rejection or hurt) by relying on beliefs about their partner's regard for them: When people feel loved and respected by their partner, that positive perceived regard gives them the "psychological insurance" to inhibit self-protection goals, and to push themselves to be good partners (Murray, 2005). Experimental studies have demonstrated that people with high and low self-esteem (presumed to differ in chronic perceptions of the extent to which their partner values them) react differently to rejection worries. People with high self-esteem tend to respond to such worries in a compensatory fashion, drawing even closer to their partner and viewing their partner even more positively. In contrast, people with low self-esteem tend to respond to relationship worries by distancing from their partner and viewing him or her negatively, protecting themselves from the potential sting of future rejection (e.g., Murray et al., 2003).

In one illustrative experiment (Murray, Rose, Bellavia, Holmes, & Kusche, 2002), high and low self-esteem participants believed that their partner, sitting behind them at another table, was writing a long list of complaints about their relationship, when the partner was actually listing the contents of his or her apartment in great detail. Participants with high and low self-esteem responded to this powerful anxiety invocation by feeling less confident about their partner's regard. However, people with high self-esteem, who had that "psychological insurance" provided by a history of positive perceived regard, responded to these rejection concerns by reporting greater closeness to their partner and enhancing their positive view of their partner's qualities. People with low self-esteem, who did not have strong resources of positive perceived regard to draw upon, responded to rejection concerns self-protectively by derogating and reporting less closeness to their partner (Murray et al., 2002). Thus, people rely on a positive sense of their partner's esteem to help them regulate their behavior in a relationship-promoting manner.

This body of research suggests that as interdependence increases within a close relationship, it presents a crucial goal content conflict. People must balance two goal end states: to be safe from rejection threat and to have a healthy relationship. The incompatibility of the content of these two goals (and the approach taken by the individual to resolve this conflict) has important consequences for relationships, determining changes in relationship satisfaction and commitment, and predicting relationship dissolution (Murray et al., 2006). For our purposes in this chapter, research on risk regulation illustrates how the content of people's close relationship goals can influence the quality of those relationships.

Personal Goal Content

While the previous section described one program of research on the content of *relationship* goals, this section describes research on the content of individuals' *personal* goals. People want things for themselves: They want to do well in school; they want a nice home; they want to relax every day after work. In this section, we describe several independent lines of research that examine the impact of such personal goals on the way people feel about their close relationship partners.

Specifically, all of these programs of research suggest that people's individual or personal goal pursuits can lead to either positive or negative relationship outcomes, depending upon whether the partner is helpful, supportive, or instrumental in bringing about those goal outcomes; that is, the way people feel about their relationship partners is shaped by the extent to which these relationships make it likelier that the self will move toward those desired outcomes.

Grounded in interdependence theory, several models of relationship functioning have noted that close relationship partners have many opportunities to facilitate or to obstruct each other's personal goal pursuits within everyday interactions, and have suggested that each of these small or large influences on goal pursuit has been theorized to generate a corresponding emotional response to the partner (Kelley, 1979). The *emotions-in-relationships model* has perhaps most clearly explicated the role of goal facilitation and obstruction in relationship well-being (Berscheid, 1983, 1991; Berscheid & Ammazzalorso, 2001; Fehr & Harasymchuk, 2005). According to this model, emotional experiences result from disruptions or synchronies in the "meshed interaction sequences" of everyday relationships, such that positive or negative emotions result when significant others affect each other's goals (Berscheid, 1983; 1991). So, when one partner wants to improve her academic performance, she will feel more positively about a partner who helps that goal end state become a likelier reality.

A recent program of research integrated interdependence theorizing about goal facilitation in interpersonal relationships with a social cognitive approach to understanding self-regulation (e.g., Bargh, Gollwitzer, Lee-Chai, Barndollar, & Troetschel, 2001; Fitzsimons & Bargh, 2003; Kruglanski et al., 2002), to examine the notion that relationship outcomes depend on the extent to which partners have positive versus negative effects on each other's personal goal progress (Fitzsimons & Fishbach, 2010; Fitzsimons & Shah, 2008, 2009). In a series of experiments, participants first nominated close others who had positive effects on their personal goal progress (i.e., *instrumental* others), and those who had no effect on their personal goal progress (i.e., *noninstrumental* others), then completed goal activation tasks (Bargh et al., 2001) designed to bring to mind important personal goals. Recently activated goals for academic achievement and fitness affected closeness to relationship partners, such that people felt closer to others whom they perceived as instrumental for achieving activated goals, and less close to others whom they perceived as noninstrumental for achieving those goals. In one study, after completing an academic achievement goal-priming task, participants reported increased closeness to achievement-instrumental friends (e.g., study partners) and decreased closeness to achievement-noninstrumental friends (e.g., hiking partners).

Follow-up studies suggest that relationship partners' instrumentality generates positive relationship outcomes (and lack of instrumentality generates negative relationship outcomes) primarily when partners are instrumental for achievement of goals currently high in *motivational priority* relative to other goals (Fitzsimons & Fishbach, 2010). When goals drop in motivational priority—that is, when they become less of a priority in terms of progress than other goals—individuals stop showing an evaluative preference for others who are instrumental in achieving those goals. Instead, individuals tend to switch allegiances, preferring others who are instrumental in achieving the goals that *are* currently high in motivational priority. Thus, the relationship benefits that accrue from being instrumental for achievement of any of a relationship partner's goals are likely to fluctuate over time, as the goal fluctuates in priority for the partner. That being said, many close relationship partners are instrumental in achieving multiple important goals, and as such, the positive relationship benefits they accrue from helping their partners make progress are unlikely to be fleeting.

Indeed, the body of research on the *Michelangelo phenomenon* has demonstrated long-term positive consequences for relationship partners who help each other make progress on *ideal-self goals* (Drigotas, Rusbult, Wieselquist, & Whitton, 1999; for a review, see Rusbult, Finkel, & Kumashiro, 2010), such as becoming more confident, more sophisticated, and closer with God. This research has found that individuals are especially likely to make progress toward achieving their ideal-self goals to the degree that partners treat them as if they already possess the desired end states. We reviewed this research in detail in our companion chapter (Finkel & Fitzsimons, Chapter 21, this volume), but we highlight one important aspect of it that is particularly relevant here: Individuals whose partners help them make progress toward their ideal self experience greater relationship well-being across time than do individuals whose partners do not (Drigotas et al., 1999; Rusbult et al., 2010; Rusbult, Kumashiro, Kubacka, & Finkel, 2009).

Thus, individuals feel more positively about partners who promote movement toward important personal goals and, over time, promoting partner growth leads to increased relationship well-being. A separate program of research examines similar ideas from a nomothetic rather than idiographic perspective on goals, demonstrating that partner instrumentality is particularly important to the extent that it helps individuals fulfill the fundamental psychological needs all humans share. According to research on *self-determination theory* (Deci & Ryan, 1991; Ryan & Deci, 2001), individuals have three basic psychological needs: (1) *relatedness*, or the need to care for others and to feel that those others care for them; (2) *autonomy*, or the need to be self-governed and agentic; and (3) *competence*, or the need to feel capable and effective. When these needs are fulfilled, individuals experience psychological well-being; when they are thwarted, individuals suffer (Reis, Sheldon, Gable, Roscoe, & Ryan, 2000). Having a partner who helps to fulfill one's basic needs (especially the needs for relatedness and autonomy) predicts greater felt security (La Guardia, Ryan, Couchman, & Deci, 2000), as well as greater relationship satisfaction and relationship commitment (Patrick, Knee, Canevello, & Lonsbary, 2007). Recent research suggests, however, that not everyone shows a preference for useful relationship partners: The relationship commitment of individuals with high attachment anxiety does not depend on a romantic partner's instrumentality for need fulfillment (Slotter & Finkel, 2009); such individuals tend to remain committed to their relationship even when it fails to advance fulfillment of their core needs.

Whether through explicit offerings of support (Brunstein, Dangelmayer, & Schultheiss, 1996), partner affirmation, role modeling, or myriad other subtle and not so subtle efforts, partners can greatly impact each other's achievement of everyday personal goals. As forecasted by interdependence theory (Kelley, 1979), empirical research on the influence of others on individuals' self-regulation has demonstrated that this influence ultimately drives relationship well-being, such that people feel most satisfied with relationship partners who promote their achievement of important personal goals.

PART 3: SELF-REGULATORY STRATEGIES

The research described in the first two sections of this chapter explained relationship behavior by looking at the strength and the content of individuals' self-regulatory pursuits. In contrast, the research described in this section focuses on the broader processes or strategies with which any goal (personal or interpersonal) can be pursued; that is, the research we discuss in this section suggests that individuals' *strategies* for self-regulation impact relationship outcomes. Specifically, we address the potential role of *general motivational orientation*—the manner, style, or fashion in which individuals approach their goal pursuits—in close relationship contexts.

Approach and Avoidance Goal Orientations

First, we describe the burgeoning literature examining the role of approach and avoidance goal pursuits in relationship contexts (see Gable, 2006). According to this research perspective, goals can be conceived of in terms of approaching a positive outcome (i.e., *approach goals*) or in terms of avoiding a negative outcome (i.e., *avoidance goals*) (Carver & White, 1994; Elliot & Covington, 2001; Gray, 1990). Thus, the self-regulatory domain of the end state or outcome is undefined: People can approach or avoid achievement, health, or financial outcomes—but what differs is the strategic orientation people take to get to that end state. For example, individuals might pursue the goal to have a successful relationship with an approach strategy (e.g., emphasizing the pursuit of positive experiences, such as bonding and intimacy) or with an avoidance strategy (e.g., emphasizing the avoidance of negative experiences in one's relationship, such as conflict and rejection) (Gable, 2006).

The degree to which individuals adopt approach and avoidance goal orientations in their relationships has wide-ranging implications for relationship dynamics. For example, when assessing how satisfied they are with their relationship, individuals with strong approach goals weight positive relationship circumstances (e.g., passion) more heavily than do individuals with weak approach goals, whereas individuals with strong avoidance goals weight negative relationship circumstances (e.g., insecurity) more heavily than do individuals with weak avoidance goals (Gable & Poore, 2008).

Individuals vary not only in the degree to which they adopt approach and avoidance motivations toward their relationship in general but also in the degree to which they adopt such motivations toward specific aspects of their relationships. For example, individuals vary in the degree to which the sacrifices they make in their relationship stem from approach or avoidance motives. Whereas approach motives for sacrifice (assessed as agreement with an item such as "I want to develop a closer relationship with my partner") predicted greater relationship adjustment, avoidance motives for sacrifice (assessed as agreement with an item such as "I do not want my partner to think negatively about me") predicted diminished relationship adjustment (Impett, Gable, & Peplau, 2005).

Individuals also vary in the degree to which their sexual behavior is motivated by approach or avoidance motives. Whereas approach motives for engaging in sexual contact with one's partner predicted greater relationship adjustment, avoidance motives for engaging in sexual contact predicted diminished relationship adjustment (Impett, Peplau, & Gable, 2005). Even general relationship goals predict sexual dynamics in relationships, with strong (vs. weak) approach goals toward the relationship buffering individuals against declines in sexual desire over time and predicting elevated sexual desire during daily sexual interactions with their partner (Impett, Strachman, Finkel, & Gable, 2008).

Promotion and Prevention Goal Orientations

Complementing this research linking approach and avoidance goals to relationship outcomes is research linking regulatory focus theory (Higgins, 1997; Molden, Lee, & Higgins, 2008) to relationship outcomes. Regulatory focus theory shares with approach and avoidance theories of motivation the idea that individuals approach pleasure and avoid pain, but it also suggests that individuals can pursue both of these end states via two different orientations: promotion focus and prevention focus. When in a *promotion focus*, individuals emphasize gains versus nongains; they eagerly pursue opportunities for advancement and strive to ensure that they do not miss out on such opportunities. When in a *prevention focus*, individuals emphasize losses versus nonlosses; they vigilantly pursue security and strive to avoid any threats to this security. Promotion and prevention orientations or foci are theoretically orthogonal to approach–avoidance orientations: People can approach gains or avoid nongains (promotion), and can approach nonlosses and avoid losses (prevention). Like approach and avoidance orientations, promotion and prevention orientations are not domain specific—people can take a promotion or prevention orientation toward any goal end state—but refer to the strategies people take to get to those end states. Within the context of close relationships, promotion goals emphasize the presence or absence of relationship growth and advancement, while prevention goals emphasize the presence or absence of relationship security and maintenance.

Scholars have only recently started to investigate the myriad implications of regulatory focus theory for relationship processes. One line of research examines the link between individual differences in regulatory focus and romantic alternatives (Finkel, Molden, Johnson, & Eastwick, 2009). Relative to predominantly prevention-focused individuals, predominantly promotion-focused individuals more readily attend to, more positively evaluate, and more vigorously pursue alternative partners. Moreover, the negative association of commitment to a particular romantic partner with evaluations of alternatives to that partner is weaker for promotion-focused than for prevention-focused individuals.

Promotion and prevention orientations also influence the forgiveness process (Molden & Finkel, 2010). Specifically, regulatory focus moderates the links between trust and forgiveness on the one hand, and commitment and forgiveness on the other. In a series of studies, *trust*, an index of expectations of positive future treatment, predicted forgiveness more strongly for individuals in a promotion focus than for those in a prevention focus, presumably because promotion-focused individuals are especially sensitive to the prospect of future gains. In contrast, *commitment*, an index of an orientation toward relationship maintenance, predicted forgiveness more strongly for individuals in a prevention focus than for those in a promotion focus, presumably because prevention-focused individuals are especially sensitive to the potential dangers of deviating from the status quo.

One additional line of research has examined how the regulatory orientations of both partners interact to predict relationship well-being (Bohns et al., 2009). Although abundant evidence (e.g., Byrne, 1971; Gonzaga, Campos, & Bradbury, 2007) suggests that similarity predicts attraction and relationship well-being more strongly than does complementarity (with the dominance–submissiveness dimension serving as an important exception; Dryer & Horowitz, 1997; Tiedens & Fragale, 2003), Bohns and colleagues (2009) tested the idea that complementary regulatory focus orientations bolster relationship adjustment because they allow the partners to coordinate their behavior in a way that allows them to pursue tasks in ways that are appealing to each of them. This division of labor lets promotion-focused individuals pursue tasks requiring eager strategies, and prevention-focused individuals pursue tasks requiring vigilant strategies. Results supported this idea, but only for relationships characterized by high levels of interdependence or goal compatibility (Bohns et al., 2009); it seems that it takes couples some time to figure out how to divide labor, but complementary couples (one promotion-oriented partner and one prevention-oriented partner) are happiest once they have had the opportunity to coordinate their goal pursuits.

Finally, research has suggested that different close relationship contexts may encourage the primacy of promotion or prevention orientations (Molden, Lucas, Finkel, Kumashiro, & Rusbult, 2009). Because of the early stage and the forward-looking aspects of dating relationships, research suggests that dating couples may primarily seek promotion goals in their relationships, such as "to take our relationship to the next step" or "to not miss out on opportunities for closeness," while married couples have a broader motivational orientation that also includes prevention goals, such as "to maintain a healthy sex life" or "to avoid getting divorced." If promotion goals are predominant in their relationships, dating couples should be most receptive to support that matches that general goal orientation. Indeed, in a longitudinal study of dating and married couples, the authors found that although perceived support for both promotion- and prevention-oriented goals was linked with positive relationship outcomes, the association was strongest when the perceived support matched the motivational context of the relationship itself; that is, participants in dating relationships felt more positively about partners who promoted their promotion goals, while married couples felt more positively about partners who supported both their promotion and their prevention goals (Molden et al., 2009).

FUTURE DIRECTIONS AND CONCLUSIONS

In this chapter, we have reviewed research on how self-regulatory strength, content, and strategies affect interpersonal relationships. Clearly, more is known about the consequences of some aspects of self-regulation than others, and the low-hanging fruit for the next decade is plentiful. For example, not much is known about the effects of different relationship goals (i.e., the content of self-regulation) on relationship outcomes. Few models of close relationship phenomena have taken a self-regulation approach (cf. Read & Miller, 1989). The body of work by Murray, Holmes, and colleagues (e.g., Murray et al., 2003) on the conflicts between self-interested and relationship-interested goals represents an important exception. Although this conflict may be fundamental, there are surely other ways to categorize the many goals people pursue in relationships. Furthermore, one exciting area for future research is the match or compatibility of goal contents between partners. Goal compatibility or coordination, on the one hand, and goal conflict, on the other, are at the core of interdependence theory (Kelley, 1979; Murray et al., 2009), yet little is known about the effects of these variables on relationships. In addition, although this chapter has reviewed the rapidly growing body of research examining the effects of self-regulation on relationship outcomes, it has neglected the nascent body of research examining the effects of *partner regulation* (when one partner tries to lead the other partner to change some aspect of his or her relationship behavior) on relationship outcomes (Overall, Fletcher, & Simpson, 2006; Overall, Fletcher, Simpson, & Sibley, 2009).

These promising future directions notwithstanding, the achievements over the past decade are impressive. For example, today's scholars understand the relationship implications of having strong versus weak self-regulatory strength, of prioritizing self-protection goals versus relationship enhancement goals, and of the strategic orientations people take toward goal pursuit. One issue is that scholars who have created the knowledge in one of these domains are sometimes unfamiliar with work taking place in the others. Our hope in writing this chapter is that linking these diverse areas of research together will alert scholars who are not experts in all of these domains to the solid foundation that now exists for increasingly integrative programs of research on the effects of self-regulation on relationships.

ACKNOWLEDGMENTS

The writing of this chapter was supported by a Social Sciences and Humanities Research Council of Canada grant awarded to Gráinne M. Fitzsimons and a National Science Foundation grant (No. 719780) awarded to Eli J. Finkel. Any opinions, findings, and conclusions or recommendations expressed in this material are those of the authors and do not necessarily reflect the views of the agencies. Authorship ordering was determined by flipping a Loonie.

REFERENCES

Ayduk, O., Mendoza-Denton, R., Mischel, W., Downey, G., Peake, P. K., & Rodriguez, M. (2000). Regulating the interpersonal self: Strategic self-regulation for coping with rejection sensitivity. *Journal of Personality and Social Psychology, 79,* 776–792.

Bandura, A. (1982). Self-efficacy mechanism in human agency. *American Psychologist, 37,* 122–147.

Bargh, J. A., Gollwitzer, P. M., Lee-Chai, A., Barndollar, K., & Troetschel, R. (2001). The auto-mated will: Nonconscious activation and pursuit of behavioral goals. *Journal of Personality and Social Psychology, 81,* 1014–1027.

Baumeister, R. F. (2005). *The cultural animal: Human nature, meaning, and social life.* New York: Oxford University Press.

Baumeister, R. F., Gailliot, M., DeWall, C. N., & Oaten, M. (2006). Self-regulation and personal-ity: How interventions increase regulatory success, and how depletion moderates the effects of trait on behavior. *Journal of Personality, 74,* 1773–1802.

Baumeister, R. F., Heatherton, T. F., & Tice, D. M. (1994). *Losing control: How and why people fail at self-regulation.* New York: Academic Press.

Baumeister, R. F., Schmeichel, B. J., & Vohs, K. D. (2007). Self-regulation and the executive func-tion: The self as controlling agent. In A. W. Kruglanski & E. T. Higgins (Eds.), *Social psy-chology: Handbook of basic principles* (2nd ed., pp. 516–539). New York: Guilford Press.

Baumeister, R. F., Vohs, K. D., & Tice, D. M. (2007). The strength model of self-control. *Current Directions in Psychological Science, 16,* 351–355.

Berscheid, E. (1983). Emotion. In H. Kelley, E. Berscheid, A. Christensen, J. Harvey, T. Huston, G. Levinger, et al. (Eds.), *Close relationships* (pp. 110–168). New York: Freeman.

Berscheid, E. (1991). The emotion-in-relationships model: Reflections and update. In W. Kessen, A. Ortony, & F. I. M. Craik (Eds.), *Memories, thoughts, and emotions: Essays in honor of George Mandler* (pp. 323–335). Hillsdale, NJ: Erlbaum.

Berscheid, E., & Ammazzalorso, H. (2001). Emotional experience in close relationships. In M. Hewstone & M. Brewer (Eds.), *Blackwell handbook of social psychology: Vol. 2. Interper-sonal processes* (pp. 308–330). Oxford, UK: Blackwell.

Bohns, V. K., Lucas, G. M., Molden, D. C., Finkel, E. J., Coolsen, M. K., Kumashiro, M., et al. (2009). *When opposites fit: Increased relationship strength from partner complementarity in regulatory focus.* Unpublished manuscript, University of Toronto, Toronto, Canada.

Brunstein, J. C., Dangelmayer, G., & Schultheiss, O. C. (1996). Personal goals and social support in close relationships: Effects on relationship mood and marital satisfaction. *Journal of Per-sonality and Social Psychology, 71,* 1006–1019.

Byrne, D. (1971). *The attraction paradigm.* New York: Academic Press.

Carver, C. S., & White, T. L. (1994). Behavioral inhibition, behavioral activation, and affective responses to impending reward and punishment: The BIS/BAS scales. *Journal of Personality and Social Psychology, 67,* 319–333.

Deci, E. L., & Ryan, R. M. (1991). A motivational approach to the self: Integration in personality. In R. Dienstbier (Ed.), *Nebraska Symposium on Motivation: Vol. 38. Perspectives on motiva-tion* (pp. 237–288). Lincoln: University of Nebraska Press.

DeWall, C. N., Baumeister, R. F., Stillman, T. F., & Gailliot, M. T. (2007). Violence restrained: Effects of self-regulation and its depletion on aggression. *Journal of Experimental Social Psychology, 43,* 62–76.

Drigotas, S. M., Rusbult, C. E., Wieselquist, J., & Whitton, S. (1999). Close partner as sculptor of the ideal self: Behavioral affirmation and the Michelangelo phenomenon. *Journal of Person-ality and Social Psychology, 77,* 293–323.

Dryer, D. C., & Horowitz, L. M. (1997). When do opposites attract?: Interpersonal complementa-rity versus similarity. *Journal of Personality and Social Psychology, 72,* 592–603.

Elliot, A. J., & Covington, M. V. (2001). Approach and avoidance motivation. *Educational Psy-chology Review, 13,* 73–92.

Emmons, R. A. (1986). Personal strivings: An approach to personality and subjective well-being. *Journal of Personality and Social Psychology, 51,* 1058–1068.

Fehr, B., & Harasymchuk, C. (2005). The experience of emotion in close relationships: Toward an integration of the emotion-in-relationships and interpersonal script models. *Personal Rela-tionships, 12,* 181–196.

Finkel, E. J., & Campbell, W. K. (2001). Self-control and accommodation in close relationships: An interdependence analysis. *Journal of Personality and Social Psychology, 81*, 263–277.

Finkel, E. J., DeWall, C. N., Slotter, E. B., Oaten, M., & Foshee, V. A. (2009). Self-regulatory failure and intimate partner violence perpetration. *Journal of Personality and Social Psychology, 97*, 483–499.

Finkel, E. J., Molden, D. C., Johnson, S. E., & Eastwick, P. W. (2009). Regulatory focus and romantic alternatives. In J. P. Forgas, R. F. Baumeister, & D. M. Tice (Eds.), *Self-regulation: Cognitive, affective, and motivational processes* (pp. 319–335). New York: Psychology Press.

Fitzsimons, G. M., & Bargh, J. A. (2003). Thinking of you: Nonconscious pursuit of interpersonal goals associated with relationship partners. *Journal of Personality and Social Psychology, 84*, 148–164.

Fitzsimons, G. M., & Fishbach, A. (2010). Shifting closeness: Interpersonal effects of personal goal progress. *Journal of Personality and Social Psychology, 98*, 535–549.

Fitzsimons, G. M., & Shah, J. Y. (2008). How goal instrumentality shapes relationship evaluations. *Journal of Personality and Social Psychology, 95*, 319–337.

Fitzsimons, G. M., & Shah, J. Y. (2009). Confusing one instrumental other for another: Goal effects on social categorization. *Psychological Science, 20*, 1468–1472.

Gable, S. L. (2006). Approach and avoidance social motives and goals. *Journal of Personality, 71*, 175–222.

Gable, S. L., & Poore, J. (2008). Which thoughts count?: Algorithms for evaluating satisfaction in relationships. *Psychological Science, 19*, 1030–1036.

Gonzaga, G. C., Campos, B., & Bradbury, T. (2007). Similarity, convergence, and relationship satisfaction in dating and married couples. *Journal of Personality and Social Psychology, 93*, 34–48.

Gray, J. A. (1990). Brain systems that mediate both emotion and cognition. *Cognition and Emotion, 4*, 269–288.

Heatherton, T. F., & Vohs, K. D. (1998). Why is it so difficult to inhibit behavior? *Psychological Inquiry, 9*, 212–216.

Higgins, E. T. (1997). Beyond pleasure and pain. *American Psychologist, 52*, 1280–1300.

Impett, E., Gable, S. L., & Peplau, L. A. (2005). Giving up and giving in: The costs and benefits of daily sacrifice in intimate relationships. *Journal of Personality and Social Psychology, 89*, 327–344.

Impett, E. A., Peplau, L. A., & Gable, S. L. (2005). Approach and avoidance sexual motivation: Implications for personal and interpersonal well-being. *Personal Relationships, 12*, 465–482.

Impett, E. A., Strachman, A., Finkel, E. J., & Gable, S. L. (2008). Maintaining sexual desire in intimate relationships: The importance of approach goals. *Journal of Personality and Social Psychology, 94*, 808–823.

Kelley, H. H. (1979). *Personal relationships: Their structure and processes.* Hillsdale, NJ: Erlbaum.

Kruglanski, A. W., Shah, J. Y., Fishbach, A., Friedman, R., Chun, W. Y., & Sleeth-Keppler, D. (2002). A theory of goal systems. *Advances in Experimental Social Psychology, 34*, 311–378.

La Guardia, J. G., Ryan, R. M., Couchman, C. E., & Deci, E. L. (2000). Within-person variation in security of attachment: A self-determination theory perspective on attachment, need fulfillment, and well-being. *Journal of Personality and Social Psychology, 79*, 367–384.

Locke, E. A., & Latham, G. P. (2002). Building a practically useful theory of goal setting and task motivation: A 35-year odyssey. *American Psychologist, 57*, 705–717.

Mischel, W. (1974). Processes in delay of gratification. In L. Berkowitz (Ed), *Advances in experimental social psychology* (Vol. 7, pp. 249–292). New York: Academic Press.

Mischel, W., Shoda, Y., & Peake, P. K. (1988). The nature of adolescent competencies predicted by preschool delay of gratification. *Journal of Personality and Social Psychology, 54,* 687–696.

Mischel, W., Shoda, Y., & Rodriguez, M. I. (1989). Delay of gratification in children. *Science, 244,* 933–938.

Molden, D. C., Lee, A. Y., & Higgins, E. T. (2008). Motivations for promotion and prevention. In J. Y. Shah & W. L. Gardner (Eds.), *Handbook of motivation science* (pp. 169–187). New York: Guilford Press.

Molden, D. C., Lucas, G. M., Finkel, E. J., Kumashiro, M., & Rusbult, C. E. (2009). Perceived support for promotion-focused and prevention-focused goals: Associations with well-being in unmarried and married couples. *Psychological Science, 20,* 787–793.

Molden, D. M., & Finkel, E. J. (2010). Motivations for promotion and prevention and the role of trust and commitment in interpersonal forgiveness. *Journal of Experimental Social Psychology, 46,* 255–268.

Muraven, M., & Baumeister, R. F. (2000). Self-regulation and depletion of limited resources: Does self-control resemble a muscle? *Psychological Bulletin, 126,* 247–259.

Murray, S. L. (2005). Regulating the risks of closeness: A relationship-specific sense of felt security. *Current Directions in Psychological Science, 14,* 74–78.

Murray, S. L., Bellavia, G., Rose, P., & Griffin, D. (2003). Once hurt, twice hurtful: How perceived regard regulates daily marital interaction. *Journal of Personality and Social Psychology, 84,* 126–147.

Murray, S. L., Holmes, J. G., & Collins, N. L. (2006). Optimizing assurance: The risk regulation system in relationships. *Psychological Bulletin, 132,* 641–666.

Murray, S. L., Pinkus, R. T., Holmes, J. G., Aloni, M., Derrick, J. T., Leder, S., et al. (2009). *Curbing risk-regulation processes in romantic relationships: The power of automatic partner attitudes.* Unpublished manuscript, University at Buffalo, State University of New York, Buffalo, NY.

Murray, S. L., Rose, P., Bellavia, G., Holmes, J. G., & Kusche, A. (2002). When rejection stings: How self-esteem constrains relationship-enhancement processes. *Journal of Personality and Social Psychology, 83,* 556–573.

Overall, N. C., Fletcher, G. J. O., & Simpson, J. A. (2006). Regulation processes in intimate relationships: The role of ideal standards. *Journal of Personality and Social Psychology, 91,* 662–685.

Overall, N. C., Fletcher, G. J. O., Simpson, J. A., & Sibley, C. G. (2009). Regulating partners in intimate relationships: The costs and benefits of different communication strategies. *Journal of Personality and Social Psychology, 96,* 620–639.

Patrick, H., Knee, C. R., Canevello, A., & Lonsbary, C. (2007). The role of need fulfillment in relationship functioning and well-being: A self-determination theory perspective. *Journal of Personality and Social Psychology, 92,* 434–456.

Pronk, T. M., Karremans, J. C., Overbeek, G., Vermulst, A. A., & Wigboldus, D. H. J. (in press). What it takes to forgive: When and why executive functioning facilitates forgiveness. *Journal of Personality and Social Psychology.*

Rawn, C. D., & Vohs, K. D. (2006). The importance of self-regulation for interpersonal functioning. In K. D. Vohs & E. J. Finkel (Eds.), *Self and relationships: Connecting intrapersonal and interpersonal processes* (pp. 15–31). New York: Guilford Press.

Read, S. J., & Miller, L. C. (1989) Inter-personalism: Toward a goal-based theory of persons in relationships. In L. Pervin (Ed.), *Goal concepts in personality and social psychology* (pp. 413–472). Hillsdale, NJ: Erlbaum.

Reis, H. T., Sheldon, K. M., Gable, S. L., Roscoe, J., & Ryan, R. M. (2000). Daily well-being: The role of autonomy, competence, and relatedness. *Personality and Social Psychology Bulletin, 26,* 419–435.

Rusbult, C. E., Finkel, E. J., & Kumashiro, M. (2009). The Michelangelo phenomenon. *Current Directions in Psychological Science, 18*, 305–309.

Rusbult, C. E., Kumashiro, M., Kubacka, K. E., & Finkel, E. J. (2009). "The part of me that you bring out": Ideal similarity and the Michelangelo phenomenon. *Journal of Personality and Social Psychology, 96*, 61–82.

Ryan, R. M., & Deci, E. L. (2001). On happiness and human potentials: A review of research on hedonic and eudaimonic well-being. *Annual Review of Psychology, 52*, 141–166.

Slotter, E. B., & Finkel, E. J. (2009). The strange case of sustained dedication to an unfulfilling relationship: Predicting commitment and breakup from attachment anxiety and need fulfillment within relationships. *Personality and Social Psychology Bulletin, 39*, 85–100.

Stroop, J. R. (1935). Studies of interference in serial verbal reactions. *Journal of Experimental Psychology, 18*, 643–662.

Tangney, J. P., Baumeister, R. F., & Boone, A. L. (2004). High self-control predicts good adjustment, less pathology, better grades, and interpersonal success. *Journal of Personality, 72*, 271–322.

Tiedens, L., & Fragale, A. (2003). Power moves: Complementarity in dominant and submissive nonverbal behavior. *Journal of Personality and Social Psychology, 84*, 558–568.

Vohs, K. D., Baumeister, R. F., & Ciarocco, N. (2005). Self-regulation and self-presentation: Regulatory resource depletion impairs impression management and effortful self-presentation depletes regulatory resources. *Journal of Personality and Social Psychology, 88*, 632–657.

von Hippel, W., & Gonsalkorale, K. (2005). "That is bloody revolting!": Inhibitory control of thoughts better left unsaid. *Psychological Science, 16*, 497–500.

CHAPTER 23

Waiting, Tolerating, and Cooperating

Did Religion Evolve to Prop Up Humans' Self-Control Abilities?

MICHAEL E. McCULLOUGH
EVAN C. CARTER

The Natufians lived 15,000–11,500 years ago on the eastern side of the Mediterranean in what is modern-day Syria, Israel, Palestine, and Jordan, and they were social pioneers in many respects. They were among the first people to make the transition to a sedentary lifestyle in which people lived in groups, including substantial numbers of nonkin. They were one of the first societies to begin the transition from foraging to agriculture—harvesting wild cereals such as wheat and barley using sickles with stone blades and wooden handles. Their society provides some of the first physical evidence for dog domestication—a marked break from the Paleolithic world, in which the world of humans was clearly separated from the world of animals. They were the first society to bury their dead in large, concentrated numbers near their own settlements (Bar-Yosef, 1998). And most important for our purposes here, the remnants of Natufian culture include the first known burial site of a shaman in the Near East.

Several years ago, anthropologists discovered a 12,000-year-old gravesite in a cave called Hilazon Tachtit, halfway between the Mediterranean and the Sea of Galilee in northern Israel. The grave contained the body of a 45-year-old woman whose pelvic and spinal deformities would have caused her to drag a leg or limp when she walked (Grosman, Munro, & Belfer-Cohen, 2008). The gravesite was prepared with care; the body was positioned deliberately and held in position by a series of large stones. The grave goods included the types of artifacts that characterize shamans' toolkits worldwide: an ox's tail, the forearm of a wild boar, the wing of an eagle, fragments from a basalt bowl, the horn core from a gazelle in association with the bowl fragments, the pelvis of a leopard, the skulls of two stone martens, 50 tortoise shells, and a fully articulated human foot (someone else's, not the shaman's). The burial—a 10-kilometer walk and a 150-meter climb up a steep escarpment from the nearest Natufian settlement—would have been time-consuming and effortful for the community. Clearly, this shaman woman was a person of great importance to her group.

Shamans were the world's first religious professionals, and they are still found almost universally in the world's extant hunter–gatherer societies (Winkelman, 1990). The Natufian shaman's grave is by no means the world's only prehistoric shaman grave, or even the oldest one (Porr & Alt, 2006), but it is tempting to view the care with which this particular shaman was treated (and the fact that she was found in association with *this* Near Eastern society, and neither an earlier Near Eastern society nor a later one) as related to the unique characteristics of Natufian society in which she lived, and the dramatic social and economic changes it was experiencing. In part due to climactic improvements, populations were growing, and their old lifestyle of seminomadic foraging, with seasonal moves in pursuit of more plentiful food, was giving way to a lifestyle characterized by permanent settlements in which wild cereals could be exploited.

To gain benefits from their new semipermanent lifestyle and to cope with their growing population base, the Natufians would have had to develop new ways of regulating group life, as is often the case when politically autonomous band-level societies are superseded by larger, more complex societies. Specifically, there would have been novel problems related to *cooperating* (i.e., engagement in personally costly actions with non-relatives to create new public and private assets such as kilns for producing lime, fences to pen livestock, or the simple gains of trade); novel problems related to *tolerating* (the emotional effects of inevitable conflicts of interest are less easily salved when the psychological affordances shaped by selection pressures for kin altruism are not activated by cues of genetic relatedness; Lieberman, Tooby, & Cosmides, 2007); and, for their descendants, who would specialize almost exclusively in animal domestication and plant cultivation (Bar-Yosef, 1998), novel problems associated with *waiting* (in agricultural societies, the problem of waiting is particularly intense because cereal cultivation requires several months between initial preparation and planting to harvest, unlike economies based on hunting and gathering, in which the time between the onset of acquisition and consumption is measured in seconds to days). And it seems that problems like these would only get more intense as societies got larger, and food economies came to involve more and more waiting. Mithen (2007) puts some of the novel problems that agriculture and sedentism introduce this way:

> The mobile hunter–gatherer lifestyle always looks far more attractive than sedentism, which creates problems of refuse disposal, hygiene and social conflict within [*sic*] one's neighbours—hunter–gatherers solve these problems by simply moving away, whether from their rubbish or other people. *That is no longer an option after one has invested in field clearance, irrigation ditches, stock fences and so forth.* (p. 710, emphasis added)

We suspect that the waiting, tolerating, and cooperating that sedentary lifestyles and agrarian economic activity necessitate draw upon specific cognitive abilities that go together under the label *self-control*. We note that Reyes-García and colleagues (2007) made a similar argument for how self-control (which they call *patience*) facilitates the accumulation of the forms of human capital (e.g., formal schooling) that enable people to transition from the economic activities that characterize life in self-sufficient societies (e.g., hunting, foraging, small-scale agriculture) to those that characterize life in market-based economies (e.g., wage earning).

Consider the following facts about how self-control influences the sorts of behavioral challenges we are outlining here. The link between animals' levels of self-control and the specific food ecologies can be viewed as something like an iron law of behavioral ecology: Animals simply cannot exploit food sources that require more waiting than they are capable of enduring, so the ability to exploit food sources that require self-control can exert selection pressure on organisms to attain higher and higher levels of self-control (Stevens, Hallinan, & Hauser, 2005). Moreover, tolerating unfair behavior from others (which is inevitable in a world in which people's interests never align perfectly) without lashing out against them draws on cortical areas associated with the top-down suppression of anger and other negative emotions (Jensen-Campbell, Knack, Waldrip, & Campbell, 2007; Tabibnia, Satpute, & Lieberman, 2008). Finally, biologists and psychologists have recently argued that self-control is a cognitive prerequisite both for the evolution of reciprocal altruism (Stevens, Cushman, & Hauser, 2005), and its proximal production (Curry, Price, & Price, 2008; Rachlin, 2000; Yi, Buchhalter, Gatchalian, & Bickel, 2007).

Our thesis here is that intensifications in human religiosity (particularly, an increasing focus on supernatural entities that (1) monitor human behavior for moral probity and moral lapses, (2) possess well-formed preferences about desirable modes of human conduct [even in the nonmoral realm], and (3) administer temporal or afterlife punishments and rewards) over the past 10,000 years reflect the efficacy of belief in these sorts of supernatural agents to increase self-control among group members, so that modern problems related to waiting, tolerating, and cooperating could be resolved without exclusive reliance on social monitoring and policing, or even expensive institutional monitoring and policing. Johnson (2005) documented how the world's distribution of "high Gods"—that is, gods with moral preferences that monitor and punish human behavior—correlates positively with a variety of indices of societal complexity, including community size, the use of money and credit, the presence of police forces, jurisdictional hierarchies above the level of the local community, taxation, and—importantly—the level of individual compliance with community norms, which suggests that the advent of moralizing gods is coincident with increasing societal concerns about adjusting to the socioemotional challenges that arise when people begin to live in large groups. Our thesis is very consistent with Johnson's—and with that of Norenzayan and Shariff, who argue that religious cognition is particularly good at facilitating prosocial behavior that is costly in the short term (Norenzayan & Shariff, 2008; Shariff & Norenzayan, 2007). We think our proposal is also congenial to Robert Wright's (2009) recent description of the connections between the social evolution of economies and the social evolution of religion.

But here is where our thesis differs from previous ideas: We want to describe the interaction between the human psychology for self-regulation and beliefs in moralizing gods because it is at this nexus of evolved cognitive hardware for self-regulation and religious innovation that people's capacities for waiting, tolerating, and cooperating might be modified by particular forms of religion. Put simply, we believe that religious cognition has been refined through cultural selection (Richerson & Boyd, 2005) because of its ability to promote self-control, which is at a premium in the large, complex, sedentary, agriculturally based societies in which most humans have increasingly lived for the past 8,000 years (Carneiro, 1978).

Human capacities for self-control were put in place by natural selection acting on neural tissue over many generations in ancestral human populations, but the parameter settings on those evolved mechanisms can be influenced by cultural inputs, such as religious parental influences (Bartkowski, Xu, & Levin, 2008) or personal involvement in religious institutions (Kenrick, McCreath, Govern, King, & Bordin, 1990) and practices (Wenger, 2007). This particular aspect of our thesis—that cultural inputs can influence the parameter settings on evolved mental mechanisms—is not particularly controversial (Tooby & Cosmides, 1992, see especially pp. 114–116).

Empirical research on the links between religion and self-control is in its infancy (McCullough & Willoughby, 2009), so we limit ourselves here to describing what is currently known about those links, even though much of that research is correlational and therefore unable to shed definitive light on religion's ability to foster self-control or self-regulation more broadly. Nevertheless, we think this research shows generally that there are reasons to believe that religion, as experienced and practiced by many people on the planet today, is indeed associated with higher levels of self-control and specific aspects of self-regulation more generally.

DEFINING RELIGION, SELF-CONTROL, AND SELF-REGULATION

Following James (1958), Pratt (1934), and Atran and Norenzayan (2004), we conceive of *religion* as a broad cultural syndrome characterized by deeply held beliefs that arise from awareness of, or perceived interaction with, supernatural agents such as gods and spirits that are presumed to play an important role in human affairs, along with the emotions and behaviors (including ritualized and socially shared practices) that arise from and support these beliefs. In research, religion is often operationalized with measures of people's self-reported religious commitment, frequency of religiously related activities (prayer, service attendance, etc.), and belief in the existence of gods or spirits (Hill & Hood, 1999).

We define *self-regulation* similarly to many other scientists (Baumeister & Vohs, 2004; Carver & Scheier, 1998) as the process by which a system uses information about its present state to change that state toward greater conformity with a desired end state or goal. Self-regulation need not be a deliberative, effortful process: Much of self-regulation occurs in a relatively effortless and automatic fashion (Fitzsimons & Bargh, 2004), and for that reason, we also wish to understand how religion might be related to automatic or implicit self-regulation (Koole, McCullough, Kuhl, & Roelofsma, 2010). We reserve the term *self-control* for situations in which people work to override a prepotent response (e.g., a behavioral tendency, an emotion, or a motivation), such as a craving for alcohol, a desire to pull one's hand out of near-freezing water, or the temptation to chase a hare instead of remaining with the group to stalk a stag (Baumeister, Vohs, & Tice, 2007). In other words, when people exert self-control, they modify their response tendencies by suppressing one goal so as to pursue another one that is more highly valued—especially when one is not actively within the thrall of that prepotent motivation to action (e.g., when we are setting an alarm clock in the evening for the next day, we value getting up early the next morning to a greater extent than we value staying in bed, but our preferences can shift when that alarm goes off at 5:30 the next morning. Self-control at 5:30 A.M. helps us to stay true to what we valued most when we set the alarm in the first place). Self-control is therefore a more specific concept than self-regulation. Not all psychological states that are self-regulated involve *self-control* as we use the term here; however, self-control may rely on a generic self-regulatory strength (Baumeister et al., 2007).

EXAMINING AND EXPLAINING THE CONNECTIONS OF RELIGION TO SELF-CONTROL AND SELF-REGULATION

We recently reviewed the extant literature on the links between religion and self-control and self-regulation (McCullough & Willoughby, 2009), and little has changed since the publication of that article. Nevertheless, we summarize some of those highlights below and emphasize how the literature has developed (and how our thinking has changed) since its publication, beginning with efforts to describe the apparent nature of the relationship of religiosity and a generic dispositional proneness toward self-control.

The General Connection of Religiosity and Self-Control

Evidence from personality research suggests that religious people tend to score higher on measures of self-control and measures of personality that subsume self-control, such as conscientiousness and agreeableness, than do their less religious counterparts (Lodi-Smith & Roberts, 2007; Saroglou, 2002). In Eysenck's model of personality, psychoticism, which can be thought of as the opposite of Big Five agreeableness and conscientiousness (Costa & McCrae, 1995) is consistently, and negatively, related to a variety of measures of religiosity for samples from a range of ages, religious denominations, and cultures (Francis, 1997; Francis & Katz, 1992; Hills, Francis, Argyle, & Jackson, 2004; Lodi-Smith & Roberts, 2007; Wilde & Joseph, 1997). With respect to Cattell's personality system, McCullough and Willoughby (2009) cited studies revealing that scale "G," also known variously as "Conformity," "Superego," and "Expedient versus Conscientious," is positively associated with church attendance, attitudes toward Christianity, and traditional Christian religious belief.

McCullough and Willoughby (2009) also summarized 12 studies that reported associations of measures of religiosity with measures of general self-control (e.g., Bouchard, McGue, Lykken, & Tellegen, 1999; Desmond, Ulmer, & Bader, 2009; French, Eisenberg, Vaughan, Purwono, & Suryanti, 2008; Walker, Ainette, Wills, & Mendoza, 2007). Of these 12 studies, 11 reported positive associations between self-report measures of religiosity and self-control, with effect size rs ranging from 0.21 to 0.38. It is worthwhile to note that in two of these studies (Bergin, Masters, & Richards, 1987; Bouchard et al., 1999), researchers found *extrinsic religious motivation*, which is a religious orientation characterized by treating religion as a means (as opposed to *intrinsic religiosity*, in which it is treated as an end; Allport & Ross, 1967) to be negatively associated with self-control. The distinction between intrinsic and extrinsic religion may be an important one to keep in mind as this research area develops.

In the United States, religious families also tend to have children with more self-control (Bartkowski et al., 2008; Brody & Flor, 1998; Brody, Stoneman, & Flor, 1996;

Lindner-Gunnoe, Hetherington, & Reiss, 1999). Parental religiosity, variously measured as church attendance, reports of the extent to which religion is discussed in the home, and self-rated importance of religion, is positively associated with parent and teacher ratings of children's self-control and lack of impulsivity. These associations do not appear to result from the confounding effects of gender, age, race, socioeconomic status, education, or religious denomination.

Confidence that the links between religion and self-control are *causally* related must be limited, in part, by the lack of appropriate longitudinal data and the limited support for the hypothesis that the (rather weak) available longitudinal data provide. McCullough and Willoughby (2009) found six longitudinal studies that reported evidence bearing on the causal nature of this relationship between religion and self-control or self-control-related personality traits, and in only one of them (Wink, Ciciolla, Dillon, & Tracy, 2007) was religiousness associated with increases in a personality trait related to self-control—agreeableness—over the life course. Moreover, this finding held only for women, and no connection between religiosity and later increases in conscientiousness was found. In contrast, five studies found that measures of self-control and relevant personality traits predicted religiosity later in life. In one study, conscientious children reliably became more religious adults, even after researchers controlled for confounds such as gender and religious upbringing (McCullough, Tsang, & Brion, 2003). In another, children who scored low in agreeableness tended to become less religious adults (McCullough, Enders, Brion, & Jain, 2005). In a third, conscientious adolescents and agreeable female adolescents experienced increases in religiousness through late adulthood, measured nearly 50 years later (Wink et al., 2007). In a fourth, religious youths who reported making decisions deliberatively and avoiding risk taking remained more religious a year later than their less religious and less controlled counterparts (Regnerus & Smith, 2005). In a fifth, high school boys whose psychoticism declined over two time points, and high school girls with increasing conscientiousness at the same two time points, reported more religiosity at a third time point (Heaven & Ciarrochi, 2007). Taken together, therefore, this body of research suggests that religion and self-control are indeed related at the level of personality. However, the longitudinal evidence that religion can *cause* increases or reductions in self-control is currently quite limited, and the evidence that changes in conscientiousness and similar constructs leads to increases in religiosity over time enjoys quite a bit more empirical support. For this reason, experimental data demonstrating that religion can create transient (or long-term) increases in self-control would be highly desirable from a scientific point of view.

Religion and the Cybernetic Model of Self-Regulation

Aside from religion's general connections to personality-level measurements of self-control, it is instructive to consider how religion might influence self-regulation via basic conceptual processes that are necessary for systems (biological systems included) to self-regulate effectively. Carver and Scheier (1998; Chapter 1, this volume) conceptualized *self-regulation* as a dynamical process by which people bring their behavior into conformity with standards, despite environmental changes that disturb equilibrium, through the operation of integrated negative feedback loops. These negative feedback loops consist of several integrated functions. The *input* function detects the system's state. In human terms, this is equivalent to one's perceptions of the self and the environment. The *com-*

parator function compares the system's state to a *reference value*. Reference values can be conceptualized as goals or standards. When a comparator indicates that the system's state matches its reference value, nothing changes, and the existing state is maintained. When the comparator notes a discrepancy between the system's state and its reference value, an *output* function is activated to reduce the discrepancy. Self-regulating systems continuously self-monitor for goal–behavior discrepancies; when discrepancies are noticed, they respond by trying to minimize them via outputs.

In other words, effective human self-regulation, as Carver and Scheier (1998) conceptualized it, requires four processes. First, it requires clear *goals* that are organized so as to permit effective management of conflict among them (Fitzsimons & Bargh, 2004). Second, it requires sufficient *self-monitoring* and/or self-directed attention, so that one can detect discrepancies between one's goals and one's actual behavior. Third, it requires sufficient motivation, or *self-regulatory strength*, to change one's behavior when discrepancies are detected. Fourth, it requires effective mechanisms, or *outputs*, for effecting behavioral change (Schmeichel & Baumeister, 2004). Presently, we consider how religion might influence these four processes and describe some of the research that is relevant to these concepts.

Religion and Goals

Religious belief encourages people to acquire specific goals and values that differ from those of nonreligious people (Roberts & Robins, 2000; Saroglou, Delpierre, & Dernelle, 2004). For instance, in meta-analytic data from 12 studies conducted in primarily Christian, primarily Muslim, and primarily Jewish nations (e.g., the United States, Turkey, and Israel), religiosity was reliably and positively correlated with the values from the Schwartz Value Survey called Tradition (described as including traits such as "responsible" and "helpful"; $r = .45$) and Conformity (including traits such as "self-discipline" and "politeness"; $r = .23$). Conversely, religiosity was negatively correlated with the values measured on scales known as Hedonism ("self-indulgent," "pleasure"; $r = -.30$), Stimulation ("exciting life"; $r = -.26$), and Self-Direction ("freedom," "independent"; $r = -.24$). These results were obtained in all three types of religious nations, suggesting that Jewish, Christian, and Muslim religious beliefs promote goals related to respect and concern for the welfare of others, while discouraging goals related to personal gratification and individuality. It seems to us no accident that religiosity is particularly good at increasing people's valuation of tradition and conformity-related values, if what religion has evolved culturally to do is increase people's ability to wait, tolerate, and cooperate.

One way in which religious thought may encourage religiously related goals at the expense of secular goals is by *sanctifying* them, or defining the source of religious goals as sacred, thereby making them more important (Emmons, 1999). For example, Mahoney et al. (1999) found that husbands and wives who characterized their marriages as "sacred" and as "manifestations of God" reported healthier marriages (better adjustment, better conflict resolution). Mahoney and colleagues (2005) also showed that college students who sanctified their bodies, believing them to be gifts from God, tended to get more sleep, wear their seat belts, and disapprove of illicit drug use. It seems that religion can be used to sanctify almost *any goal*, from getting enough exercise to killing civilians, but we anticipate that many, if not most, of the goals that people commonly sanctify through religion will be relevant (in the practitioner's eyes, at least) to waiting (e.g., being a more patient person), tolerating (e.g., being a more forgiving person), and cooperating (e.g., helping members of one's group or honoring one's debts).

Religiosity and Self-Monitoring

Awareness of an evaluative audience increases people's self-awareness. When made self-aware, they then compare their behavior to relevant behavioral standards (Carver & Scheier, 1998). Many religious belief systems posit gods or spirits that observe humans' behavior, pass judgment, then administer rewards or sanctions (Bering & Johnson, 2005), and in many of these religions, these beings can also read thoughts and are not fooled by people's attempts to deceive them. Several studies suggest that priming religious concepts produces behavioral effects on measures such as cooperation, generosity, and honesty that can be construed as prosocial in nature (Pichon, Boccato, & Saroglou, 2007; Randolph-Seng & Nielsen, 2007; Shariff & Norenzayan, 2007), and such effects could conceivably be mediated by religious cognition's effects on self-monitoring (though this remains an open question). Such speculation is also consistent with work showing that exposure to images of eyes (i.e., stimuli indicative of the fact that one is being monitored) increases generosity and honesty (Haley & Fessler, 2005). Religion could also promote self-monitoring through introspective religious rituals (e.g., prayer, meditation, reflecting on scripture) that encourage people to monitor for discrepancies between their goal states and their actual behavior (Wenger, 2007). Correlational evidence that religious people engage in more self-monitoring than do less religious people is limited, and mixed, and direct experimental work on the topic is virtually nonexistent, so we think this particular question is ripe for research (McCullough & Willoughby, 2009).

Religiosity and Self-Regulatory Strength

Once a discrepancy between a goal and one's behavior has been detected, it has been posited, people must have adequate self-regulatory strength to adjust their behavior (Schmeichel & Baumeister, 2004). Religious communities are high-constraint settings (Kenrick et al., 1990) in part because involvement in these communities exposes members to social incentives and sanctions that encourage self-regulated behavior. The presence of such incentives and sanctions may then lead people to self-regulate on a more chronic level, which, according to the muscle model of self-control (Muraven & Baumeister, 2000), should increase religious people's self-regulatory strength. Religious rituals also often involve self-control behaviors (e.g., fasting, long periods of prayer and meditation), so regular engagement in such rituals might function as a type of self-control exercise, in time increasing self-regulatory strength (McCullough & Willoughby, 2009) that can be applied toward other self-regulatory tasks.

Although we know of no experimental evidence backing this proposition, research on fasting during the month of Ramadan is a compelling case study. During Ramadan, observant fasters become more irritable and anxious (Kadri et al., 2000), experience reduced blood glucose levels (Fazel, 1998) and suffer decrements in performance on perceptual tasks (Ali & Amir, 1989), and even end up in traffic accidents and the emergency room more frequently (Fazel, 1998). These findings suggest that Ramadan observance draws on limited self-control resources (Banfield, Wyland, Macrae, Münte, & Heatherton, 2004). For this reason, Ramadan fasting may be, among other things, a month-long workout for self-regulatory strength. If that is the case, then we should also expect that people leave the month of Ramadan with more self-regulatory strength than when they entered it (although, as we noted earlier, this idea is highly speculative).

Religiosity and Outputs for Self-Change

A final requirement for effective self-regulation is the possession of a suite of effective psychological and behavioral tools for self-change. As mentioned earlier, such tools for self-change are called *outputs* (Carver & Scheier, 1998). Religious belief systems may encourage effective outputs that are not specifically religious, such as simply avoiding contact with tempting stimuli (e.g., someone to whom one is highly sexually attracted but with whom a sexual relationship would be morally off limits) (Worthington, et al., 2001), but they offer something uniquely religious as well.

For example, prayer and meditation may serve important regulatory functions (Galton, 1872; McNamara, 2002). In one study, Brefczynski-Lewis, Lutz, Schaefer, Levinson, and Davidson (2007) discovered more activation in regions of the brain associated with attention and response inhibition in experienced meditators. Also, Chan and Woollacott (2007) found that experienced meditators had less interference during a Stroop task, suggesting that they had more effective regulation of attentional processes. In addition, Koole (2007) conducted five experiments revealing that people (particularly religious people) exposed to a person in need and then instructed to pray for that person experienced more reductions in negative affect than did people instructed (1) simply to think about the person or (2) to reappraise the person's plight positively.

Other religious behaviors that may be effective outputs for self-change (especially for religious people) include religious imagery (Weisbuch-Remington, Mendes, Seery, & Blascovich, 2005; Wiech et al., 2008), and consulting religious scriptures (Wenger, 2007). Rachlin (2000) proposed that behavioral guidance gleaned from religious scripture might be a particularly effective tool for change due to its sacred nature. Wenger's (2007) experiment provides some support for this claim. Participants who were led to focus on religious shortcomings spent longer reading a passage called "How can I know when it is God who is speaking to me?" It is not a stretch to see this finding as an illustration of a self-regulating system, noting a discrepancy in behavior relative to a goal state (not following religious tenets when a goal is to be a good follower of a religious system), then reducing the discrepancy using a religiously prescribed output function (reading religious material).

Religion and Implicit Self-Regulation

As noted earlier, self-control can occur through both automatic mechanisms and deliberative ones (Fitzsimons & Bargh, 2004), so Koole, McCullough, Kuhl, and Roelofsma (2010) recently advanced a parallel view of religion's connection to self-regulation that relies on implicit or automatic routes for cognitive processing rather than conscious ones. Implicit self-regulation, as they conceptualized it, functions in three ways that might be influenced by religious cognition. First, religion might help people to form appropriate intentions that can then be translated into effective action (also known as *volitional efficiency*). Second, religion might facilitate *emotion regulation*. Third, religion might help people reconcile new experiences with what has come previously, thereby helping to create and preserve *meaning in life*.

Many studies in which religious cognition has been primed outside of conscious awareness do indeed suggest that religious cognition can foster self-regulation through implicit processes. For example, in one experiment, subliminally presented religious mental content suppressed goals related to temptation (Fishbach, Friedman, & Kruglanski, 2003). College students were subliminally primed for 50 msec with a temptation/sin-related concept (e.g., drugs, temptation, premarital sex), a religion-related concept (e.g., prayer, bible, religion, and God), or a neutral word. After each prime, participants were instructed to identify religion-related words or temptation/sin-related words as either words or nonwords as quickly as possible. Fishbach et al. found that the subliminal presentation of temptation/sin-related primes led to faster recognition of religion-relevant words than did the subliminal presentation of neutral primes. Conversely, subliminally presented religion-relevant primes slowed recognition of sin/temptation-relevant words in comparison to the neutral primes. These results suggest that people recruit religious concepts to facilitate self-control in the face of temptation and, conversely, that activating religious mental content can suppress temptation/sin-relevant content. Interestingly, these regulatory processes took place automatically, implying that the regulation was based on implicit goals that had been internalized through a religious belief system.

One important effect of implicit regulation is to stabilize people's moment-to-moment responses to emotion-inducing stimuli (Koole, 2009; Kuhl, 2000). As described previously, Koole (2007) reported the results of five experiments supporting the hypothesis that prayer can reduce negative affect. Weisbuch-Remington and colleagues (2005) found similar effects in two experiments that evaluated whether religious imagery facilitates emotion regulation. These studies revealed that subliminally exposing Christian participants to positive religious imagery (images of Christ ascending to heaven, Jesus as an infant, etc.) before they completed a stressful task caused physiological responses characterized by greater cardiac output (a so-called "challenge response"; Blascovich, Mendes, Tomaka, Salomon, & Seery, 2003). In contrast, Christians exposed to negative religious imagery (demons, satanic symbols, etc.) evinced greater total peripheral resistance (a so-called "threat" response). A threat response is thought to occur when resources are evaluated as not meeting situational demands, whereas a challenge response indicates that situational demands have been evaluated as surmountable (Blascovich et al., 2003). Taken together, these results remind us that even though self-control has traditionally been considered a conscious, effortful process, we know better now. Therefore, we should expect that many of religion's potential self-regulatory effects will occur through automatic rather than conscious cognitive processes, and research in the future should examine religion's effects on self-regulation through both of these possible routes.

CONCLUSION

Evolutionary theories of religion can be divided roughly into those that view religious belief as a by-product of more basic cognitive adaptations—for example, cognitive mechanisms for inferring both causality in the physical world and other people's mental states (Boyer, 2001), or for maintaining attachments to caregivers (Kirkpatrick, 2005)—and those positing that the capacity for religious belief results from selection for religious mental representations of reality that might facilitate within-group conformity, cooperation, or generosity (Johnson, 2005; Norenzayan & Shariff, 2008; Sosis & Ruffle, 2003; Wilson, 2002). Although these theoretical approaches differ, one can concede that the human capacity for religious belief is indeed a by-product of more basic cognitive adaptations and still hold that the effects of such a cognitive by-product (i.e., the capacity for religious belief) might have been subject to more recent regimens of cultural (if not genetic) selection (Richerson & Boyd, 2005) that have led to the diversity religious beliefs seen throughout the world from prehistory to the present day.

Within such a hybrid theoretical account, the capacity for religious belief could be conceptualized as a secondary adaptation (Andrews, Gangestad, & Matthews, 2002) that has been selected for its ability to encourage people (1) to exercise patience, or delay of gratification—that is, *to wait*; (2) to refrain from aggression or other forms of antisocial behavior when others misbehave—that is, *to tolerate*; and (3) to engage in costly prosocial behaviors that enable them to collaborate with others in generating public goods—that is, *to cooperate*.

Space does not permit a full treatment of this idea here, but we hope one illustration will suffice. Many of the mathematically plausible models of natural selection for cooperation—most notably, reciprocal altruism (Axelrod, 1984; Axelrod & Hamilton, 1981; Trivers, 1971)—imply that for cooperation to evolve, certain cognitive foundations must be in place, for example, a willingness to start transactions in a cooperative (or "nice") frame of mind, a capacity to forgive occasional defections (i.e., transform one's vindictive motivations toward a cooperation partner back into prosocial ones), and an ability to delay gratification, that is, not to discount too steeply rewards that can be obtained after a time delay (Rachlin, 2000; Stevens, Cushman, et al., 2005). Most animals lack some or most of these cognitive foundations, but humans possess them all.

We wonder whether religious cognition—activated either chronically or acutely by situational cues such as religious artifacts, linguistic symbols, or even internally generated religious cognitive material (prayers, contemplation of valued religious role models, etc.)—might be particularly good at activating or strengthening these cognitive foundations for cooperation either explicitly or implicitly. As we have described, implicit religious priming increases generosity (Pichon et al., 2007; Shariff & Norenzayan, 2007), and honesty (Randolph-Seng & Nielsen, 2007), facilitates emotion regulation (Koole, 2007; Weisbuch-Remington et al., 2005; Wiech et al., 2008), and may even reduce temporal discounting (Roelofsma, Koole, & McCullough, 2009)—the very cognitive abilities required for the evolution of reciprocal altruism. If so, then perhaps religious belief has been conserved or modified further by selection for its ability to foster self-control and self-regulation in precisely the cognitive domains upon which humans and their ultracooperative ways of life have come to depend.

Seemingly overnight, the study of religion within psychology—indeed, within many of the social, behavioral, biological sciences—has become theoretically vigorous and empirically exciting. In the foreseeable future, the effects of religion on people's individual and social lives will likely remain the subject of considerable scientific research. We think it will be fruitful for researchers interested in those effects to inquire into the extent to which religion's effects might be built on its ability to encourage self-control and self-regulation.

ACKNOWLEDGMENTS

Preparation of this chapter was supported in part by the Center for the Study of Law and Religion at Emory University and a by grant from the John Templeton Foundation.

REFERENCES

Ali, M. R., & Amir, T. (1989). Effects of fasting on visual flicker fusion. *Perceptual and Motor Skills, 69*, 627–631.

Allport, G. W., & Ross, M. J. (1967). Personal religious orientation and prejudice. *Journal of Personality and Social Psychology, 5*, 432–443.

Andrews, P. W., Gangestad, S. W., & Matthews, D. (2002). Adaptationism—how to carry out an exaptationist program. *Behavioral and Brain Sciences, 25*, 489–504.

Atran, S., & Norenzayan, A. (2004). Religion's evolutionary landscape: Counterintuition, commitment, compassion, communion. *Behavioral and Brain Sciences, 27*, 713–730.

Axelrod, R. (1984). *The evolution of cooperation.* New York: Basic Books.

Axelrod, R., & Hamilton, W. D. (1981). The evolution of cooperation. *Science, 211*, 1390–1396.

Banfield, J. F., Wyland, C. L., Macrae, C. N., Münte, T. F., & Heatherton, T. F. (2004). The cognitive neuroscience of self-regulation. In R. F. Baumeister & K. D. Vohs (Eds.), *Handbook of self-regulation: Research, theory, and applications* (pp. 62–83). New York: Guilford Press.

Bar-Yosef, O. (1998). The Natufian culture in the Levant, threshold to the origins of agriculture. *Evolutionary Anthropology, 6*, 159–177.

Bartkowski, J. P., Xu, X., & Levin, M. L. (2008). Religion and child development: Evidence from the early childhood longitudinal study. *Social Science Research, 37*, 18–36.

Baumeister, R. F., & Vohs, K. D. (2004). Self-regulation. In C. Peterson & M. E. P. Seligman (Eds.), *Character strengths and virtues: A handbook and classification* (pp. 499–516). Washington, DC/New York: American Psychological Association/Oxford University Press.

Baumeister, R. F., Vohs, K. D., & Tice, D. M. (2007). The strength model of self-control *Current Directions in Psychological Science, 16*, 351–355.

Bergin, A. E., Masters, K. S., & Richards, P. S. (1987). Religiousness and mental health reconsidered: A study of an intrinsically religious sample. *Journal of Counseling Psychology, 34*, 197–204.

Bering, J. M., & Johnson, D. D. P. (2005). "O Lord . . . You perceive my thoughts from afar": Recursiveness and the evolution of supernatural agency. *Journal of Cognition and Culture, 5*, 118–142.

Blascovich, J., Mendes, W. B., Tomaka, J., Salomon, K., & Seery, M. D. (2003). The robust nature of the biopsychosocial model of challenge and threat: A reply to Wright and Kirby. *Personality and Social Psychology Review, 7*, 234–243.

Bouchard, T. J., McGue, M., Lykken, D., & Tellegen, A. (1999). Intrinsic and extrinsic religiousness: Genetic and environmental influences and personality correlates. *Twin Research, 2*, 88–98.

Boyer, P. (2001). *Religion explained: The evolutionary origins of religious thought.* New York: Basic Books.

Brefczynski-Lewis, J. A., Lutz, A., Schaefer, H. S., Levinson, D. B., & Davidson, R. J. (2007). Neural correlates of attentional expertise in long-term meditation practitioners. *Proceedings of the National Academy of Sciences USA, 104*, 11483–11488.

Brody, G. H., & Flor, D. (1998). Maternal resources, parenting practices, and child competence in rural, single-parent African American families. *Child Development, 69*, 803–816.

Brody, G. H., Stoneman, Z., & Flor, D. (1996). Parental religiosity, family processes, and youth competence in rural, two-parent African American families. *Developmental Psychology, 32,* 696–706.

Carneiro, R. L. (1978). Political expansion of the principle of competitive exclusion. In R. Cohen & E. R. Service (Eds.), *Origins of the state: The anthropology of political evolution* (pp. 205–223). Philadelphia: Institute for the Study of Human Issues.

Carver, C. S., & Scheier, M. F. (1998). *On the self-regulation of behavior.* New York: Cambridge University Press.

Chan, D., & Woollacott, M. (2007). Effects of level of meditation experience on attentional focus: Is the efficiency of executive or orientation networks improved? *Journal of Alternative and Complementary Medicine, 13,* 651–657.

Costa, P. T., & McCrae, R. R. (1995). Primary traits of Eysenck's P-E-N system: Three- and five-factor solutions. *Journal of Personality and Social Psychology, 69,* 308–317.

Curry, O. S., Price, M. E., & Price, J. G. (2008). Patience is a virtue: Cooperative people have lower discount rates. *Personality and Individual Differences, 44,* 780–785.

Desmond, S. A., Ulmer, J. T., & Bader, C. D. (2009). *Religion, prosocial learning, self control, and delinquency.* Manuscript submitted for publication.

Emmons, R. A. (1999). *The psychology of ultimate concerns: Motivation and spirituality in personality.* New York: Guilford Press.

Fazel, M. (1998). Medical implications of controlled fasting. *Journal of the Royal Society of Medicine, 91,* 260–263.

Fishbach, A., Friedman, R. S., & Kruglanski, A. W. (2003). Leading us not into temptation: Momentary allurements elicit overriding goal activation. *Journal of Personality and Social Psychology, 84,* 296–309.

Fitzsimons, G. M., & Bargh, J. A. (2004). Automatic self-regulation. In R. F. Baumeister & K. D. Vohs (Eds.), *Handbook of self-regulation: Research, theory, and applications* (pp. 151–170). New York: Guilford Press.

Francis, L. J. (1997). Personality, prayer, and church attendance among undergraduate students. *International Journal for the Psychology of Religion, 7,* 127–132.

Francis, L. J., & Katz, Y. J. (1992). The relationship between personality and religiosity in an Israeli sample. *Journal for the Scientific Study of Religion, 31,* 153–162.

French, D. C., Eisenberg, N., Vaughan, J., Purwono, U., & Suryanti, T. A. (2008). Religious involvement and the social competence and adjustment in Indonesian Muslim adolescents. *Developmental Psychology, 44,* 597–611.

Galton, F. (1872). Statistical inquiries into the efficacy of prayer. *Fortnightly Review, 12,* 125–135.

Grosman, L., Munro, N. D., & Belfer-Cohen, A. (2008). A 12,000-year-old shaman burial from the Levant (Israel). *Proceedings of the National Academy of Sciences USA, 105,* 17665–17669.

Haley, K. J., & Fessler, D. M. T. (2005). Nobody's watching?: Subtle cues affect generosity in an anonymous economic game. *Evolution and Human Behavior, 26,* 245–256.

Heaven, P. C. L., & Ciarrochi, J. (2007). Personality and religious values among adolescents: A three-wave longitudinal analysis. *British Journal of Psychology, 98,* 681–694.

Hill, P. C., & Hood, R. W., Jr. (1999). *Measures of religiosity.* Birmingham, AL: Religious Education Press.

Hills, P., Francis, L. J., Argyle, M., & Jackson, C. J. (2004). Primary personality trait correlates of religious practice and orientation. *Personality and Individual Differences, 36,* 61–73.

James, W. (1958). *The varieties of religious experience.* New York: Penguin.

Jensen-Campbell, L. A., Knack, J. M., Waldrip, A. M., & Campbell, S. D. (2007). Do Big Five personality traits associated with self-control influence the regulation of anger and aggression? *Journal of Research in Personality, 41,* 403–424.

Johnson, D. D. P. (2005). God's punishment and public goods. *Human Nature, 26,* 410–446.

Kadri, N., Tilane, A., El-Batal, M., Taltit, Y., Tahiri, S. M., & Moussaoui, D. (2000). Irritability during the month of Ramadan. *Psychosomatic Medicine, 62,* 280–285.

Kenrick, D. T., McCreath, H. E., Govern, J., King, R., & Bordin, J. (1990). Person–environment intersections: Everyday settings and common trait dimensions. *Journal of Personality and Social Psychology, 58,* 685–698.

Kirkpatrick, L. A. (2005). *Attachment, evolution, and the psychology of religion.* New York: Guilford Press.

Koole, S. L. (2007). *Raising spirits: An experimental analysis of the affect regulation functions of prayer.* Unpublished manuscript, Vrije Universiteit, Amsterdam.

Koole, S. L., McCullough, M. E., Kuhl, J., & Roelofsma, P. H. M. P. (2010). Why religion's burdens are light: From religiosity to implicit self-regulation. *Personality and Social Psychology Review, 14,* 95–107.

Kuhl, J. (2000). A functional-design approach to motivation and self-regulation: The dynamics of personality systems interactions. In M. Bokaerts, P. R. Pintrich, & M. Zeidner (Eds.), *Handbook of self-regulation* (pp. 111–169). San Diego, CA: Academic Press.

Lieberman, D., Tooby, J., & Cosmides, L. (2007). The architecture of human kin detection. *Nature, 445,* 727–731.

Lindner-Gunnoe, M., Hetherington, E. M., & Reiss, D. (1999). Parental religiosity, parenting style, and adolescent social responsibility. *Journal of Early Adolescence, 19,* 199–225.

Lodi-Smith, J., & Roberts, B. W. (2007). Social investment and personality: A meta-analysis of the relationship of personality traits to investment in work, family, religion, and volunteerism. *Personality and Social Psychology Review, 11,* 68–86.

Mahoney, A., Carels, R. A., Pargament, K. I., Wachholtz, A., Leeper, L. E., Kaplar, M., et al. (2005). The sanctification of the body and behavioral health patterns of college students. *International Journal for the Psychology of Religion, 15,* 221–230.

Mahoney, A., Pargament, K. I., Jewell, T., Swank, A. B., Scott, E., Emery, E., et al. (1999). Marriage and the spiritual realm: The role of proximal and distal religious constructs in marital functioning. *Journal of Family Psychology, 13,* 321–338.

McCullough, M. E., Enders, C. K., Brion, S. L., & Jain, A. R. (2005). The varieties of religious development in adulthood: A longitudinal investigation of religion and rational choice. *Journal of Personality and Social Psychology, 89,* 78–89.

McCullough, M. E., Tsang, J., & Brion, S. L. (2003). Personality traits in adolescence as predictors of religiousness on early adulthood: Findings from the Terman Longitudinal Study. *Personality and Social Psychology Bulletin, 29,* 980–991.

McCullough, M. E., & Willoughby, B. L. B. (2009). Religion, self-regulation, and self-control: Associations, explanations, and implications. *Psychological Bulletin, 135,* 69–93.

McNamara, P. (2002). The motivational origins of religious practices. *Zygon, 37,* 143–160.

Mithen, S. (2007). Did farming arise from a misapplication of social intelligence? *Philosophical Transactions of the Royal Society B, 362,* 705–718.

Muraven, M., & Baumeister, R. F. (2000). Self-regulation and depletion of limited resources: Does self-control resemble a muscle? *Psychological Bulletin, 126,* 247–259.

Norenzayan, A., & Shariff, A. F. (2008). The origin and evolution of religious prosociality. *Science, 322,* 58–62.

Pichon, I., Boccato, G., & Saroglou, V. (2007). Nonconscious influences of religion on prosociality: A priming study. *European Journal of Social Psychology, 37,* 1032–1045.

Porr, M., & Alt, K. W. (2006). The burial of Bad Dürrenberg, central Germany: Osteopathology and osteoarchaeology of a Late Mesolithic shaman's grave. *Journal of Osteoarchaeology, 16,* 395–406.

Pratt, J. B. (1934). *The religious consciousness: A psychological study.* New York: Macmillan.

Rachlin, H. (2000). *The science of self-control.* Cambridge, MA: Harvard University Press.

Randolph-Seng, B., & Nielsen, M. E. (2007). Honesty: One effect of primed religious representations. *International Journal for the Psychology of Religion, 17*, 303–315.

Regnerus, M. D., & Smith, C. (2005). Selection effects in studies of religious influences. *Review of Religious Research, 47*, 23–50.

Reyes-García, V., Godoy, R., Huanca, T., Leonard, W. R., McDade, T., Tanner, S., et al. (2007). The origins of monetary income inequality: Patience, human capital, and division of labor. *Evolution and Human Behavior, 28*, 37–47.

Richerson, P. J., & Boyd, R. (2005). *Not by genes alone: How culture transformed human evolution*. Chicago: University of Chicago Press.

Roberts, B. W., & Robins, R. W. (2000). Broad dispositions, broad aspirations: The intersection of personality traits and major life goals. *Personality and Social Psychology Bulletin, 26*, 1284–1296.

Roelofsma, P. H., Koole, S. L., & McCullough, M. E. (2009). *Religion and time discounting.* Unpublished manuscript, VU University, Amsterdam.

Saroglou, V. (2002). Religion and the five factors of personality: A meta-analytic review. *Personality and Individual Differences, 32*, 15–25.

Saroglou, V., Delpierre, V., & Dernelle, R. (2004). Values and religiosity: A meta-analysis of studies using Schwartz's model. *Personality and Individual Differences, 37*, 721–734.

Schmeichel, B. J., & Baumeister, R. F. (2004). Self-regulatory strength. In R. F. Baumeister & K. D. Vohs (Eds.), *Handbook of self-regulation: Research, theory, and applications* (pp. 84–98). New York: Guilford Press.

Shariff, A. F., & Norenzayan, A. (2007). God is watching you: Supernatural agent concepts increase prosocial behavior in an anonymous economic game. *Psychological Science, 18*, 803–809.

Sosis, R., & Ruffle, B. J. (2003). Religious ritual and cooperation: Testing for a relationship on Israeli religious and secular kibbutzim. *Current Anthropology, 44*, 713–722.

Stevens, J. R., Cushman, F. A., & Hauser, M. D. (2005). Evolving the psychological mechanisms for cooperation. *Annual Review of Ecology, Evolution, and Systematics, 36*, 499–518.

Stevens, J. R., Hallinan, E. V., & Hauser, M. D. (2005). The ecology and evolution of patience in two New World monkeys. *Biology Letters, 1*, 223–226.

Tabibnia, G., Satpute, A. B., & Lieberman, M. D. (2008). The sunny side of fairness: Preference for fairness activates reward circuitry (and disregarding unfairness activates self-control circuitry). *Psychological Science, 19*, 339–347.

Tooby, J., & Cosmides, L. (1992). Psychological foundations of culture. In J. Barkow, L. Cosmides, & J. Tooby (Eds.), *The adapted mind: Evolutionary psychology and the generation of culture* (pp. 19–136). New York: Oxford University Press.

Trivers, R. L. (1971). The evolution of reciprocal altruism. *Quarterly Review of Biology, 46*, 35–57.

Walker, C., Ainette, M. G., Wills, T. A., & Mendoza, D. (2007). Religiosity and substance use: Test of an indirect-effect model in early and middle adolescence. *Psychology of Addictive Behaviors, 21*, 84–96.

Weisbuch-Remington, M., Mendes, W. B., Seery, M. D., & Blascovich, J. (2005). The nonconscious influence of religious symbols in motivated performance situations. *Personality and Social Psychology Bulletin, 31*, 1203–1216.

Wenger, J. L. (2007). The implicit nature of intrinsic religious pursuit. *International Journal for the Psychology of Religion, 17*, 47–60.

Wiech, K., Farias, M., Kahane, G., Shackel, N., Tiede, W., & Tracey, I. (2008). An fMRI study measuring analgesia enhanced by religion as a belief system. *Pain, 139*, 467–476.

Wilde, A., & Joseph, S. (1997). Religiosity and personality in a Moslem context. *Personality and Individual Differences, 29*, 899–900.

Wilson, D. S. (2002). *Darwin's cathedral: Evolution, religion, and the nature of society.* Chicago: University of Chicago Press.

Wink, P., Ciciolla, L., Dillon, M., & Tracy, A. (2007). Religiousness, spiritual seeking and personality: Findings from a longitudinal study. *Journal of Personality, 75,* 1051–1070.

Winkelman, M. J. (1990). Shamans and other "magico-religious" healers: A cross-cultural study of their origins, nature, and social transformations. *Ethos, 18,* 308–352.

Worthington, E. L., Bursley, K., Berry, J. T., McCullough, M. E., Baier, S. N., Berry, J. W., et al. (2001). Religious commitment, religious experiences, and ways of coping with sexual attraction. *Marriage and Family: A Christian Journal, 4,* 411–423.

Wright, R. (2009). *The evolution of God.* New York: Little, Brown.

Yi, R., Buchhalter, A. R., Gatchalian, K. M., & Bickel, W. K. (2007). The relationship between temporal discounting and the prisoner's dilemma game in intranasal abusers of prescription opioids. *Drug and Alcohol Dependence, 87,* 94–97.

PART V

PERSONALITY AND SELF-REGULATION

CHAPTER 24

Temperament and Self-Regulation

MARY K. ROTHBART
LESA K. ELLIS
MICHAEL I. POSNER

Concepts of temperament have ancient roots, linking observations of individual differences to an underlying physiology. Many of us are familiar with the Greco-Roman typology of temperament based on the body humors, in which the melancholic person is described as anxious and moody, with a predominance of black bile; the sanguine person as cheerful and good natured, with a predominance of blood; the choleric as prone to anger and irritability, with a predominance of yellow bile; and the phlegmatic as slow to arousal, with a predominance of phlegm. The ancient typology demonstrated approaches to temperament that persist to the present day. First, the typology reflected observed consistencies in individual emotions and behavior; second, these individual differences could be observed early in life. Third, temperament types were linked to the individual's physiology as it was understood at the time, in terms of the bodily humors. In modern times, attempts to relate temperament to an underlying physiology have continued, with recent links to physiology in brain imaging studies and molecular genetics (Hariri, 2009). Fourth, the typology was associated with the development of psychopathology, especially in the melancholic and choleric types.

The ancient typology also focused on the primary emotions and the self-regulatory action tendencies related to them: positive affect and sociability in the sanguine person; fear and sadness in the melancholic; anger, irritability, and aggression in the choleric; and a general slowness to emotion and action in the phlegmatic. We have defined *temperament* as constitutionally based individual differences in reactivity and self-regulation, as seen in the emotional, motor, and attentional domains (Rothbart & Bates, 2006; Rothbart & Derryberry, 1981). By *constitutional*, we refer to the biological bases of temperament, influenced over time by genes, environment, and experience. By *reactivity*, we mean the onset, intensity, and duration of emotional, motor, and attentional reactions.

Reactivity may apply to quite general dispositions, as in negative emotional reactivity, or to more specific physiological reactions, such as heart rate reactivity. Although some current definitions of temperament limit the temperament domain to the emotions, we also include activity level, orienting and effortful control, with these variables establishing even stronger connections with self-regulation (Rothbart, 2007; Rothbart, Sheese, & Posner, 2007).

Self-regulation, defined as processes that serve to modulate reactivity, is a major contributor to the organization of temperament. Self-regulating processes include orienting, fearful inhibition, angry attack, surgent or extraverted approach, and the effortful control of behavior based on the executive attention system. Whereas some aspects of attention are almost entirely self-regulatory, as in effortful control, the reactive emotions also include behavior tendencies with self-regulatory aspects. Fear, for example, involves regulation of motor and autonomic circuits in the support of avoidance or inhibition of action, as well as modulation of perceptual pathways to enhance information about locations of safety and threat (Derryberry & Rothbart, 1997). Thus, fear is a reactive system, but it also involves motivational systems of self-regulation. As we describe some of the recent history of temperament theory, the special contributions of attention to self-regulation will, we hope, become apparent.

TEMPERAMENT AND PERSONALITY

Temperament involves evolutionarily conserved systems seen in both humans and other animals (Strelau, 1983). These systems are commonly shared by all humans, but individuals differ in the strength and sensitivity of their emotional and behavioral dispositions, and the efficiency of the attentional capacities. Temperament can be seen as part of the broader domain of personality, with *personality* defined as patterns of thought and behavior that show consistency across situations and stability over time, and affect the individual's adaptation to the internal and social environment. In addition to temperamental dispositions, personality includes many additional characteristics, including self-concept, perceptions of others, personal values, morals, expectations, defenses, coping strategies, attitudes, and beliefs. Many of these characteristics are strongly self-regulatory, as in the influences of self-related thought on emotion (Beck, 1976). Temperament can be seen as forming the evolutionarily conserved core from which personality develops. *Temperament* also refers to individual differences in personality of the infant and young child before many of the more cognitive aspects of personality have developed.

MODELS OF TEMPERAMENT AND SELF-REGULATION

Theoretical approaches to temperament have often included strong self-regulative components. Temperamental self-regulation, however, has almost always been seen as driven by individual differences in arousal or emotional reactivity. Two examples of this approach are the theories of Eysenck (1967) and Gray (1970; Gray & McNaughton, 1996). In Eysenck's (1967) theory of temperament, three major dimensions were identified. The first, Extraversion (vs. Introversion), was tied to self-regulation through a theory of arousal and its relation to pleasure and distress. Eysenck postulated that the introvert is more sensitive and arousable to stimulation than the extravert. As stimulation increases in quantity, intensity, or duration, the introvert more rapidly reaches a level of pleasant stimulation. Introverts are seen to enjoy lower-intensity pleasures than extraverts, who are likely to be bored with low levels of stimulation. The introvert, however, will reach and then exceed an optimal level of stimulation at lower levels than the extravert, experiencing distress in reaction to overstimulation. The extravert is thus a stimulation seeker, whereas the introvert seeks to avoid overstimulation. In Strelau's (1983) theory, based on extensive research in Russia and Eastern Europe, people are seen to engage in self-regulatory activity in order to add or decrease stimulation, depending on their reactivity or arousability.

Eysenck's dimension of Neuroticism (vs. Emotional Stability), seen as orthogonal to Extraversion–Introversion, is less closely tied to self-regulation. By crossing the axes of Extraversion and Neuroticism dimensions, Eysenck generated the ancient fourfold typology. Eysenck's third dimension of Psychoticism includes aspects of psychopathy or disinhibition and is related to the ability to inhibit action (Watson & Clark, 1993).

Jeffrey Gray (1970) followed in Eysenck's general tradition, but his model modified Eysenck's structure: He rotated the axes of Eysenck's Extraversion–Neuroticism structure and postulated an approach system labeled *Impulsivity* that ranged from the combination of low Extraversion and low Neuroticism to high Extraversion and high Neuroticism. He also postulated a behavioral inhibition system (BIS) labeled *Anxiety*, ranging from the combination of high Extraversion and low Neuroticism to low Extraversion and high Neuroticism. More impulsive individuals were seen as having a more reactive approach system, with underlying brain circuits involving the medial forebrain bundle and the lateral hypothalamus, and a greater sensitivity to reward or nonpunishment. An individual high in behavioral inhibition or anxiety was hypothesized to have a more reactive orbitofrontal cortex, medial septal area, and hippocampus, and to be more sensitive to punishment or nonreward. The approach (behavioral activation system; BAS) and anxiety (BIS) systems were both seen as having a positive input into the arousal system, increasing the behavioral intensity of the selected response and related at high levels to negative affect.

Gray (1981) postulated that when a mismatch between expectation and outcome is detected, the control mode of the BIS comes into play, interrupting the current execution of behavioral programs, and identifying stimuli to mentally resolve the mismatch. Gray further postulated a fight-versus-flight system. Gray's dimensions, like Eysenck's, are reactive, although they also include aspects of attention. Similar models, all based on reactive systems and identifying underlying physiology of temperament, have been developed by Zuckerman (1991), Depue and Iacono (1989), and Panksepp (1998).

TEMPERAMENT IN INFANCY AND CHILDHOOD

Thomas and Chess's (1977) pioneering work described individual differences in temperament during infancy. Content analyses of parental interviews describing their infants' reactions to a number of different stimuli and situations yielded nine temperament dimensions: Activity Level, Approach–Withdrawal, Mood, Attention Span–Persistence, Intensity, Distractibility, Adaptability, Threshold, and Rhythmicity (Thomas & Chess, 1977). Thomas and Chess's nine dimensions have not held up well in factor analysis (Rothbart

& Bates, 2006). In addition, item-level factor analyses of New York Longitudinal Study (NYLS)–based questionnaires, and other factor-analytic and rational approaches to scale development yielded a smaller number of dimensions in infancy (Rothbart & Mauro, 1990). These included Activity Level, Positive Affect and Approach, Fear, Frustration or Irritability, and Attentional Persistence. These dimensions involve emotional and attentional systems that, as early as infancy, demonstrate self-regulative properties.

Gartstein and Rothbart (2003) have further investigated the factor structure of parent-reported infant temperament, adding several dimensions derived from research on temperament in childhood. Three broad dimensions were revealed in factor analysis of these scales: Surgency/Extraversion, with loadings for approach, vocal reactivity, high-intensity pleasure, smiling and laughter, activity level and perceptual sensitivity; Negative Affectivity, with loadings for sadness, frustration, fear, and, loading negatively, falling reactivity; and Orienting/Regulation, with loadings for low-intensity pleasure, cuddliness, duration of orienting and soothability, and a secondary loading for smiling and laughter.

At Oregon, we have also developed a comprehensive and highly differentiated parent report instrument called the Children's Behavior Questionnaire, or CBQ, for children 3–7 years of age (Ahadi, Rothbart, & Ye, 1993; Rothbart, Ahadi, Hershey, & Fisher, 2001). Over a number of studies in several laboratories, three broad factors of children's temperament have emerged from studies using the CBQ. The first factor is called Surgency or Extraversion. It is defined by scales assessing positive emotionality and approach, including positive anticipation, high-intensity pleasure (sensation seeking), impulsivity and activity level, with a negative loading for shyness. The second broad factor, called Negative Affectivity, is defined by discomfort, fear, anger/frustration, and sadness, with a secondary loading for shyness, and a negative loading for soothability/falling reactivity. The third broad factor, Effortful Control, is defined by scales assessing inhibitory control, attentional focusing, low-intensity pleasure, and perceptual sensitivity. Discovery of the Effortful Control factor was interesting and important because it identified a latent variable related to the inhibition or activation of behavior that was either orthogonal to, or negatively related to, fearfulness, another system linked to inhibitory control.

In the United States, and in both child and adult samples, Effortful Control was also inversely related to Negative Affectivity, and independent of Surgency. In a Chinese sample of children, however, these relations were not found (Ahadi et al., 1993). Effortful Control in the Chinese sample was instead negatively related to measures of Surgency and independent of Negative Affectivity, suggesting that Effortful Control might serve to enhance or suppress reactive behavior in keeping with the values of the culture (for a more extended discussion of temperament, culture and self-regulation, see Rothbart, in press).

ORIENTING AND REGULATION

As early as infancy, there is thus evidence for a broad dimension of positive reactivity and approach, negative emotionality, and a regulative factor with contributions from both caregiver soothing and infant orienting. Infants' orienting to distractors presented by the caregiver offers an early example of this kind of regulation of emotion. Harman, Rothbart, and Posner (1997) showed that infants were soothed while orienting their attention to a visual and/or auditory stimulus, but when infants' orienting was broken, they returned to the prior level of distress, even though the distressing event was no longer present. Orienting of attention thus appears to block the expression of emotion, while the level of distress activation appears to remain stored, likely in limbic areas.

For young infants, the control of orienting is at first largely in the hands of caregiver presentations. By age 4 months, however, infants have gained considerable control over disengaging their gaze from one visual location and moving it to another, and greater orienting skill in the laboratory has been associated with lower parent-reported negative affect and greater soothability (Johnson, Posner, & Rothbart, 1991). Relatively automatic shifts of orienting can be seen later in development, for example, when we look away from horrific movie scenes. Not until early childhood do we see signs of another attention regulation dimension that we call *effortful control*. Effortful control of orienting in older children and adults provides an important aspect of self-regulation, to be discussed later in this chapter. Adults and adolescents who report themselves as having good ability to focus and shift attention also say they experience less negative emotion, and high negative emotion is related to low Effortful Control in parent reports of temperament in toddlers and school-age children (Putnam, Ellis, & Rothbart, 2001).

In our infant laboratory research, we used parent report and laboratory measures in a longitudinal study of infants at ages 3, 6½, 10, and 13½ months (Rothbart, Derryberry, & Hershey, 2000). Infants' reactions were videotaped during presentation of nonsocial- and social-eliciting stimuli. For example, smiling and laughter in response to visual and auditory stimuli was coded for its latency, intensity, and duration, then aggregated into positive affect measures. Approach was assessed in infants' latency to grasp low-intensity toys, such as small squeeze toys, blocks, and a cup, and activity level was assessed in children's movement among toys distributed across a grid-lined floor.

We also observed a number of changes in emotion regulation between ages 3 months and 13 months (Rothbart, Ziaie, & O'Boyle, 1992). With age, infants increasingly looked to their mothers during presentation of arousing stimuli, such as masks and unpredictable mechanical toys. Infants' disengagement of attention from arousing stimuli by looking away was also related to lower levels of negative affect in the laboratory at 13 months. We found stability from ages 10 months to 13 months in infants' use of disengaging attention, as well as other coping strategies such as mouthing, hand to mouth (e.g., thumb sucking), approach, and withdrawing the hand. These data suggested that some of the infants' self-regulation strategies, including attention disengagement, were becoming habitual in the laboratory situation.

More recent studies have found direct links between infants' self-regulated disengagement of attention and decreases in their negative affect (Stifter & Braungart, 1995), and there is also support for the idea that early mechanisms for coping with negative emotion may later be transferred to the control of cognition and behavior, as suggested by Posner and Rothbart (1998). In support of this hypothesis, infants' use of self-regulation in anger-inducing situations predicted their preschool ability to delay responses (Calkins & Williford, 2003). In research by Mischel and his colleagues (Sethi, Mischel, Aber, Shoda, & Rodriguez, 2000), toddlers' higher use of distraction strategies in an arousing situation positively predicted their delay of gratification at age 5. In this study, the use of toddler attentional distraction was viewed as an attempt at self-regulating the child's distress. Indeed, lower levels of negative affect were found in children who used these strategies.

APPROACH

At 7 years, parents of a subset of our infants filled out the CBQ (Rothbart et al., 2001), describing their temperamental tendencies in childhood. Smiling and laughter in infancy positively predicted both infants' and 7-year-olds' approach tendencies. Infant approach at 6, 10, and 13 months also positively predicted later mother-reported high approach, impulsivity, anger and aggression, and low sadness at age 7. These findings suggest that approach tendencies may contribute to externalizing negative emotionality, as well as to positive emotionality. The findings are also consistent with the observation that more active children are more frequently frustrated; indeed, positive relations between anger and activity level are found throughout infancy (Rothbart, 1981, 1986; Rothbart et al., 2001).

Questionnaire measures of approach have shown stability from the toddler to early childhood years (Pedlow, Sanson, Prior, & Oberklaid, 1993), and both approach and activity level have demonstrated stability from 2 to 12 years (Guerin & Gottfried, 1994). Caspi and Silva (1995) found that children high on confidence or approach at age 3–4 years were high on social potency and impulsiveness at age 18.

FEAR AND SELF-REGULATION

Late in the first year, some infants begin to demonstrate fear in their inhibited approach to unfamiliar and intense stimuli (Rothbart, 1988; Schaffer, 1974), and this inhibition can be predicted by a measure of crying and motor reactivity to stimulation at 4 months (Calkins, Fox, & Marshall, 1996; Kagan, 1994). Fear-related inhibition also shows considerable stability across childhood and into adolescence (Kagan, 1998) and allows inhibitory control of behavior.

Stability of fearful inhibition has been found from 2 years onward in childhood (e.g., Lemery, Goldsmith, Klinnert, & Mrazek, 1999), and between ages 8–12 years and early adulthood (17–24 years; Gest, 1997). In our longitudinal work, infant fear in the laboratory predicted the internalizing emotions of fear, sadness, and shyness, as well as low-intensity pleasure at 7 years (Rothbart et al., 2001). Fear did not predict later frustration/anger, and was negatively related to later approach, impulsivity, and aggression, suggesting the involvement of fear in the regulation of those tendencies.

More fearful infants also showed greater empathy, guilt, and shame in childhood (Rothbart, Ahadi, & Hershey, 1994). These findings suggest that fear might be involved in the early development of conscience, and indeed Kochanska (1995, 1997) has found that greater temperamental fearfulness predicts greater early conscience development. Fearful children whose mothers made use of gentle socialization techniques also developed particularly highly internalized conscience, demonstrating an interaction between temperament and socialization in the development of internal control. Later in development, attentionally based effortful control becomes particularly influential in the operation of children's conscience (Kochanska, Murray, & Harlan, 2000).

Other studies indicate the further regulative influence of fearfulness. Children with concurrent attention-deficit/hyperactivity disorder (ADHD) and anxiety show lower impulsivity than do children with ADHD alone (Pliszka, 1989), and children with internalizing patterns of behavior show decreases in aggressiveness between kindergarten and first grade (Bates, Pettit, & Dodge, 1995). Raine, Reynolds, Venables, Mednick, and Farrington (1998) also found that lack of fear at age 3 predicted higher aggression at age 11. At age 15, the high autonomic arousal and electrodermal orienting typically associated with fearfulness were protective factors against the development of criminal behavior by age 29 (Raine, Venables, & Williams, 1995).

When high approach is linked with low fear, approach may not be inhibited under circumstances that could lead to punishment. Children with strong approach tendencies who are also fearful, on the other hand, can inhibit approach tendencies when they might lead to negative outcomes. Because anxiety is linked to enhanced attention to threats (Derryberry & Reed, 1998), fear may enhance sensitivity to potential negative events and allow the child to avoid problems. On the other hand, extreme fear can lead to problems with rigid overcontrol of behavior, as reflected in Block and Block's (1980) description of overcontrolled patterns that can limit positive experiences. Thus, fearfulness within the first year of life allows a reactive control system of behavior, opposing the reactive system of approach.

EFFORTFUL CONTROL AND SELF-REGULATION

A behavior system developing late in infancy and continuing to develop through the early years, which we have labeled *effortful control*, allows voluntary control of behavior and emotion. Effortful control, defined as the ability to inhibit a dominant response in order to perform a subdominant response, was identified in parent-report measures of temperament in childhood (Rothbart & Bates, 1998) and in a review of the literature on temperament and development (Rothbart, 1989). Kochanska and colleagues (2000) characterized the construct of effortful control as being "situated at the intersection of the temperament and behavioral regulation literatures" (p. 220).

In further study of the link between self-regulatory temperament and the ability to consciously focus attention, we hypothesized that brain networks of executive attention might underlie effortful control (Posner & Rothbart, 1998). This hypothesis was also influenced by positive correlations found among attentional focusing, attentional shifting, and inhibitory control in self-reports of adults (Derryberry & Rothbart, 1988). The resulting hypothesis led to studies in Oregon on the early development of attentional control under conditions of conflict between one response and another (Gerardi-Caulton, 2000; Posner & Rothbart, 2007). A basic measure of executive attention is the Stroop task, in which subjects are asked to report the color of ink in which a word is written, when the color word (e.g., red) might conflict with the ink color (e.g., blue). A variety of Stroop-like tasks have been found to activate a midline brain structure in the anterior cingulate gyrus that has been associated with other executive attention activities (Bush, Luu, & Posner, 2000). We developed a marker task to assess executive attention in young children by creating conflict between the identity of an object and its location, called the *spatial conflict task*. Children's performance on this task demonstrated considerable improvement between 27 and 36 months of age (Gerardi-Caulton, 2000). Children who performed well on the task were also described by their parents as more skilled at attentional control, less impulsive, and less prone to frustration reactions.

As described in another chapter, we also developed and tested a Child Attention Network Test (see Rueda, Posner, & Rothbart, Chapter 15, this volume). Employing this measure, we found that the executive attention network developed strongly between 4 and 7 years of age. Diamond and Taylor (1996), who also evaluated performance of children between 3½ and 7 years in the tapping test developed by Luria, found steady improvement in both accuracy and speed on the tapping test. Most of the improvement occurred by age 6 years, with the 7-year-old group showing an accuracy rate close to 100%.

We assessed toddlers at 24, 30, and 36 months of age using the spatial conflict task, and replicated a significant improvement on the task with increasing age (Rothbart, Ellis, Rueda, & Posner, 2003). Children with higher spatial conflict performance were also rated by their parents as having higher levels of effortful control and lower levels of negative affectivity. The children in this study also completed a task involving anticipatory eye movements to ambiguous locations (Clohessy, Posner, & Rothbart, 2001), which is thought to involve the executive attention system (Rothbart, Posner, Rueda, Sheese, & Tang, 2009). Higher performance on the anticipation task was also related to higher performance on the spatial conflict task and to greater parent-reported effortful control (Rothbart et al., 2003).

Finally, the children completed a block tower–building task and a nested cup-stacking task, both of which involve volitional skills such as task orientation, error detection and correction, and goal completion. Scores for the two tasks were combined to form a composite measure of volitional skills and compared to parent-reported temperament scores within each age group. At age 24 months, volitional skill was positively related to parent-reported effortful control, and negatively related to surgency and negative affectivity. At 30 months, children's skill was negatively related to impulsivity and, at a trend level, to low surgency. At 36 months, the skills composite was positively related to attention focusing at a trend level. These results suggest that emerging self-regulation at 24 months may allow a child greater control as he or she waits or searches for appropriate opportunities to act, resists distractions, detects and corrects errors, overcomes obstacles, and attains a goal (Rothbart & Rueda, 2005). As these skills become more practiced and automated with age, effortful self-regulation may play a lesser role in their deployment.

TEMPERAMENT AND KOPP'S MODEL OF THE DEVELOPMENT OF SELF-REGULATION

In Claire Kopp's (1982) analysis of the development of self-regulation, she notes that during the first 3 months, genetically programmed physiological mechanisms and preadapted action systems regulate the physiological state of the infant. During the next phase (about 3 to 9 months), infants engage in sensorimotor activities shaped by the environment that allow them to make contact with others, and from 9 to 12 months, infants become better able to engage in goal-directed action and respond to commands from others.

During the second year, language and increasing impulse control become available to the child. There is also increased understanding of the self as an independent being in potential control of events, with toddlers attempting to influence objects and others. Children of this age, however, have few self-regulatory skills and little patience, and when their expectations are not met, they frequently respond with anger, crying, or temper tantrums (Kopp, 1992, 2009).

In Kopp's model, true self-control does not emerge until age 3 to 4 years, when children are able to comply with the requests of caregivers and show control in the absence of adult monitoring. We have suggested that changes occurring during this period are related to development of the executive attention system and evidenced in the child's effortful control (Posner & Rothbart, 2007; Rothbart, in press). Individual differences in effortful control allow the child to consciously inhibit dominant responses and to perform subdominant responses.

DEVELOPMENT OF EFFORTFUL CONTROL

Kochanska and her associates (2000) developed a battery of effortful control tasks used in the laboratory between ages 22 months and 5 years. Beginning at age 2½ years, children's performance showed considerable consistency across tasks, supporting the existence of a common underlying capacity of effortful control. Children showed improvements in their performance on the battery but were also remarkably stable in their individual performance over time, with correlations ranging from .44 for the youngest children (ages 22 to 33 months) to .59 (ages 32 to 46 months), and .65 (ages 46 to 66 months) (Kochanska et al., 2000).

Additional evidence for stability of effortful control constructs has been found in research by Mischel, Shoda, and Peake (1988). Preschoolers were measured on their ability to wait for a delayed treat rather than choosing a readily available but less preferred treat. Delay of gratification in seconds predicted higher parent-reported attentiveness, concentration, competence, planfulness, and intelligence during adolescence. In addition, adolescents who as preschoolers were better able to delay gratification showed better self-control and an increased ability to deal with stress, frustration, and temptation. Seconds of preschool delay also predicted Scholastic Aptitude Test (SAT) scores, even when researchers controlled for intelligence. In additional follow-up studies, preschool ability to delay predicted higher goal-setting and self-regulatory abilities when the participants reached their early 30s (Ayduk et al., 2000), suggesting extensive continuity in self-regulatory capacities.

To examine the possibility that effortful control and executive attention remain correlated during adolescence, Ellis (2002) measured executive attention in 100 adolescents, using two Stroop-like computerized tasks. Effortful control and other temperament variables were measured with parent- and self-report versions of the Early Adolescent Temperament Questionnaire—Revised (Ellis, Rothbart, & Posner, 2004). Performance on the computerized measures related positively to adolescents' parent- reported effortful control and inversely to negative affectivity. Teacher reports of risk for deviant behaviors were also inversely related to adolescents' scores on these tasks. Derryberry and Reed (1998), in a similar spatial conflict task with adults, found that participants with poor performance tended to describe themselves as low on self-reported attentional control and high on anxiety.

EFFORTFUL CONTROL, PARENTING, AND SOCIOEMOTIONAL OUTCOMES

Effortful control plays an important role in the development of conscience, with children high in effortful control displaying greater internalized conscience (Kochanska & Knaack, 2003; Kochanska et al., 2000). Thus, both the reactive control system of fear and the attentionally based system of effortful control appear to regulate the development of conscientious thought and behavior, with the influence of fear seen earlier in development. At Oregon, we found that children 6 to 7 years old who were high in effortful control were also high in empathy and guilt/shame, and low in aggressiveness (Rothbart et al., 1994). Effortful control may support empathy by allowing children to attend to the other people's emotional states instead of focusing on their own sympathetic distress. Eisenberg and colleagues (1994) found that 4- to 6-year-old boys with good attentional control dealt with anger using nonhostile verbal methods rather than overt aggression.

Effortful control has become an important element in models of child development (Rothbart, in press). Eisenberg and Fabes (1992), for example, proposed a model in which emotionality and regulation combine or interact to affect social behavior. Their model suggests that children high in negative affectivity and low in regulation are most likely to exhibit externalizing behavior problems. Eisenberg and colleagues (1996) examined kindergarten through third-grade children, measuring negative emotionality and attentional regulation. As predicted, children high in negative emotionality and low in regulation were most likely to have externalizing behavior problems. Lack of regulation also more strongly predicted behavior problems in children with higher levels of negative affectivity.

In a 2-year longitudinal follow-up study (Eisenberg, Fabes, Guthrie, & Reiser, 2004), children were assessed for behavioral regulation during a puzzle box task. Replicating the results of the previous study, attentional control predicted fewer behavioral problems in children with higher levels of negative emotionality. Children who were low in negative emotionality were generally low in externalizing behaviors and showed no effect of attentional control on problems.

In the years since the first edition of this book, numerous studies have supported the relation between low effortful control and greater externalizing (e.g., Kochanska & Knaack, 2003; Muris, Meesters, & Blijlevens, 2007; Spinrad et al., 2007). There is also evidence for interactions between temperament and parenting in predicting problems. Negative emotionality typically heightens effects of poor parenting, whereas effortful control appears to protect or buffer the child against poor parenting (see review by Rothbart & Bates, 2006). Morris and colleagues (2002), for example, found that children rated by their mothers as high in effortful control showed less influence of mothers' hostility on their development of externalizing problems. Rubin, Burgess, Dwyer, and Hastings (2003) found that when parenting was poor, children's self-regulation at age 2 predicted lower externalizing problems at age 4; when parenting was good, however, children's earlier self-regulation was not related to their development of problems.

Greater internalizing symptoms are also predicted in children with low effortful control (Eisenberg et al., 2001, 2009; Lengua, 2003; Muris et al., 2007; Murray & Kochanska, 2002; Oldehinkel, Hartman, DeWinter, Veenstra, & Ormel, 2004), but here the data are more mixed (e.g., Rydell, Berlin, & Bohlin, 2003). While these relations may result chiefly from attentional rather than behavioral inhibitory control (Eisenberg et al., 2005), Eisenberg, Shepard, Fabes, Murphy, and Guthrie (1998) found a relation between internalizing and inhibitory control, and children's shyness. In another study, children high in parent-reported fear, sadness, anxiety, and autonomic reactivity, combined with poor regulation, were seen as high in shyness by both parents and teachers (Eisenberg et al., 2001). Children high in internalizing behaviors were lower in impulsivity and higher in inhibitory control than were children high in externalizing behaviors. However, there was little relation with attentional regulation.

Eisenberg and her colleagues (2009) recently used effortful control, impulsivity, and negative emotionality to predict concurrent externalizing and internalizing symptoms and also changes in children's problem status over a 4-year period. Low effortful control, high impulsivity, and negative emotionality predicted concurrent externalizing problems and were also related to changes in externalizing problems over time. Low attentional control predicted change only in signs of internalizing problems. Overall, effortful control was associated with lower and decreasing behavior problems in children.

Effortful control is also related to the development of socially appropriate and prosocial behavior (Eisenberg et al., 1997). Children high in self-regulation exhibited higher levels of social competence, and the relationship was strongest for children higher in general emotional intensity. High attentional control was also related to greater ego resiliency, and was particularly important in predicting positive outcomes for those children who were prone to negative affect. Again, further support of a positive relation between effortful control and social competence and/or prosocial behavior has been found since the first edition of this book (e.g., Checa, Rodríguez-Bailón, & Rueda, 2008; Lengua, 2006; Rotenberg, Michalik, Eisenberg, & Betts, 2008). Effortful control also contributes to children's school readiness and success (Blair & Razza, 2007; Checa et al., 2008; Valiente, Lemery-Chalfant, Swanson, & Reiser, 2008).

Ellis and colleagues (2004) found links between poor effortful control and both externalizing (aggression) and internalizing problems (depressive mood) in a group of young adolescents. Low effortful control and high approach tendencies best predicted aggression, whereas low effortful control and high levels of affiliative needs, combined with gender (being female), best predicted depressive mood. In a study involving both early and late adolescent samples (Ellis, 2002), both low effortful control and high frustration predicted aggression, and low effortful control and high affiliation predicted depressive mood.

Children's effortful control may be particularly linked to the development of *resiliency*, that is, the ability to withstand difficult or stressful situations. Gardner, Dishion, and Connell (2008), for example, found that effortful control protected against effects of deviant peer groups on antisocial behavior in young people. Lengua and Long (2002) found that children with low self-regulation showed a stronger relation between family stress and internalizing behavior problems than did children with high self-regulation. Effortful control also promotes prosocial behavior, even when parenting is not ideal (Valiente et al., 2004).

Can parenting compensate for deficiencies in children's effortful control? There is some evidence that it can. For highly impulsive adolescents, high levels of parent control and support are associated with lower antisocial behavior (Stice & Gonzales, 1998). Parent management may also lessen the likelihood that children's low self-control will lead to problem behavior. However, high levels of parent control may not be ideal for all children: High maternal control has been linked to greater externalizing problems in more highly manageable children (Bates, Pettit, Dodge, & Ridge, 1998).

MECHANISMS FOR THE INFLUENCE OF EFFORTFUL CONTROL

Earlier, we discussed the role of orienting in regulation of emotion, as seen in infancy. With the development of effortful control, orienting comes under the influence of executive attention (Posner & Raichle, 1994). Regulation of orienting, however, may not always be enough to manage emotional reactions and motivationally driven behavior. We may, for example, look away from the cake on the kitchen counter, but even so, we continue to know it is there. With development, conceptual processing and memory allow us to maintain internal representations of stimuli over time. These internal representations may both trigger and maintain the activation of affective systems, and the regulation of internal representations becomes an important avenue for the regulation of emotional responding (Rothbart & Sheese, 2008). The same general network involved in control of emotions is also active during the manipulation of internal representations, such as generating word associations (Posner & Raichle, 1994), although the ventral rather than the dorsal part of the anterior cingulate cortex tends to be involved (see Rueda et al., Chapter 15, this volume).

It is also possible to exclude, at least for the moment, representations we wish to avoid. The executive attention system allows monitoring and resolution of conflict among brain networks, permitting the selection of one representation over another. By literally thinking about something other than the thought we wish to avoid, we engage in thought suppression. However, thought suppression seems to have limited utility and can lead to long-term negative consequences for those who use it (Gross, 2002).

The executive attention network also supports another strategy for altering representations through the process of *reappraisal*, in which the person reinterprets the meaning or value of a representation (Gross, 2002). Reappraisal can be seen as involving a competition among alternate internal representations, in which the executive attention system facilitates selection of a secondary representation over the prepotent representation. Prefrontal and anterior cingulate regions are involved in the modulation of emotion processing through reappraisal (Ochsner, 2004), indicating another means for the executive attention system to regulate emotion and action.

Effortful control and executive attention also allow the activation of behavior that would otherwise not be performed, such as when a young child provides a polite smile when he or she has just received a disappointing gift (Simonds, Kieras, Rueda, & Rothbart, 2007). In this situation, the child needs both to inhibit a negative expression and to activate the expression of positive emotion. Effortful control is not itself a basic motivation, but it provides the means to satisfy desired ends effectively. It is similar to the attentional capacities underlying Block's (2002) construct of *ego resiliency*, the ability to shift levels of control flexibly depending on the situation. The ends achieved through effortful control may or may not be adaptive ones, however, and when control results in rigid responses to social situations, the outcomes may not be favorable ones. The use of effortful control can also result in disconnections between thought and behavior, emotion and its expression, leading to feelings of a less authentic self (Rothbart, in press).

Effortful control can also support the internalization of competence-related goals (e.g., being kind to others, performance in school) and their achievement, and is involved in the inhibition of immediate approach with the goal of attaining a larger reward later, as in the Mischel and colleagues (1988) research and Block's (2002) "hedonism of the future." In general, it allows the person to act "on principle." It can also support the compassionate support of others even when our perceived self-interest does not agree with the chosen action.

Effortful control adds the capacity for self-control to the domain of temperament. Going beyond the models described at the beginning of this chapter that see us as moved chiefly by affect or arousal, effortful control allows us to resist the immediate influence of emotion, to flexibly approach situations we fear and to resist actions we desire. We expect, however, that the efficiency of effortful control will depend on the strength of the prepotent or dominant response. Our only predictor of effortful control from infancy, given that we were not directly measuring this system during the early months, was the speed with which children grasped high-intensity toys in the laboratory (Rothbart et al., 2000). Children who grasped the toys more quickly showed higher impulsivity, anger/frustration, and aggression at 7 years, and tended to be lower in attentional and inhibitory control. We have suggested that strong approach tendencies may limit the effects of effortful control (Rothbart et al., 2000). If we use an analogy of approach tendencies as the "accelerator" and inhibitory tendencies, both fear and effortful control, as the "brakes" on behavior and emotional expression, we would expect stronger acceleration resulting from approach to weaken the braking influence of fear and effortful inhibitory control.

Because effortful control is so important to adaptive development, Lengua has studied environmental and parenting events that may influence its development (Lengua, Honorado, & Bush, 2007). In 8- to 12-year-olds, she found that risk factors, including family income, parent education, neighborhood, negative life events, family conflict, maternal depression and quality of parenting, were concurrently related to lower effortful control, but they did not predict the growth in effortful control that took place between ages 8 to 12 years (Lengua, 2003, 2008; Lengua, Bush, Long, Trancik, & Kovacs, 2008). During the preschool years (between approximately age 3 and 3½ years), however, environmental and parenting risk factors were related to lower effortful control, and they also predicted less growth in effortful control over this period (Lengua et al., 2007). Mothers' appropriate limit setting and support of 3-year-olds' autonomy were also related to increases in effortful control. Further analysis showed that environmental risk was mediated through the mothers' behavior.

Effortful control may thus be particularly sensitive to the environment, as reflected in parental behavior during the preschool years, and this is also a time when some of the greatest increases in effortful control are taking place (Rothbart & Rueda, 2005). Spinrad and colleagues (2007) found that the impact of mothers' behavior on children's externalizing behavior decreased with toddlers' age, suggesting that "as children's regulation skills become more sophisticated, the relations between parenting and externalizing problems may become more fully mediated through toddlers' effortful control" (p. 1183).

TRAINING ATTENTION

In our laboratory, we have trained attention in 4- and 6-year-old children over a 5-day period (Rueda, Rothbart, McCandliss, Saccomanno, & Posner, 2007). The details of this training are included in Rueda and colleagues (Chapter 15, this volume). Effects of training, in comparison with controls who viewed child-appropriate videos, included increases in IQ scores and patterns of brain activation that were more like those of adults. Rueda, Checa, and Santonja (2008) have replicated and extended this work in a Spanish preschool. Several exercises were added to the training, leading to 10 days' training for the experimental group and videos for the control group. Children were also followed up 2 months after the training. Once again, trained children showed improvement in IQ, as well as improved performance on conflict tasks. Both the training and control groups showed increases in attention task performance immediately after training, but only the trained children sustained their improvement over the follow-up period. Attention training also positively influenced tasks that required emotional self-regulation.

Research on the effects of other training programs has also indicated that executive attention can be trained in preschool and kindergarten children (e.g., Diamond, Barnett, Thomas, & Munro, 2007). Taken together with Lengua and colleagues' (2007) findings of social influences on young children's development of effortful control, the preschool and kindergarten years may prove to be a periods of particular plasticity for executive attention and effortful control. Additional research in this area will be of great importance in fostering effective early education (Posner & Rothbart, 2007).

SUMMARY

Effortful control provides a voluntary basis for self-regulation that goes beyond the earlier inhibitory influences of fear and orienting. Differences among individuals in the degree to which they can exercise effortful control have a dramatic influence on behavior, particularly in later childhood, adolescence, and adulthood. The ability to measure and study the correlates and outcomes of these individual differences by questionnaire, observation, and laboratory tasks provides a strong basis for future understanding of the developing mechanisms of self-regulation.

REFERENCES

Ahadi, S. A., Rothbart, M. K., & Ye, R. (1993). Children's temperament in the U.S. and China: Similarities and differences. *European Journal of Personality, 7,* 359–378.

Ayduk, O., Mendoza-Denton, R., Mischel, W., Downey, G., Peake, P., & Rodriguez, M. (2000). Regulating the interpersonal self: Strategic self-regulation for coping with rejection sensitivity. *Journal of Personality and Social Psychology, 79,* 776–792.

Bates, J. E., Pettit, G. S., & Dodge, K. A. (1995). Family and child factors in stability and change in children's aggressiveness in elementary school. In J. McCord (Ed.), *Coercion and punishment in long-term perspectives* (pp. 124–138). New York: Cambridge University Press.

Bates, J. E., Pettit, G. S., Dodge, K. A., & Ridge, B. (1998). Interaction of temperamental resistance to control and restrictive parenting in the development of externalizing behavior. *Developmental Psychology, 34*(5), 982–995.

Beck, A. T. (1976). *Cognitive therapy and the emotional disorders.* New York: International Universities Press.

Blair, C., & Razza, R. P. (2007). Relating effortful control, executive function, and false belief understanding to emerging math and literacy ability in kindergarten. *Child Development, 78*(2), 647–663.

Block, J. H. (2002). *Personality as an affect-processing system.* Mahwah, NJ: Erlbaum.

Block, J. H., & Block, J. (1980). The role of ego-control and ego-resiliency in the organization of behavior. In W. A. Collins (Ed.), *Minnesota Symposium on Child Psychology* (Vol. 13, pp. 39–101). Hillsdale, NJ: Erlbaum.

Bush, G., Luu, P., & Posner, M. I. (2000). Cognitive and emotional influences in anterior cingulate cortex. *Trends in Cognitive Sciences, 4*(6), 215–222.

Calkins, S. D., Fox, N. A., & Marshall, T. R. (1996). Behavioral and psychological antecedents of inhibition in infancy. *Child Development, 67,* 523–540.

Calkins, S. D., & Williford, A. (2003, April). *Anger regulation in infancy: Correlates and consequences.* Paper presented at the biennial meeting of the Society for Research in Child Development, Tampa, FL.

Caspi, A., & Silva, P. A. (1995). Temperamental qualities at age three predict personality traits in young adulthood: Longitudinal evidence from a birth cohort. *Child Development, 66,* 486–498.

Checa, P., Rodríguez-Bailón, R., & Rueda, M. R. (2008). Neurocognitive and temperamental systems of self-regulation and early adolescents' social and academic outcomes. *Mind, Brain, and Education, 2*(4), 177–187.

Clohessy, A. B., Posner, M. I., & Rothbart, M. K. (2001). Development of the functional visual field. *Acta Psychologica, 106*(1–2), 51–68.

Depue, R. A., & Iacono, W. G. (1989). Neurobehavioral aspects of affective disorders. In M. R. Rosenzweig & L. Y. Porter (Eds.), *Annual review of psychology* (Vol. 40, pp. 457–492). Palo Alto, CA: Annual Reviews.

Derryberry, D., & Reed, M. A. (1998). Anxiety and attentional focusing: Trait, state and hemispheric influences. *Personality and Individual Differences, 25,* 745–761.

Derryberry, D., & Rothbart, M. K. (1988). Arousal, affect, and attention as components of temperament. *Journal of Personality and Social Psychology, 55,* 958–966.

Derryberry, D., & Rothbart, M. K. (1997). Reactive and effortful processes in the organization of temperament. *Development and Psychopathology, 9,* 633–652.

Diamond, A., Barnett, W. S., Thomas, J., & Munro, S. (2007). Preschool program improves cognitive control. *Science, 318,* 1387–1388.

Diamond, A., & Taylor, C. (1996). Development of an aspect of executive control: Development of the abilities to remember what I said and to "Do as I say, not as I do." *Developmental Psychobiology, 29,* 315–334.

Eisenberg, N., Cumberland, A., Spinrad, T. L., Fabes, R. A., Shepard, S. A., Reiser, M., et al. (2001). The relations of regulation and emotionality to children's externalizing and internalizing problem behavior. *Child Development, 72*(4), 1112–1134.

Eisenberg, N., & Fabes, R. A. (Eds.). (1992). *Emotion and its regulation in early development* (New Directions for Child Development, No. 55). San Francisco: Jossey-Bass.

Eisenberg, N., Fabes, R. A., Guthrie, I. K., Murphy, B. C., Maszk, P., Holmgren, R., et al. (1996). The relations of regulation and emotionality to problem behavior in elementary school children. *Development and Psychopathology, 8*(1), 141–162.

Eisenberg, N., Fabes, R. A., Guthrie, I. K., & Reiser, M. (2004). The relations of effortful control and impulsivity to children's resiliency and adjustment. *Child Development, 75,* 25–46.

Eisenberg, N., Fabes, R. A., Murphy, B., Karbon, M., Maszk, P., Smith, M., et al. (1994). The role of emotionality and regulation in children's social functioning: A longitudinal study. *Child Development, 66,* 1360–1384.

Eisenberg, N., Fabes, R. A., Shepard, S. A., Murphy, B. C., Guthrie, I. K., Jones, S., et al. (1997). Contemporaneous and longitudinal prediction of children's social functioning from regulation and emotionality. *Child Development, 68,* 642–664.

Eisenberg, N., Sadovsky, A., Spinrad, T. L., Fabes, R. Q., Losoya, S., Valiente, C., et al. (2005). The relations of problem behavior status to children's negative negative emotionality, effortful control, and impulsivity: Concurrent relations and prediction of change. *Developmental Psychology, 41,* 193–211.

Eisenberg, N., Shepard, S. A., Fabes, R. A., Murphy, B. C., & Guthrie, I. K. (1998). Shyness and children's emotionality, regulation, and coping: Contemporaneous, longitudinal, and across-context relations. *Child Development, 69,* 767–790.

Eisenberg, N., Valiente, C., Spinrad, T., Cumberland, A., Liew, J., Reiser, M., et al. (2009). Longitudinal relations of children's effortful control, impulsivity and negative emotionality to their externalizing, internalizing and co-occurring behavior problems. *Developmental Psychology, 45,* 988–1008.

Ellis, L. K. (2002). *Individual differences and adolescent psychosocial development.* Unpublished doctoral dissertation, University of Oregon, Eugene.

Ellis, L. K., Rothbart, M. K., & Posner, M. I. (2004). Individual differences in executive attention predict self-regulation and adolescent psychosocial behaviors. *Annals of the New York Academy of Sciences, 1021,* 337–340.

Eysenck, H. J. (1967). *The biological basis of personality.* Springfield, IL: Thomas.

Gardner, T. W., Dishion, T. J., & Connell, A. M. (2008). Adolescent self-regulation as resilience: Resistance to antisocial behavior within the deviant peer context. *Journal of Abnormal Child Psychology, 36*(2), 273–284.

Gartstein, M., & Rothbart, M. K. (2003). Studying infant temperament via a revision of the Infant Behavior Questionnaire. *Infant Behavior and Development, 26*(1), 64–86.

Gerardi-Caulton, G. (2000). Sensitivity to spatial conflict and the development of self-regulation in children 24–36 months of age. *Developmental Science, 3*(4), 397–404.

Gest, S. D. (1997). Behavioral inhibition: Stability and associations with adaptation from childhood to early adulthood. *Journal of Personality and Social Psychology, 72*(2), 467–475.

Gray, J. A. (1970). The psychophysiological basis of introversion–extraversion. *Behaviour Research and Therapy, 8,* 249–266.

Gray, J. A. (1981). A critique of Eysenck's theory of personality. In H. J. Eysenck (Ed.), *A model for personality* (pp. 246–276). Berlin: Springer-Verlag.

Gray, J. A., & McNaughton, N. (1996). The neuropsychology of anxiety: Reprise. In D. A. Hope (Ed.), *Nebraska Symposium on Motivation: Perspectives on anxiety, panic, and fear* (Vol. 43, pp. 61–134). Lincoln: University of Nebraska Press.

Gross, J. J. (2002). Emotion regulation: Affective, cognitive, and social consequences. *Psychophysiology, 39*(3), 281–291.

Guerin, D. W., & Gottfried, A. W. (1994). Temperamental consequences of infant difficultness. *Infant Behavior and Development, 17*(4), 413–421.

Hariri, A. R. (2009). The neurobiology of individual differences in complex behavioral traits. *Annual Review of Neuroscience, 32,* 225–247.

Harman, C., Rothbart, M. K., & Posner, M. I. (1997). Distress and attention interactions in early infancy. *Motivation and Emotion, 21,* 27–43.

Johnson, M. H., Posner, M. I., & Rothbart, M. K. (1991). Components of visual orienting in early infancy: Contingency learning, anticipatory looking, and disengaging. *Journal of Cognitive Neuroscience, 3*(4), 335–344.

Kagan, J. (1994). *Galen's prophecy: Temperament in human nature.* New York: Basic Books.

Kagan, J. (1998). Biology and the child. In W. S. E. Damon & N. V. E. Eisenberg (Eds.), *Handbook of child psychology: Vol. 3. Social, emotional and personality development* (5th ed., pp. 177–235). New York: Wiley.

Kochanska, G. (1995). Children's temperament, mothers' discipline, and security of attachment: Multiple pathways to emerging internalization. *Child Development, 66,* 597–615.

Kochanska, G. (1997). Multiple pathways to conscience for children with different temperaments: From toddlerhood to age five. *Developmental Psychology, 33* 228–240.

Kochanska, G., & Knaack, A. (2003). Effortful control as a personality characteristic of young children: Antecedents, correlates and consequences. *Journal of Personality, 71*, 1087–1112.

Kochanska, G., Murray, K. T., & Harlan, E. (2000). Effortful control in early childhood: Continuity and change, antecedents, and implications for social development. *Developmental Psychology, 36*, 220–232.

Kopp, C. B. (1982). Antecedents of self-regulation: A developmental perspective. *Developmental Psychology, 18*, 199–214.

Kopp, C. B. (1992). Emotional distress and control in young children. In N. Eisenberg & R. A. Fabes (Eds.), *Emotion and its regulation in early development* (New Directions for Child Development, No. 55, pp. 41–56). San Francisco: Jossey-Bass.

Kopp, C. B. (2009). Emotion-focused coping in young children: Self and self-regulatory processes. In E. A. Skinner & M. J. Zimmer-Gembeck (Eds.), *Coping and the development of regulation* (New Directions for Child and Adolescent Development, No. 124, pp. 33–46). San Francisco: Jossey-Bass.

Lemery, K. S., Goldsmith, H. H., Klinnert, M. D., & Mrazek, D. A. (1999). Developmental models of infant and childhood temperament. *Developmental Psychology, 35*, 189–204.

Lengua, L. J. (2003). Associations among emotionality, self-regulation, adjustment problems, and positive adjustment in middle childhood. *Journal of Applied Developmental Psychology, 24*, 595–618.

Lengua, L. J. (2008, October). *Effortful control in the context of socioeconomic and psychosocial risk.* Paper presented at the American Psychological Association's fourth annual Science Leadership Conference Designing the Future: Innovations in Knowledge Dissemination for Psychological Science, Tempe, AZ.

Lengua, L. J., Bush, N., Long, A. C., Trancik, A. M., & Kovacs, E. A. (2008). Effortful control as a moderator of the relation between contextual risk and growth in adjustment problems. *Development and Psychopathology, 20*, 509–528.

Lengua, L. J., Honorado, E., & Bush, N. R. (2007). Contextual risk and parenting as predictors of effortful control and social competence in preschool children. *Journal of Applied Developmental Psychology, 28*(1), 40–55.

Lengua, L. J., & Long, A. C. (2002). The role of emotionality and self-regulation in the appraisal-coping process: Tests of direct and moderating effects. *Journal of Applied Developmental Psychology, 23*(4), 471–493.

Mischel, W., Shoda, Y., & Peake, P. (1988). The nature of adolescent competencies predicted by preschool delay of gratification. *Journal of Personality and Social Psychology, 54*, 687–696.

Morris, A. S., Silk, J. S., Steinberg, L., Sessa, F. M., Avenevoli, S., & Essex, M. J. (2002). Temperamental vulnerability and negative parenting as interacting predictors of child adjustment. *Journal of Marriage and Family, 64*, 461–471.

Muris, P., Meesters, C., & Blijlevens, P. (2007). Self-reported reactive and regulative temperament in early adolescence: Relations to internalizing and externalizing problem behavior and "Big Three" personality factors. *Journal of Adolescence, 30*(6), 1035–1049.

Murray, K. T., & Kochanska, G. (2002). Effortful control: Factor structure and relation to externalizing and internalizing behaviors. *Journal of Abnormal Child Psychology, 30*, 503–513.

Ochsner, K. N. (2004). Current directions in social cognitive neuroscience. *Current Opinion in Neurobiology, 14*(2), 254–258.

Oldehinkel, A. J., Hartman, C. A., De Winter, A. F., Veenstra, R., & Ormel, J. (2004). Temperament profiles associated with internalizing and externalizing problems in preadolescence. *Development and Psychopathology, 16*, 421–440.

Panksepp, J. (1998). *Affective neuroscience: The foundations of human and animal emotions.* New York: Oxford University Press.

Pedlow, R., Sanson, A., Prior, M., & Oberklaid, F. (1993). Stability of maternally reported temperament from infancy to 8 years. *Developmental Psychology, 29,* 998–1007.

Pliszka, S. R. (1989). Effect of anxiety on cognition, behavior, and stimulant response in ADHD. *Journal of the American Academy of Child and Adolescent Psychiatry, 28,* 882–887.

Posner, M. I., & Raichle, M. E. (1994). *Images of mind.* New York: Scientific American Library/ Scientific American Books.

Posner, M. I., & Rothbart, M. K. (1998). Attention, self-regulation, and consciousness. *Philosophical Transactions of the Royal Society of London B, 353,* 1915–1927.

Posner, M. I., & Rothbart, M. K. (2007). *Educating the human brain.* Washington, DC: American Psychological Association.

Putnam, S. P., Ellis, L. K., & Rothbart, M. K. (2001). The structure of temperament from infancy through adolescence. In A. Eliasz & A. Angleitner (Eds.), *Advances in research on temperament* (pp. 165–182). Lengerich, Germany: Pabst Science.

Raine, A., Reynolds, C., Venables, P. H., Mednick, S. A., & Farrington, D. P. (1998). Fearlessness, stimulation-seeking, and large body size at age 3 years as early predispositions to childhood aggression at age 11 years. *Archives of General Psychiatry, 55,* 745–751.

Raine, A., Venables, P. H., & Williams, M. (1995). High autonomic arousal and electrodermal orienting at age 15 years as protective factors against criminal behavior at age 29 years. *American Journal of Psychiatry, 152,* 1595–1600.

Rotenberg, K. J., Michalik, N., Eisenberg, N., & Betts, L. R. (2008). The relations among young children's peer-reported trustworthiness, inhibitory control, and preschool adjustment. *Early Childhood Research Quarterly, 23,* 288–298.

Rothbart, M. K. (1981). Measurement of temperament in infancy. *Child Development, 52,* 569–578.

Rothbart, M. K. (1986). Longitudinal observation of infant temperament. *Developmental Psychology, 22,* 356–365.

Rothbart, M. K. (1988). Temperament and the development of inhibited approach. *Child Development, 59,* 1241–1250.

Rothbart, M. K. (1989). Temperament in childhood: A framework. In G. Kohnstamm, J. Bates, & M. K. Rothbart (Eds.), *Temperament in childhood* (pp. 59–73). Chichester, UK: Wiley.

Rothbart, M. K. (2007). Temperament, development, and personality. *Current Directions in Psychological Science, 16,* 207–212.

Rothbart, M. K. (in press). *Becoming who we are: Temperament and personality in development.* New York: Guilford Press.

Rothbart, M. K., Ahadi, S. A., & Hershey, K. L. (1994). Temperament and social behavior in childhood. *Merrill–Palmer Quarterly, 40,* 21–39.

Rothbart, M. K., Ahadi, S. A., Hershey, K. L., & Fisher, P. (2001). Investigations of temperament at three to seven years: The Children's Behavior Questionnaire. *Child Development, 72,* 1394–1408.

Rothbart, M. K., & Bates, J. E. (1998). Temperament. In W. Damon & N. Eisenberg (Eds.), *Handbook of child psychology: Social, emotional and personality development* (5th ed., Vol. 3, pp. 105–176). New York: Wiley.

Rothbart, M. K., & Bates, J. E. (2006). Temperament. In W. Damon, R. Lerner, & N. Eisenberg (Eds.), *Handbook of child psychology: Vol. 3. Social, emotional, and personality development* (6th ed., pp. 99–106). New York: Wiley.

Rothbart, M. K., & Derryberry, D. (1981). Development of individual differences in temperament. In M. E. Lamb & A. L. Brown (Eds.), *Advances in developmental psychology* (pp. 37–86). Hillsdale, NJ: Erlbaum.

Rothbart, M. K., Derryberry, D., & Hershey, K. (2000). Stability of temperament in childhood: Laboratory infant assessment to parent report at seven years. In V. J. Molfese & D. L. Molfese

(Eds.), *Temperament and personality development across the life span* (pp. 85–119). Hillsdale, NJ: Erlbaum.

Rothbart, M. K., Ellis, L. K., Rueda, M. R., & Posner, M. I. (2003). Developing mechanisms of temperamental effortful control. *Journal of Personality, 71*(6), 1113–1143.

Rothbart, M. K., & Mauro, J. A. (1990). Questionnaire approaches to the study of infant temperament. In J. W. Fagen & J. Colombo (Eds.), *Individual differences in infancy: Reliability, stability, and prediction* (pp. 411–429). Hillsdale, NJ: Erlbaum.

Rothbart, M. K., Posner, M. I., Rueda, M. R., Sheese, B. E., & Tang, Y. Y. (2009). Enhancing self-regulation in school and clinic. In D. Cicchetti & M. R. Gunnar (Eds.), *Minnesota Symposium on Child Psychology: Meeting the challenge of translational research in child psychology* (Vol. 35, pp. 115–158). New York: Wiley.

Rothbart, M. K., & Rueda, M. R. (2005). The development of effortful control. In U. Mayr, E. Awh, S. W. Keele, U. Mayr, E. Awh, & S. W. Keele (Eds.), *Developing individuality in the human brain: A tribute to Michael I. Posner* (pp. 167–188). Washington, DC: American Psychological Association.

Rothbart, M. K., & Sheese, B. (2007). Temperament and emotion regulation. In J. J. Gross (Ed.), *Handbook of emotion regulation* (pp. 331–350). New York: Guilford Press.

Rothbart, M. K., Sheese, B., & Posner, M. I. (2007). Executive attention and effortful control: Linking temperament, brain networks, and genes. *Child Development Perspectives, 1*(1), 2–7.

Rothbart, M. K., Ziaie, H., & O'Boyle, C. G. (1992). Self-regulation and emotion in infancy. In N. Eisenberg & R. A. Fabes (Eds.), *Emotion and its regulation in early development* (New Directions for Child Development, No. 55, pp. 7–23). San Francisco: Jossey-Bass.

Rubin, K. H., Burgess, K. B., Dwyer, K. M., & Hastings, P. D. (2003). Predicting preschoolers' externalizing behaviors from toddler temperament, conflict, and maternal negativity. *Developmental Psychology, 39*, 164–176.

Rueda, M. R., Checa, P., & Santonja, M. (2008, April). *Training executive attention in preschoolers: Lasting effects and transfer to affective self-regulation.* Paper presented at the annual meeting of the Cognitive Neuroscience Society, San Francisco.

Rueda, M. R., Rothbart, M. K., McCandliss, B. D., Saccomanno, L., & Posner, M. I. (2005). Training, maturation, and genetic influences on the development of executive attention. *Proceedings of the National Academy of Sciences of the United States of America, 102*, 14931–14936.

Rueda, M. R., Rothbart, M. K., Saccomanno, L., & Posner, M. I. (2007). Modifying brain networks underlying self-regulation. In D. Romer & E. F. Walker (Eds.), *Adolescent psychopathology and the developing brain: Integrating brain and prevention science* (pp. 401–419). New York: Oxford University Press.

Rydell, A.-M., Berlin, L., & Bohlin, G. (2003). Emotionality, emotion regulation, and adaptation among 5- to 8-year-old children. *Emotion, 3*, 30–47.

Schaffer, H. R. (1974). Cognitive components of the infant's response to strangeness. In M. Lewis & L. A. Rosenblum (Eds.), *The origins of fear* (pp. 11–24). New York: Wiley.

Sethi, A., Mischel, W., Aber, J. L., Shoda, Y., & Rodriguez, M. L. (2000). The role of strategic attention deployment in development of self-regulation: Predicting preschoolers' delay of gratification from mother–toddler interactions. *Developmental Psychology, 36*(6), 767–777.

Simonds, J., Kieras, J. E., Rueda, M. R., & Rothbart, M. K. (2007). Effortful control, executive attention, and emotional regulation in 7- to 10-year-old children. *Cognitive Development, 22*(4), 474–488.

Spinrad, T. L., Eisenberg, N., Gaertner, B., Popp, T., Smith, Kupfer, A., et al. (2007). Relations of maternal socialization and toddlers' effortful control to children's adjustment and social competence. *Developmental Psychology, 43*(5), 1170–1186.

Strelau, J. (1983). *Temperament personality activity.* New York: Academic Press.

Stice, E., & Gonzales, N. (1998). Adolescent temperament moderates the relation of parenting to antisocial behavior and substance use. *Journal of Adolescent Research, 13*(1), 5–31.

Stifter, C. A., & Braungart, J. M. (1995). The regulation of negative reactivity in infancy: Function and development. *Developmental Psychology, 31*(3), 448–455.

Thomas, A., & Chess, S. (1977). *Temperament and development.* New York: Brunner/Mazel.

Valiente, C., Eisenberg, N., Fabes, R. A., Shepard, S. A., Cumberland, A., & Losoya, S. (2004). Prediction of children's empathy-related responding from their effortful control and parents' expressivity. *Developmental Psychology, 40,* 911–926.

Valiente, C., Lemery-Chalfant, K., Swanson, J., & Reiser, M. (2008). Prediction of children's academic competence from their effortful control, relationships, and classroom participation. *Journal of Educational Psychology, 100*(1), 67–77.

Watson, D., & Clark, L. A. (1993). Behavioral disinhibition versus constraint: A dispositional perspective. In D. M. Wegner & J. W. Pennebaker (Eds.), *Handbook of mental control* (pp. 506–527). Englewood Cliffs, NJ: Prentice-Hall.

Zuckerman, M. (1991). *Psychobiology of personality.* New York: Cambridge University Press.

CHAPTER 25

Self-Efficacy Beliefs and the Architecture of Personality
On Knowledge, Appraisal, and Self-Regulation

DANIEL CERVONE
NILLY MOR
HEATHER OROM
WILLIAM G. SHADEL
WALTER D. SCOTT

This chapter addresses the role of self-efficacy beliefs in the process of self-regulation. We begin by addressing the meaning of the two key terms we have just used: *self-regulation* and *self-efficacy* beliefs. We then review research documenting the contribution of beliefs in personal efficacy to the successful self-regulation of behavior and experience.

SELF-REGULATION AND THE CONTROL OF BEHAVIOR

Human beings do a lot of different things. A variety of them are termed acts of *self-regulation* or *self-control*. A challenge to self-regulation researchers is to recognize the full range of phenomena referenced by the term. One must avoid the "blind men and an elephant problem," in which different investigators explore parts of the whole, each thinking that he or she is studying the whole thing.

To this end, psychologists can recruit the assistance of people trained to explore the nuances of conceptually complex phenomena: philosophers. Horstkötter (2009) explains that questions of self-control encompass, yet go beyond, phenomena explored under the heading of *willpower* (e.g., Gailliot & Baumeister, 2007). There exist "varieties of self-control that we cannot analyze in terms of weakness of will" (Horstkötter, 2009, p. 49) including, for example, cases of "psychological incapacity" (p. 57), in which a relative lack of skills and task strategies induces self-regulatory failure. Mele (1990) distinguishes self-control that results from a "brute" overcoming of impulses (i.e., a deliberate, effortful exertion of willpower) from "skilled" self-control, in which a person executes an effective coping strategy.

As Horstkötter (2009) emphasizes, delineating varieties of self-control has implications for an issue much discussed in social psychology, namely, the relation between self-control and the automaticity of cognition. The distinction between control and uncontrolled action cannot be equated with the distinction between deliberate and automatic cognitive processes, she notes, since in skilled self-control the skill may be automatized. The "automatic" behavior then is an act of successful self-control. Alternatively, people may deliberate on future actions yet fail to act in a manner that is consistent with personal goals and values. "Whether or not any behavior is conducted in an automatic fashion," then, "is a totally different question" (Horstkötter, 2009, p. 23) than the question of whether a person is exerting self-control. Judgment of whether a person has exerted self-control rests on normative considerations. If one person consumes two ice-cream cones and another consumes two low-fat protein shakes, we may judge that the former but not the latter person failed to regulate his or her behavior. This judgment rests not on the distinction between automatic and deliberate cognitive processes, but on social norms regarding the acts.

These points bear on the rest of our chapter in the following way. The beings who are self-regulating—human beings—have two particularly defining qualities. People think about (1) not only the present but also the future, and (2) not only the world around them but themselves as actors in that world. Given this combination of attributes, it is inevitable that people will contemplate a question that is central to self-regulation: the (in)capacity of the self to cope with prospective challenges that the world may present (Horstkötter, 2009; Mele, 1990), or *self-efficacy beliefs* (Bandura, 1997, 2001).

SELF-EFFICACY WITHIN THE ARCHITECTURE OF PERSONALITY

When the self-efficacy literature began, self-efficacy processes were analyzed in relative isolation. Bandura (1977) identified one specific psychological mediator of the effects of psychotherapeutic interventions. Today, decades later, it is best to adopt a broader analysis (as has Bandura; 1986, 1999). Self-efficacy processes can be understood within a broader analysis of the design and functioning, or *architecture* (Cervone, 2005), of social cognitive systems in personality.

Personality architecture refers to the within-person design and operating characteristics of those psychological systems that underlie individual personality functioning and differences among individuals (cf. Anderson, 1983). Critically, a model of personality architecture is designed to capture *within*-person psychological structure and dynamics—a different goal than describing between-person variability in psychological tendencies in the population at large (e.g., Ashton & Lee, 2007).

A recently proposed model of the cognitive architecture of personality is the knowledge-and-appraisal personality architecture (KAPA) model, which proposes two key distinctions (Cervone, 2005). One differentiates knowledge from appraisal (cf. Lazarus, 1991). *Knowledge* refers to enduring mental representations of a typical attribute or attributes of oneself, other persons, or the physical or social world. An *appraisal*, in contrast, is a "continuing evaluation[s] of the significance of what is happening for one's personal well-being" (Lazarus, 1991, p. 144), with evaluations performed by relating features of the self to features of the world. Within this personality architecture, self-efficacy perceptions are appraisals—specifically, of one's capacity to execute actions to cope with challenges the world presents. The second distinction (Cervone, 2005), grounded in both psychological considerations and work in philosophy of mind (Searle, 1998), differentiates (1) beliefs about the nature of the world, (2) goals for bringing about a state of the world, or (3) standards for evaluating the goodness or worth of an entity. Self-efficacy appraisals are beliefs that are conceptually distinct from—yet empirically may be systematically related to—personal goals and standards.

Knowledge and appraisal mechanisms play different roles in intentional self-regulation. Knowledge structures are distal determinants that influence self-regulated action through their effects on appraisals (Cervone, 1997, 2005; cf. Lazarus, 1991). For example, if one is deciding whether to participate in a group discussion on a challenging topic, and if one possesses enduring mental representations involving knowledge that one is a "smart person" or is "good with words," that knowledge may prove influential in the encounter. However, the knowledge would not be influential unless it came to mind and influenced appraisals of the encounter.

On a general note, although we discuss *the effects of perceived self-efficacy*, the phrase should be understood as useful shorthand. The entity that "affects" the psychological outcomes of interest is the whole person. It is Stern's (1935) *unitas multiplex* that has the capacity to act as a causal, self-regulating agent (Harré, 1998). "We have to make a reference to the agent's personality, to who she is as a whole, to what she knows and to how she allocates appraisals" (Horstkötter, 2009, p. 130).

High versus low perceived self-efficacy should not be interpreted as "levels of a property of a person, like their weight, which has different magnitudes in different people" (as Harré [1998, p. 130] aptly characterized traditional treatments of self-esteem). *Perceived self-efficacy* refers to a class of thought, namely, people's thoughts about their capabilities for performance. In any given setting, different people may think differently about their capabilities. When referring to persons who "have high perceived self-efficacy," we merely are referencing individuals whose confidence regarding the level or type of performance they can accomplish in that setting exceeds the norm.

PERCEIVED SELF-EFFICACY: DEFINITION AND ASSESSMENT

Definition

Perceived self-efficacy is a person-in-context construct. It refers to people's thoughts about their capabilities for performance within a particular encounter, or types of encounters. Perceived capabilities to perform socially skilled behaviors (Hill, 1989), control eating (Glynn & Ruderman, 1986; Goodrick et al., 1999), resist peer pressure (Bandura, Barbaranelli, Caprara, & Pastorelli, 1996; Caprara et al., 1998), or engage in safe-sex practices (Dilorio, Maibach, O'Leary, & Sanderson, 1997; Montoya, 1998) exemplify the class of thinking referred to as *self-efficacy appraisal*.

The construct, then, differs from others with which it is sometimes confused. Self-efficacy appraisals differ from self-esteem; appraising capabilities for performance is not the same as judging the overall value of the self. Perceived self-efficacy also does not refer to mental representations of abstract, situation-free personal attributes. Statements such as "I am a good person" or "I have poor social skills" are not person-in-context appraisals; they are aspects of self-knowledge (see Cervone, 2004).

Other distinctions are noteworthy. Bandura (1977) distinguished self-efficacy judgments from outcome expectations, the latter being beliefs about consequences that may follow an act. Skinner (1996) distinguished among *agents* (the entity taking action to control events), *means* (the actions to be performed to gain control), and *ends* (desired and undesired outcomes); in this framework, self-efficacy perceptions are agents–means relations. Finally, Oettingen (1996) distinguished realistic appraisals, such as self-efficacy, from fantasies; highly optimistic fantasies may be associated with goal setting and self-regulation in a manner that is distinct from efficacy judgments (Oettingen, Pak, & Schnetter, 2001).

Assessment

Requirements for self-efficacy assessment follow naturally from its definition. To assess perceived self-efficacy, one needs to tap people's appraisals of the level or type of performance they believe they can achieve when facing designated challenges.

This generally is done via structured self-report measures (Bandura, 1977, 1997, 2006). People indicate either the level of performance they believe they can achieve on a task (*level of self-efficacy*) or their degree of confidence in attaining designated levels of achievement (*strength of self-efficacy*), or both. Scales are tailored to the performance domain of interest; they tap people's appraisals of performance capabilities in the face of specific challenges in those domains. Investigators might, for example, determine the social and interpersonal settings in which it is particularly difficult for individuals to resist the urge to smoke (Gwaltney et al., 2001), or the workplace challenges employees face (Saks, 1995), and formulate items that tap people's confidence in executing behaviors to cope with these settings.

A well-crafted self-efficacy scale can gauge not only between-person differences but also within-person variations across contexts. In the "microanalytic" research strategy of self-efficacy theory (Bandura, 1977; Cervone, 1985), self-efficacy measures assess people's appraisals of their ability to cope with each of a wide variety of different challenges. This enables prediction of those intraindividual patterns of cognition and action that often define an individual's personality (Mischel & Shoda, 1995).

Structured self-report questionnaires are not the only means of assessing efficacy appraisals. The Articulated Thoughts in Simulated Situations paradigm (ATSS; see Davison, Robins, & Johnson, 1983; Davison, Vogel, & Coffman, 1997) exposes individuals (usually via audiotape) to a relevant situation (e.g., an anger-arousing situation; see Eckhardt & Crane, 2008) and instructs them periodically to speak aloud their thoughts. Raters, who are unaware of the stimuli presented, code responses. Research supports the ATSS's validity. Davison, Haaga, Rosenbaum, Dolezal, and Weinstein (1991) exposed undergraduates to supportive and to stressful situations, and examined their articulated thoughts in response to those situations. ATSS-based self-efficacy ratings were associated significantly with self-reports and behavioral observations of anxiety in response to stressful situations (Davison et al., 1991). In ATSS research on smokers' and nonsmokers' responses to simulated situations that pose risk for relapse (Haaga, Davison, McDermut,

Hillis, & Twomey, 1993), more positive outcome expectancies of smoking during the simulated situation prospectively predicted increased chances of relapse at 3, but not 12, months (Haaga, 1989), and moderate self-efficacy levels to recover abstinence following a lapse predicted were associated with increased chances of abstinence (Haaga & Stewart, 1992).

PERCEIVED SELF-EFFICACY: CAUSES AND CONSEQUENCES

That self-efficacy perceptions are central to self-regulation is not surprising. It is difficult to envision an organism that possesses the capacity to reflect on its capabilities for action but does not incorporate those self-reflections into its decision-making calculus. Self-efficacy theory moves beyond the obvious by providing analytical tools for conceptualizing causes and consequences of self-efficacy appraisals.

Bandura (1977) outlined four sources of self-efficacy information, that is, four types of psychosocial experiences that influence perceptions of efficacy for coping with encounters: (1) firsthand behavioral experience, or mastery experience; (2) observation of others' experiences, that is, vicarious information conveyed via modeling; (3) evaluation of one's own emotional and physiological states, which is important because physical state is commonly of much relevance to one's immediately subsequent capabilities; and (4) verbal persuasion, that is, speech acts by others that may boost or lower one's own self-appraisals. Firsthand mastery experiences generally have the greatest influence on self-efficacy appraisals (Bandura, 1997; Williams & Cervone, 1998).

Bandura (1997) also identified four processes through which efficacy beliefs influence behavioral outcomes. First, self-efficacy perceptions influence decisions about which activities to pursue; people commonly avoid activities they judge to be beyond their capacities (e.g., Hackett & Betz, 1995). Second, once one undertakes an activity, self-efficacy perceptions affect effort and task persistence. Decisions about how long to persevere are based partly on self-reflections on one's capabilities (e.g., Cervone & Peake, 1986). Third, self-efficacy contributes to affective experience. People with a high sense of self-efficacy experience less anxiety when facing threats (e.g., Bandura, Cioffi, Taylor, & Brouillard, 1988; Bandura, Taylor, Williams, Mefford, & Barchas, 1985). People with a low sense of self-efficacy for accomplishing important life tasks are vulnerable to depression (Bandura, Pastorelli, Barbaranelli, & Caprara, 1999; Cutrona & Troutman, 1986). Finally, efficacy beliefs influence the quality of analytical cognitive performance. People with a higher sense of self-efficacy display superior performance on cognitively complex laboratory tasks (Cervone, Jiwani, & Wood, 1991; Cervone & Wood, 1995), everyday problem-solving tasks (Artistico, Cervone, & Pezzuti, 2003), and tests of memory performance (Berry, West, & Dennehey, 1989). The impact of self-efficacy appraisals on cognitive performance is partly mediated by cognitive interference (Sarason, Pierce, & Sarason, 1996); people with a low sense of self-efficacy may dwell on not only task demands but also on their personal experiences during task performance (Elliott & Dweck, 1988).

By affecting people's acceptance of challenges, persistence despite setbacks, execution of complex cognitive strategies, and anxiety versus calmness in the face of threat, higher self-efficacy perceptions generally promote superior self-regulation and achievement. The data here are quite strong. A veritable mountain of evidence (reviewed in Bandura, 1997; Caprara & Cervone, 2000) documents the influence of self-efficacy appraisals on subsequent behavior. This includes not only correlational data but also studies that manipulate self-efficacy beliefs experimentally (e.g., Cervone, 1989; Cervone & Peake, 1986; Peake & Cervone, 1989), or that relate self-efficacy perceptions to future performance, while statistically controlling for the effects of past performance (e.g., Cervone et al., 1991).

Meta-analytic reviews provide particularly valuable evidence of the predictive strength of self-efficacy measures. Stajkovic and Luthans (1998) synthesized studies relating contextualized self-efficacy assessments to work performance and found mean correlations in the .4–.5 range (with results varying somewhat as a function of task complexity). Even this result may underestimate the real-world impact of efficacy self-appraisals, in that people with a particularly low sense of efficacy may self-select out of activities rather than merely display inferior performance once an activity has begun.

In addition to their direct effect on behavioral and emotional processes, self-efficacy perceptions influence other personality processes that come into play as people strive to regulate their actions. Goal setting is one such variable. Performance on both achievement and interpersonal tasks is greatly influenced by the nature of the personal goals that people set for themselves (e.g., Grant & Dweck, 1999). People who set explicit, challenging goals and receive feedback on their progress generally outperform others (Locke & Latham, 1990) and often enjoy activities as well (Csikszentmihalyi, 1990). People commonly reflect on their capabilities when establishing personal goals. High self-efficacy induces the adoption of, and commitment to, challenging task goals (Bandura, 1997; Cervone, 1993).

Another pathway from self-efficacy perception to self-regulation involves skills. When low self-efficacy causes people to avoid activities, they fail to acquire knowledge and skills they might have learned had they attempted them. For example, among U.S. college students, women often have a lower sense of self-efficacy for mathematics than do men; differences are found even when researchers control for students' tested ability (Betz & Hackett, 1981; also see Betz, 2001). As a result, women less frequently enroll in upper-level math courses. The decision not to enroll then deprives them of the skills development they might have experienced.

SELF-EFFICACY IN CONTEXT

Self-efficacy perceptions should be assessed contextually. The construct refers to people's perceptions of their capabilities for performance, and performances, of necessity, occur in a social or environmental context. Pragmatic considerations also motivate contextualism. A global approach can obscure psychological phenomena that might be understood via contextualized assessment. We consider here two illustrations of this point that serve also to illustrate the general role of self-efficacy appraisal in behavioral self-regulation. The first concerns cognitive performance among older adults. The second addresses the generalization of the effects of psychosocial interventions.

Cognitive Performance among Older Adults

As the human lifespan increases, enhancing older adults' capacity to function effectively becomes increasingly important. Biologically based declines in cognitive performance occur with age (Willott, 1999), accompanied by increasing knowledge and expertise (Baltes, 1997; Baltes & Baltes, 1990) that may sustain well-being.

Because expertise generally is grounded in contextually linked knowledge structures, age-related expertise may reveal itself primarily in specific performance contexts, such as those in which older adults invest personal effort (Baltes & Lang, 1997; Baltes & Staudinger, 2000). In research on aging, then, investigators cannot merely present laboratory tasks that lack ecological validity but must incorporate everyday problem-solving tasks of personal relevance to the older adult (Willis, 1999). Everyday problems often are amenable to multiple solutions; the ability to generate alternative solutions is thus an index of performance capabilities (e.g., Allaire & Marsiske, 2002).

Generating multiple solutions to problems requires cognitive effort that may in turn require a strong sense of efficacy for problem solving. People who possess knowledge but doubt their personal efficacy may fail to exert the effort required for optimal cognitive achievement. A contextual analysis is needed in this domain because older adults may have relatively high efficacy perceptions and performance in select domains of problem solving that are ecologically representative of challenges they face in everyday life (Berry & West, 1993; Lachman & Jelalian, 1984).

In research, Artistico and colleagues (2003) presented younger and older adults with alternative problem-solving tasks representative of activities commonly confronted by younger adults, older adults, or both age groups. They also attempted a laboratory task, the Tower of Hanoi problem. On both self-efficacy and performance measures, age group and task characteristics interacted (Figure 25.1). Young participants had higher efficacy beliefs and displayed superior performance on both the Tower of Hanoi problem and everyday tasks common to both older and younger adults. Looking merely at these three tasks, one might conclude, as a general rule, that young adults have higher self-efficacy and outperform older adults in cognitive problem solving. However, on everyday problems that were ecologically relevant to their age group, older adults had higher self-efficacy perceptions and outperformed young adults (Figure 25.1).

The findings suggest that older adults are fully capable of superior cognitive performance in particular contexts in which everyday experience has instilled in them a robust sense of problem-solving efficacy. This important result would have been overlooked had we assessed efficacy beliefs in a global, decontextualized manner.

Generalization in the Effects of Psychosocial Interventions

Another question of both theoretical and practical significance is whether the effects of a given psychosocial intervention generalize. Practitioners generally hope that interventions produce widespread effects that generalize beyond the domain in which treatment is conducted (Smith, 1989).

There are two ways to address generalization in self-efficacy perceptions. One is to employ a generalized self-efficacy scale (e.g., Schwarzer, Babler, Kwiatek, & Shrooder, 1997; Sherer et al., 1982). Interventions may alter the degree to which people see themselves as being, in general, competent, efficacious individuals (e.g., Smith, 1989; Weitlauf, Smith, & Cervone, 2000). However, a drawback to this strategy is that people's self-reports of personal attributes tend to change slowly, or may fail to change despite novel life experiences (Mischel, 1968; cf. Klein & Loftus, 1993). Thus, global self-reports may fail to reveal psychological changes that would be evident if one applied a more focused assessment strategy. The second strategy, then, involves contextualized measures that tap self-efficacy beliefs across each of a variety of contexts. In this approach, one can ask whether an intervention in one domain changes self-efficacy beliefs in others.

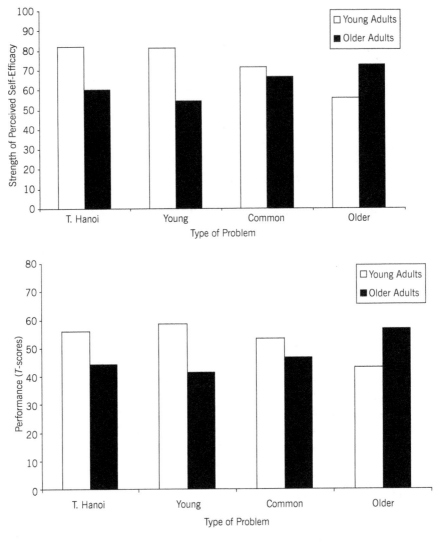

FIGURE 25.1. Mean levels of perceived self-efficacy (top panel) and problem-solving performance (bottom panel) among young and older adults on three types of everyday problems and one traditional laboratory task (see text). From Artistico, Cervone, and Pezzuti (2003). Copyright 2003 by the American Psychological Association. Adapted by permission.

Building on earlier research by Ozer and Bandura (1990), Weitlauf, Cervone, Smith, and Wright (2001) examined generalization in treatment effects stemming from an intervention of significance in the lives of many women, namely, self-defense training. Women took part in a 16-hour, physical self-defense class that taught verbal and physical resistance to rape, and martial arts. Before and after self-defense training, two types of self-efficacy assessments were employed: a measure of general self-efficacy (Sherer et al., 1982) and a 32-item, situation-specific self-efficacy index that tapped perceived capabilities in a variety of specific domains, including athletics, academics, work, interpersonal encounters, and coping with life stressors of relevance to this population. Analyses of the multidomain self-efficacy questionnaire revealed that the effects of self-defense training generalized (Weitlauf et al., 2001). Self-defense training boosted efficacy beliefs in domains beyond those involving physical self-defense (e.g., interpersonal assertiveness). The generalization effects detected by our multidomain, contextualized self-efficacy measure were not replicated on the measure of general self-efficacy or self-esteem. Thus, contextualized assessment had practical benefits. An exclusive use of global self-report measures would have obscured the actual generalization effects that were detectable only when we assessed efficacy appraisals for specific challenges in specific contexts.

THE ROLE OF SELF-EFFICACY WITHIN GOAL SYSTEMS

As we have emphasized, self-efficacy perceptions do not operate in a vacuum. They are aspects of an overall architecture of knowledge structures and appraisal processes that underlie behavioral self-regulation. Another critical aspect of this architecture involves goals. Here, we present an overview of the different types of interactions among self-efficacy processes and goal systems that are indicated by contemporary theory and research on self-regulation.

In addressing this issue, it is important to recognize that the psychological phenomena referenced by the term *goals* include both enduring knowledge structures and dynamic appraisal processes. As knowledge structures, goals can be conceptualized as interlinked nodes in a semantic network (Shah & Kruglanski, 2000). Indeed, goals have been demonstrated to possess features characteristic of other knowledge structures with interlinked informational structures (Kruglanski et al., 2002; Kruglanski & Kopetz, 2009), including the interconnectedness of goals and the means to attain those goals; variation in the strength of those interconnections; the transfer of properties (e.g., affect and beliefs) from one goal to another, or between goals and their means of attainment; the subconscious impact of goals on each other; and contextual dependence, whereby the relations between goals change across contexts (Kruglanski & Kopetz, 2008, 2009).

The term *goals* also aptly applies to dynamic appraisal processes that occur as people evaluate their relation to ongoing encounters and activities. When engaged in such activities, people formulate and reformulate aims for action, as well as strategies for achieving those aims. People devise and discard goals as they evaluate their successes and failures, and try to move from a present state to a desired future state.

Self-efficacy perceptions are linked both to enduring goal structures and to dynamic goal processes. To best understand the diverse ways in which efficacy beliefs and goals may be linked, one should recognize qualitative distinctions among aspects of goals and the ways that self-efficacy perceptions relate to these distinctions. In outlining distinctions among goals, one may focus on differences in the content represented by goals; in particular, some activities are pursued with the goal of accomplishing a positive outcome, whereas others are pursued to avoid a negative outcome, as many theorists have recognized (e.g., Carver & Scheier, 1998). A second distinction involves the process of pursuing the goals, in which processes can be construed in terms of different stages or phases of goal pursuit, such as weighing alternatives versus maximizing yield once an alternative is chosen (Gollwitzer, 1996; Gollwitzer & Sheeran, 2006; Parks-Stamm & Gollwitzer, 2009). Content and process may interact; that is, different goal contents may be associated with devoting greater or lesser attention to different processes of attainment. We now review the extensive work that has related goal structures and processes to self-efficacy perceptions.

Self-Efficacy Perceptions and Enduring Goal Structures

Goals differ from one another both quantitatively and qualitatively. Quantitative distinctions include difficulty level, specificity, and proximity. For example, a person may aim to complete a marathon versus a 10-kilometer race (*variations in goal difficulty*), volunteer at a homeless shelter versus "do something to help the homeless" (*goal specificity*), or read one book chapter for class each week versus reading four chapters by the end of the month (*goal proximity*). Variations along these goal dimensions differentially influence motivation and performance; these effects are mediated in part by self-efficacy perceptions (Bandura, 1997; Locke & Latham, 1990). For example, when people set proximal goals, they more quickly and frequently receive feedback on their progress; thus, they tend to have higher self-efficacy perceptions and in turn higher interest in, and performance of, the activities as hand (Bandura & Cervone, 1983; Latham & Brown, 2006; Stock & Cervone, 1990; see also Garland, 1985; Houser-Marko & Sheldon, 2008; Manderlink & Harackiewicz, 1984).

Goals also can be differentiated according to several qualitative distinctions. One such distinction is goal orientation. When pursuing a given task, different individuals may be oriented toward different types of goals; some may pursue the activity for the purpose of demonstrating or evaluating their abilities, whereas others may by trying to learn and to hone their skills (Elliott & Dweck, 1988). These two different orientations are commonly referred to as *performance* and *learning* goals (Dweck & Leggett, 1988), or similarly, as *judgment* versus *development* goal orientations (Grant & Dweck, 1999). People who possess high levels of self-efficacy are more likely to endorse learning-oriented goals (e.g., Baird, Scott, Dearing, & Hamill, 2009; see Payne, Youngcourt, & Beaubien, 2007, for a meta-analytic review). Similarly, a learning orientation, as opposed to a performance orientation, has been shown to promote self-efficacy even in the face of failure (Button, Mathieu, & Zajac, 1996) and is related to better performance (e.g., Bell & Kozlowski, 2002). Failure on performance goals induces negative self-evaluation and helplessness, and is often coupled with general beliefs about one's deficiencies (Grant & Dweck, 1999).

Another qualitative distinction differentiates between goals that involve an approach to positive outcomes and goals that entail avoidance of a negative outcome (e.g., Emmons, 1989, 1999). Avoidance goals have often been associated with negative outcomes and poor well-being (Elliott & Sheldon, 1997; Emmons & Kaiser, 1996). Self-efficacy appraisals may play a role here as well (e.g., Sins, van Joolingen, Savelsbergh, van Hout-Wolters, 2008). People have been found to view avoidance goals as less clear than approach goals (i.e., as involving less clearly defined strategies and outcomes) and to have a relatively lower sense of self-efficacy for the accomplishment of avoidance goals (Mor & Cervone, 2002). Goal clarity and self-efficacy may be linked; self-efficacy perceptions may be higher when pathways to goal pursuit come to mind clearly (cf. Cervone, 1989). Furthermore, compromised goal clarity in avoidance goals may result in maladaptive persistence despite failure (e.g., Lench & Levine, 2008) and to decreased self-efficacy.

Higgins (1997, 1999) has distinguished two forms of regulatory focus through which goals can be pursued: promotion and prevention. *Promotion focus* refers to sensitivity to positive outcomes. Individuals in a promotion focus aim to attain or to avoid loss of positive outcomes. *Prevention focus*, in contrast, involves an aim to avoid or to "gain the absence" of negative outcomes. Because a prevention focus involves regulation of necessary duties and obligations, expectancies play a more minor role in goal pursuit (Shah & Higgins, 1997). This raises an interesting general point about self-efficacy and goal systems: Different goals differentially engage self-efficacy processes (Bandura & Cervone, 1983); that is, they moderate the role of self-efficacy processes in the self-regulation of behavior. Efficacy appraisals play a relatively larger role when people are promotion-oriented (Shah & Higgins, 1997), and when they receive clear, easy-to-interpret feedback on performance goals (Bandura & Cervone, 1983; Cervone & Wood, 1995; Cervone et al., 1991).

Goals differ also in the extent to which the motivation for their pursuit is externally versus autonomously controlled (e.g., Ryan & Deci, 2000). People pursue autonomous goals because of a sense of personal volition and choice, whereas they pursue controlled goals because of external or internal pressure to accomplish the goal (Williams, Gagné, Ryan, & Deci, 2002). Autonomous motivation predicts higher task interest, persistence, and performance (Deci & Ryan, 1991; Sheldon, Ryan, Rawsthorne, & Ilardi, 1997), even when people have the same level of perceived competence—a construct generally associated with autonomous motivation (Deci, 1992) that relates closely to self-efficacy, though it constitutes a more general self-evaluation. A direct link between self-efficacy beliefs and intrinsically motivated goals was recently demonstrated in a sample of American Indian youth (Scott et al., 2008). However, inconsistent findings are reported regarding the joint effect of efficacy beliefs and autonomous versus external goal pursuit on motivation and performance. For example, although autonomous goal pursuit and self-efficacy were found to predict both behavioral adherence to a goal and general life satisfaction, autonomous goal pursuit was a more powerful predictor of life satisfaction, whereas self-efficacy was a more potent predictor of behavioral adherence (Sene'cal, Nouwen, & White, 2000). A different picture emerged in Scott and colleagues' (2008) study, in which higher self-efficacy predicted intrinsic goal orientation, which in turn was positively related to depression. In interpreting these findings, it should be remembered that self-efficacy theory is not a "unifactor" theory. As we have stressed, efficacy perceptions are one of a number of personal determinants of human motivation and achievement (see Bandura, 1986, 1999), and the interaction between efficacy perceptions and goal characteristics may depend on sample characteristics, as well as motivational and behavioral outcomes.

Self-Efficacy and Nonconscious Goals

Work on perceived self-efficacy primarily has addressed the role of conscious self-reflection in self-regulation. In contrast, a large body of research on goal processes indicates that nonconscious processes also are significant (e.g., Ferguson, Hassin, & Bargh, 2008). Goals can be primed and activated by environmental cues outside of awareness (e.g., Bargh & Chartrand, 1999; Bargh & Gollwitzer, 1994; Moskowitz & Gesundheit, 2009). Once activated, these goals can enhance performance, persistence in the face of failure, and the resumption of disrupted goal-directed behavior in the presence of alternatives (Bargh, Lee-Chai, Barndollar, Gollwitzer, & Trotschel, 2001). Thus, in these ways, nonconscious goals operate in a manner similar to that of conscious goals, despite their being relative "automatic" cognitions (Bargh & Huang, 2009).

A question that arises, then, is the role of self-efficacy perceptions when goals are activated automatically by environmental stimuli (Bargh et al., 2001) rather than as a result of conscious deliberation. One view is that, under certain conditions, perceptions of agency and control arise from nonconsciously activated goals (Aarts, Custers, & Marien, 2009). Extant findings on automatic goal activation provide an "existence proof"; there clearly do exist cases in which goal activation and subsequent behavioral effects occur outside of conscious awareness. These findings, however, should not obscure from view the many cases in which difficult tasks or personal setbacks prompt people to dwell on their efficacy for coping with life's challenges. A challenge for future research on self-efficacy processes is to understand better the social contexts and personal factors that prompt individuals to contemplate their efficacy beliefs and personal goals rather than act in accord with goals that are activated nonconsciously.

Self-Efficacy and Hindrance of Goal Pursuit

Self-efficacy perceptions may also hinder goal attainment. Under some circumstances, highly self-efficacious persons may be overly persistent in pursuing unattainable goals (Brandtstadter & Renner, 1990; Janoff-Bulman & Brickman, 1982) or may undertake risky endeavors they should avoid (Haaga & Stewart, 1992; see also Baumeister & Scher, 1988). Later in life, when resources become scarce (e.g., a deterioration in health, lesser physical capacities, a shorter remaining lifespan), optimal goal pursuit involves calibration of goals to the available resources and selection of manageable goals (Freund & Baltes, 2002), whereby an inflated sense of efficacy may interfere with goal attainment.

High self-efficacy beliefs, then, are not always beneficial. Rather than asking whether high self-efficacy beliefs are good, it is better to examine specific functional relations among self-appraisal, experience, and action. The ultimate utility of the experiences and actions that are self-regulated via efficacy beliefs, of course, may vary from one context to another.

Mood, Goals, and Standards for Performance

The previous discussion of self-regulatory processes was relatively "cold"; that is, it involved cognitive mechanisms rather than affective states. Recent work has examined the effects of affect on self-regulatory processes, with a focus on the impact of dysphoric mood (Scott & Cervone, 2002; Tillema, Cervone, & Scott, 2001).

This work has focused in particular on the relation between self-efficacy perceptions (i.e., beliefs about what one can do) and personal standards for performance (i.e., criteria that specify what one would have to achieve to be satisfied with oneself). Personal standards, of course, have long been recognized as critical to self-regulation (e.g., Lewin, Dembo, Festinger, & Sears, 1944). Correlational studies indicate that people who chronically experience dysphoric moods tend to hold relatively stringent performance standards that exceed the performances that, in their judgment, they actually can attain (Ahrens, 1987). Experimental studies indicate that affect plays a direct role in this tendency to adopt relatively perfectionistic standards. People in experimentally induced negative moods were found to display relatively high standards for performance; because negative mood did not raise efficacy beliefs, such persons exhibited the discrepancies between standards and efficacy perceptions that are typical of chronically depressed individuals (Cervone, Kopp, Schaumann, & Scott, 1994).

TABLE 25.1. Adjusted Mean Minimal Performance Standards and Evaluative Judgments for Semester GPA by Condition

Experimental condition	Minimal performance standard for semester GPA	Evaluative judgment for semester GPA
Nonsalient–negative	8.34 (2.34)	5.45 (2.91)
Salient–negative	7.16 (2.09)	6.86 (3.03)
Nonsalient–neutral	7.10 (2.73)	6.67 (3.04)

Note. Standard derivations are in parentheses. From Scott and Cervone (2002, Experiment 2). Copyright 2002 by Kluwer Academic/Plenum Press. Adapted by permission.

Research suggests that affect-as-information processes (Schwarz & Clore, 1983, 1988) account for this result. A unique affect-as-information prediction is that mood will not influence judgment when people attribute it to a source unrelated to the target of judgment. Scott and Cervone (2002) induced negative mood experimentally, then asked participants to completed a survey with measures of self-efficacy perceptions and personal standards for daily activities. Before completing the survey, the prior mood induction was made salient to some participants; they were briefly reminded of the procedure that had induce negative mood. In two studies, participants' standards for performance were similar to their self-efficacy perceptions; that is, they felt they could achieve their minimal standards for performance—*unless* they experienced a negative mood induction *and* that mood induction was not salient to them at the time of judgment (Scott & Cervone, 2002). When negative mood was made salient, participants no longer reported perfectionistic standards that exceeded their efficacy beliefs (Table 25.1), as anticipated by affect-as-information theory (Schwarz & Clore, 1983, 1988).

KNOWLEDGE STRUCTURES AND SELF-EFFICACY APPRAISAL

In the self-efficacy literature, investigators have long asked whether different types of experience differentially influence people's subjective beliefs about their capabilities for performance; Bandura's (1977) taxonomy of sources of efficacy information (reviewed earlier) valuably guided much of this work. Results robustly indicated that experiences of personal mastery are the most powerful influence on efficacy beliefs (Bandura, 1997).

A different question about determinants of self-efficacy beliefs, however, concerns not external influences but internal cognitive structures and processes. The question, as we have phrased it elsewhere (Cervone et al., 2008), is "What underlies appraisals?" What, in other words, are the personality dynamics underlying an individual's appraisal of his or her coping potential in a given situation? This question has been curiously neglected not only in the self-efficacy literature but also throughout personality, social, and clinical psychology studies of appraisal processes. Investigators have devoted more attention to the consequences of cognitive appraisal—the influence of appraisal processes on emotion, behavior, and self-regulatory efforts (e.g., John & Gross, 2004; Witkiewitz & Marlatt, 2004)—than to their causes.

We have addressed this issue by drawing on both the KAPA model of personality architecture (Cervone, 2004) and basic principles of social cognition (e.g., Higgins & Kruglanski, 1996). The KAPA model was outlined earlier. Regarding social cognition, Higgins (1996) valuably delineated factors that determine whether a given element of knowledge influences judgment. Knowledge is used in appraising circumstances to the degree (1) to which a person has that knowledge *available*, that is, encoded in memory; (2) to which the knowledge is *applicable* to the given situation; and (3) to which it is easily retrieved and used, or *accessible*. Different elements of knowledge possessed by the individual vary in the ease with which they come to mind (Higgins & King, 1981). Social judgments may become automatized when people's chronically accessible constructs are applicable, as evidence by research on beliefs about personality attributes (e.g., Higgins, King, & Mavin, 1982), goals (Grant & Dweck, 1999; Sanderson & Cantor, 1995), significant others (Andersen & Chen, 2002), and the self (Green & Sedikides, 2001).

We have applied these lessons from social cognition to the question of how rich bodies of knowledge about the self, or *self-schemas* (Markus, 1977; Markus, Crane, Bernstein, & Siladi, 1982), shape self-efficacy appraisals (Cervone, 1997, 2004; Orom & Cervone, 2009). The guiding idea is that a given self-schema may come to mind in multiple situations and, as a result, foster a consistent pattern of self-efficacy appraisal in those situations. The individual, then, may have a *personality style*—a consistent tendency evident across multiple situations—that derives from the influence of self-schemas on appraisal processes.

We study this possibility by employing an idiographic assessment strategy (Cervone, Shadel, & Jencius, 2001). We assess participants' beliefs about their personal attributes through open-ended procedures, and assess beliefs about the ways in which these attributes bear upon everyday situations through a structured sorting task in which participants relate situations to personal attributes. The combination of assessments yields a kind of "map" of the way in which a given individual relates elements of the self to everyday contexts. Finally, in subsequent laboratory sessions, participants are asked to appraise their self-efficacy for handling everyday challenges in specific situations. Our map of social and self-knowledge is used to predict self-efficacy appraisal.

Multiple studies indicate that people consistently display high and low self-efficacy appraisals in situations that they subjectively link to positively and negatively valenced self-schemas. When asking themselves, "Can I handle this situation?", positive and negative beliefs about the self come to mind and, respectively, raise and lower self-appraisals across self-relevant situations. This pattern is found among college students appraising their efficacy for everyday interpersonal and academic challenges (Cervone, 2004; Orom & Cervone, 2009), and smokers struggling to cope with urges to smoke that arise is specific life contexts (Cervone et al., 2007, 2008).

Note how these results argue against a "generalized" self-efficacy approach. There is substantial within-person, across-situation variability in efficacy appraisals. On this point, our results are consistent with other research testing the KAPA model (Wise, 2007, 2009) as well as with experience sampling studies of self-efficacy appraisals in context (Gwaltney, Shiffman, Balabanis, & Paty, 2005).

We have tested KAPA model predictions about knowledge and appraisal experimentally by manipulating the accessibility of elements of self-knowledge. We used priming procedures to manipulate the accessibility of "personal strengths" and "personal weaknesses," that is, elements of self-knowledge about attributes that participants judged as personal strengths and weaknesses. Self-efficacy appraisals were assessed subsequent to priming. As predicted, priming exerted a situation-specific effect (see Figure 25.2). The cognitive priming of knowledge about attributes that people considered to be personal strengths increased self-efficacy appraisals—but only when people were appraising their efficacy for coping with situations that they earlier had judged to be relevant to those attributes (Cervone et al., 2008). Our idiographic "maps" of personal and situational beliefs, then, allowed used to predict the contexts in which priming would influence judgment.

Related work with smokers has used priming to manipulate smokers' knowledge of themselves as smokers and potential ex-smokers. Self-efficacy to quit smoking is stronger when thoughts of the self as an ex-smoker are activated compared to when thoughts of the self as a smoker are activated (Shadel & Cervone, 2006).

The idea that chronically accessible self-schemas influence self-efficacy appraisal suggests that, in addition to affecting the content of self-efficacy beliefs, self-knowledge should affect the speed with which people judge their efficacy for performance. Self-appraisals should be faster in situations relevant to positive self-schemas (cf. Markus, 1977). To explore this possibility, we supplemented standard questionnaire assessments of self-efficacy perceptions with reaction time measures (Cervone et al., 2007; Orom & Cervone, 2009). People judged the relevance of their salient and highly self-representative attributes to various challenging social situations. They also judged whether they could perform challenging behaviors in these situations, while the time it took to make these judgments was assessed. Finally, they rated their confidence on a 10-point self-efficacy scale typical of the literature. As predicted, people appraised their capabilities more quickly for situations perceived as relevant to an *important* personal strength than for situations irrelevant to the same strength or relevant to a common positive attribute not descriptive of themselves.

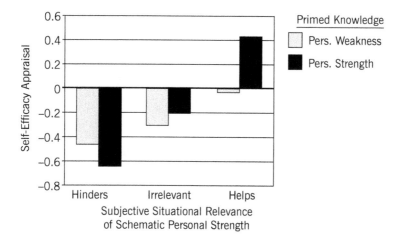

FIGURE 25.2. Mean self-efficacy appraisals plotted as a function of subjective situational beliefs (specifically, each participants' beliefs about the relation between their schematic personal strength and the present set of high-risk smoking situations) and priming condition. Black bars are self-efficacy appraisals subsequent to the priming of personal strengths; white bars are self-efficacy appraisals in the same situations subsequent to the priming of personal weaknesses. From Cervone et al. (2008). Copyright 2008 by John Wiley & Sons, Inc. Reprinted by permission.

Results confirmed that reaction time measures are useful for bringing to light information-processing differences between self-efficacy appraisals for schema-relevant and -irrelevant targets, which are especially notable because these judgments are more complex than the types of decisions to which reaction times have often been applied. One possible implication is that people can take different routes to get to the same self-efficacy rating. Which route they take may depend on the accessibility of relevant information. When situations activate chronically accessible self-beliefs, people may make "snap" judgments about their efficacy for performance.

An advantage of our idiographic methods becomes apparent when one recalls that self-regulatory efforts are made in social contexts. We find that people—even those who describe themselves in a similar manner when asked about their personal weaknesses and strengths—differ in the contexts in which their personal qualities are most relevant. Consider Figure 25.3 (from Cervone et al., 2007), which depicts three smokers who each said that their personal strength is their "willpower." (Note here that we are not claiming to have assessed, for these people, an inner quality of willpower; instead, our assessments indicate merely that these people held subjective beliefs about themselves that they summarized with the term *willpower*.) As shown in Figure 25.3, different people believed their willpower to be relevant to different situations involving different interpersonal settings and emotional states. There is idiosyncrasy, then, in both beliefs about the self and beliefs about the relevance of personal attributes to the social world (also see Orom & Cervone, 2009).

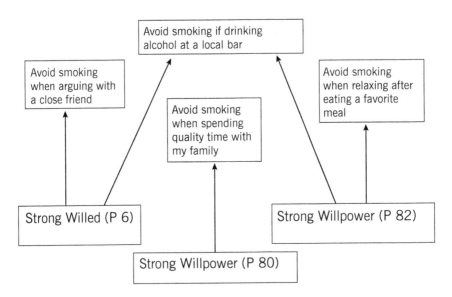

FIGURE 25.3. Representation of three participants whose schematic personal strength was "strong willed" or "has strong will," and situations in which individuals believed this strength would strongly help them avoid smoking. Presence (absence) of arrows indicates that the participant judged that his or her willpower did (not) bear on the ability to resist smoking urges in the given situation. P 6, Participant 6; P 80, Participant 80; P 82, Participant 82. From Cervone, Orom Artistico, Shadel, and Kassel (2007). Copyright 2007 by the American Psychological Association. Reprinted by permission.

This last point suggests that this chapter's opening, which encouraged investigators to think open-mindedly about the diversity of psychological systems that contribute to self-regulation, may have been an understatement. Researchers need to study not only the inner psychological systems of personality but also the outer social world in which individuals regulate their actions. Building a science of self-regulation might be a relatively straightforward matter if people did not vary—if a given individual were consistently good or bad, strong or weak, confident or doubtful, or skilled or unskilled in self-regulation. But our results, and others throughout personality science (e.g., Mischel, 2004), paint a more complex portrait. Individuals possess "pockets" of skill and incapability, of self-confidence and self-doubt. The challenge for research is to embrace the complexity and ultimately to explain the idiosyncratic patterns of belief, skills, and self-regulatory success and failure that mark the life of the individual.

ACKNOWLEDGMENT

During the preparation of this chapter, the work of Daniel Cervone and William G. Shadel was supported by Grant No. R01CA127491 from the National Cancer Institute.

REFERENCES

Aarts, H., Custers, R., & Marien, H. (2009). Priming and authorship ascription: When nonconscious goals turn into conscious experiences of self-agency. *Journal of Personality and Social Psychology, 96,* 967–979.

Ahrens, A. H. (1987). Theories of depression: The role of goals and the self-evaluation process. *Cognitive Therapy and Research, 11,* 665–680.

Allaire, J. C., & Marsiske, M. (2002). Well- and ill-defined measures of everyday cognition: Relationship to older adults' intellectual ability and functional status. *Psychology and Aging, 17,* 101–115.

Andersen, S. M., & Chen, S. (2002). The relational self: An interpersonal social-cognitive theory. *Psychological Review, 109,* 619–645.

Anderson, J. R. (1983). *The architecture of cognition.* Cambridge, MA: Harvard University Press.

Artistico, D., Cervone, D., & Pezzuti, L. (2003). Perceived self-efficacy and everyday problem solving among young and older adults. *Psychology and Aging, 18,* 68–79.

Ashton, M. C., & Lee, K. (2007). Empirical, theoretical, and practical advantages of the HEXACO model of personality structure. *Personality and Social Psychology Review, 11,* 150–166.

Baird, G. L., Scott, W. D., Dearing, E., & Hamill, S. K. (2009). Cognitive self-regulation in youth with and without learning disabilities: Academic self-efficacy, theories of intelligence, learning vs. performance goal preferences, and effort attributions. *Journal of Social and Clinical Psychology, 28,* 881–908.

Baltes, M. M., & Lang, F. R. (1997). Everyday functioning and successful aging: The impact of resources. *Psychology and Aging, 12,* 433–443.

Baltes, P. B. (1997). On the incomplete architecture of human ontogeny: Selection, optimization, compensation as foundation of developmental theory. *American Psychologist, 52,* 366–380.

Baltes, P. B., & Baltes, M. M. (1990). *Successful aging: Perspective from the behavioral sciences.* Cambridge, UK: Cambridge University Press.

Baltes, P. B., & Staudinger, U. M. (2000). Wisdom: A metaheuristic (pragmatic) to orchestrate mind and virtue toward excellence. *American Psychologist, 55,* 122–136.

Bandura, A. (1977). Self-efficacy: Toward a unifying theory of behavioral change. *Psychological Review, 84*, 191–215.

Bandura, A. (1986). *Social foundations of thought and action.* Englewood Cliffs, NJ: Prentice-Hall.

Bandura, A. (1997). *Self-efficacy: The exercise of control.* New York: Freeman.

Bandura, A. (1999). Social-cognitive theory of personality. In D. Cervone & Y. Shoda (Eds.), *The coherence of personality: Social-cognitive bases of consistency, variability, and organization* (pp. 185–241). New York: Guilford Press.

Bandura, A. (2001). Social cognitive theory: An agentic perspective. *Annual Review of Psychology, 52*, 1–26.

Bandura, A. (2006). Guide for constructing self-efficacy scales. In F. Pajares & T. Urdan (Eds.), *Self-efficacy beliefs of adolescents* (Vol. 5, pp. 307–337). Greenwich, CT: Information Age.

Bandura, A., Barbaranelli, C., Caprara, G. V., & Pastorelli, C. (1996). Mechanisms of moral disengagement in the exercise of moral agency. *Journal of Personality and Social Psychology, 71*, 364–374.

Bandura, A., & Cervone, D. (1983). Self-evaluative and self-efficacy mechanisms governing the motivational effects of goal systems. *Journal of Personality and Social Psychology, 45*, 1017–1028.

Bandura, A., Cioffi, D., Taylor, C. B., & Brouillard, M. E. (1988). Perceived self-efficacy in coping with cognitive stressors and opioid activation. *Journal of Personality and Social Psychology, 55*, 479–488.

Bandura, A., Pastorelli, C., Barbaranelli, C., & Caprara, G. V. (1999). Self-efficacy pathways to childhood depression. *Journal of Personality and Social Psychology, 76*, 258–269.

Bandura, A., Taylor, C. B., Williams, S. L., Mefford, I. N., & Barchas, J. D. (1985). Catecholamine secretion as a function of perceived coping self-efficacy. *Journal of Consulting and Clinical Psychology, 53*, 406–414.

Bargh, J. A., & Chartrand, T. L. (1999). The unbearable automaticity of being. *American Psychologist, 54*, 462–479.

Bargh, J. A., & Gollwitzer, P. M. (1994). Environmental control of goal-directed action: Automatic and strategic contingencies between situations and behavior. *Nebraska Symposium on Motivation, 41*, 71–124.

Bargh, J. A., & Huang, J. Y. (2009). The selfish goal. In G. B. Moskowitz & H. Grant (Eds.), *The psychology of goals* (pp. 127–150). New York: Guilford Press.

Bargh, J. A., Lee-Chai, A., Barndollar, K., Gollwitzer, P. M., & Trotschel, R. (2001). The automated will: Nonconscious activation and pursuit of behavioral goals. *Journal of Personality and Social Psychology, 81*, 1014–1027.

Baumeister, R. F., & Scher, S. J. (1988). Self-defeating behavior patterns among normal individuals: Review and analysis of common self-destructive tendencies. *Psychological Bulletin, 104*, 3–22.

Bell, B. S., & Kozlowski, S. W. J. (2002). Goal orientation and ability: Interactive effects on self-efficacy, performance, and knowledge. *Journal of Applied Psychology, 87*, 497–505.

Berry, J. M., & West, R. L. (1993). Cognitive self-efficacy in relation to personal mastery and goal setting across the life span. *International Journal of Behavioral Development, 16*, 351–379.

Berry, J. M., West, R. L., & Dennehey, D. M. (1989). Reliability and validity of the memory self-efficacy questionnaire. *Developmental Psychology, 25*, 701–713.

Betz, N. E. (2001). Career self-efficacy. In F. Leong & A. Barak (Eds.), *Contemporary models in vocational psychology: A volume in honor of Samuel H. Osipow* (pp. 55–77). Mahwah, NJ: Erlbaum.

Betz, N. E., & Hackett, G. (1981). The relationship of career-related self-efficacy expectations to perceived career options in college women and men. *Journal of Counseling Psychology, 23*, 399–410.

Brandtstadter, J., & Renner, G. (1990). Tenacious goal pursuit and flexible goal adjustment: Explication and age-related analysis of assimilative and accommodative strategies of coping. *Psychology and Aging, 5,* 58–67.

Button, S. B., Mathieu, J. E., & Zajac, D. M. (1996). Goal orientation in organizational research: A conceptual and empirical foundation. *Organizational Behavior and Human Decision Processes, 67,* 26–48.

Caprara, G. V., & Cervone, D. (2000). *Personality: Determinants, dynamics, and potentials.* New York: Cambridge University Press.

Carver, C. S., & Scheier, M. F. (1998). *On the self-regulation of behavior.* New York: Cambridge University Press.

Cervone, D. (1985). Randomization tests to determine significance levels for microanalytic congruences between self-efficacy and behavior. *Cognitive Therapy and Research, 9,* 357–365.

Cervone, D. (1989). Effects of envisioning future activities on self-efficacy judgments and motivation: An availability heuristic interpretation. *Cognitive Therapy and Research, 13,* 247–261.

Cervone, D. (1993). The role of self-referent cognitions in goal setting, motivation, and performance. In M. Rabinowitz (Ed.), *Cognitive science foundations of instruction* (pp. 57–96). Hillsdale, NJ: Erlbaum.

Cervone, D. (1997). Social-cognitive mechanisms and personality coherence: Self-knowledge, situational beliefs, and cross-situational coherence in perceived self-efficacy. *Psychological Science, 8,* 43–50.

Cervone, D. (2004). The architecture of personality. *Psychological Review, 111,* 183–204.

Cervone, D., Caldwell, T. L., Fiori, M., Orom, H., Shadel, W. G., Kassel, J., et al. (2008). What underlies appraisals?: Experimentally testing a knowledge-and-appraisal model of personality architecture among smokers contemplating high-risk situations. *Journal of Personality, 76,* 929–967.

Cervone, D., Jiwani, N., & Wood, R. (1991). Goal-setting and the differential influence of self-regulatory processes on complex decision-making performance. *Journal of Personality and Social Psychology, 61,* 257–266.

Cervone, D., Kopp, D. A., Schaumann, L., & Scott, W. D. (1994). Mood, self-efficacy, and performance standards: Lower moods induce higher standards for performance. *Journal of Personality and Social Psychology, 67,* 499–512.

Cervone, D., Orom, H., Artistico, D., Shadel, W. G., & Kassel, J. (2007). Using a knowledge-and-appraisal model of personality architecture to understand consistency and variability in smokers' self-efficacy appraisals in high-risk situations. *Psychology of Addictive Behaviors, 21,* 44–54.

Cervone, D., & Peake, P. K. (1986). Anchoring, efficacy, and action: The influence of judgmental heuristics on self-efficacy judgments and behavior. *Journal of Personality and Social Psychology, 50,* 492–501.

Cervone, D., Shadel, W. G., & Jencius, S. (2001). Social-cognitive theory of personality assessment. *Personality and Social Psychology Review, 5,* 33–51.

Cervone, D., & Wood, R. (1995). Goals, feedback, and the differential influence of self-regulatory processes on cognitively complex performance. *Cognitive Therapy and Research, 19,* 521–547.

Csikszentmihalyi, M. (1990). *Flow: The psychology of optimal experience.* New York: Harper & Row.

Cutrona, C. E., & Troutman, B. R. (1986). Social support, infant temperament, and parenting self-efficacy: A mediational model of postpartum depression. *Child Development, 57,* 1507–1518.

Davison, G., Robins, C., & Johnson, M. (1983). Articulated thoughts in simulated situations: A paradigm for studying cognition in emotion and behavior. *Cognitive Therapy and Research, 7,* 17–40.

Davison, G., Vogel, R., & Coffman, S. (1997). Think-aloud approaches to cognitive assessment and the articulated thoughts in simulated situations paradigm. *Journal of Consulting and Clinical Psychology, 65*, 950–958.

Davison, G. C., Haaga, D. A., Rosenbaum, J., Dolezal, S. L., & Weinstein, K. L. (1991). Assessment of self-efficacy in articulated thoughts: "States of mind" analysis and association with speech-anxious behavior. *Journal of Cognitive Psychotherapy, 5*, 83–93.

Deci, E. L. (1992). On the nature and functions of motivation theories. *Psychological Science, 3*, 167–171.

Deci, E. L., & Ryan, R. M. (1991). A motivational approach to self: Integration in personality. In R. Dienstbier (Ed.), *Nebraska Symposium on Motivation: Vol. 38. Perspectives on motivation* (pp. 237–288). Lincoln: University of Nebraska Press.

Dilorio, C., Maibach, E., O'Leary, A., & Sanderson, C. A. (1997). Measurement of condom use self-efficacy and outcome expectancies in a geographically diverse group of STD patients. *AIDS Education and Prevention, 9*, 1–13.

Dweck, C., & Leggett, E. (1988). A social-cognitive approach to motivation and personality. *Psychological Review, 95*, 256–273.

Eckhardt, C., & Crane, C. (2008). Effects of alcohol intoxication and aggressivity on aggressive verbalizations during anger arousal. *Aggressive Behavior, 34*, 428–436.

Elliott, A. J., & Dweck, C. S. (1988). Goals: An approach to motivation and achievement. *Journal of Personality and Social Psychology, 54*, 5–12.

Elliott, A. J., & Sheldon, K. M. (1997). Avoidance achievement motivation: A personal goals analysis. *Journal of Personality and Social Psychology, 73*, 171–185.

Emmons, R. A. (1989). The personal striving approach to personality. In L. A. Pervin (Ed.), *Goal constructs in personality and social psychology* (pp. 87–126). Hillsdale, NJ: Erlbaum.

Emmons, R. A. (1999). *The psychology of ultimate concerns: Motivation and spirituality in personality*. New York: Guilford Press.

Emmons, R. A., & Kaiser, H. A. (1996). Goal orientation and emotional well-being: Linking goals and affect through the self. In L. L. Martin & A. Tesser (Eds.), *Striving and feeling: Interactions among goals, affect, and self-regulation* (pp. 79–98). Mahwah, NJ: Erlbaum.

Ferguson, M. J., Hassin, R., & Bargh, J. A. (2008). Implicit motivation: Past, present, and future. In J. Y. Shah & W. L. Gardner (Eds.), *Handbook of motivation science* (pp. 150–166). New York: Guilford Press.

Freund, A. M., & Baltes, P. B. (2002). Life-management strategies of selection, optimization, and compensation: Measurement by self-report and construct validity. *Journal of Personality and Social Psychology, 82*, 642–662.

Gailliot, M. T., & Baumeister, R. F. (2007). The physiology of willpower: Linking blood glucose to self-control. *Personality and Social Psychology Review, 11*, 303–327.

Garland, H. (1985). A cognitive mediation theory of task goals and human performance. *Motivation and Emotion, 9*, 345–367.

Glynn, S. M., & Ruderman, A. J. (1986). The development and validation of an eating self-efficacy scale. *Cognitive Therapy and Research, 10*, 403–420.

Gollwitzer, P. M. (1996). The volitional benefits of planning. In P. M. Gollwitzer & J. A. Bargh (Eds.), *The psychology of action: Linking cognition and motivation to behavior* (pp. 287–312). New York: Guilford Press.

Gollwitzer, P. M., & Sheeran, P. (2006). Implementation intentions and goal achievement: A meta-analysis of effects and processes. *Advances of Experimental Social Psychology, 38*, 69–119.

Goodrick, G. K., Pendleton, V. R., Kimball, K. T., Poston, W. S. C., Reeves, R. S., & Foreyt, J. P. (1999). Binge eating severity, self-concept, dieting, self-efficacy and social support during treatment of binge eating disorder. *International Journal of Eating Disorders, 26*, 295–300.

Grant, H., & Dweck, C. S. (1999). A goal analysis of personality and personality coherence. In D.

Cervone & Y. Shoda (Eds.), *The coherence of personality: Social-cognitive bases of consistency, variability, and organization* (pp. 345–371). New York: Guilford Press.

Green, J. D., & Sedikides, C. (2001). When do self-schemas shape social perception?: The role of descriptive ambiguity. *Motivation and Emotion, 25*, 67–83.

Gwaltney, C., Shiffman, S., Balabanis, M. H., & Paty, J. A. (2005). Dynamic self-efficacy and outcome expectancies: Prediction of smoking lapse and relapse. *Journal of Abnormal Psychology, 114*, 661–675.

Gwaltney, C. J., Shiffman, S., Norman, G. J., Paty, J. A., Kassel, J. D., Gnys, M., et al. (2001). Does smoking abstinence self-efficacy vary across situations?: Identifying context specificity within the Relapse Situation Efficacy Questionnaire. *Journal of Consulting and Clinical Psychology, 69*, 516–527.

Haaga, D. A. F. (1989). Articulated thoughts and endorsement procedures for cognitive assessment in the prediction of smoking relapse. *Psychological Assessment, 1*, 112–117.

Haaga, D. A. F., Davison, G., McDermut, W., Hillis, S., & Twomey, H. (1993). "State of mind" analysis of the articulated thoughts of ex-smokers. *Cognitive Therapy and Research, 17*, 427–439.

Haaga, D. A. F., & Stewart, B. L. (1992). Self-efficacy for recovery from a lapse after smoking cessation. *Journal of Consulting and Clinical Psychology, 60*, 24–28.

Hackett, G., & Betz, N. E. (1995). Self-efficacy and career choice. In J. Maddux (Ed.), *Self-efficacy, adaptation, and adjustment: Theory, research, and application* (pp. 249–280). New York: Plenum Press.

Harré, R. (1998). *The singular self: An introduction to the psychology of personhood.* London: Sage.

Higgins, E. T. (1996). Knowledge activation: Accessibility, applicability, and salience. In E. T. Higgins & A. W. Kruglanski (Eds.), *Social psychology: Handbook of basic principles* (pp. 133–168). New York: Guilford Press.

Higgins, E. T. (1997). Beyond pleasure and pain. *American Psychologist, 52*, 1280–1300.

Higgins, E. T. (1999). Persons and situations: Unique explanatory principles or variability in general principles? In D. Cervone & Y. Shoda (Eds.), *The coherence of personality: Social-cognitive bases of consistency, variability, and organization* (pp. 61–93). New York: Guilford Press.

Higgins, E. T., & King, G. A. (1981). Accessibility of social constructs: Information-processing consequences of individual and contextual variability. In N. Cantor & J. Kihlstrom (Eds.), *Personality, cognition, and social interaction* (pp. 69–121). Hillsdale, NJ: Erlbaum.

Higgins, E. T., King, G. A., & Mavin, G. H. (1982). Individual construct accessibility and subjective impressions and recall. *Journal of Personality and Social Psychology, 43*, 35–47.

Higgins, E. T., & Kruglanski, A. W. (Eds.). (1996). *Social psychology: Handbook of basic principles.* New York: Guilford Press.

Hill, G. J. (1989). An unwillingness to act: Behavioral appropriateness, situational constraint, and self-efficacy in shyness. *Journal of Personality, 57*, 871–890.

Horstkötter, D. (2009). *Self-control revisited: Varieties of normative agency.* Nijmegen, The Netherlands: Radboud University.

Houser-Marko, L., & Sheldon, K. M. (2008). Eyes on the prize or nose to the grindstone?: The effects of level of goal evaluation on mood and motivation. *Personality and Social Psychology Bulletin, 34*, 1556–1569.

Janoff-Bulman, R., & Brickman, P. (1982). Expectations and what people learn from failure. In N. T. Feather (Ed.), *Expectations and action: Expectancy–value models in psychology* (pp. 207–272). Hillsdale, NJ: Erlbaum.

John, O. P., & Gross, J. J. (2004). Healthy and unhealthy emotion regulation: Personality processes, individual differences, and life span development. *Journal of Personality, 72*, 1301–1334.

Klein, S. B., & Loftus, J. (1993). The mental representation of trait and autobiographical knowledge about the self. In T. K. Srull & R. S. Wyer (Eds.), *Advances in social cognition* (Vol. 5, pp. 1–49). Hillsdale, NJ: Erlbaum.

Kruglanski, A. W., & Kopetz, C. (2008). The role of goal-systems in self-regulation. In E. Morsella, J. A. Bargh, & P. M. Gollwitzer (Eds.), *The psychology of action: Vol. 2. The mechanisms of human action* (pp. 350–367). New York: Oxford University Press.

Kruglanski, A. W., & Kopetz, C. (2009). What is so special (and non-special) about goals?: A view from the cognitive perspective. In G. B. Moskowitz & H. Grant (Eds.), *The psychology of goals* (pp. 27–55). New York: Guilford Press.

Kruglanski, A. W., Shah, J. Y., Fishbach, A., Friedman, R., Chun, W. Y., & Sleeth-Keppler, D. (2002). A theory of goal-systems. In M. Zanna (Ed.), *Advances in experimental social psychology* (pp. 331–378). San Diego, CA: Academic Press.

Lachman, M. E., & Jelalian, E. (1984). Self-efficacy and attributions for intellectual performance in young and elderly adults. *Journal of Gerontology, 39,* 577–582.

Latham, G. P., & Brown, T. C. (2006). The effect of learning vs. outcome goals on self-efficacy, satisfaction and performance in an MBA program. *Applied Psychology: An International Review, 55,* 606–623.

Lazarus, R. S. (1991). *Emotion and adaptation.* New York: Oxford University Press.

Lench, H. C., & Levine, L. J. (2008). Goals and response to failure: Knowing when to hold them and when to fold them. *Motivation and Emotion, 32,* 127–140.

Lewin, K., Dembo, T., Festinger, L., & Sears, P. S. (1944). Level of aspiration. In J. M. Hunt (Ed.), *Personality and the behavior disorders* (Vol. 1, pp. 333–378). New York: Ronald Press.

Locke, E. A., & Latham, G. P. (1990). *A theory of goal setting and task performance.* Englewood Cliffs, NJ: Prentice-Hall.

Manderlink, G., & Harackiewicz, J. M. (1984). Proximal versus distal goal setting and intrinsic motivation. *Journal of Personality and Social Psychology, 47,* 918–928.

Markus, H. (1977). Self-schemata and processing information about the self. *Journal of Personality and Social Psychology, 35,* 63–78.

Markus, H., Crane, M., Bernstein, S., & Siladi, M. (1982). Self-schemas and gender. *Journal of Personality and Social Psychology, 42,* 38–50.

Mele, A. R. (1990). Irresistible desires. *Nous, 24,* 455–472.

Mischel, W. (1968). *Personality and assessment.* New York: Wiley.

Mischel, W. (2004). Toward an integrative science of the person. *Annual Review of Psychology, 55,* 1–22.

Mischel, W., & Shoda, Y. (1995). A cognitive-affective system theory of personality: Reconceptualizing situations, dispositions, dynamics, and invariance in personality structure. *Psychological Review, 102,* 246–286.

Montoya, I. D. (1998). Social network ties, self-efficacy and condom use among women who use crack cocaine: A pilot study. *Substance Use and Misuse, 33,* 2049–2073.

Mor, N., & Cervone, D. (2002, January). *Approach and avoidance goals and subgoal mediation of the relationship between goal orientation and negative affect.* Poster presented at the annual meeting of the Society for Personality and Social Psychology, Savannah, GA.

Moskowitz, G. B., & Gesundheit, Y. (2009). Goal priming. In G. B. Moskowitz & H. Grant (Eds.), *The psychology of goals* (pp. 203–233). New York: Guilford Press.

Oettingen, G. (1996). Positive fantasy and motivation. In P. M. Gollwitzer & J. A. Bargh (Eds.), *The psychology of action: Linking cognition and motivation to behavior* (pp. 236–259). New York: Guilford Press.

Oettingen, G., Pak, H., & Schnetter, K. (2001). Self-regulation of goal-setting: Turning free fantasies about the future into binding goals. *Journal of Personality and Social Psychology, 80,* 736–753.

Orom, H., & Cervone, D. (2009). Personality dynamics, meaning, and idiosyncrasy: Identifying cross-situational coherence by assessing personality architecture. *Journal of Research in Personality, 43,* 228–240.

Ozer, E. M., & Bandura, A. (1990). Mechanisms governing empowerment effects: A self-efficacy analysis. *Journal of Personality and Social Psychology, 58,* 472–486.

Parks-Stamm, E. J., & Gollwitzer, P. M. (2009). Goal implementation: The benefits and costs of if-then planning. In G. B. Moskowitz & H. Grant (Eds.), *The psychology of goals* (pp. 362–391). New York: Guilford Press.

Payne, S. C., Youngcourt, S. S., & Beaubien, J. M. (2007). A meta-analytic examination of the goal orientation nomological net. *Journal of Applied Psychology, 92,* 128–150.

Peake, P. K., & Cervone, D. (1989). Sequence anchoring and self-efficacy: Primacy effects in the consideration of possibilities. *Social Cognition, 7,* 31–50.

Ryan, R. M., & Deci, E. L. (2000). Self-determination theory and the facilitation of intrinsic motivation, social development, and well-being. *American Psychologist, 55,* 68–78.

Saks, A. M. (1995). Longitudinal field investigation of the moderating and mediating effects of self-efficacy on the relationship between training and newcomer adjustment. *Journal of Applied Psychology, 80,* 639–654.

Sanderson, C. A., & Cantor, N. (1995). Social dating goals in late adolescence: Implications for safer sexual activity. *Journal of Personality and Social Psychology, 68,* 1121–1134.

Sarason, I. G., Pierce, G. R., & Sarason, B. R. (1996). *Cognitive interference: Theories, methods, and findings.* Mahwah, NJ: Erlbaum.

Schwarz, N., & Clore, G. L. (1983). Mood, misattribution, and judgments of well-being: Informative and directive functions of affective states. *Journal of Personality and Social Psychology, 45,* 513–523.

Schwarz, N., & Clore, G. L. (1988). How do I feel about it?: Informative functions of affective states. In K. Fiedler & J. Forgas (Eds.), *Affect, cognition, and social behavior* (pp. 44–62). Toronto: Hogrefe International.

Schwarzer, R., Babler, J., Kwiatek, P., & Shrooder, K. (1997). The assessment of optimistic self-beliefs: Comparison of the German, Spanish, and Chinese versions of the General Self-Efficacy Scale. *Applied Psychology: An International Review, 46,* 69–88.

Scott, W. D., & Cervone, D. (2002). The impact of negative affect on performance standards: Evidence for an affect-as-information mechanism. *Cognitive Therapy and Research, 26,* 19–37.

Scott, W. D., Dearing, E., Reynolds, W. R., Lindsay, J. E., Baird, G. L., & Hamill, S. (2008). Cognitive self-regulation and depression: Examining academic self-efficacy and goal characteristics in youth of a northern plains tribe. *Journal of Research on Adolescence, 18,* 379–394.

Searle, J. R. (1998). *Mind, language, and society: Philosophy in the real world.* New York: Basic Books.

Sene'cal, C., Nouwen, A., & White, D. (2000). Motivation and dietary self-care in adults with diabetes: Are self-efficacy and autonomous self-regulation complementary or competing constructs? *Health Psychology, 19,* 452–457.

Shadel, W. G., & Cervone, D. (2006). Evaluating social cognitive mechanisms that regulate self-efficacy in response to provocative smoking cues: An experimental investigation. *Psychology of Addictive Behaviors, 20,* 91–96.

Shah, J. Y., & Higgins, E. T. (1997). Expectancy × value effects: Regulatory focus as a determinant of magnitude and direction. *Journal of Personality and Social Psychology, 73,* 447–458.

Shah, J. Y., & Kruglanski, A. W. (2000). Aspects of goal networks: Implication for self-regulation. In M. Boekaerts, P. R., Pintrich, & M. Zeidner (Eds.), *Handbook of self-regulation* (pp. 85–110). San Diego, CA: Academic Press.

Sheldon, K. M., Ryan, R. M., Rawsthorne, L., & Ilardi, B. (1997). Trait self and true self: Cross-role variation in the Big Five traits and its relations with authenticity and subjective well-being. *Journal of Personality and Social Psychology, 73,* 1380–1393.

Sherer, M., Maddux, J. E., Mercandante, B., Prentice-Dunn, S., Jacobs, B., & Rogers, R. W. (1982). The Self-Efficacy Scale: Construction and validation. *Psychological Reports, 51,* 663–671.

Sins, P. H. M., van Joolingen, W. R., Savelsbergh, E. R., & van Hout-Wolters, B. (2008). Motivation and performance within a collaborative computer-based modeling task: Relations between students' achievement goal orientation, self-efficacy, cognitive processing, and achievement. *Contemporary Educational Psychology, 33,* 58–77.

Skinner, E. A. (1996). A guide to constructs of control. *Journal of Personality and Social Psychology, 71,* 549–570.

Smith, R. E. (1989). Effects of coping skills training on generalized self-efficacy and locus of control. *Journal of Personality and Social Psychology, 56,* 228–233.

Stajkovic, A. D., & Luthans, F. (1998). Self-efficacy and work-related performance: A meta-analysis. *Psychological Bulletin, 124,* 240–261.

Stern, W. (1935). *Allgemeine Psychologie auf personalisticher grundlage.* Dordrecht, The Netherlands: Nijoff.

Stock, J., & Cervone, D. (1990). Proximal goal-setting and self-regulatory processes. *Cognitive Therapy and Research, 14,* 483–498.

Tillema, J., Scott, W. D., & Cervone, D. (2001). Dysphoric mood, perceived self-efficacy, and personal standards for performance: The effects of attributional cues on self-defeating patterns of cognition. *Cognitive Therapy and Research, 25,* 535–549.

Weitlauf, J., Cervone, D., Smith, R. E., & Wright, P. M. (2001). Assessing generalization in perceived self-efficacy: Multidomain and global assessments of the effects of self-defense training for women. *Personality and Social Psychology Bulletin, 27,* 1683–1691.

Weitlauf, J., Smith, R. E., & Cervone, D. (2000). Generalization of coping skills training: Influence of self-defense instruction on women's efficacy beliefs, assertiveness, and aggression, task-specific and generalized self-efficacy, aggressiveness, and personality. *Journal of Applied Psychology, 85,* 625–633.

Williams, G. C., Gagné, M., Ryan, R. M., & Deci, E. L. (2002). Facilitating autonomous motivation for smoking cessation. *Health Psychology, 21,* 40–50.

Williams, S. L., & Cervone, D. (1998). Social cognitive theories of personality. In D. F. Barone, M. Hersen, & V. B. Van Hasselt (Eds.), *Advanced personality* (pp. 173–207). New York: Kluwer.

Willis, S. L. (1999). Everyday problem solving. In J. E. Birren & K. W. Schaie (Eds.), *Handbook of the psychology of aging* (4th ed., pp. 287–307). San Diego, CA: Academic Press.

Willott, J. F. (1999). *Neurogerontology: Aging and the nervous system.* New York: Springer.

Wise, J. B. (2007). Testing a theory that explains how self-efficacy beliefs are formed: Predicting self-efficacy appraisals across recreation activities. *Journal of Social and Clinical Psychology, 26,* 841–846.

Wise, J. B. (2009). Using the knowledge-and-appraisal personality architecture to predict physically active leisure self-efficacy in university students. *Journal of Applied Social Psychology, 39,* 1913–1927.

Witkiewitz, K., & Marlatt, G. A. (2004). Relapse prevention for alcohol and drug problems: That was Zen, this is Tao. *American Psychologist, 59,* 224–235.

CHAPTER 26

Impulsivity as a Personality Trait

COLIN G. DeYOUNG

mpulsivity is one of the most frequently examined constructs in psychology, and rightly so. Perhaps nothing better characterizes the dilemmas of human existence than the difficulty of balancing long-term goals against immediate impulses. No other species appears capable of planning explicitly for a distant future; humans, however, routinely adapt their behavior to goals that will not be obtained for weeks, months, or even years. Humans, therefore, are uniquely vulnerable to impulses that disrupt their plans. When human functioning goes wrong, impulsivity is often at the heart of dysfunction. No symptom, other than subjective distress, appears more often than impulsivity as a diagnostic criterion in the American Psychiatric Association's *Diagnostic and Statistical Manual of Mental Disorders* (Whiteside & Lynam, 2001).

Given the vast literature on impulsivity, a brief review cannot possibly be comprehensive. Following a discussion of definitions of impulsivity, this chapter focuses on impulsivity as a *personality trait*—that is, a dimension of relatively stable individual differences in the tendency to be impulsive, roughly normally distributed in the general population. After developing a working definition of impulsivity, the chapter considers methods of measuring impulsivity as a trait, then reviews research on different conceptions of impulsivity and the relation of impulsivity to broad taxonomies of personality, focusing primarily on the five-factor model, or the Big Five (John, Naumann, & Soto, 2008). Consideration is given to the psychological and biological mechanisms that underlie trait impulsivity in relation to a theory of the substrates of the Big Five and their higher-order factors (DeYoung & Gray, 2009), with the goal of developing hypotheses about how and why people differ in their predisposition toward impulsivity.

DEFINING IMPULSIVITY

For a trait so important, impulsivity exhibits surprisingly little consistency or coherence in definition and measurement within psychology. Many authors have noted the heterogeneity that exists in descriptions of impulsivity as a trait (Depue & Collins, 1999; Evenden, 1999; Parker, Bagby, & Webster, 1993; Whiteside & Lynam, 2001; Zuckerman, 2005). What constitutes a single impulsive action may be easier to specify than the attributes of an impulsive person. In every impulsive action, two elements must be present: (1) an impulse—an urge, motivation, or desire—to act in some way, and (2) a lack of inhibition, restraint, or control of that impulse (cf. Carver, Johnson, & Joormann, 2009; Hofmann, Friese, & Strack, 2009). Without the impulse there would be no need for restraint; with sufficient restraint, the impulse would not be expressed in action.

The fact that impulsive action logically requires these two components suggests one reason for the existence of multiple conceptions of trait impulsivity: Individual differences either in the strength of impulses or in the ability and tendency to restrain impulses could influence individual differences in impulsivity. Before proceeding to a more thorough examination of the various conceptions of impulsivity, however, let us consider some additional definitional issues that stem from the question of when and why impulses should be restrained.

The International Society for Research on Impulsivity (ISRI) offers three definitions of *impulsivity* (*impulsivity.org*; retrieved September 2, 2009):

1. Behavior without adequate thought.
2. The tendency to act with less forethought than do most individuals of equal ability and knowledge.
3. A predisposition toward rapid, unplanned reactions to internal or external stimuli, without regard to the negative consequences of these reactions.

The first of these defines individual instances of impulsive behavior rather than a trait, and begs the question "Adequate for what?" The implication is that impulsive behavior must be inadequate to achieve some goal. The second definition avoids the question of whether the behavior is desirable; any action undertaken with less than average forethought is considered impulsive. The third is most specific and implies that impulsive action entails negative consequences or at least some possibility of negative consequences, which would serve as the reason that impulses should be restrained.

One important question, therefore, is how crucial is the existence of negative consequences for a definition of impulsivity? Does impulsivity, as two of the ISRI definitions imply, necessarily involve action that is in conflict with the longer-term well-being of the individual? This question is not often considered explicitly. Unsurprisingly, given the clinical focus of much research on impulsivity, negative consequences for impulsivity are usually assumed as a given. However, Dickman (1990) proposed the existence of both "functional" and "dysfunctional" forms of impulsivity, suggesting that impulsivity may be beneficial in some circumstances. The scale he devised to measure functional impulsivity assesses comfort with acting, talking, and making decisions quickly, with little or no deliberation, when the situation calls for it, such as in fast-paced conversation or sport, or in the presence of fleeting opportunity. Block (2002) has similarly argued that some degree of "undercontrol" is not detrimental because it allows spontaneous exploration and utilization of unforeseen opportunities. Although impulsivity has typically been considered only as a dysfunctional tendency, the possibility of an adaptive form or level of impulsivity is worth keeping in mind when examining the association of impulsivity with other personality traits.

A more complex set of issues surrounds the question of how negative consequences of impulsive action are to be specified as such. Must they be negative for the individual committing the action, or might they be positive for that individual but negative for others? For example, someone might often steal impulsively, without getting caught, and never regret the action, though it would have negative consequences for others. This example raises a related question: Must the consequences of the action for the impulsive individual be judged as negative by that individual, or might they be judged as negative for that individual by others exclusively? A person who often steals impulsively, without getting caught, might not feel this to be a bad habit, though others might feel that he or she was taking unnecessary risks. Perhaps the most general claim that can be made about negative consequences of impulsivity is that impulsive action is inherently risky, regardless of its evaluation as positive or negative by anyone, because it involves acting on a present desire that might interfere with longer-term goals. Dickman (1990) acknowledged that even functional impulsivity is risky (though, by definition, usually worth the risk), in that the rapid responding it entails is likely to be error-prone.

One final definitional issue to consider is whether impulsive action must be rapid, as asserted by the third ISRI definition. What if someone experiences the urge to steal something, wanders around the store for 20 minutes, weighing the desire to steal against the fact that stealing would be risky and unnecessary, then decides to steal the item and does so; is this impulsive? Ainsley (2001) would argue that whether this action should be deemed impulsive is related to whether the person's decision is stable—that is, whether he or she (1) would have made the same decision, prospectively, before actually being at the store and (2) would regret the decision at some later time. An unstable choice, one that is rejected in advance and regretted in retrospect, is typically considered impulsive, even if it does not involve the rapid response and lack of deliberation that some definitions of impulsivity require. Such a choice does follow the pattern of an action based on an impulse that one fails to restrain.

This kind of impulsivity with deliberation appears to be possible because people typically discount rewards proportionally to their distance in time from the present (Ainsley, 2001). This allows for the situation in which a person considering a trip to the store the next day might value freedom from legal punishment above the thrill of shoplifting but, then, when faced in the store with the immediate possibility of theft, would decide that the reward of shoplifting was great enough to proceed, and, finally, might change his or her mind again after the theft, feeling that the action had been foolish, not worth the risk. When both the short- and long-term rewards were discounted (the day before), the long-term reward was perceived as greater than the short-term reward. When the short-term reward was immediate, however, and thus not discounted, its value spiked above that of the long-term reward, which remained discounted. This spike in value led to the impulsive action, even though the action was previously undesired and subsequently regretted.

This chapter offers a working definition of impulsivity that encompasses both rapid impulsivity without deliberation and this slower form of impulsivity with deliberation. *As a personality trait, impulsivity is the tendency to act on immediate urges, either before consideration of possible negative consequences or despite consideration of likely negative consequences.*

MEASUREMENT OF IMPULSIVITY

Many instruments have been designed specifically to measure impulsivity. The best established of these are questionnaires, including the Barratt Impulsiveness Scale, Version 11 (BIS-11; Patton, Stanford, & Barratt, 1995), the I_7 Impulsiveness Scale (Eysenck, Pearson, Easting, & Allsopp, 1985), the UPPS (Urgency, Premeditation, Perseverance, Sensation Seeking) Impulsive Behavior Scale (Whiteside & Lynam, 2001), the Control versus Impulsivity scale of the Multidimensional Personality Questionnaire (MPQ; Tellegen & Waller, 2008), and the Impulsiveness scale of the Revised NEO Personality Inventory (NEO PI-R; Costa & McCrae, 1992). Additionally, impulsivity is a central feature of attention-deficit/hyperactivity disorder (ADHD), and ADHD symptoms have been used as the basis for questionnaire assessment of trait impulsivity in nonclinical populations (Avila, Cuenca, Felix, Parcet, & Miranda, 2004; Kuntsi et al., 2004).

Impulsivity is one of the few traits for which the number of performance tests devised may rival the number of questionnaires. Currently, the major problem with performance tests of impulsivity is that much psychometric work remains to be done to ensure that they function properly as reliable measures of a trait. We need to know the degree to which they are stable over time and what proportion of their variance is indicative of latent impulsivity rather than task-specific performance. An informative comparison is with IQ tests, which are perhaps the most well-developed and validated tests psychometrically in all of psychology, and in which the majority of variance is due to a general intelligence factor rather than to abilities specific to individual tests (Deary, 2001). Research on impulsivity would benefit greatly from a well-validated battery of impulsivity tests that would yield summary scores, much like an IQ score. To justify a single summary score would require that all the tests load on a single factor, and the few investigations that have factor-analyzed multiple putative impulsivity tests have found that impulsivity seems to comprise multiple dimensions, some of which are only weakly, if at all, correlated (Avila et al., 2004; Reynolds, Ortengren, Richards, & de Wit, 2006). Nonetheless, a battery of impulsivity tests might yield useful scores for multiple impulsivity factors, just as IQ tests often provide separate scores for Verbal IQ and Performance IQ, in addition to Total IQ.

Although the available evidence is still slim, two factors appearing in batteries of impulsivity tests may correspond to the distinction, made earlier, between impulsivity with and without deliberation (Reynolds et al., 2006). These two types of performance test have been described as measuring, respectively, "rapid-response impulsivity," which lacks "adequate assessment of context," and "reward-discounting," which involves "inability to wait for a larger reward" (Swann, Bjork, Moeller, & Dougherty, 2002, p. 988). Many of the rapid-response tests require inhibiting prepotent responses (e.g., the Stroop, go/no-go, and stop-signal tasks). In the go/no-go task, for example, subjects must respond quickly with a button press to a set of frequent stimuli (e.g., letters other than X) but inhibit responding to a set of infrequent stimuli (e.g., the letter X). Impulsivity is measured as individual differences in failures of inhibition (though variability in response times has also proven to be an important indicator of impulsivity in this and other paradigms, perhaps because the impulsive person is easily distracted from the task at hand;

Leth-Steensen, King Elbaz, & Douglas, 2000). Reward discounting is often assessed by asking people to choose, without time pressure, between smaller rewards sooner, and larger rewards later. These paradigms are a rare case in the impulsivity literature, in which task performance has been demonstrated to have the long-term stability necessary to validate a trait measure (Kirby, 2009). Stable individual differences exist in the degree to which people discount the future, and these should logically be associated with the frequency with which individuals succumb to temptation, despite not intending to beforehand and regretting it afterward.

Another problem regarding performance tests of impulsivity is posed by the fact that the degree to which they correlate with questionnaire measures of impulsivity is still highly uncertain, varying depending on the instruments and samples involved (Avila et al., 2004; Edmonds, Bogg, & Roberts, 2009; Keilp, Sackeim, & Mann, 2005; Logan, Schachar, & Tannock, 1997; Reynolds et al., 2006; Spinella, 2004; Swann et al., 2002). Many studies find only weak to moderate correlations. A lack of reliable correlation between questionnaire and performance measures of impulsivity does not necessarily indicate inadequacy of the latter. Indeed, various impulsivity tests have shown predictive validity for relevant behavior in many studies, and one study pitting questionnaires against performance tests as predictors of health behaviors found that the two types of measure served as independent predictors, each accounting for variance that the other did not (Edmonds et al., 2009). Nonetheless, given that the questionnaire measures are better established and understood psychometrically, I consider only questionnaires in exploring the relations of impulsivity to broader models of personality.

As with the performance tests, questionnaire measures of impulsivity or traits that have been deemed closely related to impulsivity appear to load on multiple factors that vary greatly in the degree to which they are correlated. Understanding the nature of the different factors contributing variance to impulsivity questionnaires can be facilitated by mapping these factors onto broad structural models of personality. Such a mapping reveals that impulsivity is a highly complex trait, with a number of different underlying dispositions contributing to it.

IMPULSIVITY IN PERSONALITY TRAIT TAXONOMIES

Understanding the consequences of impulsivity is relatively straightforward. Impulsive people are more likely than others to overeat, overspend, abuse drugs, interrupt, get in fights, break the law, gamble, engage in risky sexual behavior, say things they regret, and so forth (Cyders & Smith, 2008; Krueger, Markon, Patrick, Benning, & Kramer, 2007). What is more difficult to understand are the causes of impulsivity. What predisposes some people to act impulsively even when it runs counter to their own interests? Why are some people consistently so much more impulsive than others? One approach to investigating these questions is to locate the trait of impulsivity within a hierarchical taxonomy of personality traits. Important clues about the nature of impulsivity may be revealed by its association with other traits.

Psychologists have long known that personality can be represented as a hierarchy, with specific, lower-level traits (e.g., talkativeness, sociability, assertiveness) varying together, such that one can deduce the existence of broader, higher-level traits (e.g., Extraversion, for the three traits just mentioned) that account for the covariation of the lower-level traits. A major project in personality psychology over the last 60 years has been the development of trait taxonomies that use correlations among the multitude of specific traits to identify a limited number of broader factors that represent the most important dimensions of personality. The fundamental challenge for this project is to find a sufficiently broad and unbiased pool of trait measurements in which to identify structure. A reasonably representative sample from the universe of all possible traits must be used to ensure unbiased results in factor analysis. No approach ensures a complete lack of bias in the pool of traits, but two of the most promising strategies are the lexical approach, which samples trait-descriptive words from natural language (Saucier & Goldberg, 2001), and the use of trait measurements from many existing questionnaires designed to capture a variety of different personality traits and structures (Markon, Krueger, & Watson, 2005). These two strategies have produced considerable evidence for a five-factor structure, known as the five-factor model, or Big Five, which includes dimensions of Extraversion, Neuroticism, Agreeableness, Conscientiousness, and Openness/Intellect (John et al., 2008).[1]

In order to understand the location of impulsivity in the Big Five, it is helpful first to examine the development of Eysenck's personality taxonomy, which was perhaps the dominant model of trait structure prior to the emergence of the Big Five. Eysenck (1947) originally assigned traits to two "superfactors," Extraversion and Neuroticism, and located impulsivity within Extraversion. Eysenck later revised his model with the addition of a third superfactor labeled "Psychoticism," though this label is widely considered misleading because the trait encompasses antisocial rather than psychotic tendencies (Zuckerman, 2005). In this revised model, Eysenck located impulsivity within Psychoticism, though "venturesomeness" and "sensation seeking," which he considered aspects of impulsivity, were retained within Extraversion (Eysenck & Eysenck, 1977).

Eysenck's three superfactors are largely compatible with the Big Five because Extraversion and Neuroticism are very similar in both systems, and Psychoticism (reversed) represents a blend of Agreeableness and Conscientiousness (Golberg & Rosolack, 1994; Markon et al., 2005). The major addition in the Big Five is a fifth factor, Openness/Intellect, encompassing imagination, creativity, intellectual engagement, and aesthetic and artistic interests.

Eysenck located impulsivity in two different traits; the Big Five model adds a third. In the NEO PI-R, a widely used measure of the Big Five that divides each broad trait into six lower-level traits, called "facets," Impulsiveness is a facet of Neuroticism (Costa & McCrae, 1992). Similarly, another measure, the Abridged Big Five Circumplex for the International Personality Item Pool (AB5C-IPIP; Goldberg, 1999), locates Impulse Control as a facet of Emotional Stability, which is Neuroticism reversed. However, the location of impulsivity within the Big Five is not necessarily incompatible with Eysenck's scheme: In the lexical version of the AB5C (Hofstee, de Raad, & Goldberg, 1992), the adjective *impulsive* has its primary loading on Conscientiousness, which would fall within Eysenck's Psychoticism, and Excitement Seeking, a facet of Extraversion in the NEO PI-R, is very similar in content to sensation seeking and venturesomeness. The Big Five thus appears to spread impulsivity across multiple dimensions, which may explain why impulsivity has been difficult to measure consistently.

Whiteside and Lynam (2001) have substantially clarified the diversity of conceptions of trait impulsivity and their relation to the Big Five. In factor analysis of many of the most common impulsivity questionnaires, they found four factors, each of which was strongly marked by a facet of the NEO PI-R. Their labels for these factors are listed below, followed by their corresponding NEO PI-R facet and Big Five dimension:

1. <u>U</u>rgency (Impulsiveness, Neuroticism)
2. (lack of) <u>P</u>remeditation (Deliberation, Conscientiousness)
3. (lack of) <u>P</u>erseverance (Self-Discipline, Conscientiousness)
4. <u>S</u>ensation Seeking (Excitement Seeking, Extraversion)

Thus, there appear to be at least four different types of impulsivity. The items that best marked these four factors were used to create the four subscales of the UPPS Impulsive Behavior Scale. A follow-up study analyzing the latent structure of the scale found that Premeditation and Perseverance were strongly correlated and could best be described as separable but related facets of one broader trait (Smith et al., 2007)—hardly surprising, given that both are facets of Conscientiousness. Other factor analyses of smaller numbers of impulsivity questionnaires have found smaller numbers of factors, which are recognizable as subsets of the UPPS factors (Flory et al., 2006; Parker et al., 1993).

The UPPS model demonstrates that, in the Big Five, the traits most directly related to impulsivity are located in Conscientiousness, Neuroticism, and Extraversion. Consideration of the psychobiological mechanisms underlying these three traits, in conjunction with the two elements of impulsive action (discussed earlier), suggests why all three traits would be associated with impulsivity. Conscientiousness appears to reflect the ability and tendency to use effortful, top-down control to follow rules and pursue long-term plans (DeYoung & Gray, 2009; Van Egeren, 2009), and it is associated with volume in the brain region (lateral prefrontal cortex) most strongly implicated in that form of control (DeYoung et al., 2010). Thus, increased Conscientiousness should lead to more frequent restraint of impulses that are disruptive of rules and plans.[2] However, unless an impulse emerges in the first place, there will be nothing for the conscientious individual to restrain. Impulses are reactions to motivationally salient internal or external stimuli—rewards and punishments, or predictors thereof—and a large body of self-report, behavioral, and neurobiological evidence suggests that Extraversion and Neuroticism reflect the primary manifestations in personality of sensitivity to reward and punishment, respectively (Clark & Watson, 2008; DeYoung & Gray, 2009). Extraversion involves positive affect and approach behavior, whereas Neuroticism involves negative affect and reactivity to threat. At any level of Conscientiousness, increased Extraversion or Neuroticism would be associated with increases in the strength and frequency of urges to approach rewards or react to threats, respectively, and this should in turn lead to more instances in which the individual's effortful control is insufficient to restrain impulses. Thus, Extraversion and Neuroticism may influence impulsivity independently of Conscientiousness (and of each other). Of course, this model also suggests the possibility of interactions. Increased Extraversion or Neuroticism may be particularly likely to lead to increased impulsivity in those with low Conscientiousness.

PREMEDITATION, PERSEVERANCE, SENSATION SEEKING, AND URGENCY

Because a tendency toward impulsive behavior is associated with four different factors, falling within three Big Five dimensions, Whiteside and Lynam (2001, p. 687) argued that *impulsivity* is "an artificial umbrella term" that should no longer be used as a trait descriptor. In subsequent articles, however, they softened this argument because the correlations among the UPPS subscales (even outside the Premeditation–Perseverance pair) tend to be moderate, "suggesting that in general the scales measure overlapping yet distinct constructs" (Whiteside, Lynam, Miller, & Reynolds, 2005, p. 564).[3] This overlap among the UPPS traits does suggest the existence of a general tendency toward impulsivity, even if that general tendency is influenced by variability in multiple, distinct traits and their associated psychobiological systems. Nonetheless, discriminant validity has been demonstrated for each of the four UPPS scales, in relation to a variety of impulsivity-related criteria, such as aggression, psychopathology, and drug use (Cyders & Smith, 2008; Miller, Flory, Lynam, & Leukefeld, 2003). Treating these four different impulsivity-related traits as if they are interchangeable is inadvisable and may result in contradictory or ambiguous findings. Thus, it is worth considering each UPPS trait in more depth.

Premeditation reflects "the tendency to think and reflect on the consequences of an act before engaging in that act," and lack of Premeditation appears to be the most common conceptualization of impulsivity in personality psychology (Whiteside & Lynam, 2001, p. 685). The working definition of *impulsivity*, presented earlier, described two modes of failure to restrain impulses: (1) failure to consider possible negative consequences before acting and (2) succumbing to temptation despite considering negative consequences. Lack of Premeditation clearly indicates the former.

Premeditation has a complicated status in the Big Five. Although it is a facet of Conscientiousness, it is less central to this broad dimension than Perseverance or most other Conscientiousness facets. Deliberation (the NEO PI-R equivalent of Premeditation) shows the weakest loading on Conscientiousness of any facet of that domain in the normative data for the NEO PI-R (Costa & McCrae, 1992), and it loads relatively weakly on both Industriousness and Orderliness, the two major subfactors within Conscientiousness (DeYoung, Quilty, & Peterson, 2007). Perhaps the most informative demonstration of what is different about Premeditation/Deliberation relative to other Conscientiousness facets is a factor analysis of many traits conceptually related to Conscientiousness (Roberts, Chernyshenko, Stark, & Goldberg, 2005). In this analysis, Deliberation was the only NEO PI-R facet to load primarily on a factor other than Industriousness and Orderliness, and this factor was also marked by two scales that have their primary loading on Extraversion (in the AB5C system), and their secondary loadings on Conscientiousness (Johnson, 1994). In the AB5C system, Deliberation loads primarily on Conscientiousness but has a secondary, negative loading on Extraversion (Johnson, 1994). These findings suggest that Premeditation, as a latent trait, may represent a roughly equal blend of high Conscientiousness and low Extraversion. This conclusion echoes that of Depue and Collins (1999), who argued that impulsivity is a compound trait reflecting the conjunction of high Extraversion and low Conscientiousness. Indeed, rapid action without deliberation should be potentiated by Extraversion, which has been described as the "energizer" of behavior (Van Egeren, 2009), and Extraversion is positively correlated with reaction time in many behavioral tasks (Zeidner & Matthews, 2000). Nonetheless, Conscientiousness seems the most appropriate primary location for Premeditation, from a conceptual standpoint, because planning is related to effortful control and the functions of lateral prefrontal cortex (Miller & Cohen, 2001). However, when considering research using impulsivity scales that primarily tap lack of Premeditation (such as the BIS-11; Whiteside & Lynam, 2001), one must remember that effects may be attributable to variance shared with Conscientiousness or to variance shared with Extraversion.

Perseverance reflects the "ability to remain focused on a task that may be boring or difficult" (Whiteside & Lynam, 2001, p. 685). A major factor in the ability to work at a task that is not immediately rewarding is the ability to avoid succumbing to the temptation to do something more immediately rewarding instead. Unlike Premeditation, Perseverance is quite central to Conscientiousness. Self-Discipline, the NEO PI-R equivalent of Perseverance, loads strongly on Conscientiousness generally and on its Industriousness subfactor specifically (Costa & McCrae, 1992; DeYoung et al., 2007). Working hard requires the ability to restrain impulses that would conflict with an ongoing plan, and people low in Perseverance are likely to act on such impulses, even when they are aware of the negative consequences for their longer-term goals. Perhaps the existence of Perseverance and Premeditation as two separable but closely related traits reflects the difference between impulsivity with and without deliberation. Both traits seem likely to rely on prefrontal effortful control systems, but perhaps they emphasize different components of those systems or interact differently with additional systems. These possibilities should be explored in future research.

Sensation Seeking reflects "willingness to take risks for the sake of excitement or novel experiences" (Zuckerman, Kuhlman, Joireman, Teta, & Kraft, 1993, p. 759). One could argue that high levels of Sensation Seeking need not be associated with impulsivity at all because those who decide to take risks for fun (e.g., hang gliding, mountain climbing, gambling, taking drugs) may do so with full consideration of possible negative consequences, may often take steps to ensure that the risk is not higher than they wish it to be (e.g., safety equipment for the mountain climber, a limited amount of money in the wallet of the gambler), and may have a stable preference for their behavior, eagerly anticipating the experience beforehand and having no regret afterward. Indeed, when Sensation Seeking has been used as a predictor while controlling for the other UPPS traits, "it consistently predicts, both concurrently and prospectively, the frequency of engaging in risky behaviors (such as drinking and gambling), but it does not relate to problem levels of involvement in those behaviors" (Cyders & Smith, 2008, p. 810). Notably, the Functional Impulsivity scale (Dickman, 1990) loads on the Sensation Seeking factor (Whiteside & Lynam, 2001). Nonetheless, Sensation Seeking is associated with the other UPPS traits (except Perseverance; Miller et al., 2003; Whiteside et al., 2005), and Zuckerman found that it correlated strongly enough with other measures of impulsivity to indicate a single Impulsive Sensation Seeking dimension (Zuckerman et al., 1993; Zuckerman, 2005).[4] Sensation Seeking's location in Extraversion suggests that it reflects a strong sensitivity to the possibility of reward, which should make impulsive action more likely, by increasing the strength and frequency of reward-seeking urges. Thus, although Sensation Seeking may not be inherently impulsive, it is associated with impulsivity. As one might expect, it appears to be those high in Sensation Seeking and also low in Premeditation who are especially likely to take risks with negative outcomes, in addition to risks with positive outcomes (Fischer & Smith, 2004).

Urgency, in Whiteside and Lynam's (2001, p. 685) original conception, reflects "the tendency to experience strong impulses, frequently under conditions of negative affect," which lead to "impulsive behaviors in order to alleviate negative emotions despite the long-term harmful consequences of these actions" (e.g., overeating, abusing drugs, or speaking or arguing rashly). That Urgency is associated with Neuroticism is in keeping with its emphasis on negative emotion as the trigger for rash action. However, since the original publication of the UPPS model, Cyders and colleagues (2007) have developed a measure of Positive Urgency (renaming the original scale Negative Urgency), based on evidence that strong positive emotion can also lead to rash action with harmful consequences (e.g., celebratory binge drinking by college students or resumption of gambling by pathological gamblers). Like Premeditation and Perseverance, Positive and Negative Urgency appear to be distinct facets of a single broader trait (Cyders & Smith, 2008). This general Urgency trait appears to describe dysfunctional impulsivity in which emotions are particularly salient, whereas lack of Premeditation and Perseverance appears to describe impulsivity in which emotions are less salient.

One might expect that Positive Urgency would be primarily associated with Extraversion and Sensation Seeking given that positive affect is a central component of Extraversion. Instead, however, Positive Urgency displays a profile of correlations with the Big Five similar to that of Negative Urgency (Cyders & Smith, 2008). Closer inspection of this pattern provides an additional insight into the nature of impulsivity as a personality trait. Despite the fact that Impulsiveness (the NEO PI-R equivalent of Negative Urgency) is a facet of Neuroticism, it has the lowest loading on Neuroticism (.49) of any facet of that domain (Costa & McCrae, 1992). The trait that the general Urgency dimension most strongly reflects does not appear to be Neuroticism. Rather, it appears to be one of the higher-order factors of the Big Five.

IMPULSIVITY AND THE HIGHER-ORDER FACTORS OF THE BIG FIVE

The Big Five were originally conceived as orthogonal dimensions and the broadest level of personality description. However, measures of the Big Five display a consistent pattern of intercorrelation, which reveals the existence of two higher-order factors or meta-traits, labeled *Alpha*, or *Stability*, and *Beta*, or *Plasticity* (DeYoung, 2006; DeYoung, Peterson, & Higgins, 2002; Digman, 1997; Markon et al., 2005; McCrae et al., 2008). Stability comprises the shared variance of Conscientiousness, Agreeableness, and Neuroticism (reversed), whereas Plasticity comprises the shared variance of Extraversion and Openness/Intellect. Stability appears to reflect a general tendency toward restraint and lack of disruption in emotion, motivation, and social relationships, whereas Plasticity appears to reflect a general tendency toward exploration and engagement with novel phenomena (DeYoung, 2006; Hirsh, DeYoung, & Peterson, 2009). Stability, therefore, seems likely to be associated with impulsivity generally, whereas Plasticity seems particularly likely to be associated with Sensation Seeking (indeed, Sensation Seeking is related to Openness/Intellect, as well as Extraversion; Aluja, García, & García, 2003; Flory et al., 2006).

In a factor analysis of the 30 facets of the NEO PI-R and the two Urgency scales, Cyders and Smith (2008) found that both Positive (PU) and Negative Urgency (NU) showed a similar pattern of factor loadings in a five-factor solution, with each loading on Neuroticism (PU = .28, NU = .58), Conscientiousness (PU = −.39, NU = −.40), and Agreeableness (PU = −.30, NU = −.37). Additionally, in both their sample and the normative data for the NEO PI-R, a similar pattern of factor loadings is evident for the NEO PI-R Impulsiveness facet (Costa & McCrae, 1992; Cyders & Smith, 2008). Cyders and Smith also examined a two-factor solution and found that PU and NU and Impulsiveness strongly marked the Stability factor. Urgency, therefore, appears to be a form of impulsivity that is most clearly described in personality taxonomies as a manifestation of low levels of the meta-trait Stability.

Another scale that exhibited this pattern of correlations with the Big Five is the Self-Control Scale (SCS; Tangney, Baumeister, & Boone, 2004), in which nearly all items are face valid as markers of three of the four UPPS factors (the SCS does not appear to include

Sensation Seeking items). One item especially, "People would describe me as impulsive," highlights the fact that this is a reversed impulsivity scale. The SCS was correlated almost equally with Neuroticism ($r = -.50$), and Conscientiousness ($r = -.54$), and somewhat more weakly with Agreeableness ($r = .29$) (Tangney et al., 2004). In this context, it is interesting to note that "Self-Control" has been suggested as an alternative label for Stability (Olson, 2005).

Finally, another variable, even broader in scope than impulsivity and clearly related to a lack of self-control, is associated with the same three Big Five dimensions and with the meta-trait Stability (DeYoung, Peterson, Séguin, Pihl, & Tremblay, 2008; Miller & Lynam, 2001). This is *externalizing behavior*, a broad category of behaviors that tend to be correlated, including aggression, impulsivity, antisocial behavior, and drug abuse (Krueger et al., 2002, 2007). Behavior genetics research indicates that the various types of externalizing behavior share a single underlying factor that is strongly genetically influenced and accounts for their correlation (Krueger et al., 2002). This factor appears to represent a continuous trait that is normally distributed in the general population (Markon & Krueger, 2006). Associations with broad personality models offer one approach to understanding the sources of this externalizing factor. In a sample of adolescent males, Stability was a strong predictor of externalizing behavior, as measured by both self- and teacher reports (DeYoung et al., 2008). Additionally, Plasticity predicted externalizing behavior positively, but only when the researchers controlled for Stability. In other words, if one compares two groups or individuals of equal Stability, the one with more of the exploratory tendency described by Plasticity will be likely to express higher levels of externalizing behavior.

The association of the meta-traits with various types of impulsivity and with externalizing behavior more generally is consistent with a theory of the neurobiological substrates of personality that links Stability to the neurotransmitter serotonin and Plasticity to the neurotransmitter dopamine (DeYoung et al., 2002, 2008; DeYoung & Gray, 2009). Although many brain systems have been implicated in impulsivity, one consistent set of findings is that impulsivity and other forms of externalizing behavior are associated with serotonergic and dopaminergic function (Carver et al., 2009; Chambers, Taylor, & Potenza, 2003; Congdon & Canli, 2008; Cyders & Smith, 2008; Depue & Collins, 1999; Kruesi et al., 1990; Zuckerman, 2005).

Serotonin acts very widely in the brain as a neuromodulator, with regulatory or inhibiting effects on mood, behavior, and cognition (Spoont, 1992). Serotonin not only potentiates the function of effortful control processes that allow the top-down restraint of impulses (Carver et al., 2009), but it also serves to suppress the bottom-up hypothalamic and brainstem systems (including the dopaminergic system) that generate impulses in the first place (Chambers et al., 2003; Gray & McNaughton, 2000). Serotonin acts to limit negative affect and aggression, while maintaining behavioral and motivational stability, and it has been directly linked to Conscientiousness, Agreeableness, and low Neuroticism, the traits constituting Stability (e.g., Jang et al., 2001; Manuck et al., 1998). Increasing serotonergic function thus appears to modulate both elements of impulsive action—the impulses and the lack of restraint—so as to reduce impulsivity. Individual differences in serotonergic function are therefore likely to be a key substrate of all impulsivity-related traits, perhaps most strongly related to the dimension labeled Urgency because this dimension explicitly describes strong impulses as well as weak restraint of those impulses.

Dopamine is another important neuromodulator, but one with primarily activating effects on behavior and cognition. Dopaminergic circuitry modulates exploration and approach behavior, sensitivity to possible rewards, desire, and curiosity, as well as cognitive control and flexibility (Berridge & Robinson, 1998; Braver & Barch, 2002; Panksepp, 1998). Considerable evidence links Extraversion to variation in dopaminergic function (Depue & Collins, 1999; Wacker, Chavanon, & Stemmler, 2006), and a smaller body of evidence suggests that Openness/Intellect may also be related to dopamine (DeYoung, Peterson, & Higgins, 2005; Harris et al., 2005). The association of Extraversion, a trait reflecting sensitivity to reward, with various aspects of impulsivity is consistent with the role of dopamine in potentiating impulses and increasing the subjective value of temptations. Interestingly, dopamine plays complementary and potentially conflicting roles in different brain areas: In the striatum, it potentiates impulses, whereas in the prefrontal cortex, it enhances the ability to control attention (up to a point—either too little or too much dopamine disrupts prefrontal function) (Arnsten & Robbins, 2002; Depue & Collins, 1999). Associations of dopamine with impulsivity, therefore, may be more complex than those of serotonin. In summary, both biological and psychometric considerations indicate that the meta-traits and their biological substrates should be investigated in conjunction with impulsivity.

CONCLUSION

As a personality trait, impulsivity has been conceived in many different and often competing ways, but personality psychology is beginning to clarify the different varieties of impulsivity. The development of the UPPS model (Whiteside & Lynam, 2001) has provided a set of dimensions, emerging from many questionnaire measures of impulsivity, that provides an excellent jumping-off point for research on individual differences in impulsive behavior. (Eventually, similar clarity may be brought to performance tests of impulsivity, though much additional psychometric work will be necessary.) The complex set of associations, reviewed in this chapter, between UPPS traits and the Big Five and their meta-traits is likely to be indicative of multiple underlying processes that determine impulsive behavior, including multiple systems that generate impulses and multiple processes that restrain impulses. Individual differences in any of these processes are likely to affect the general tendency toward *impulsivity*, defined as acting on immediate urges, either before consideration of possible negative consequences or despite consideration of likely negative consequences.

As it becomes feasible to develop theories of the neurobiological sources of basic personality traits like the Big Five and their meta-traits (DeYoung & Gray, 2009; DeYoung et al., 2010), these theories may provide a useful lens to help us understand individual traits of interest, particularly traits as complex as impulsivity. Systems responsible for sensitivity to reward and punishment and for effortful control are likely sources of individual differences in impulsivity that can be mapped onto specific Big Five traits. Additionally, the association of impulsivity with the functions of the serotonin and dopamine systems (which overlap with the three systems just mentioned but act more broadly than any one of them) may help to explain the relation of different forms of impulsivity to the meta-traits Stability and Plasticity, which represent shared variance among the Big Five.

Although Whiteside and Lynam (2001) made an excellent case for considering Conscientiousness, Extraversion, and Neuroticism in relation to impulsivity, the evidence reviewed earlier suggests that we should cast our net even more widely. One limitation of the analysis that produced the UPPS model is that it did not include measures of Agreeableness and Openness/Intellect. Both traits have important links to impulsivity. Agreeableness predicts the tendency to restrain aggressive impulses (Meier, Robinson, & Wilkowski, 2006), and impulsive aggression is a major concern in research on impulsivity. Openness/Intellect has been positively associated with substance use disorders (Trull & Sher, 1994). Additionally, both Agreeableness and Openness/Intellect are of interest because of their role in the meta-traits, which appear to be associated with impulsivity and externalizing behavior.[5] All of the Big Five should be included in any future research on the relation of impulsivity to personality taxonomies.

The study of impulsivity as a personality trait cannot shrink from complexity, either in the traits that may be related to impulsivity or in the behaviors that are considered impulsive. One might question the wisdom of introducing the construct of externalizing behavior into this investigation given that it is an even broader construct than impulsivity. However, externalizing behavior is highly relevant to research on impulsivity because antisocial behavior, aggression, and drug abuse are among the most common criteria for prediction by trait measures of impulsivity. Conceiving of the general externalizing behavior factor as a target for research on impulsivity may help researchers identify the shared mechanisms influencing the great variety of behaviors that are likely to be performed impulsively.

Human impulsivity reveals the fundamental struggle between phylogenetically old brain systems that drive us to pursue immediate gratification of simple desires and the newer brain systems that evolved to restrain those systems in order to pursue complex and distant goals. On both sides of this conflict, these systems are multiple and complex; an effective explanatory model cannot be boiled down to a monolithic restraint system in conflict with a monolithic impulse system. Individual differences in impulsivity reflect this complexity, as is evident in the multiple dimensions of impulsivity as a personality trait. In this chapter I have attempted to describe trait impulsivity in a manner that respects the complexity of the systems involved, while rendering the logic of their manifestation in personality more comprehensible.

NOTES

1. Recently, lexical research has discovered a six-factor solution that appears to be more widely replicable across languages than the Big Five (Ashton et al., 2004); however, this model appears to be only a minor variation on the Big Five, splitting Agreeableness into two factors (DeYoung et al., 2007). Social salience is likely to be a biasing factor in lexical studies, and traits within Agreeableness are highly socially salient because Agreeableness reflects cooperation as opposed to antagonism in social relationships.
2. The kind of restraint or inhibition of impulsive behaviors associated with Conscientiousness, which has been described as "nonaffective constraint" (Depue & Lenzenweger, 2005), must be distinguished from behavioral inhibition associated with anxiety. Gray and McNaughton (2000) posited a behavioral inhibition system (BIS) that detects threats to the accomplishment of goals (regardless of whether they are immediate or distant goals) and generates anxiety that inhibits ongoing behavior, in order to avoid or resolve conflicts with one's goals. However, this

inhibition is automatic and emotional rather than voluntary and effortful, and is not controlled by the prefrontal cortex. Someone who is anxious may well be less impulsive in relation to potential rewards (due to detection of conflicts between the distracting reward and longer-term goals) but more impulsive in relation to threats because the BIS automatically triggers threat-related impulses.

3. Aside from the correlation between Perseverence and Premeditation, Smith and colleagues (2007) found that correlations among the four UPPS traits were weak or nonexistent, but there are two reasons to question the reliability of this finding. First, Whiteside and Lynam (2001) used an orthogonal factor rotation, which artificially forces factors to be uncorrelated, even when they would be correlated if an oblique rotation were used. The UPPS scales based on these orthogonal factors might be less correlated than they should be. Second, Smith and colleagues used an undergraduate sample. In a large community sample, another study found that the correlations among UPPS scales ranged from .29 to .56, with the exception of the correlation between Sensation Seeking and lack of Perseverance, which was .06 (Miller et al., 2003). A very similar pattern of correlations was found in a sample with high rates of borderline personality disorder, pathological gambling, and alcohol abuse (Whiteside et al., 2005), suggesting that populations with higher levels of impulsivity than college undergraduates may tend to show stronger associations between distinct impulsivity-related traits.

4. Note that Zuckerman's (1979) earlier Sensation-Seeking scale (SSS) is broader than the UPPS Sensation-Seeking scale or the NEO PI-R Excitement-Seeking scale. In addition to Thrill- and Adventure-Seeking and Experience-Seeking subscales, Zuckerman's SSS also includes Disinhibition and Boredom Susceptibility scales. Whiteside and Lynam (2001) found Disinhibition to load equally on Sensation Seeking and lack of Perseverance, whereas Boredom Susceptibility loaded primarily on lack of Perseverance. In keeping with these findings, the SSS is associated with low Conscientiousness at least as strongly as with high Extraversion (Zuckerman, 2005; Zuckerman et al., 1993).

5. The association of impulsivity and externalizing behavior with Openness/Intellect is likely to be complex because, in addition to being associated with Extraversion, Openness/Intellect is the only Big Five trait consistently associated positively with intelligence (DeYoung et al., 2005). Intelligence, however, is negatively associated with impulsivity and externalizing behavior (DeYoung et al., 2008; Kuntsi et al., 2004). The apparent paradox can be resolved by the observation that Openness/Intellect is associated with intelligence independently of its association with Extraversion (DeYoung et al., 2005, 2008). Thus, there are two distinct pools of variance in Openness/Intellect, and we found them to be associated in opposite directions with externalizing behavior (DeYoung et al., 2008). This suggests that, to the degree that Openness/Intellect entails being exploratory, it may increase impulsivity, or at least sensation seeking, whereas, to the degree that it entails being intelligent, it reduces impulsivity.

REFERENCES

Ainsley, G. (2001). *Breakdown of will*. New York: Cambridge University Press.

Aluja, A., García, O., & García, L. F. (2003). Relationships among extraversion, openness to experience, and sensation seeking. *Personality and Individual Differences, 35*, 671–680.

Arnsten, A. F. T., & Robbins, T. W. (2002). Neurochemical modulation of prefrontal cortical function. In D. T. Stuss & R. T. Knight (Eds.), *Principles of frontal lobe function* (pp. 51–84). New York: Oxford University Press.

Ashton, M. C., Lee, K., Perugini, M., Szarota, P., de Vries, R. E., Blas, L. D., et al. (2004). A six-factor structure of personality descriptive adjectives: Solutions from psycholexical studies in seven languages. *Journal of Personality and Social Psychology, 86*, 356–366.

Avila, C., Cuenca, I., Felix, V., Parcet, M. A., & Miranda, A. (2004). Measuring impulsivity in school-aged boys and examining its relationship with ADHD and ODD ratings. *Journal of Abnormal Child Psychology, 32,* 295–304.

Berridge, K. C., & Robinson, T. E. (1998). What is the role of dopamine in reward?: Hedonic impact, reward learning, or incentive salience? *Brain Research Reviews, 28,* 309–369.

Block, J. (2002). *Personality as an affect-processing system: Toward an integrative theory.* Mahwah, NJ: Erlbaum.

Braver, T. S., & Barch, D. M. (2002). A theory of cognitive control, aging cognition, and neuromodulation. *Neuroscience and Biobehavioral Review, 26,* 809–817.

Carver, C. S., Johnson, S. L., & Joormann, J. (2009). Two-mode models of self-regulation as a tool for conceptualizing effects of the serotonin system in normal behavior and diverse disorders. *Current Directions in Psychological Science, 18,* 195–199.

Chambers, R. A., Taylor, J. R., & Potenza, M. N. (2003). Developmental neurocircuitry of motivation in adolescence: A critical period of addiction vulnerability. *American Journal of Psychiatry, 160,* 1041–1052.

Clark, L. A., & Watson, D. (2008). Temperament: An organizing paradigm for trait psychology. In O. P. John, R. W. Robins, & L. A. Pervin (Eds.), *Handbook of personality: Theory and research* (pp. 265–286). New York: Guilford Press.

Congdon, E., & Canli, T. (2008). A neurogenetic approach to impulsivity. *Journal of Personality, 76,* 1447–1483.

Costa, P. T., Jr., & McCrae, R. R. (1992). *NEO PI-R professional manual.* Odessa, FL: Psychological Assessment Resources.

Cyders, M. A., & Smith, G. A. (2008). Emotion-based dispositions to rash action: Positive and Negative Urgency. *Psychological Bulletin, 134,* 807–828.

Cyders, M. A., Smith, G. T., Spillane, N. S., Fischer, S., Annus, A. M., & Peterson, C. (2007). Integration of impulsivity and positive mood to predict risky behavior: Development and validation of a measure of positive urgency. *Psychological Assessment, 19,* 107–118.

Deary, I. (2001). Human intelligence differences: A recent history. *Trends in Cognitive Sciences, 5,* 127–130.

Depue, R. A., & Collins, P. F. (1999). Neurobiology of the structure of personality: Dopamine, facilitation of incentive motivation, and extraversion. *Behavioral and Brain Sciences, 22,* 491–569.

Depue, R. A., & Lenzenweger, M. F. (2005). A neurobehavioral dimensional model of personality disturbance. In M. F. Lenzenweger & J. Clarkin (Eds.), *Theories of personality disorders* (2nd ed., pp. 391–454). New York: Guilford Press.

DeYoung, C. G. (2006). Higher-order factors of the Big Five in a multi-informant sample. *Journal of Personality and Social Psychology, 91,* 1138–1151.

DeYoung, C. G., & Gray, J. R. (2009). Personality neuroscience: Explaining individual differences in affect, behavior, and cognition. In P. J. Corr & G. Matthews (Eds.), *The Cambridge handbook of personality psychology* (pp. 323–346). New York: Cambridge University Press.

DeYoung, C. G., Hirsh, J. B., Shane, M. S., Papademetris, X., Rajeevan, N., & Gray, J. R. (2010). Testing predictions from personality neuroscience: Brain structure and the Big Five. *Psychological Science, 21,* 820–828.

DeYoung, C. G., Peterson, J. B., & Higgins, D. M. (2002). Higher-order factors of the Big Five predict conformity: Are there neuroses of health? *Personality and Individual Differences, 33,* 533–552.

DeYoung, C. G., Peterson, J. B., & Higgins, D. M. (2005). Sources of Openness/Intellect: Cognitive and neuropsychological correlates of the fifth factor of personality. *Journal of Personality, 73,* 825–858.

DeYoung, C. G., Peterson, J. B., Séguin, J. R., Pihl, R. O., & Tremblay, R. E. (2008). Externalizing behavior and the higher-order factors of the Big Five. *Journal of Abnormal Psychology, 117,* 947–953.

DeYoung, C. G., Quilty, L. C., & Peterson, J. B. (2007). Between facets and domains: 10 aspects of the Big Five. *Journal of Personality and Social Psychology, 93,* 880–896.

Dickman, S. J. (1990). Functional and dysfunctional impulsivity: personality and cognitive correlates. *Journal of Personality and Social Psychology, 58,* 95–102.

Digman, J. M. (1997). Higher-order factors of the Big Five. *Journal of Personality and Social Psychology, 73,* 1246–1256.

Edmonds, G. W., Bogg, T., & Roberts, B. W. (2009). Are personality and behavioral measures of impulse control convergent or distinct predictors of health behaviors? *Journal of Research in Personality, 43,* 806–814.

Evenden, J. L. (1999). Varieties of impulsivity. *Psychopharmacology, 146,* 348–361.

Eysenck, H. J. (1947). *Dimensions of personality.* New York: Methuen.

Eysenck, S. B., & Eysenck, H. J. (1977). The place of impulsiveness in a dimensional system of personality description. *British Journal of Social and Clinical Psychology, 16*(1), 57–68.

Eysenck, S. B. G., Pearson, P. R., Easting, G., & Allsopp, J. F. (1985). Age norms for impulsiveness, venturesomeness and empathy in adults. *Personality and Individual Differences, 6,* 613–619.

Fischer, S., & Smith, G. T. (2004). Deliberation affects risk taking beyond sensation seeking. *Personality and Individual Differences, 36,* 527–537.

Flory, J. D., Harvey, P. D., Mitropoulou, V., New, A. S., Silverman, J. M., Siever, L. J., et al. (2006). Dispositional impulsivity in normal and abnormal samples. *Journal of Psychiatric Research, 40,* 438–447.

Goldberg, L. R. (1999). A broad-bandwidth, public domain, personality inventory measuring the lower-level facets of several five-factor models. In I. Mervielde, I. Deary, F. De Fruyt, & F. Ostendorf (Eds.), *Personality psychology in Europe* (Vol. 7, pp. 7–28). Tilburg, The Netherlands: Tilburg University Press.

Goldberg, L. R., & Rosolack, T. K. (1994). The Big Five factor structure as an integrative framework: An empirical comparison with Eysenck's P-E-N model. In C. F. Halverson, Jr., G. A. Kohnstamm, & R. P. Martin (Eds.), *The developing structure of temperament and personality from infancy to adulthood* (pp. 7–35). Hillsdale, NJ: Erlbaum.

Gray, J. A., & McNaughton, N. (2000). *The neuropsychology of anxiety: An enquiry into the functions of the septo-hippocampal system.* New York: Oxford University Press.

Harris, S. E., Wright, A. F., Hayward, C., Starr, J. M., Whalley, L. J., & Deary, I. J. (2005). The functional COMT polymorphism, Val158Met, is associated with logical memory and the personality trait intellect/imagination in a cohort of healthy 79 year olds. *Neuroscience Letters, 385,* 1–6.

Hirsh, J. B., DeYoung, C. G., & Peterson, J. B. (2009). Metatraits of the Big Five differentially predict engagement and restraint of behavior. *Journal of Personality, 77,* 1085–1102.

Hofmann, W., Friese, M., & Strack, F. (2009). Impulse and self-control from a dual-systems perspective. *Perspectives on Psychological Science, 4,* 162–176.

Hofstee, W. K., de Raad, B., & Goldberg, L. R. (1992). Integration of the Big Five and circumplex approaches to trait structure. *Journal of Personality and Social Psychology, 63,* 146–163.

Jang, K. L., Hu, S., Livesley, W. J., Angleitner, A., Riemann, R., Ando, J., et al. (2001). Covariance structure of Neuroticism and Agreeableness: A twin and molecular genetic analysis of the role of the serotonin transporter gene. *Journal of Personality and Social Psychology, 81,* 295–304.

John, O. P., Naumann, L. P., & Soto, C. J. (2008). Paradigm shift to the integrative Big Five trait taxonomy: History, measurement, and conceptual issues. In O. P. John, R. W. Robins, & L. A. Pervin (Eds.), *Handbook of personality: Theory and research* (pp. 114–158). New York: Guilford Press.

Johnson, J. A. (1994). Clarification of factor five with the help of the AB5C model. *European Journal of Personality, 8,* 311–334.

Keilp, J. G., Sackeim, H. A., & Mann, J. J. (2005) Correlates of trait impulsiveness in performance measures and neuropsychological tests. *Psychiatry Research, 135,* 191–201.

Kirby, K. N. (2009). One-year temporal stability of delay-discount rates. *Psychonomic Bulletin and Review, 16,* 457–462.

Krueger, R. F., Hicks, B. M., Patrick, C. J., Carlson, S. R., Iacono, W. G., & McGue, M. (2002). Etiologic connections among substance dependence, antisocial behavior, and personality: Modeling the externalizing spectrum. *Journal of Abnormal Psychology, 111,* 411–424.

Krueger, R. F., Markon, K. E., Patrick, C. J., Benning, S. D., & Kramer, M. D. (2007). Linking antisocial behavior, substance use, and personality: An integrative quantitative model of the adult externalizing spectrum. *Journal of Abnormal Psychology, 116,* 645–666.

Kruesi, M., Rapoport, J., Hamburger, S., Hibbs, E., Potter, W., Levane, M., et al. (1990). Cerebrospinal fluid monoamine metabolites, aggression, and impulsivity in disruptive behavior disorders of children and adolescents. *Archives of General Psychiatry, 47,* 419–426.

Kuntsi, J., Eley, T. C., Taylor, A., Hughes, C., Ascheron, P., Caspi, A., et al. (2004). Co-occurrence of ADHD and low IQ has genetic origins. *American Journal of Medical Genetics, 124B,* 41–47.

Leth-Steensen, C., King Elbaz, Z., & Douglas, V. I. (2000). Mean response times, variability, and skew in the responding of ADHD children: A response time distributional approach. *Acta Psychologica, 104,* 167–190.

Logan, G. D., Schachar, R. J., & Tannock, R. (1997). Impulsivity and inhibitory control. *Psychological Science, 8,* 60–64.

Manuck, S. B., Flory, J. D., McCaffery, J. M., Matthews, K. A., Mann, J. J., & Muldoon, M. F. (1998). Aggression, impulsivity, and central nervous system serotonergic responsivity in a nonpatient sample. *Neuropsychopharmacology, 19,* 287–299.

Markon, K. E., & Krueger, R. F. (2006). Categorical and continuous models of liability to externalizing disorders: A direct comparison in NESARC. *Archives of General Psychiatry, 62,* 1352–1359.

Markon, K. E., Krueger, R. F., & Watson, D. (2005). Delineating the structure of normal and abnormal personality: An integrative hierarchical approach. *Journal of Personality and Social Psychology, 88,* 139–157.

McCrae, R. R., Jang, K. L., Ando, J., Ono, Y., Yamagata, S., Riemann, R., et al. (2008). Substance and artifact in the higher-order factors of the Big Five. *Journal of Personality and Social Psychology, 95,* 442–455.

Meier, B. P., Robinson, M. D., & Wilkowski, B. M. (2006). Turning the other cheek: Agreeableness and the regulation of aggression-related primes. *Psychological Science, 17,* 136–142.

Miller, E. K., & Cohen, J. D. (2001). An integrative theory of prefrontal cortex function. *Annual Review of Neuroscience, 24,* 167–202.

Miller, J. D., Flory, K., Lynam, D. R., & Leukefeld, C. (2003). A test of the four-factor model of impulsivity-related traits. *Personality and Individual Differences, 34,* 1403–1418.

Miller, J. D., & Lynam, D. R. (2001). Structural models of personality and their relation to antisocial behavior: A meta-analytic review. *Criminology, 39,* 765–798.

Olson, K. R. (2005). Engagement and self-control: Superordinate dimensions of Big Five traits. *Personality and Individual Differences, 38,* 1689–1700.

Panksepp, J. (1998). *Affective neuroscience: The foundations of human and animal emotion.* New York: Oxford University Press.

Parker, J. D. A., Bagby, R. M., & Webster, C. D. (1993). Domains of the impulsivity construct: A factor analytic investigation. *Personality and Individual Differences, 15,* 267–274.

Patton, J. H., Stanford, M. S., & Barratt, E. S. (1995). Factor structure of the Barratt Impulsiveness Scale. *Journal of Clinical Psychology, 6,* 768–774.

Reynolds, B., Ortengren, A., Richards, J. B., & de Wit, H. (2006). Dimensions of impulsive behavior: Personality and behavioral measures. *Personality and Individual Differences, 40,* 305–315.

Roberts, B. W., Chernyshenko, O. S., Stark, S., & Goldberg, L. R. (2005). The structure of Conscientiousness: An empirical investigation based on seven major personality questionnaires. *Personnel Psychology, 58,* 103–139.

Saucier, G., & Goldberg, L. R. (2001). Lexical studies of indigenous personality factors: Premises, products, and prospects. *Journal of Personality, 69,* 847–879.

Smith, G. T., Fischer, S., Cyders, M. A., Annus, A. M., Spillane, N. S., & McCarthy, D. M. (2007). On the validity of discriminating among impulsivity-like traits. *Assessment, 14,* 155–170.

Spinella, M. (2004). Neurobehavioral correlates of impulsivity: Evidence of prefrontal involvement. *International Journal of Neuroscience, 114,* 95–104.

Spoont, M. R. (1992). Modulatory role of serotonin in neural information processing: Implications for human psychopathology. *Psychological Bulletin, 112,* 330–350.

Swann, A. C., Bjork, J. M., Moeller, F. G., & Dougherty, D. M. (2002). Two models of impulsivity: Relationship to personality traits and psychopathology. *Biological Psychiatry, 51,* 988–994.

Tangney, J. P., Baumeister, R. F., & Boone, A. L. (2004). High self-control predicts good adjustment, less pathology, better grades, and interpersonal success. *Journal of Personality, 72,* 271–324.

Tellegen, A., & Waller, N. G. (2008). Exploring personality through test construction: Development of the Multidimensional Personality Questionnaire. In G. J. Boyle, G. Matthews, & D. H. Saklofske (Eds.), *Handbook of personality theory and testing: Vol. II. Personality measurement and assessment* (pp. 261–292). London: Sage.

Trull, T. J., & Sher, K. J. (1994). Relationship between the five-factor model of personality and Axis I disorders in a nonclinical sample. *Journal of Abnormal Psychology, 103,* 350–360.

Van Egeren, L. F. (2009). A cybernetic model of global personality traits. *Personality and Social Psychology Review, 13,* 92–108.

Wacker, J., Chavanon, M.-L., & Stemmler, G. (2006). Investigating the dopaminergic basis of Extraversion in humans: A multilevel approach. *Journal of Personality and Social Psychology, 91,* 171–187.

Whiteside, S. P., & Lynam, R. W. (2001). The five factor model and impulsivity: Using a structural model of personality to understand impulsivity. *Personality and Individual Differences, 30,* 669–689.

Whiteside, S. P., Lynam, D. R., Miller, J. D., & Reynolds, S. K. (2005). Validation of the UPPS Impulsive Behavior Scale: A four-factor model of impulsivity. *European Journal of Personality, 19,* 559–574.

Zeidner, M., & Matthews, G. (2000). Intelligence and personality. In R. Sternberg (Ed.), *Handbook of intelligence* (pp. 581–610). New York: Cambridge University Press.

Zuckerman, M. (1979). *Sensation seeking: Beyond the optimal level of arousal.* Hillsdale, NJ: Erlbaum.

Zuckerman, M. (2005). *Psychobiology of personality* (2nd ed., revised and updated). New York: Cambridge University Press.

Zuckerman, M., Kuhlman, D. M., Joireman, J., Teta, P., & Kraft, M. (1993). A comparison of three structural models of personality: The Big Three, the Big Five, and the Alternative Five. *Journal of Personality and Social Psychology, 65,* 757–768.

PART VI

COMMON PROBLEMS WITH SELF-REGULATION

CHAPTER 27

Self-Regulatory Failure and Addiction

MICHAEL A. SAYETTE
KASEY M. GRIFFIN

Since the publication of *Losing Control: How and Why People Fail at Self-Regulation* (Baumeister, Heatherton, & Tice, 1994) there has been a proliferation of research examining self-regulatory processes and addiction (see Hull & Slone, 2004; Sayette, 2004). Borrowing from Baumeister et al. (1994), in our chapter in the first edition of this volume, we considered self-regulation to refer generally to any effort by a human being to alter his or her own responses (Sayette, 2004). With respect to addiction, self-regulation often refers to an attempt to override a well-learned drug use behavior or habit in order to realize a positive long-term outcome. As outlined by Baumeister and colleagues (1994), the constituent actions required for drug use (e.g., asking a friend for a cigarette, holding it, lighting it) are voluntary behaviors that can be controlled. Accordingly, drug use is a particularly interesting domain for examining self-regulation failure.

Self-regulation failure can be subdivided into failures of *underregulation* and *misregulation*. The former refers to a failure to exert control over oneself, whereas the latter refers to exerting control in a way that fails to produce the desired result (Baumeister et al., 1994). Both types of self-regulation failures likely contribute to addictive behavior and are addressed herein.

This chapter summarizes and updates our previous review of the relation between nicotine addiction (more specifically, cigarette smoking) and self-regulation (Sayette, 2004). There are several reasons why smoking presents an ideal model for considering the relation between self-regulation and addiction. First, although millions of Americans try to quit smoking each year, 81% of these attempts fail within the first month (Hughes et al., 1992), suggesting that nicotine is an especially good drug to consider when examining self-regulatory failure. Second, the public health implications of nicotine dependence dwarf those of all other drugs (U.S. Department of Health and Human Services [USD-HHS], 1989), highlighting the importance of studying self-regulatory processes related to smoking. Third, compared to other substances, such as alcohol, nicotine is an especially addictive drug, and the majority of regular users become dependent. Fourth, because withdrawal states can be induced via robust deprivation manipulations in a medically safe manner, a substantial amount of research has examined smoking motivation and self-regulatory processes.

Smokers may require self-regulation under two different circumstances. During periods of abstinence–avoidance, one desires to smoke but cigarettes are unavailable (e.g., while watching a film in a theater). Self-regulation here may reflect a need to override temporary urges. In contrast, during periods of abstinence seeking, one wishes to abstain. As noted by Tiffany (1990), in either case, a smoker may experience cravings. Effective self-regulation typically requires overriding the craving to smoke. Accordingly, research protocols that provoke cigarette cravings provide a suitable environment for investigating self-regulation.

Research interest in craving has intensified in recent years [e.g., see special issue of *Addiction* (2000) devoted to craving]. *Craving*, a term often used interchangeably with *urge*, is provoked using a variety of manipulations, including drug deprivation, drug use imagery, and drug cue exposure (Niaura et al., 1988; Sayette et al., 2000; Tiffany, 1992).

This chapter addresses research examining self-regulation difficulties faced by smokers who have already developed the habit. (Readers interested in the role of self-regulation in the initiation of smoking are referred elsewhere; e.g., Baumeister et al., 1994; Rawn & Vohs, Chapter 20, this volume). Misregulation failures are discussed first, followed by an analysis of the role of underregulation in smoking.

MISREGULATION

Most discussion of self-regulation failure and addiction has centered on underregulation. Many problems linked to addiction, however, also can be conceived of as misregulation, in which one exerts control in a way that fails to bring about the desired result (Baumeister et al., 1994). Rather than assuming that a person who experiences a smoking lapse (i.e., an initial violation of abstinence) does so due to a breakdown in impulse control, it is possible that the act of smoking represents an attempt, albeit misguided, to address a critical problem for the smoker.

One example of misregulation among smokers is the belief that quitting smoking will lead to weight gain (Baumeister et al., 1994; Levine, Marcus, Kalarchian, Weissfeld, & Qin, 2006). Although quitting often is linked to an increase of 5 or 10 pounds, there is overwhelming evidence that the harmful effects of continuing to smoke override this short-term weight gain (Baumeister et al., 1994). Thus, smoking is mistakenly viewed as a "reasonable" method for controlling weight.

A second example of misregulation is the use of cigarettes to improve mood (Conklin & Perkins, 2005). A fundamental question regarding nicotine addiction concerns why a smoker who appears to be committed to quitting will suffer a smoking lapse. It often is assumed that such a lapse indicates a breakdown in impulse control. Alternatively, a lapse may represent a strategic attempt to regulate affect. Tice, Bratslavsky, and Baumeister (2001) found that after a negative affect induction, impulsive behaviors—such as eating fattening, tasty snacks—occurred only when participants believed that their mood was modifiable. When they believed that their negative affective state was "frozen," participants' desire to engage in impulsive behaviors was not enhanced. Tice and colleagues concluded that regardless of the ultimate success of these actions, the "impulsive" behavior may be viewed as a rational attempt to address a pressing concern.

The research by Tice and colleagues (2001) suggests that a former smoker who is under stress may lapse because the short-term need to alleviate negative affect becomes particularly salient. This begs a question that has interested addiction researchers for years: Just how often does a lapse or relapse occur during moments of distress? Early models of addiction articulated by Wikler (1948) and Conger (1956), for example, posited that drugs and alcohol were consumed by addicts to alleviate negative affective states. These initial negative reinforcement models have been challenged (see Tiffany, 1990). It has been suggested, for instance, that smokers who lapse or relapse often do not report experiencing negative affect (Shiffman et al., 2002), and that many "absentminded lapses" seem to occur outside of awareness (Tiffany, 1990).

Nevertheless, updated versions of negative reinforcement models assert that the chief component of the withdrawal response is negative affect, and that with some modifications to original formulations, "escape and avoidance of negative affect is the prepotent motive for addictive drug use" (Baker, Piper, McCarthy, Majeskie, & Fiore, 2004, p. 33). These authors examined a diverse set of animal and human studies to address many of the criticisms leveled against negative reinforcement models. Their review suggests that, construed broadly, the alleviation or prevention of negative affect can motivate some, if not most, lapses (see also Brownell, Marlatt, Lichtenstein, & Wilson, 1986; Piper et al., 2008).

If smoking a cigarette is viewed as an attempt to improve mood, then treatments that focus on mood regulation may prove effective. Consistent with this position is the success of the antidepressant bupropion (e.g., McCarthy et al., 2008). In addition, as argued by Baker and colleagues (2004), even nicotine replacement products suppress negative affect. From a psychological perspective, smoking cessation treatments that ignore concerns related to negative affect are unlikely to succeed.

UNDERREGULATION

As noted earlier, much of the smoking research on self-regulation failure has emphasized underregulation. Baumeister and colleagues (1994) discussed three basic features of self-regulation that may fail and lead to underregulation: (1) setting proper standards; (2) monitoring oneself in relation to these standards, and (3) altering one's responses to conform to these standards. Though not all the findings addressed below fit cleanly into just one of these categories, it nevertheless remains heuristic to retain this structure.

Setting Standards

Difficulty setting proper standards may interfere with smoking cessation. Most smokers believe that smoking is a bad habit that they would like to break (Baumeister et al., 1994). Yet smokers may hold distorted standards related to smoking and health (Kunda, 1990). In a prospective study of smokers attempting to quit, Gibbons and Eggleston (1996) found that a smoker's perception of the "typical smoker" at the outset of treatment was a reliable predictor of relapse. Specifically, those vulnerable to relapse were more likely to view typical smokers in a positive light than were those who successfully quit. Thus, people who continue to smoke may construct a standard of what it means to be a smoker that protects them from feeling irrational for maintaining their habit. Research from a social learning perspective may shed light on how such standards may develop (Marlatt & Gordon, 1985).

Rather than viewing standards solely as stable character traits, it may be useful to consider standards as being subject to momentary fluctuations. Specifically, when smokers crave a cigarette, the way that they think about smoking may change. In her theory of motivated reasoning, Kunda (1990) suggested that motivation could bias how one generates and evaluates information related to the topic of interest. The degree of change in generation and evaluation of information may be a function of one's momentary level of smoking motivation (Sayette, 2004).

As detailed in Sayette (2004) we have tested the effects of craving on the generation of smoking-related information in a study that required smokers to attend two (counterbalanced) laboratory sessions within 10 days of each other (Sayette & Hufford, 1997). While in high- and low-urge conditions, smokers listed as many positive, then negative, characteristics of smoking as they could. Smokers generated significantly more positive items about smoking during the high-urge session than they did during the low-urge assessment. Although craving increased generation of positive smoking-related information, it did not have this effect on negative information. Indeed, craving led to a nonsignificant drop in the generation of negative smoking-related information. Thus, while craving, smokers generated a list of smoking characteristics that was positively biased, relative to when they were not craving.

Craving also may be associated with the way that smoking-related information is evaluated. Sayette, Martin, Wertz, Shiffman, and Perrott (2001) examined the effects of craving on the evaluation of smoking consequences. While holding a lit cigarette, abstinent and nonabstinent smokers were asked to rate the probability that a list of smoking consequences would occur. Abstinent smokers tended to judge positive consequences to be more probable, relative to negative ones, than did nonabstinent smokers. As suggested by Marlatt (1985), craving may distort outcome expectancies, such that positive outcomes appear more likely than negative ones.

These studies suggest that standards related to smoking may be viewed differently when one is in a craving state than when one is in a neutral state (Sayette, 2004). Consequently, measuring one's views about smoking may require careful consideration of the assessment context. A clinician who learns that a smoker holds a negative view of smoking and is motivated to quit may be surprised to learn of a quick relapse. Had these standards been assessed while the smoker was in a craving state (or perhaps while intoxicated) (Kirchner & Sayette, 2007), the information might have revealed that the smoker was ambivalent about giving up the habit. After all, it takes only a single moment of weakness during a high-risk situation for a committed quitter to reconsider and smoke a cigarette.

In addition to appreciating the importance of momentary shifts in attitudes, another complicating factor when considering standards is that smokers may simultaneously hold conflicting standards. For instance, they may believe it is foolish to risk their health by continuing to smoke, yet also believe that because life is uncertain, they might as well enjoy the moment (Stritzke, Breiner, Curtin, & Lang, 2004). Which of these standards predominates may switch moment to moment and when craving, a standard that promotes smoking may emerge.

In summary, there are myriad ways that one's standards regarding smoking may contribute to underregulation. The concept of smoking or being a smoker may shift over time as a smoker becomes more committed to the habit. Furthermore, at particular moments, such as when motivation to smoke is high, one's standards may tilt even more toward a smoking promotion position.

Monitoring

Research also has focused on the adverse consequences of failing to monitor one's thoughts, feelings, and actions with respect to one's standards. Even if one holds standards that promote smoking cessation, it remains important to monitor oneself in relation to these standards. The need to monitor oneself vigilantly is thought to be instrumental in preventing relapse (Brownell et al., 1986).

Attention plays a critical role in monitoring. Baumeister and colleagues (1994) argued that managing attention may be the most effective approach to self-regulation. An individual can exercise self-regulation by attending to information that reaches beyond the immediate stimulus environment, what Baumeister and colleagues label *transcendence*. Rather than merely focusing on the immediate object of desire, one engages in high-level thinking that recognizes the standards that promote self-regulation. Such perspective is needed to override impulses. In contrast, transcendence failure occurs when an individual attends only to the immediate present and does not monitor discrepancies between current interests and long-term goals.

Monitoring requires self-awareness, which is often compromised during high-risk moments. Social cues (e.g., celebrations) have been implicated in smoking relapse (Brownell et al., 1986). Presumably these situations do not provide fertile ground for self-reflection and monitoring. Similarly, monitoring may prove difficult during highly emotional states. Baumeister and colleagues (1994) posit that affectively charged moments may focus attention on immediate stimuli, leaving little attention available for self-reflection. Consistent with these findings, we recently found that craving increased mindwandering, while reducing the likelihood of noticing that one's mind has wandered (Sayette, Schooler, & Reichle, 2010).

It also is likely that monitoring of standards related to smoking will be inhibited following alcohol consumption. There is evidence that drinking alcohol increases smoking behavior and smoking motivation (see Piasecki, McCarthy, Fiore, & Baker, 2008; Sayette, Martin, et al., 2005). Moreover, relapse to smoking occurs more often after drinking alcohol than after any other identified situational variable (Shiffman & Balabanis, 1995). Several models of the effects of alcohol suggest that drinking impairs cognitive processes (Hull & Slone, 2004). Whether due to an impaired ability to encode information in terms of self-relevance (Hull, 1987), difficulty monitoring internal processes (Sayette, Reichle, & Schooler, 2009), or a reduced capacity to focus on information other than immediate smoking cues (Steele & Josephs, 1990), alcohol intoxication may impede self-regulation by compromising the ability to monitor performance relative to standards (Baumeister et al., 1994). (If cues that inhibit smoking are salient, however, then intoxication might even support self-regulation [MacDonald, Fong, Zanna, & Martineau, 2000].) Research that addresses directly the effects of alcohol on the monitoring of standards and norms would be useful.

One final danger related to monitoring is that smokers may have developed unrealistic expectations about the impact of quitting. Smokers may assume, for example, that quitting will influence all aspects of their lives. Although quitting is likely to improve health, it may not substantially affect one's personality. When cessation fails to produce such global change, monitoring may have the unfortunate effect of revealing a substandard outcome and may precipitate a relapse. This process has been referred to as the "false hope syndrome" (Polivy, 2000). (For a review of behavioral health change models and possible reasons for relapse, see Rothman, Baldwin, and Hertel [2004].)

Altering Responses

Smokers may recognize that smoking conflicts with their standards, and they may be able to monitor a discrepancy between their smoking behavior and their standards, yet still experience a lapse. Indeed, the bulk of research on self-regulation failure centers on an inability to exercise the necessary control or discipline to resist a temptation to smoke. Baumeister and colleagues (1994) have conceived of this control in terms of *strength*. From this perspective, a smoker requires sufficient "muscle" to resist the impulse to smoke (see Baumeister, Vohs, & Tice, 2007; Muraven & Baumeister, 2000). These authors propose that repeated encounters with high-risk situations over a particular time interval may deplete muscle strength, leaving one vulnerable to a lapse.

The concept of self-regulation strength has been examined from three perspectives. The first relates to stable individual differences. Certain people may be "weak" and lack the inhibition necessary to resist succumbing to temptation. This person-level analysis of smoking is likely to yield important individual-difference markers for relapse risk (Shiffman & Balabanis, 1995).

A second approach to examining strength involves situational constraints that deplete the limited capacity resources needed to resist a temptation to smoke (Baumeister et al., 1994; Tiffany, 1990). Given the effort required to override a temptation to smoke, factors that undermine limited capacity processing resources should hamper self-regulation. For instance, fatigue may prevent effective self-regulatory behavior in the face of a smoking urge. Accordingly, Baumeister and colleagues (1994) suggest that smokers attempt smoking cessation at a time when other demands requiring self-control are relatively low. Recent naturalistic studies using ecological momentary assessment have, however, yielded mixed findings (cf. Muraven, Collins, Shiffman, & Paty, 2005; O'Connell, Schwartz, & Shiffman, 2008). In theory, while under stress, a person may be too exhausted to combat a strong urge to smoke. Stressors that threaten one's self-concept or that require self-monitoring may be especially exhausting.

Related to stress is tobacco withdrawal. It has been suggested that subtle effects of tobacco withdrawal can begin to occur even after very brief periods of abstinence (Hughes, 1991). Furthermore, it has been argued that the cardinal feature of withdrawal is negative affect, or stress (Baker et al., 2004). From a self-regulatory strength perspective, people may smoke when distressed because they cannot cope simultaneously with the stressors and their cravings.

Because alcohol demands limited capacity, nonautomatic resources (Josephs & Steele, 1990), presumably there would be insufficient cognitive capacity to override a well-learned smoking routine during intoxication (Sayette, Martin, et al., 2005; Tiffany, 1990). Moreover, because alcohol can cue smoking (e.g., Erblich, Montgomery, & Bovbjerg, 2009), drinking may initiate automatized smoking behavior (Burton & Tiffany, 1997). Thus, like fatigue and stress, drinking alcohol is likely to compromise one's ability to alter responses in the service of self-regulation.

Another area of cognition that may affect self-regulation is time perception. Data suggest that while waiting to smoke, time may seem to pass more rapidly when subjects are not craving than when they are in a craving state (Klein, Corwin, & Stine, 2003; Sayette, Loewenstein, Kirchner, Travis, 2005). These data are in accord with recent findings that the act of self-regulation changes the subjective experience of time, such that time feels more extended than it really is, and this state leads to subsequent failures in self-regulation (Vohs & Schmeichel, 2003).

The third approach to examining strength involves temporary states influenced by appetitive cues. Smokers may lack the strength to resist an urge due not only to a weakness—whether it be chronic or temporary—but also because of powerful appetitive stimuli. Studies reveal that craving disrupts limited capacity processes (see Sayette, 2004). In several studies across multiple laboratories, exposure to smoking cues, for example, led smokers to respond more slowly during a secondary-response time probe than during exposure to control cues, suggesting that limited capacity nonautomatic processing resources were diverted during the craving manipulation (see Sayette, 2004). These performance deficits suggest a demand on processing resources during craving.

If smoking does represent a well-learned routine, then it will likely take considerable effort, requiring limited capacity, nonautomatic resources to refrain from completing the smoking action sequence once it has been initiated (Tiffany, 1990). Indeed, the ability to override a well-learned habitual behavior is the central feature of self-regulation (Baumeister et al., 1994). Baumeister and colleagues (1994) also suggest that the further into the routine, the more difficult (i.e., the more cognitive resources will be required) it is to terminate. Thus, it is far easier to resist smoking when one first sees a friend smoking than after lighting and holding the cigarette that is offered, a process they label *psychological inertia*.

After a smoking routine is activated, limited capacity cognitive resources are likely directed toward several other functions, in addition to struggling to resist completing the routine (Sayette, Martin, Hull, Wertz, & Perrott, 2003). Resources may be directed toward monitoring: the level of motivation or desire to use the drug (e.g., "I really want a cigarette"); the drug cues themselves (e.g., thoughts of how the cigarette will feel in one's hand); anticipated positive effects of smoking (e.g., "If I smoke this cigarette, then I will feel better"); feelings associated with the event (e.g., frustration that one's friend lit a cigarette in one's presence); as well as problem-solving cognitions associated with completing the smoking action plan (e.g., "How can I hide this cigarette from my spouse?"). Resources directed toward any of these cognitions leave less resources available for successful self-regulation involved in maintaining abstinence.

Addiction researchers have used measures other than secondary response time probes to examine shifts in attention and cognitive processing during high-risk situations (Waters & Sayette, 2006). An increasingly popular measure of attentional bias is the *color-naming task*, also called the emotional Stroop task. In this task, participants name the color of words while ignoring word content. When words are personally or emotionally relevant, individuals are thought to be drawn to them automatically, and the latency period required to name the color of the word generally increases. A number of emotional Stroop studies has shown that smokers display greater response interference when presented with smoking-related words during withdrawal than when they were permitted to smoke normally (for reviews, see Cox, Fadardi, & Pothos, 2006; Field, Munafò, & Franken, 2009; Waters & Sayette, 2006). These data are consistent with models of addiction emphasizing shifts in the incentive salience of drug cues, such that these cues "grab attention" and cue the addict to engage in further drug use (Robinson & Berridge, 1993, p. 261).

Recently, we found that performance on a version of the emotional Stroop task on quit day predicted subsequent relapse, even after we controlled for self-reported urge (Waters et al., 2003). Thus, during moments of temptation, attention appears to be biased toward smoking-related stimuli. Such a drift may hamper the ability to produce regulating responses, also known as *coping responses*. Indeed, recently there have been attempts to train smokers and drinkers to overcome their automatic distraction for alcohol- and smoking-related stimuli (Attwood, O'Sullivan, Leonards, Mackintosh, & Munafo, 2008; Wiers, Houben, Smulders, Conrod, & Jones, 2006).

The issue of coping is particularly important when we discuss self-regulation. Smokers who relapse often fail to use coping skills (Shiffman, 1982). In many cases, relapsers fail despite having obtained relevant coping skills (Brandon, Tiffany, Obremski, & Baker, 1990). As reviewed in the first edition of this volume (Sayette, 2004) studies suggest a direct connection between temptation and the ability to cope with temptation, such that high-urge situations are associated with weak coping responses.

As cravings emerge, coping resources may become inaccessible or coping resources may remain accessible but smokers may just choose not to engage them, or both (Sayette, 2004). Regardless, the motivation to smoke may fundamentally influence the way coping-related information is processed. Thus, we might expect a smoker to generate and employ an impressive array of coping resources while experiencing a mild urge but fail to do so during a strong urge. From this perspective, it may be wiser to teach coping skills in a high-urge environment than in a sterile, low-urge context.

Related to coping is Bandura's (1997) concept of self-efficacy, which has been applied to a range of addictive behaviors (for a review of self-regulation and self-efficacy, see Cervone, Mor, Orom, Shadel, & Scott, 2004). The most prominent conceptualization of self-efficacy in the smoking literature involves *abstinence self-efficacy*, or the confidence in one's ability to abstain from smoking (Gwaltney et al., 2001). Individuals with greater confidence in their ability to abstain should be more likely to maintain abstinence (Marlatt & Gordon, 1985; Niaura et al., 1988). As we noted previously, however, pretreatment abstinence self-efficacy judgments do not always predict relapse (Sayette, 2004). Furthermore, abstinence self-efficacy does not appear to mediate the effect of concurrent smoking on future smoking (see Sayette, 2004). One reason may be that initial efficacy judgments usually are made in a neutral state, whereas the temptation periods that one must overcome to remain abstinent are typically affectively charged.

Persons in an affectively neutral "cold" state often underestimate the impact of being in an affectively charged "hot" state on their own future behavior, referred to by Loewenstein (1999) as the "cold-to-hot empathy gap." Consistent with this proposition, a disproportionate number of subjects inaccurately report maximum self-efficacy scores (for review, see Forsyth & Carey, 1998). We recently observed that smokers in a cold "low craving" state, but not those in a hot "high-craving" state, underpredicted the value of smoking during a subsequent "high craving" session (Sayette, Loewenstein, Griffin, & Black, 2008). Were initial self-efficacy assessments recorded in a craving state, which more closely approximates high-risk situations, they might prove more accurate than they typically are in prediction of quitting.

To test the relation between abstinence self-efficacy and cigarette craving we used Ecological Momentary Assessment in a sample of smokers who participated in a smoking cessation treatment (Gwaltney, Shiffman, & Sayette, 2005). Smokers reported their urge to smoke and abstinence self-efficacy using palm-top computers during multiple temptation and nontemptation periods. When smokers reported high urges, they tended to report less abstinence self-efficacy than when they were reporting weaker craving states. Thus, both laboratory and field research supports the notion that smokers' ability, and confidence in their ability, to cope with temptation diminishes during the precise moments they are most needed. In summary, there is converging evidence that cravings brought about by nicotine deprivation, smoking cue exposure, or both, may alter cognitive processes such that the ability to resist smoking may be compromised.

ACQUIESCENCE

A strength model implies that self-regulation will fail only when an individual lacks sufficient strength and is "powerless" to exert self-control. A provocative issue raised by Baumeister and colleagues (1994) was "whether people actually acquiesce in their own self-regulation failures" (p. 29). The idea is that people may sometimes, perhaps unconsciously, cooperate in their failure to self-regulate. These authors suggest that acquiescence may be common, and that few impulsive behaviors are truly involuntary. MacAndrew and Edgerton (1969), in their cross-cultural analysis of drinking behavior, posited that most societies need periods of time-out from typical standards of conduct, and that drinking alcohol implicitly permits group members to relax their behavioral norms. Similarly, Baumeister and colleagues (1994) suggested that there are times when individuals may want to loosen up and relax their level of self-awareness, which is likely to reduce further the monitoring necessary for successful self-regulation.

Although the notion that smokers may indulge their cravings has rarely been studied, indirect evidence suggests that people may sometimes acquiesce to their urges. Data across multiple substance-abusing samples indicate that exposure to drug cues leads to elevated urge ratings (see Carter &Tiffany, 1999). What is surprising is the variability in the magnitude of this effect. Addicts who are conflicted about drug use may experience their urges in a variety of ways. If they attempt to exert self-control in the situation, then they are likely motivated to suppress their urge. In contrast, were addicts at some level inclined to acquiesce and consume their drug, they would no longer be motivated to suppress their urge. Indeed, they might even wish to embellish their urge to justify drug use: "I had no real choice but to smoke. Anyone with a craving as strong as mine would have smoked." Consistent with this position, a review of cue exposure studies found that, across substances, participants who perceived an opportunity to use reported significantly higher urges than those who did not anticipate use (Wertz & Sayette, 2001).

All of the smoking cue exposure studies included in Wertz and Sayette (2001) used smokers who were not currently interested in quitting. Because these participants were still active smokers, they presumably could cope with urges by simply smoking a cigarette. Accordingly, they would be expected to report strong cigarette urges during cue exposure. Consistent with this hypothesis, these studies reveal that participants report high levels of craving (about 74% of maximum value on scales) (see Table 1 in Wertz & Sayette, 2001). In contrast, when smokers are attempting cessation, they may be motivated to cope with urges by suppressing rather than indulging them. Smokers undergoing a cue exposure assessment at the beginning of a quit attempt do report relatively low urges (Shiffman et al., 2003). We also have observed across multiple studies different neurobiological responses to drug cues based on treatment-seeking status (see Wilson, Sayette, & Fiez, 2004).

In addition to influencing the magnitude of craving, acquiescence may affect the emotional valence of a craving experience. Typically the affect associated with craving is assumed to be negative (Tiffany, 1992). When a smoker expects to satisfy an urge rather than resist it, however, he or she actually may experience positive affect. The moments just prior to use and even the beginning of consumption may be particularly positive. It is often difficult, however, to capture brief experiences of positive affect in the laboratory. Self-report measures are not ideally suited to assess moment-to-moment fluctuations in emotion response that occur over time. When participants complete self-report measures, they aggregate their experience over time. Moreover, after their responses are filtered through consciousness, they must impose language on what may be a nonverbal experience (Nisbett & Wilson, 1977).

Analysis of expressive behavior may prove to be a nice complement to more traditional measures (Sayette, Wertz, et al., 2003). The most sophisticated and established system for assessing facial expression is the Facial Action Coding System (FACS; Ekman & Friesen, 1978), an anatomically based system derived from 7,000 different expressions decomposed into 44 action units (AUs) that can be combined to describe all possible visible movements of the face. FACS has proven to be reliable and to provide accurate and specific information across a range of emotional experiences (Ekman & Rosenberg, 2005; Sayette, Cohn, Wertz, Perrott, & Parrott, 2001).

Studies using FACS indicate that manipulating instructions (i.e., informing smokers that they will or will not be able to smoke a lit cigarette) influence the probability of evincing AUs associated with either positive or negative affect (Sayette & Hufford, 1995; Sayette, Wertz, et al., 2003); that is, under certain conditions, craving may even be linked to positive affect (see also Carter & Tiffany, 2001). Similarly, Zinser, Fiore, Davidson, and Baker (1999) used an electrophysiological assessment that suggested a pattern of activation associated with approach motivation during craving. Together, these data suggest that some of the perceived reward generally associated with drug use may actually precede drug consumption. Such a proposition is consistent with recent neurobiological evidence indicating that dopamine is released during presentations of cues predictive of drug, food, and alcohol use (see Weiss et al., 2000). Thus, craving itself may be rewarding, particularly to those who anticipate using the drug very soon (Kavanagh, Andrade, & May, 2005). Loewenstein (1987) has described *savoring* as the "positive utility derived from anticipation of future consumption" (p. 667). Children who hoard their stash of Halloween candy rather than eating it, for example, may prefer savoring their candy to actually consuming it. In summary, under certain conditions, smokers may in fact acquiesce or indulge their cravings.

One further implication of acquiescence is that poor coping may not cause lapses but rather may be a reflection of an intended lapse; that is, once individuals decide, perhaps unconsciously, that they are going to indulge their craving, then it stands to reason that they will fail to employ coping skills, even those skills they have mastered. This proposition is at odds with most models of temptation and coping, which, as noted earlier, imply that poor coping causes temptations to become lapses. Alternatively, coping may be a reflection of urges, such that low urges provide opportunities to employ coping responses, while high urges, or at least urges associated with an intention to use, may to some extent preclude coping.

This alternative resembles Lazarus and Folkman's (1984) conception of stress and coping. Their three-stage appraisal model holds that an experience of stress reflects a primary appraisal of loss, threat, or harm, coupled with a secondary appraisal of coping resources available to counter the stressor. A third "reappraisal" stage, which takes into account both the primary and secondary appraisals, ultimately determines the degree of stress response. Importantly, these three appraisal processes blend together seamlessly.

In the context of craving, this model suggests that, in an instant, an "urge appraisal" can emerge that actually is a function of (1) a primary appraisal of a desire to smoke; (2) a secondary appraisal of whether one will acquiesce or attempt to resist the desire; and (3) an urge reappraisal that may reveal a high urge along with weak efforts to cope, or less intense urges accompanied by strong attempts to cope. Future research is needed to determine specifically the utility of this conceptualization of urges and coping, and more generally to explore the possible role of acquiescence in self-regulation failure.

CONCLUSIONS AND FUTURE DIRECTIONS

This chapter considered several aspects of self-regulation failure in smokers. The self-regulation framework proposed by Baumeister and colleagues (1994) continues to provide a useful structure for examining a diverse set of findings related to smoking urges and lapse. Studies suggest that misregulation may play a critical role in understanding smoking motivation. As proposed by Baker and colleagues (2004), the possibility that smoking represents an attempt to attenuate, or perhaps ward off negative moods, is a model that still warrants serious attention.

Recognition of the potential role of acquiescence in self-regulation failure highlights the need to develop multiple methods and a wide range of measures to capture processes that may not always be available to conscious awareness (Wiers & Stacy, 2006). Use of implicit cognitive measures may improve understanding of mechanisms underlying self-regulation failure and help generate predictions regarding relapse risk. As noted earlier, use of the emotional Stroop task to predict relapse highlights the importance of attentional processes in self-regulation (Waters et al., 2003).

As with cognition, improved understanding of self-regulatory process in addiction requires development of new approaches for assessing affect. The use of nonverbal measures (e.g., FACS, functional magnetic resonance imaging, electroencephalography) that are conceptually linked to theories of craving and self-regulation may prove especially useful. It remains to be seen whether particular facial expressions during cue exposure assessment might predict relapse in addiction (see Griffin & Sayette, 2008). Future research also is needed to better understand the link between affect and cognition. More generally, addiction research that accounts for affective, motivational, as well as cognitive changes, will likely prove especially useful.

Most laboratory research on self-regulatory failure in addiction uses designs in which subjects participate individually. Yet it is clear that many lapses occur in group settings. Investigations that incorporate theory and methods from social psychology will help to provide an important context for examining self-regulation (Sayette, Kirchner, Moreland, Levine, & Travis, 2004). Social comparison, group formation, and peer pressure are just a few examples of the kinds of social processes that may influence self-regulation.

Drug use requires a series of voluntary actions; thus, it is fair to claim that addiction is a failure of self-regulation (Baumeister et al., 1994; Marlatt & Gordon, 1985). Yet the studies examined in this chapter do show that during affectively charged moments, the information available to smokers may shift in a manner that promotes smoking. Given the disappointing relapse rates among smokers attempting cessation, it is imperative that researchers begin to translate these laboratory observations into clinical interventions that help smokers recognize and undermine these biases.

This chapter has not addressed individual differences that influence self-regulation processes. This area of great interest from biological, psychological, and social perspectives relates to initiation of smoking, as well as to maintenance and relapse. Indeed, it is likely that future efforts will cut across these perspectives to provide a richer understanding of self-regulation processes. Clearly, imaging research already being conducted is an illustration of such integration (Ochsner & Gross, 2007). Instead, this chapter has focused on momentary changes that may affect self-regulation. Research examining changes in cognitive processing during cigarette cravings provides insight into the role of underregulation in addiction.

Clinical Implications

The research described in this chapter also has suggested clinical applications. Cognitive-behavioral therapies emphasize that people's cognitive biases and distortions can contribute to a range of psychopathological behaviors. Often treatment involves helping patients uncover and modify these biases. In the field of addiction, preventing relapse has been the greatest clinical challenge (Brownell et al., 1986; Marlatt & Gordon, 1985). Consider the challenges awaiting smokers who have only recently quit. Data from cognitive studies suggest that when they walk down the street, there appears to be much that reminds them of a cigarette. Every cigarette butt that has been dropped on the pavement grabs their attention like a billboard. Even ambiguous cues may remind them of their habit (Sayette, 2004).

In a clinic setting, patients may be warned that they will face these temptations and will need to dispute rationally their distorted perceptions and the judgments that follow. Perhaps writing down the pros and cons and of resumption of smoking may help them to regain perspective. Yet if this list is generated while they experience craving, it may not resemble one generated in a noncraving state. While craving, the balance of pros and cons may shift, and the reinforcing consequences of drug use might be strengthened. Suddenly, the decision to resume drinking or smoking may not appear to be such a bad idea (Sayette, 2004).

Pavlov's research suggested the potential of cue exposure/response prevention to extinguish previously conditioned appetites. Yet only recently have addiction researchers focused on the clinical implications of this research (Conklin & Tiffany, 2002). Poulos,

Hinson, and Siegel (1981) suggest that treatment programs would fare better if they altered their sterile environments to include the types of drug cues likely to elicit cravings. In addition to conditioning models, cognitive theories also may account for the utility of cue exposure treatment (e.g., Marlatt, 1985). Treatment should include helping patients prepare to refrain from drinking in the context of the often powerful cognitive shifts that occur outside the clinic. Craving induction treatments in which smoking is prevented may help patients learn to cope with temptations and better handle powerful craving-related changes in cognitive processing while they are experiencing them. Coping skills taught in the context of a craving manipulation may be especially effective (e.g., Monti et al., 1993). In addition to developing skills to deal with high-risk situations, patients also may enhance their self-efficacy that they will be able to cope, which also may prove important for preventing relapse (Wilson, 1987).

In summary, this chapter has aimed to highlight the importance of self-regulation in the context of addiction. By using cigarette smoking as a model, we presented data to illustrate the multiple domains in which craving might contribute to self-regulation failure (e.g., underregulation, misregulation, acquiescence). Using a self-regulation framework, future work is indicated that promises to provide both conceptual and clinical advances in the understanding of drug craving.

REFERENCES

Attwood, A. S., O'Sullivan, H., Leonards, U., Mackintosh, B., & Munafo, M. R. (2008). Attentional bias training and cue reactivity in cigarette smokers. *Addiction, 103,* 1875–1882.

Baker, T. B., Piper, M. E., McCarthy, D. E., Majeskie, M. R., & Fiore, M. C. (2004). Addiction motivation reformulated: An affective processing model of negative reinforcement. *Psychological Review, 111,* 33–51.

Bandura, A. (1997). *Self-efficacy: The exercise of control.* New York: W. H. Freeman.

Baumeister, R. F., Heatherton, T. F., & Tice, D. M. (1994). *Losing control: How and why people fail at self-regulation.* San Diego, CA: Academic Press.

Baumeister, R. F., Vohs, K. D., & Tice, D. M. (2007). The strength model of self-control. *Current Directions in Psychological Science, 16,* 351–355.

Brandon, T. H., Tiffany, S. T., Obremski, K. M., & Baker, T. B. (1990). Postcessation cigarette use: The process of relapse. *Addictive Behaviors, 15,* 105–114.

Brownell, K. D., Marlatt, G. A., Lichtenstein, E., & Wilson, G. T. (1986). Understanding and preventing relapse. *American Psychologist, 41,* 765–782.

Burton, S. M., & Tiffany, S. T. (1997). The effect of alcohol consumption on craving to smoke. *Addiction, 92,* 15–26.

Carter, B. L., & Tiffany, S. T. (1999). Meta-analysis of cue reactivity in addiction research. *Addiction, 94,* 327–340.

Carter, B. L., & Tiffany, S. T. (2001). The cue-availability paradigm: Impact of cigarette availability on cue reactivity in smokers. *Experimental and Clinical Psychopharmacology, 9,* 183–190.

Cervone, D., Mor, N., Orom, H., Shadel, W. G., & Scott, W. D. (2004). Self-efficacy beliefs on the architecture of personality: On knowledge, appraisal, and self-regulation. In R. F. Baumeister & K. D. Vohs (Eds.), *Handbook of self-regulation* (pp. 188–210). New York: Guilford Press.

Conger, J. (1956). Reinforcement theory and the dynamics of alcoholism. *Quarterly Journal of Studies on Alcohol, 17,* 296–305.

Conklin, C. A., & Perkins, K. A. (2005). Subjective and reinforcing effects of smoking during negative mood induction. *Journal of Abnormal Psychology, 114*, 153–164.

Conklin, C. A., & Tiffany, S. T. (2002). Applying extinction research and theory to cue-exposure addiction treatments. *Addiction, 97*, 155–167.

Cox, W. B., Fadardi, J. S., & Pothos, E. M. (2006). The addiction-Stroop test: Theoretical considerations and procedural recommendations. *Psychological Bulletin, 132*, 443–476.

Ekman, P., & Friesen, W. V. (1978). *Facial Action Coding System*. Palo Alto, CA: Consulting Psychologists Press.

Ekman, P., & Rosenberg, E. L. (Eds.). (2005). *What the face reveals: Basic and applied studies of spontaneous expression using the Facial Action Coding System (FACS)*. New York: Oxford University Press.

Erblich, J., Montgomery, G. H., & Bovbjerg, D. H. (2009). Script-guided imagery of social drinking induces both alcohol and cigarette craving in a sample of nicotine-dependent smokers. *Addictive Behaviors, 34*, 164–170.

Field, M., Munafo, M. R., & Franken, I. H. A. (2009). A meta-analytic investigation of the relationship between attentional bias and subjective craving in substance abuse. *Psychological Bulletin, 135*, 589–607.

Forsyth, A., & Carey, M. (1998). Measuring self-efficacy in the context of HIV risk reduction: Research challenges and recommendations. *Health Psychology, 17*, 559–568.

Gibbons, F. X., & Eggleston, T. J. (1996). Smoker networks and the "typical smokers": A prospective analysis of smoking cessation. *Health Psychology, 15*, 469–477.

Griffin, K. M., & Sayette, M. A. (2008). Facial reactions to smoking cues relate to ambivalence about smoking. *Psychology of Addictive Behaviors, 22*, 551–556.

Gwaltney, C. J., Shiffman, S., Norman, G. J., Paty, J. A., Kassel, J. D., & Gnys, M. (2001). Does smoking abstinence self-efficacy vary across situations?: Identifying context-specificity within the Relapse Situation Efficacy Questionnaire. *Journal of Consulting and Clinical Psychology, 69*, 516–527.

Gwaltney, C. J., Shiffman, S., & Sayette, M. A. (2005). Situational correlates of abstinence self-efficacy. *Journal of Abnormal Psychology, 114*, 649–660.

Hughes, J. R. (1991). Distinguishing withdrawal relief and direct effects of smoking. *Psychopharmacology, 104*, 409–410.

Hughes, J. R., Gulliver, S. B., Fenwick, J. W., Valliere, W. A., Cruser, K., Pepper, S., et al. (1992). Smoking cessation among self-quitters. *Health Psychology, 11*, 331–334.

Hull, J. G. (1987). Self-awareness model. In H. T. Blane & K. E. Leonard (Eds.), *Psychological theories of drinking and alcoholism* (pp. 272–304). New York: Guilford Press.

Hull, J. G., & Slone, L. (2004). Alcohol and self-regulation. In R. F. Baumeister & K. D. Vohs (Eds.), *Handbook of self-regulation* (pp. 466–491). New York: Guilford Press.

Josephs, R. A., & Steele, C. M. (1990). The two faces of alcohol myopia: Attentional mediation of psychological stress. *Journal of Abnormal Psychology, 99*, 115–126.

Kavanagh, D. J., Andrade, J., & May, J. (2005). Imaginary relish and exquisite torture: The elaborated intrusion theory of desire. *Psychological Review, 112*, 446–467.

Kirchner, T. R., & Sayette, M. A. (2007). Effects of smoking abstinence and alcohol consumption on smoking-related outcome expectancies in heavy smokers and tobacco chippers. *Nicotine and Tobacco Research, 9*, 365–376.

Klein, L. C., Corwin, E. J., & Stine, M. M. (2003). Smoking abstinence impairs time estimation accuracy in cigarette smokers. *Psychopharmacology Bulletin, 37*, 90–95.

Kunda, Z. (1990). The case for motivated reasoning. *Psychological Bulletin, 108*, 480–498.

Lazarus, R. S., & Folkman, S. (1984). *Stress, appraisal, and coping*. New York: Springer.

Levine, M. D., Marcus, M. D., Kalarchian, M. A., Weissfeld, L., & Qin, L. (2006). Weight concerns affect motivation to remain abstinent from smoking postpartum. *Annals of Behavioral Medicine, 32*, 147–153.

Loewenstein, G. (1987). Anticipation and the valuation of delayed consumption. *Economic Journal, 97,* 666–684.

Loewenstein, G. (1999). A visceral account of addiction. In J. Elster & O.-J. Skog (Eds.), *Getting hooked: Rationality and addiction* (pp. 235–264). Cambridge, UK: Cambridge University Press.

MacAndrew, C., & Edgerton, R. B. (1969). *Drunken comportment: A social explanation.* Chicago: Aldine.

MacDonald, T., Fong, G. T., Zanna, M. P., & Martineau, A. M. (2000). Alcohol myopia and condom use: Can alcohol intoxication be associated with more prudent behavior? *Journal of Personality and Social Psychology, 78,* 605–619.

Marlatt, G. A. (1985). Cognitive factors in the relapse process. In G. A. Marlatt & J. R. Gordon (Eds.), *Relapse prevention: Maintenance strategies in the treatment of addictive behaviors* (pp. 128–200). New York: Guilford Press.

Marlatt, G. A., & Gordon, J. R. (Eds.). (1985). *Relapse prevention: Maintenance strategies in the treatment of addictive behaviors.* New York: Guilford Press.

McCarthy, D. E., Piasecki, T. M., Lawrence, D. L., Jorenby, D. E., Shiffman, S., Fiore, M. C., et al. (2008). A randomized controlled clinical trial of bupropion SR and individual smoking cessation counseling. *Nicotine and Tobacco Research, 10,* 717–729.

Monti, P. M., Rohsenow, D. J., Rubonis, A. V., Niaura, R. S., Sirota, A. D., Colby, S. M., et al. (1993). Cue exposure with coping skills treatment for male alcoholics: A preliminary investigation. *Journal of Consulting and Clinical Psychology, 61,* 1011–1019.

Muraven, M., & Baumeister, R. F. (2000). Self-regulation and depletion of limited resources: Does self-control resemble a muscle? *Psychological Bulletin, 126,* 247–259.

Muraven, M., Collins, R. L., Shiffman, S., & Paty, J. A. (2005). Daily fluctuations in self-control demands and alcohol intake. *Psychology of Addictive Behaviors, 19,* 140–147.

Niaura, R. S., Rohsenow, D. J., Binkoff, J. A., Monti, P. M., Pedraza, M., & Abrams, D. B. (1988). Relevance of cue reactivity to understanding alcohol and smoking relapse. *Journal of Abnormal Psychology, 97,* 133–152.

Nisbett, R., & Wilson, T. D. (1977). Telling more than we know: Verbal reports on mental processes. *Psychological Review, 84,* 231–259.

Ochsner, K. N., & Gross, J. J. (2007). The neural architecture of emotion regulation. In J. J. Gross (Ed.), *Handbook of emotion regulation* (pp. 87–109). New York: Guilford Press.

O'Connell, K. A., Schwartz, J. E., & Shiffman, S. (2008). Do resisted temptations during smoking cessation deplete or augment self-control resources? *Psychology of Addictive Behaviors, 22,* 486–495.

Piasecki, T. M., McCarthy, D. E., Fiore, M. C., & Baker, T. B. (2008). Alcohol consumption, smoking urge, and the reinforcing effects of cigarettes: An ecological study. *Psychology of Addictive Behaviors, 22,* 230–239.

Piper, M. E., Federman, E. B., McCarthy, D. E., Bolt, D. M., Smith, S. S., Fiore, M. C., et al. (2008). Using meditational models to explore the nature of tobacco motivation and tobacco treatment effects. *Journal of Abnormal Psychology, 117,* 94–105.

Polivy, J. (2000). The false hope syndrome: Unfulfilled expectations of self-change. *Current Directions in Psychological Science, 9,* 128–131.

Poulos, C. X., Hinson, R. E., & Siegel, S. (1981). The role of Pavlovian processes in drug tolerance and dependence: Implications for treatment. *Addictive Behaviors, 6,* 205–211.

Robinson, T. E., & Berridge, K. C. (1993). The neural basis of drug craving: An incentive-sensitization theory of addiction. *Brain Research Reviews, 18,* 247–291.

Rothman, A. J., Baldwin, A. S., & Hertel, A. W. (2004). Self-regulation and behavior change: Disentangling behavioral initiation and behavioral maintenance. In R. F. Baumeister & K. D. Vohs (Eds.), *Handbook of self-regulation: Research, theory, and applications* (pp. 130–150). New York: Guilford Press.

Sayette, M. A. (2004). Self-regulatory failure and addiction. In R. F. Baumeister & K. D. Vohs (Eds.), *Handbook of self-regulation: Research, theory, and applications* (pp. 466–491). New York: Guilford Press.

Sayette, M. A., Cohn, J. F., Wertz, J. M., Perrott, M. A., & Parrott, D. J. (2001). A psychometric evaluation of the Facial Action Coding System for assessing spontaneous expression. *Journal of Nonverbal Behavior, 25,* 167–186.

Sayette, M. A., & Hufford, M. R. (1995). Urge and affect: A facial coding analysis of smokers. *Experimental and Clinical Psychopharmacology, 3,* 417–423.

Sayette, M. A., & Hufford, M. R. (1997). Effects of smoking urge on generation of smoking-related information. *Journal of Applied Social Psychology, 27,* 1395–1405.

Sayette, M. A., Kirchner, T. R., Moreland, R. L., Levine, J. M., & Travis, T. (2004). The effects of alcohol on risk-seeking behavior: A group-level analysis. *Psychology of Addictive Behaviors, 18,* 190–193.

Sayette, M. A., Loewenstein, G., Griffin, K. M., & Black, J. (2008). Exploring the cold-to-hot empathy gap in smokers. *Psychological Science, 19,* 926–932.

Sayette, M. A., Loewenstein, G., Kirchner, T. R., & Travis, T. (2005). Effects of smoking urge on temporal cognition. *Psychology of Addictive Behaviors, 19,* 88–93.

Sayette, M. A., Martin, C. S., Hull, J. G., Wertz, J. M., & Perrott, M. A. (2003). The effects of nicotine deprivation on craving response covariation in smokers. *Journal of Abnormal Psychology, 112,* 110–118.

Sayette, M. A., Martin, C. S., Wertz, J. M., Perrott, M. A., & Peters, A. R. (2005). The effects of alcohol consumption on cigarette craving in heavy smokers and tobacco chippers. *Psychology of Addictive Behaviors, 19,* 263–270.

Sayette, M. A., Martin, C. S., Wertz, J. M., Shiffman, S., & Perrott, M. A. (2001). A multidimensional analysis of cue-elicited craving in heavy smokers and tobacco chippers. *Addiction, 96,* 1419–1432.

Sayette, M. A., Reichle, E. D., & Schooler, J. W. (2009). Lost in the sauce: The effects of alcohol on mind-wandering. *Psychological Science, 20,* 747–752.

Sayette, M. A., Schooler, J. W., & Reichle, E. D. (2010). Out for a smoke: The impact of cigarette craving on zoning-out during reading. *Psychological Science, 21,* 26–30.

Sayette, M. A., Shiffman, S., Tiffany, S. T., Niaura, R. S., Martin, C. S., & Shadel, W. G. (2000). The measurement of drug craving. *Addiction, 95,* S189–S210.

Sayette, M. A., Wertz, J. M., Martin, C. S., Cohn, J. F., Perrott, M. A., & Hobel, J. (2003). Effects of smoking opportunity on cue-elicited urge: A facial coding analysis. *Experimental and Clinical Psychopharmacology, 11,* 218–227.

Shiffman, S. (1982). Relapse following smoking cessation: A situational analysis. *Journal of Consulting and Clinical Psychology, 50,* 71–86.

Shiffman, S., & Balabanis, M. (1995). Associations between alcohol and tobacco. In J. B. Fertig & J. P. Allen (Eds.), *Alcohol and tobacco: From basic science to clinical practice* (Research Monograph No. 30). Bethesda, MD: National Institute on Alcohol Abuse and Alcoholism.

Shiffman, S., Gwaltney, C. J., Balabanis, M. K., Liu, K. S., Paty, J. A., Kassel, J. D., et al. (2002). Immediate antecedents of cigarette smoking: An analysis from ecological momentary assessment. *Journal of Abnormal Psychology, 111,* 535–545.

Shiffman, S., Shadel, W. G., Niaura, R., Khayrallah, M. A., Jorenby, D. E., Ryan, C. F., et al. (2003). Efficacy of acute administration of nicotine gum in relief of cue-provoked cigarette craving. *Psychopharmacology, 166,* 343–350.

Steele, C. M., & Josephs, R. A. (1990). Alcohol myopia: Its prized and dangerous effects. *American Psychologist, 45,* 921–933.

Stritzke, W. G. K., Breiner, M. J., Curtin, J. J., & Lang, A. R. (2004). Assessment of substance cue reactivity: Advances in reliability, specificity, and validity. *Psychology of Addictive Behaviors, 18,* 148–159.

Tice, D. M., Bratslavsky, E., & Baumeister, R. F. (2001). Emotional distress regulation takes precedence over impulse control: If you feel bad, do it! *Journal of Personality and Social Psychology, 80,* 53–67.

Tiffany, S. T. (1990). A cognitive model of drug urges and drug-use behavior: Role of automatic and nonautomatic processes. *Psychological Review, 97,* 147–168.

Tiffany, S. T. (1992). A critique of contemporary urge and craving research: Methodological, psychometric, and theoretical issues. *Advances in Behaviour Research and Therapy, 14,* 123–139.

U.S. Department of Health and Human Services (USDHHS). (1989). *Reducing the health consequences of smoking: 25 years of progress: A report of the Surgeon General.* Rockville, MD: Public Health Service, Office on Smoking and Health.

Vohs, K. D., & Schmeichel, B. J. (2003). Self-regulation and the extended now: Controlling the self alters the subjective experience of time. *Journal of Personality and Social Psychology, 85,* 217–230.

Waters, A. J., & Sayette, M. A. (2006). Implicit cognition and tobacco addiction. In R. W. Wiers & A. W. Stacy (Eds.), *Handbook of implicit cognition and addiction* (pp. 309–338) London: Sage.

Waters, A. J., Shiffman, S., Sayette, M. A., Paty, J., Gwaltney, C., & Balabanis, M. (2003). Attentional bias predicts outcome in smoking cessation. *Health Psychology, 22,* 378–387.

Weiss, F., Maldonado-Vlaar, C. S., Parsons, L. H., Kerr, T. M., Smith, D. L., & Ben-Shahar, O. (2000). Control of cocaine-seeking behavior by drug associated stimuli in rats: Effects on recovery of extinguished operant-responding and extracellular dopamine levels in amygdala and nucleus accumbens. *Proceedings of the National Academy of Sciences USA, 97,* 4321–4326.

Wertz, J. M., & Sayette, M. A. (2001). A review of the effects of perceived drug use opportunity on self-reported urge. *Experimental and Clinical Psychopharmacology, 9,* 3–13.

Wiers, R. W., Houben, K., Smulders, F. T. Y., Conrod, P. J., & Jones, B. T. (2006). To drink or not to drink: The role of automatic and controlled cognitive processes in the etiology of alcohol-related problems. In R. W. Wiers & A. W. Stacy (Eds.), *Handbook on implicit cognition and addiction* (pp. 339–361). Thousand Oaks, CA: Sage.

Wiers, R. W., & Stacy, A. W. (Eds.). (2006). *Handbook of implicit cognition and addiction.* London: Sage.

Wikler, A. (1948). Recent progress in research on the neurophysiological basis of morphine addiction. *American Journal of Psychiatry, 105,* 329–338.

Wilson, G. T. (1987). Cognitive processes in addiction. *British Journal of Addiction, 82,* 343–353.

Wilson, S. J., Sayette, M. A., & Fiez, J. A. (2004). Prefrontal responses to drug cues: A neurocognitive analysis. *Nature Neuroscience, 7,* 211–214.

Zinser, M., Fiore, M., Davidson, R., & Baker, T. B. (1999). Manipulating smoking motivation: Impact on an electrophysiological index of approach motivation. *Journal of Abnormal Psychology, 108,* 240–254.

CHAPTER 28

The Self-Regulation of Eating
Theoretical and Practical Problems

C. PETER HERMAN
JANET POLIVY

In this chapter, we attempt to impose a self-regulatory framework on eating. Eating is normally regarded as a highly regulated activity, as it must be if it is to serve its biological function. Of course, closer examination reveals that eating is not as well-regulated as one might imagine. Moreover, it turns out that the regulation of eating is often opposed by the self-regulation of eating, which naturally creates all sorts of personal and theoretical problems. The bulk of this chapter is devoted to self-regulation, successful and unsuccessful, including a survey of the empirical evidence and a consideration of various models of self-regulation and self-regulation failure. We conclude that there is still much to be learned.

SELF-REGULATION OF EATING *QUA* WEIGHT LOSS

The self-regulation of eating refers to deliberate attempts to override natural regulatory processes. Our experiences of hunger and satiety reflect our bodies' natural concern with (1) short-term regulation of energy and (2) maintaining a reserve of energy for emergencies. For many people, though, these natural concerns are sacrificed to the project of eating in an unnatural, mindful way designed to achieve (or perhaps maintain) weight loss.

Deliberately eating less than what the body demands has several consequences. For one thing, it means that one may become chronically hungry. Although even a diet meal will satisfy immediate hunger, it will not do so for long, so hunger is likely to reappear sooner; and chronic hunger is only one consequence of dieting. Weight loss induces in the body various defensive reactions designed to counteract the attempt to reduce weight. Such defenses—most notably, changes in metabolism—make it increasingly difficult to continue to lose weight, even with the same spartan diet that initially produced weight loss. Some of the defensive changes experienced by dieters are more subtle: Fatigue makes it more difficult to maintain one's customary activity level, and changes in taste make certain high-calorie foods more attractive. For example, for people who have lost weight, postmeal sweets taste better than they do for people who have not lost weight. These defensive adjustments, then, occur at both physiological and behavioral levels. In either case, they force the dieter to impose an even tighter self-regulatory regimen if further weight loss is to be accomplished. Of course, one could try to lose weight by other means (e.g., acupuncture, food combining, exercise, drugs), but the most frequently used method is caloric restriction. Indeed, many of these "alternative" methods are really just other ways of making it easier for one to eat less.

SOCIAL NORMS AND SELF-REGULATION

One can set self-regulatory goals by reference to calories or to specific foods; such goals are matters for the individual to decide, either in isolation or in consultation with a diet coach, book, or some other authority. In practice, however, the particular intake choices that one makes may depend less on the rules prescribed by authorities than on the behavior of one's eating companions. Our analysis of social influences on eating (Herman, Roth, & Polivy, 2003) indicates, first, that social influences are extremely powerful, often overriding other influences on eating, including one's prior intentions or goals. Second, the influence exerted by one's eating companions is of a specifically regulatory sort; that is, people appear to use the intake of their eating companions as a regulatory guide. Studies of modeling, in which an experimental confederate (i.e., someone who is taking part in the experiment ostensibly as a naive participant but actually is in cahoots with the experimenter) eats more or less, and the naive participant eats correspondingly more or less, suggest that we regulate our intake with reference to the intake of others. Note that using the behavior of others as a guide for regulating one's intake does not make much sense in terms of satisfying one's own specific physiological needs; nor does it make much sense for dieters to abandon their caloric or other regulatory scheme and simply follow the example of others. Yet people, dieters and nondieters alike, do follow the example of others.

Although people do follow others' example, they tend to follow at a slight distance. The modeling that occurs is not simply a matter of matching one's intake to that of the companion; closer examination suggests that the naive participant often tends to eat slightly less than does the confederate. It is as if the goal of the eater is to eat less than the other person; accomplishing this goal may be all that is required to convince the eater that he or she has consumed an appropriate amount. Herman and colleagues (2003; Herman & Polivy, 2005) suggest that for some people, the real (regulatory) goal is to avoid excessive intake, and that *excessive* is defined situationally as more than the companion eats. Eating less than (or no more than) the confederate eats therefore serves as a socially based regulatory strategy. Insufficient attention has been paid to the behavior of other people as the basis for regulation of eating, possibly because it makes so little biological sense—either for dieters or for normal eaters—to allow others to dictate their intake. Traditional views of the regulation of eating have long been confined to models in which people regulate on the basis of either their internal physiological signals or their own cognitive calculations of appropriate foods (or amounts of foods) to eat. We must expand our view to include the role of others' intake as a regulatory force and recognize that self-regulation may often be tantamount to regulation by others.

Before leaving this topic, we should add that using the intake of others as a standard may "regulate" our intake not just by providing intake guidelines. Extensive research (see Herman et al., 2003, for a review) suggests that when we eat in the presence of noneating observers, our intake is suppressed (e.g., Polivy, Herman, Hackett, & Kuleshnyk, 1986). Obviously, we cannot eat less than someone who is not eating at all, but we certainly do "down-regulate."

SELF-REGULATORY FAILURE

The seeds of conflict have already been sown. If we consider the models of self-regulation of intake that we have already introduced, it is evident that the goals implicit in the various models may not coincide. The demands of the formal diet, for instance, may not coincide with the intake norms of our eating companions. If we stick to our diet, we may offend our companion (Leone, Herman, & Pliner, 2008). (Remember, the more we eat, the more our companion can eat without eating excessively, so we are likely to be pressured by our companion to "just have a little more.") But if we adhere to the social norm, then the limits imposed by the weight-loss diet may well be exceeded. Only in the case of "dieters" whose diets consist of eating no more than do their eating companions can these two self-regulatory principles be reconciled satisfactorily.

Although the potential exists for conflict between competing self-regulatory principles, the most common and well-appreciated threat to self-regulation arises when a single self-regulatory principle is challenged and defeated by circumstances. Our research program over the past three decades has documented the difficulties of dieting (see Polivy & Herman, 2002).

Our very first study of dieters (Herman & Mack, 1975) forced us to start thinking in terms of self-regulation and self-regulatory failure. We had not begun with the intention of studying these phenomena; we had been looking for parallels between the behavior of normal-weight sorority girls and the obese males Schachter had been studying (see Schachter & Rodin, 1974, for a review). Schachter had demonstrated that whereas normal-weight individuals were responsive to preload size (i.e., eating more after a small preload, and less after a large preload), obese individuals were relatively unresponsive to preload size and seemingly oblivious to this "internal cue." When we tested the effects of preloading experimental participants with 0, 1, or 2 milkshakes (7.5-ounces each), we found that whereas many of them "regulated," subsequently eating in inverse proportion to preload size, others (who eventually came to be known as *restrained eaters*) ate more after the 1- or 2-milkshake preload than after no preload at all. This result did not conform to our expectation, namely, that this latter group (like the obese group) would display an absence of regulation by not responding differentially to preload size. Instead, we had uncovered a new pattern, "counterregulation," that demanded a new interpretation. Eventually, we concluded that members of this anomalous group must have been attempting to inhibit their intake (hence the label *restrained eaters*), and that the forced milkshake consumption had disrupted this attempt.

We argued at the time that the forced preload had undermined the restrained eaters' motivation to diet. The rich milkshake had exceeded their caloric quota for the day, and once the diet was ruined, further attempts to restrict intake served no purpose. (We called it the "what-the-hell effect.") In short, our interpretation of self-regulatory failure was motivational: We assumed that the restrained eaters could have continued (i.e., maintained the ability) to exert self-control when confronted with palatable food, but after the forced preload, there was no point in doing so. Only much later (see later discussion) did we begin to entertain other interpretations.

Note some of the perplexities raised by our interpretation, even accepting a motivational perspective. For one thing, it is absurd to argue that once one's diet has been broken, there is no point in exercising further self-control. Even if one's caloric quota for the day has been exceeded, does it not make sense to compensate for this excess rather than to abandon all self-control? If one exceeds one's quota by 200 calories, is that not better than exceeding it by 2,000 calories? According to the perverse logic of the dieter, apparently not. The dieter tends to think in all-or-none terms: Once the diet is broken, it matters little whether one has exceeded it by a lot or a little. At least in part, this irrational calculation stems from the fact that dieters are aware of how much they should eat to satisfy the diet, but they do not have a self-regulatory plan for what happens if and when the diet is broken. A single self-regulatory failure could, in principle, trigger a secondary or "backup" self-regulatory plan, but dieters are generally so invested in the initial plan that no contingency plans are ever developed.

A second perplexity, related to the first, is raised by the assumption that diets should operate diurnally. As we saw earlier, diurnal self-regulation appears to be the norm for dieting (as for many other self-regulatory human activities), but ultimately, it is arbitrary. Excess calories consumed today still "count" tomorrow, in the sense that they contribute to one's continuing weight problem. As long as one has not achieved one's weight-loss goal, one should remain motivated toward it. Why does a milkshake undermine that motivation, especially when everyone knows that the diet will be resumed tomorrow morning, and the consequences of today's post–milkshake binge must be "tacked on" to the diet, probably extending the need to diet for several days? We conclude that if dieters act as if their motivation to diet has been undermined, it may be more than the milkshake per se that contributes to this undermining.

Finally, and again related to the foregoing issues, the milkshake preload, rich as it may be, does not necessarily exceed the caloric quota for the day. An 8-ounce milkshake does not contain *that* many calories, and if it is consumed early in the day, it is quite likely that it is still mathematically possible, by restricting one's subsequent intake, to adhere to the daily allowance. Maybe something else is going on, in addition to quota busting.

VARIATIONS ON THE THEME OF SELF-REGULATORY FAILURE

Preload Studies

Much of our research has been devoted to exploring various other experimental conditions that lead restrained eaters to (temporarily) abandon their restraint. Some of these variations are extensions of the preloading paradigm; others attack restraint from entirely different angles.

The first preload variation study (Polivy, 1976) demonstrated that it was not the actual number of calories in the preload that determined whether dieters would "lose control"; rather, it was what they *believed* about the richness of the preload. Participants' beliefs about whether the preload (in this case, pudding) was high or low in calories were manipulated orthogonally to the actual caloric content of the pudding. Perceived calories exerted more control than did actual calories, and restrained eaters who believed that they had consumed a high-calorie preload were more likely to become disinhibited, whether or not that belief was correct. This finding, which has been replicated (Knight & Boland, 1989; Spencer & Fremouw, 1979; Woody, Costanzo, Liefer, & Conger, 1981), indicates that the preload operates through a cognitive (not physiological) mechanism; the dieter is making a calculation pertaining to calories.

We speculated that a rich preload produces disinhibition and subsequent overeating because the preload precludes success at adhering to the daily diet requirements. In most of the studies, that failure is induced by a prior forced preload. If the forced preload were merely anticipated, rather than already consumed, how might that affect the dieter? If the dieter were assured that the impending preload would sabotage the diet before the day was done, then the chances of dietary success would be as negligible as if the preload were already ingested. And, indeed, such appears to be the case. Some studies (Ruderman, Belzer, & Halperin, 1985; Tomarken & Kirschenbaum, 1984) have found that anticipating a preload later in the day produces disinhibition and overeating in restrained eaters.

The vulnerability of dietary restraint to disruption by caloric considerations seems to know no bounds. Urbszat, Herman, and Polivy (2002) demonstrated that anticipation of a weeklong diet, starting first thing tomorrow, leads dieters to overeat today. In this case, these researchers argued, the anticipated deprivation may "justify" the prediet overindulgence; another possibility is that, among dieters, the connection between overindulgence today and compensatory deprivation planned for tomorrow is so strong that it may operate reciprocally, with deprivation planned for tomorrow triggering (compensatory) overindulgence today.

Yet another variation on the disinhibitory power of the preload is evident in situations in which the preload is merely encountered rather than consumed. When dieters are exposed to rich, palatable food but not required (or even allowed) to eat it, and when this exposure to attractive food cues (including smell and indulgent thoughts) extends for several minutes, dieters become more likely to overeat when subsequently given access to palatable food. These studies (Fedoroff, Polivy, & Herman, 1997, 2003; Jansen & van den Hout, 1991) are typically interpreted as evidence of craving as a precipitant of disinhibition. It is not that the diet has been (or will necessarily be) broken; rather, the urge to eat, stimulated by focused concentration on food cues, becomes overwhelming. Note that, in this case, exposure to the preload does not ruin the diet by exceeding the caloric quota for the day; rather, this exposure undermines the diet by making the prospect of eating more attractive than the prospect of not eating. Normally, dieters' self-regulatory inhibitions are enough to allow them to resist temptation; but sometimes, either because of the sustained power of the tempting food cues, or because of cue-induced cravings at the physiological level, or both, self-regulatory inhibitions fail. Later, we consider more systematically how these various interpretations map onto various models of how self-regulation works in dieters.

One question that may be fairly asked at this point is: What is the smallest preload that will produce disinhibited eating? It may be that a very small amount of food, if the food is of a "forbidden" type, will suffice to break a diet. This diet-breaking hinges on the (somewhat magical) notion that some foods, in any quantity, are intolerable. If a diet does not allow a certain type of food, then any amount of that food ruins the diet, and disinhibition will ensue.

Finally, it is important to recognize that self-regulation-failure-induced disinhibited eating may proceed in a fashion devoid of self-regulation, but it is not necessarily immune to other (more reliable) regulatory influences. Herman, Polivy, and Esses (1987) showed that whereas a large, rich preload disinhibited eating in restrained eaters, an extra-large preload (twice as large as the large preloads used in prior studies) did not cause restrained eaters to eat any more than they did in the control (no-preload) condition. We believe that in the extra-large preload condition, restrained eaters were disinhibited, in the sense that they were no longer adhering to their original self-regulatory plans; but because the preload was so huge, they were near the limit of physical capacity and literally could not eat much more. Physical capacity, of course, is a "natural" regulator of intake and should not be confused with self-regulation, which is an "unnatural" regulator not grounded in—and usually opposed to—one's automatic physiological processes.

Other Studies

Several studies have explored the role of emotional arousal as a disrupter of dietary restraint. (Interestingly, just as preloading suppresses eating in unrestrained eaters, while disinhibiting eating in restrained eaters, distress suppresses eating in unrestrained eaters, while disinhibiting eating in restrained eaters.) Distress has been manipulated in many ways, most often in the form of fear (e.g., McKenna, 1972) or anxiety (e.g., Herman, Polivy, Lank, & Heatherton, 1987), but also in the form of acute depression (e.g., Baucom & Aiken, 1981). Anxiety obviously does not exert its effect on self-regulation by ruining the diet; the anxious dieter has not eaten any more than the nonanxious dieter before encountering whatever food is available for subsequent overeating. From the beginning, we (Herman & Polivy, 1975) assumed that anxiety undermines the diet through a different mechanism, that the anxious dieter rearranges priorities: Whereas adhering to the diet successfully remains calorically possible, the dieter no longer cares so much about dietary success; coping with distress is more important, and eating is one way to cope with distress. The notion that emotion regulation is the basis for overeating is nicely captured by Tice, Bratslavsky, and Baumeister (2001), who demonstrated that overeating can be prevented if one is convinced that eating will not improve one's emotional state. Nevertheless, it remains possible that distress may induce disinhibited eating without engaging distress-management mechanisms (see later discussion). Also, the phenomenon has been refined empirically (Heatherton, Herman, & Polivy, 1991), with the discovery that certain types of distress (e.g., ego threat) are more effective than others (e.g., physical threat) in inducing disinhibition. Whatever the underlying mechanism may be, distress does interfere with self-regulation, just as preloading does; these disrupters of self-regulation can substitute for each other, such that if the dieter is preloaded, then anxiety does not produce any additional overeating, and if the dieter is anxious, preloading does not produce any additional overeating (Herman, Polivy, Lank, & Heatherton, 1987).

Finally, we have found that alcohol, at least under certain circumstances, can produce self-regulatory failure (Polivy & Herman, 1976a, 1976b; see also Hofmann &

Friese, 2008). It will come as no surprise to the reader that alcohol leads to disinhibition (see Sayette & Griffin, Chapter 27, this volume), but the precise mechanism underlying the effect remains in dispute despite millennia of human experience of the phenomenon. Intoxicants, emotional distress, and diet-threatening preloads all interfere with the self-regulation on which the dieter depends. Empirically, the disruption of self-control by exposure to these conditions or situations is well established, with only some minor details unresolved. What remains to be established, however, is precisely how these experimental (or natural) manipulations exert their effects. We have casually alluded to some interpretations of how these disrupters undermine and often defeat self-regulatory strategies. We now focus on this question more systematically.

MODELS OF SELF-REGULATION AND SELF-REGULATION FAILURE

Attempts to impose self-regulation on eating, which in most cases amount to attempts to restrict intake, can be understood most simply as the exercise of self-control. We have argued (Herman & Polivy, 1980) that the advent of research on restrained eating represents a significant change in our understanding of controls on eating. Prior research focused on *internal* (physiological) and *external* (environmental) controls but ignored self-control. Obviously, restrained eaters, insofar as they are successful, are resisting both internal and external cues promoting intake; even if they are not successful, or are successful only for a while, dieters are attempting to exercise self-control. Our introduction of self-control as an oppositional force in eating, however, was intuitive and did not specify exactly how self-control operated.

General Self-Regulatory Models

Formal models of self-regulation (e.g., Carver & Scheier, Chapter 1, this volume) specify the goal, assessment of progress toward the goal, and adjustments implemented when progress toward the goal is inadequate. Such models help to explain how dieters approach the long-term goal of weight loss (or possibly weight maintenance), but they are not very helpful when it comes to the more proximate goal of intake regulation in the short term. Recently, however, some interesting models have addressed themselves specifically to the issues involved in restricting food intake.

Stroebe (2008; Stroebe, Mensink, Aarts, Schut, & Kruglanski, 2008) has recently proposed a "goal conflict" theory of eating that describes the competing motives of the dieter. On the one hand, the dieter's overriding (and defining) goal is to restrict food intake, yet dieters share with everyone else the goal of eating enjoyment. (Everyone enjoys palatable food.) Stroebe (2008) analyzes the dieter's conflict in terms of the accessibility and/or activation of competing goals. These goals, or *knowledge structures*, are typically measured in terms of reaction times to stimuli representing the goals. In Stroebe's view, the dieter begins with a commitment to the diet goal, but repeated exposure to attractive food cues activates the eating-enjoyment goal, which eventually trumps the diet goal and leads to overeating. This view of the cognitive dynamics of dieting is consistent with our own view of restrained eating, and with Jansen's (1998) cue-reactivity model, but it is inconsistent with a starkly different view championed by Fishbach, Friedman, and Kruglanski (2003; see also Fishbach & Converse, Chapter 13, this volume). Their counteractive-control model posits that exposure to attractive food stimuli automatically activates the dieter's diet goals (rather than the dieter's eating goals). Fishbach et al.'s dieters had faster reaction times to diet-related stimuli and were more likely to choose a healthy snack after exposure to tempting food-related stimuli.

Fishbach and colleagues (2003, p. 297) argued that "over the course of their life, individuals learn to resist temptations by activating the higher priority goals these temptations threaten to undermine." This assertion suggests that counteractive control is an acquired process associated with success in resisting temptation; in short, it is a phenomenon that should characterize successful dieters. Papies, Stroebe, and Aarts (2008; see also Papies & Aarts, Chapter 7, this volume) pursued this suggestion explicitly, proposing that success or failure at dieting "moderates the effect of food cues on restrained eaters such that food cues activate the dieting goal in successful restrained eaters and inhibit the dieting goal in unsuccessful restrained eaters" (p. 1290). Their study demonstrated such moderation: "For successful restrained eaters, food primes led to the facilitation of the dieting goal compared to baseline, whereas for unsuccessful restrained eaters, food primes caused the inhibition of the dieting goal" (p. 1295). In other words, successful dieters react to temptations with enhanced adherence to their diet goals, whereas unsuccessful dieters react to temptations by abandoning their diet goals. This formulation serves to reconcile the conventional view of restrained eating and cue-reactivity (e.g., Fedoroff et al., 1997, 2003) with the counteractive-control model (Fishbach et al., 2003), but not without a trace of circularity. Is it being a successful dieter that renders one more likely to react to temptations with greater dietary resolve, or is it greater dietary resolve in the face of temptation that renders one a successful dieter?

A similar analysis is provided by construal-level theory (Trope & Liberman, 2003; see also Ledgerwood & Trope, Chapter 12, this volume), wherein it is argued that thinking about situations in a more abstract way (consistent with long-term goals) leads to greater self-control than does thinking about the same situation in a more concrete way (emphasizing short-term temptations that conflict with the long-term self-regulatory goal). Fujita, Trope, Liberman, and Levin-Sagi (2006), for instance, found that people rated food temptations more positively (and would thus presumably be more prone to self-control failure) when the situation in which the temptation appeared was described in specific detail than when it was described abstractly. Likewise, Fujita and Han (2009) found greater negativity toward tempting candy bars (and reduced selection of candy bars) when people performed a task, unrelated to food or eating, requiring them to think at a relatively high level of abstraction.

Delay of Gratification

Another approach to self-control—one that appears to map quite directly onto the dieter's situation—is represented by Mischel's work on delay of gratification (Mischel, Cantor, & Feldman, 1996; see Mischel & Ayduk, Chapter 5, this volume). Mischel's research appears to be especially pertinent in that it is concerned with acute influences on consummatory behavior. Obviously, we all (try to) delay gratification in the service of long-term goals, but the gratifications that we deny ourselves present themselves in the here and now, and the task boils down to a series of proximate challenges. In Mischel's laboratory studies, success (delay) or failure (capitulation to temptation) is a single-episode phenomenon. The fact that the temptation often takes the form of palatable food brings the parallel closer.

Mischel has focused on factors that enhance or impede delay. For instance, we all know that resistance to temptation may be enhanced if the tempting object is rendered less salient; indeed, ancient behavior therapy recommendations for dieting (e.g., Stuart, 1967) have emphasized distancing oneself from the tempting stimulus, either by removing the temptation from one's environment (e.g., keeping tempting snacks out of sight) or removing oneself from the tempting environment (e.g., staying out of the kitchen). A simple extension of this notion is to reduce the "temptingness" of the stimulus by psychological means, even while staying in close proximity to it. Mischel demonstrates that delay can be enhanced if the object of temptation is construed in such a way as to reduce its sensory allure (Mischel, Shoda, & Rodriguez, 1992). A chocolate bar can be construed as a log (or something worse). Such reconstrual appears to be effective, but we have to wonder how long it can be sustained; a chocolate bar, to paraphrase Freud, is sometimes (in fact, always) a chocolate bar. An alternative tactic to enhance resistance to temptation (Herman & Polivy, 1993) does not require denying that a chocolate bar is what it is, nor does it require denying that it would be delicious; it simply requires making salient the equally true proposition that a chocolate bar represents a significant caloric threat: "It tastes good, but it's not good for me." If the dieter can focus on the negative aspects of the stimulus, while perhaps still acknowledging that the stimulus instantiates both positive and negative features, then perhaps the angel on one shoulder will win the argument with the devil on the other, even though the devil has a good argument. The real threat here, we believe, arises when the dieter's ability to attend to the angel's argument ("Watch out for those calories!") is reduced by distraction. If the dieter's mental energy is depleted or devoted to some more urgent task, the devil is likely to win the argument, if only because the argument can then proceed on a noncognitive level. The distracted dieter does not *think* about the food but merely reacts to its sensory properties in an almost decorticate way. At the sensory level, temptation will always triumph. Although everyone responds to normative cues regarding eating (e.g., portion size, modeling), dieters appear to be particularly responsive to sensory cues (Herman & Polivy, 2008).

Eating Hijacked by Salient External Cues

The conflict between sensory control and self-control of behavior is articulated clearly in Heatherton and Baumeister's (1991) analysis of binge eating. They postulate that distress—particularly those forms of distress that pose a threat to one's ego or self-esteem—renders self-awareness aversive (because it is aversive to contemplate a besieged self) and prompts the individual to "escape" from self-awareness. Aspects of the "self" that are discarded during this escape include one's long-range goals (e.g., weight loss, in the case of dieters). Not only is the goal of weight loss (temporarily) abandoned, but the escape from self is a flight into the not-self, more specifically, the immediate environment of sensory stimuli. It is almost as though the individual descends to a lower level of consciousness, devoid of abstract ideals and goals, and dominated by salient cues demanding an unmediated, reflexive response. In the presence of palatable food, and having lost sight of long-range objectives, the distressed dieter is easy prey for forbidden food.

The idea that distress renders the individual more vulnerable to the sensory allure of food was proposed earlier by Slochower (1983), although she restricted her prescient analysis to the obese and did not focus on distress-induced externality as a threat to self-regulatory control.

Other models pertinent to self-regulation have emphasized conditions under which behavior is "captured" by salient cues. Steele and Josephs (1990) proposed that alcohol narrows the individual's attentional field, so that behavior comes under the control of most salient cues in the immediate environment. Ward and Mann (2000) extended the "alcohol myopia" model and proposed that a cognitive load of any sort will reduce available cognitive resources and have the net effect of focusing attention more narrowly on salient stimuli (e.g., palatable, forbidden food that is enticingly available to dieters). Ward and Mann found that imposition of a memory task led to disinhibition of eating among restrained eaters.

The Role of Cognition and Memory in Self-Regulation

We often try to eat in an appropriate manner and regulate our intake in terms of what we consider to be an appropriate amount to eat, considering the circumstances. Thus, if we have recently eaten a high-calorie meal or snack, then we might eat less at our next eating opportunity than if the prior meal or snack had been lower in calories. Of course, our ability to assess how many calories we have consumed recently depends at least as much on our cognitive abilities as on feedback from the gut (Herman & Polivy, 2005). Thus, as we discussed earlier under the heading of "Preload Studies," if we are told that a particular preload is high in calories, we react differently than if we are told that it is low in calories. Our self-regulatory calculations, then, are based on fallible beliefs, cognitions, and memories. Higgs (2002, 2005) has explored the contribution of memory to the self-regulation of food intake. Insofar as we remember that we have recently eaten, we are less likely to indulge ourselves further. Higgs (2002, 2005; Higgs, Williamson, & Attwood, 2008) has demonstrated that enhancing memory of recent intake, by having participants actively recall a meal, tends to suppress further intake (holding recent intake constant). Watching television while eating lunch increases subsequent intake (Higgs & Woodward, 2009). Apparently, watching television interferes with encoding the lunch experience in memory, and in the absence of a strong memory of a recent meal, further intake becomes more likely.

Self-Regulatory Strength

A somewhat different rendition of the impairment of self-regulatory ability is the self-regulatory strength model (Baumeister, Bratslavsky, Muraven, & Tice, 1998; Baumeister, Vohs, & Tice, 2007; Muraven, Tice, & Baumeister, 1998), which proposes that effective self-regulation demands a certain degree of self-regulatory strength. Like muscular strength, self-regulatory strength can be depleted in the short term by exertions of self-control, although in the long term, repeated exertions of self-control (like regular exercise) supposedly increase one's self-regulatory strength. This metaphor can explain why having to exert self-control in one situation may impair self-regulation in another immediately thereafter.

Some evidence (Kahan, Polivy, & Herman, 2003; Vohs & Heatherton, 2000) suggests that such may be the case for restrained eaters: Exertions of self-control, whether or not they are related to inhibiting eating, may make it more difficult to inhibit eating immediately thereafter. Hofmann, Rauch, and Gawronski (2007; see also Hofmann, Friese, Schmeichel, & Baddeley, Chapter 11, this volume) examined the effect of self-regulatory-strength depletion on intake of candy, as moderated by dietary restraint and automatic attitudes toward candy (i.e., a cognitive assessment of one's favorability toward candies). When not depleted, people's candy intake was an inverse function of dietary restraint; that is, restrained eaters were able to suppress their intake (irrespective of their liking of candies). When depleted, however (because they had been instructed to suppress their emotional reactions to a film), people's candy intake was a direct function of their automatic attitude toward candy; that is, dieters no longer suppressed their intake, and everyone ate as a direct function of how much they liked candy. This pattern of results was replicated by Friese, Hofmann, and Wänke (2008), with explicit attitudes replacing dietary restraint. More generally, Hofmann and colleagues have emphasized that variations in self-control capacities and in the strength of temptations must be jointly considered in predictions of self-regulatory outcomes (Hofmann, Friese, & Strack, 2009).

Gailliot and Baumeister (2007) have proposed that glucose mediates self-control processes, and that self-control efforts deplete brain glucose stores (especially in the prefrontal cortex), making further self-control efforts less likely to succeed. Glucose beverages enhance success in self-control tasks more so than do control beverages. This analysis is intriguing, but Gailliot and Baumeister do not address our preload paradigm, in which rich preloads (containing plenty of sugar) undermine self-control in restrained eaters. One possibility is that these high-calorie preloads provoke a "paradoxical" hypoglycemic reaction in restrained eaters, making them more vulnerable to the lure of forbidden treats. Maybe individuals who have a hypoglycemic reaction to sugar loads tend to become restrained eaters, in an attempt to deal with the problem of the positive feedback loop (eating → hypoglycemia → eating). This interpretation is not easy to reconcile with the findings that calorically identical preloads lead to opposing outcomes in restrained eaters depending on how the preloads are labeled (high vs. low in calories) (e.g., Polivy, 1976); but it remains remotely possible that believing a preload is high in calories may induce hypoglycemia in affected individuals, whereas believing that the preload is low in calories will not. More generally, the "glucose hypothesis" should alert us to the possibility that restrained eaters, insofar as they deprive themselves of operating glucose, may be highly susceptible to self-control failures.

Desire

Most of the attempts to account for self-regulatory failure in dieters that we have examined locate the main source of the problem in the dieter's impaired capacity to resist temptation. Owing to a lapse in motivation, attention, or self-regulatory strength (willpower) and/or perhaps to temporarily losing sight of long-range goals, the dieter can no longer summon the resources necessary to fend off the desire for palatable food. This analysis of the problem seems reasonable as far as it goes; but, as Hofmann and colleagues have argued (Hofmann, Friese, & Strack, 2009), more than one element in the equation predicts successful resistance to temptation. Obviously, the fewer the resources one brings to the resistance effort, the less likely it is to succeed, but by the same token, not all temptations demand the same amount of resistance. Some temptations are more tempting than others, and the prediction of self-regulatory success should take that fact into consideration. Loewenstein's analysis of self-control (e.g., Hoch & Loewenstein, 1991; Loewenstein, 1996) emphasizes fluctuations in desire, with the probability of self-control success varying inversely with the intensity of desire at the visceral level. If the hungry individual displays less resistance to forbidden food, is it because hunger depletes the resources necessary for resistance, or because hunger renders the forbidden food even sweeter? It may be that the "resistance resources" remain constant but the temptation to be resisted becomes more desirable, overwhelming the resources that formerly were capable of sustaining resistance to less intense temptations. A rich dessert is easier to resist when it is merely described verbally on the menu than when it is glistening right in front of you on your plate. This analysis finds empirical support in the previously described studies by Fedoroff and colleagues (1997, 2003).

CONCLUSIONS

Consideration of the magnitude or intensity of temptation simply reminds us that resistance to temptation is a dynamic process, and that success at a task depends on both our ability and the difficulty of the task, either of which can in principle be manipulated independently. This perspective, although obvious in a way, also makes clear that we have not yet achieved a truly comprehensive analysis of self-regulatory success and failure. The final model will have to include both the state of the dieter and the power of the tempting stimulus. Neither factor is easy to measure independently; most models assume that the "other" factor is held constant, while the factor of interest is varied. Hofmann and his colleagues appear to be addressing this challenge effectively.

We have come a long way in understanding self-regulation in the past few decades, although one cannot help thinking that some ancient Greek philosophers must have known all of this. Still, we clearly have a long way to go in terms of establishing the relative merits of the competing theories (or even the extent to which the competing theories are not just saying the same thing in different words). Eating provides a nice crucible for testing models of self-regulation and self-regulatory failure. As our survey indicates, several intriguing models have been developed specifically in the context of eating, whereas others have been developed elsewhere and imported into the domain of eating. The next steps, we believe, will be to identify and articulate more clearly the empirically testable differences among these models, and to do the sort of research that will help us to decide which models best account for the data.

REFERENCES

Baucom, D. H., & Aiken, P. A. (1981). Effect of depressed mood on eating among obese and nonobese dieting and nondieting persons. *Journal of Personality and Social Psychology, 41,* 577–585.

Baumeister, R. F., Bratslavsky, E., Muraven, M., & Tice, D. M. (1998). Ego depletion: Is the active self a limited resource? *Journal of Personality and Social Psychology, 74,* 1252–1265.

Baumeister, R. F., Vohs, K. D., & Tice, D. M. (2007). The strength model of self-control. *Current Directions in Psychological Science, 16,* 351–355.

Fedoroff, I., Polivy, J., & Herman, C. P. (2003). The specificity of restrained versus unrestrained eaters' responses to food cues: General desire to eat, or craving for the cued food? *Appetite, 41*, 7–13.

Fedoroff, I. C., Polivy, J., & Herman, C. P. (1997). The effect of pre-exposure to food cues on the eating behavior of restrained and unrestrained eaters. *Appetite, 28*, 33–47.

Fishbach, A., Friedman, R. S., & Kruglanski, A. W. (2003). Leading us not unto temptation: Momentary allurements elicit overriding goal activation. *Journal of Personality and Social Psychology, 84*, 296–309.

Friese, M., Hofmann, W., & Wänke, M. (2008). When impulses take over: Moderated predictive validity of implicit and explicit attitude measures in predicting food choice and consumption behavior. *British Journal of Social Psychology, 47*, 397–419.

Fujita, K., & Han, H. A. (2009). Moving beyond deliberative control of impulses: The effect of construal levels on evaluative associations in self-control conflicts. *Psychological Science, 20*, 799–804.

Fujita, K., Trope, Y., Liberman, N., & Levin-Sagi, M. (2006). Construal levels and self-control. *Journal of Personality and Social Psychology, 90*, 351–367.

Gailliot, M. T., & Baumeister, R. F. (2007). The physiology of willpower: Linking blood glucose to self-control. *Personality and Social Psychology Review, 11*, 303–327.

Heatherton, T. F., & Baumeister, R. F. (1991). Binge eating as escape from self-awareness. *Psychological Bulletin, 110*, 86–108.

Heatherton, T. F., Herman, C. P., & Polivy, J. (1991). Effects of physical threat and ego threat on eating behavior. *Journal of Personality and Social Psychology, 60*, 138–143.

Herman, C. P., & Mack, D. (1975). Restrained and unrestrained eating. *Journal of Personality, 43*, 647–660.

Herman, C. P., & Polivy, J. (1975). Anxiety, restraint, and eating behavior. *Journal of Abnormal Psychology, 84*, 666–672.

Herman, C. P., & Polivy, J. (1980). Restrained eating. In A. J. Stunkard (Ed.), *Obesity* (pp. 208–225). Philadelphia: Saunders.

Herman, C. P., & Polivy, J. (1993). Mental control of eating: Excitatory and inhibitory food thoughts. In D. M. Wegner & J. W. Pennebaker (Eds.), *Handbook of mental control* (pp. 491–505). Englewood Cliffs, NJ: Prentice-Hall.

Herman, C. P., & Polivy, J. (2005). Normative influences on food intake. *Physiology and Behavior, 86*, 762–772.

Herman, C. P., & Polivy, J. (2008). External cues in the control of food intake in humans: The sensory–normative distinction. *Physiology and Behavior, 94*, 722–728.

Herman, C. P., Polivy, J., & Esses, V. M. (1987). The illusion of counter-regulation. *Appetite, 9*, 161–169.

Herman, C. P., Polivy, J., Lank, C., & Heatherton, T. F. (1987). Anxiety, hunger, and eating behavior. *Journal of Abnormal Psychology, 96*, 264–269.

Herman, C. P., Roth, D. A., & Polivy, J. (2003). Effects of the presence of others on food intake: A normative interpretation. *Psychological Bulletin, 129*, 873–886.

Higgs, S. (2002). Memory for recent eating and its influence on subsequent food intake. *Appetite, 39*, 159–166.

Higgs, S. (2005). Memory and its role in appetite regulation. *Physiology and Behavior, 85*, 67–72.

Higgs, S., Williamson, A. C., & Attwood, A. S. (2008). Recall of recent lunch and its effect on subsequent snack intake. *Physiology and Behavior, 94*, 454–462.

Higgs, S., & Woodward, M. (2009). Television watching during lunch increases afternoon snack intake of young women. *Appetite, 52*, 39–43.

Hoch, S. J., & Loewenstein, G. F. (1991). Time-inconsistent preferences and consumer self-control. *Journal of Consumer Research, 17*, 492–507.

Hofmann, W., & Friese, M. (2008). Impulses got the better of me: Alcohol moderates the influence of implicit attitudes toward food cues on eating behavior. *Journal of Abnormal Psychology, 117,* 420–427.

Hofmann, W., Friese, M., & Strack, F. (2009). Impulse and self-control from a dual-systems perspective. *Perspectives on Psychological Science, 4,* 162–176.

Hofmann, W., Rauch, W., & Gawronski, B. (2007). And deplete us not into temptation: Automatic attitudes, dietary restraint, and self-regulatory resources as determinants of eating behavior. *Journal of Experimental Social Psychology, 43,* 497–504.

Jansen, A. (1998). A learning model of binge eating: Cue reactivity and cue exposure. *Behaviour Research and Therapy, 36,* 257–272.

Jansen, A., & van den Hout, M. (1991). On being led into temptation: "Counterregulation" of dieters after smelling a "preload." *Addictive Behaviors, 16,* 247–253.

Kahan, D., Polivy, J., & Herman, C. P. (2003). Conformity and dietary disinhibition: A test of the ego-strength model of self-regulation. *International Journal of Eating Disorders, 33,* 165–171.

Knight, L. J., & Boland, F. J. (1989). Restrained eating: An experimental disentanglement of the disinhibiting variables of perceived calories and food type. *Journal of Abnormal Psychology, 98,* 499–503.

Leone, T., Herman, C. P., & Pliner, P. (2008). Perceptions of undereaters: A matter of perspective? *Personality and Social Psychology Bulletin, 34,* 1737–1746.

Loewenstein, G. (1996). Out of control: Visceral influences on behavior. *Organizational Behavior and Human Decision Processes, 65,* 272–292.

McKenna, R. J. (1972). Some effects of anxiety level and food cues on the eating behavior of obese and normal subjects: A comparison of the Schachterian and psychosomatic conceptions. *Journal of Personality and Social Psychology, 22,* 311–319.

Mischel, W., Cantor, N., & Feldman, S. (1996). Principles of self-regulation: The nature of willpower and self-control. In E. T. Higgins & A. W. Kruglanski (Eds.), *Social psychology: Handbook of basic principles* (pp. 329–360). New York: Guilford Press.

Mischel, W., Shoda, Y., & Rodriguez, M. L. (1992). Delay of gratification in children. In G. Loewenstein & J. Elster (Eds.), *Choice over time* (pp. 147–164). New York: Russell Sage Foundation.

Muraven, M., Tice, D. M., & Baumeister, R. F. (1998). Self-control as limited resource: Regulatory depletion patterns. *Journal of Personality and Social Psychology, 74,* 774–789.

Papies, E. K., Stroebe, W., & Aarts, H. (2008). Healthy cognition: Processes of self-regulatory success in restrained eating. *Personality and Social Psychology Bulletin, 34,* 1290–1300.

Polivy, J. (1976). Perception of calories and regulation of intake in restrained and unrestrained subjects. *Addictive Behaviors, 1,* 237–243.

Polivy, J., & Herman, C. P. (1976a). Effects of alcohol on eating behavior: Disinhibition or sedation? *Addictive Behaviors, 1,* 121–125.

Polivy, J., & Herman, C. P. (1976b). Effects of alcohol on eating behavior: Influences of mood and perceived intoxication. *Journal of Abnormal Psychology, 85,* 601–606.

Polivy, J., & Herman, C. P. (2002). If at first you don't succeed: False hopes of self-change. *American Psychologist, 57,* 677–689.

Polivy, J., Herman, C. P., Hackett, R., & Kuleshnyk, I. (1986). The effects of self-attention and public attention on eating in restrained and unrestrained subjects. *Journal of Personality and Social Psychology, 50,* 1253–1260.

Ruderman, A. J., Belzer, L. J., & Halperin, A. (1985). Restraint, anticipated consumption, and overeating. *Journal of Abnormal Psychology, 94,* 547–555.

Schachter, S., & Rodin, J. (Eds.). (1974). *Obese humans and rats.* Potomac, MD: Erlbaum.

Slochower, J. A. (1983). *Excessive eating: The role of emotions and environment.* New York: Human Sciences Press.

Spencer, J. A., & Fremouw, W. J. (1979). Binge eating as a function of restraint and weight classification. *Journal of Abnormal Psychology, 88,* 262–267.

Steele, C. M., & Josephs, R. A. (1990). Alcohol myopia: Its prized and dangerous effects. *American Psychologist, 45,* 921–933.

Stroebe, W. (2008). *Dieting, overweight, and obesity: Self-regulation in a food-rich environment.* Washington, DC: American Psychological Association Press.

Stroebe, W., Mensink, W., Aarts, H., Schut, H., & Kruglanski, A. W. (2008). Why dieters fail: Testing the goal conflict model of eating. *Journal of Experimental Social Psychology, 44,* 26–36.

Stuart, R. B. (1967). Behavioral control of overeating. *Behaviour Research and Therapy, 5,* 357–365.

Tice, D. M., Bratslavsky, E., & Baumeister, R. F. (2001). Emotional distress regulation takes precedence over impulse control: If you feel bad, do it! *Journal of Personality and Social Psychology, 80,* 53–67.

Tomarken, A. J., & Kirschenbaum, D. S. (1984). Effects of plans for future meals on counter regulatory eating by restrained eaters. *Journal of Abnormal Psychology, 93,* 458–472.

Trope, Y., & Liberman, N. (2003). Temporal construal. *Psychological Review, 110,* 403–421.

Urbszat, D., Herman, C. P., & Polivy, J. (2002). Eat, drink and be merry, for tomorrow we diet: Effects of anticipated deprivation on food intake in restrained and unrestrained eaters. *Journal of Abnormal Psychology, 111,* 396–401.

Vohs, K. D., & Heatherton, T. F. (2000). Self-regulatory failure: A resource-depletion approach. *Psychological Science, 11,* 249–254.

Ward, A., & Mann, T. (2000). Don't mind if I do: Disinhibited eating under cognitive load. *Journal of Personality and Social Psychology, 78,* 753–763.

Woody, E. Z., Costanzo, P. R., Liefer, H., & Conger, J. (1981). The effects of taste and caloric perceptions on the eating behavior of restrained and unrestrained subjects. *Cognitive Therapy and Research, 5,* 381–390.

CHAPTER 29

Self-Regulation and Spending
Evidence from Impulsive and Compulsive Buying

RONALD J. FABER
KATHLEEN D. VOHS

Controlling the self is a crucial aspect of human life, with researchers unearthing even more situations in which self-regulation and the executive function serve to guide people in their behavioral choices (Baumeister & Vohs, 2003; Higgins, 1996). One area that has begun to receive attention in the self-regulation literature is buying impulses and decisions (Baumeister, 2002). In Western society, people are constantly encountering tempting products, goods, or services that they may elect to acquire. If the economic crisis of 2008–2009 has highlighted anything, it is that regardless of what people may wish to believe, they clearly cannot have it all. A conflict between "having now" versus "having later" requires the person to engage in self-regulation.

Self-regulation has been characterized as having three component parts: (1) establishing a goal; (2) engaging in actions that lead to obtaining this goal; and (3) monitoring progress toward the goal (Baumeister & Vohs, 2003). For example, one may set a goal of putting at least $50 a week into savings. To achieve this goal, the person may need to cut back on spending, while monitoring whether the savings that result from these behaviors meet the goal. If not, further cutbacks are enacted and more assessments are made until finally the goal of saving $50 a week is reached.

Unfortunately, self-regulation efforts are not always successful. Baumeister and Heatherton (1996) identified three causes of self-control failure: (1) conflicting goals, (2) failure to track one's own behavior, and (3) depletion of the resources that permit self-control to operate. From our perspective, purchasing behaviors can both contribute to the failure to exert self-regulation and be a response to such failures.

Certainly, most people have numerous goals or plans that compete for their financial resources. People may save for a house; their children's education; retirement; a vacation; a particular good, such as a couch or new car; or any of a number of other things.

These items often compete with each other, in that acquiring one item may necessitate not obtaining another.

Failure to track behavior is also evident in the way people engage in spending. People often resolve to make a budget and stick with it, but not many succeed in doing so. Oftentimes it is difficult to monitor behavior, which makes accurate assessments of spending significantly less likely. At the point of making a purchase decision, rarely do people have their monthly spending balance clearly in mind. In short, keeping track of where one's money goes is a difficult task. Consequently, reaching one's goals regarding purchases becomes less likely.

The last factor influencing self-control in purchasing is resource depletion. This model states that self-regulation is a function of the amount of a person's psychic energy, and that engaging in self-regulation takes away some of that energy. Hence, controlling behavior after engaging in laborious prior self-regulation efforts is more likely to fail (Baumeister, Vohs, & Tice, 2007).

Our purpose in this chapter is to demonstrate how the literatures on two types of purchasing fit what is known about self-control. The purchasing behaviors we highlight are impulsive and compulsive buying. We demonstrate how these behaviors may be used in support of self-regulatory goals, how other factors can affect the success of purchase-related goals, and how resource depletion can explain these various types of buying behavior.

IMPULSE BUYING

It has been estimated that impulse purchases account for $4.2 billion dollars in store sales (Mogelonsky, 1998). One study concluded that over one-third (38.7%) of department store purchases are impulse buys (Bellenger, Robertson, & Hirschman, 1978). With shop-at-home television networks multiplying, direct marketing techniques becoming more ubiquitous, and the proliferation of Internet stores, opportunities to engage in impulse buying continue to grow. The likelihood of people succumbing to impulsive purchases may in many cases be traced back to temporary failures in exercising self-control.

Recent definitions of *impulse buying* have pointed out some important characteristics of impulse purchases. Included among these is the notion that the decision to buy is a relatively rapid one (Kacen & Lee, 2002); that there is a diminished concern for consequences of the action (Beatty & Ferrell, 1998; Rook, 1987); and that the decision to buy emerges from a conflict between *affect* (desire) and *cognition* (control) (Hoch & Loewenstein, 1991). These characteristics can also be seen as basic elements of a failed attempt at self-regulation.

Most people attempt to exert self-control to avoid buying everything they desire. Simply put, unless one has an unlimited budget, excessive purchasing conflicts with other goals, such as saving money or buying more desirable items. A serious challenge to the exercise of self-regulation thus occurs when one is faced with an urge to buy. This urge may stem from spotting a desirable brand, other elements of the store environment, or an internal state experienced by the consumer.

It has been hypothesized that factors such as proximity can increase the strength of desire for goods (Hoch & Lowenstein, 1991). Research in self-regulation also points to the role of proximity in producing failures of self-control. Walter Mischel and colleagues (e.g., Mischel & Ebbesen, 1970; see also Mischel & Ayduk, Chapter 5, this volume) have spent over 30 years showing that children seated near a desired object fare significantly worse in their delay of gratification attempts than do children who are not placed close to such objects. Thus, the temptation of inviting products or goods is more difficult to overcome when the desired product is proximal to the person.

There are two types of proximity that can influence desire (Hoch & Lowenstein, 1991). One is physical proximity, which allows a person to have a sensory experience with an item. Seeing a beautiful watch in the store, touching a cashmere sweater, tasting a free sample at the supermarket, smelling perfume sprayed by a store clerk, or test-driving a car are all ways in which consumers may experience sensory stimuli through physical proximity. A second method of boosting desire for a product is via temporal proximity. The closer in time one is to having a possession, the more difficult it is to delay gratification. In support of this notion, consumers describe impulse buying as an unexpected, immediate, and intense urge to buy (Rook, 1987; Rook & Hoch, 1985). It appears that the initial desire might be the most difficult to control.

Technological and marketing innovations, such as TV shopping channels, the Internet, and credit cards, have served to alter proximity and increase desire. However, purchasing urges, even if they are very powerful, do not always lead to action (Rook & Fisher, 1995). In fact, the urge to buy was found to account for just 20% of the variance in impulse buying (Beatty & Ferrell, 1998).

Consumers can utilize various strategies to decrease desire and thereby reduce the likelihood of impulse buying. Control of buying impulses requires willpower. This involves utilizing cognitive effort to exert self-control. As with desire, a number of factors can enhance or diminish this ability. The most common form of exerting willpower is to focus mentally on the costs involved in making a purchase (Puri, 1996; Rook & Hoch, 1985). This may involve considering other uses for the money one is about to spend or reminding oneself of the negative impact of buying the specific item (e.g., "The candy bar will make me fat"; "Buying a martini now means I won't go home and work tonight"; "My spouse will be angry if I bring home another new outfit").

Through interviews with consumers, Rook and Hoch (1985) identified a number of other strategies people use to exert willpower over an impulse buying urge. These included delay strategies, bargaining, and guilt. Delay involves efforts to postpone making a purchase. For example, consumers may say to themselves that they will not make a purchase until they have looked at other items, or that after waiting for some period of time, if they still want the item, then they can come back and buy it. Bargaining strategies involve promising oneself a small reward if the immediate desire is denied (e.g., thinking one can buy the relatively inexpensive, cute earrings if one doesn't buy the expensive purse right now). Finally, to boost resistance, consumers might remind themselves of the guilt they will feel later for making a purchase.

Researchers have demonstrated that cognitive considerations do indeed modify impulse buying behavior (Puri, 1996; Rook & Fisher, 1995). Rook and Fisher (1995), for example, found that normative evaluations of impulse buying moderated the relationship between respondents' own impulsiveness (measured as a personality trait) and what they thought a hypothetical character in a story should do when faced with the desire to make an impulse purchase. For respondents who viewed impulse buying favorably, there was a significant relationship between their own impulsiveness and thinking the character should buy impulsively. However, for respondents who held a negative evaluation of impulse buying, the relationship between trait impulsiveness and recommendations for others' hypothetical behavior disappeared. A second study replicated these relationships for consumers' actual purchasing behavior. It would thus appear that norms affect resistance and therefore influence the likelihood of impulse buying.

Willpower may help to improve self-control over buying impulses, but there are situations in which it may be difficult to exert willpower. Several researchers have noted the role of mood as an antecedent of impulse buying (Beatty & Ferrell, 1998; Rook & Gardner, 1993; Weinberg & Gottwald, 1982). Impulse buying has been found to occur more frequently when people feel positively than when they are distressed or in a bad mood (Beatty & Ferrell, 1998). Rook and Gardner (1993) reported that 85% of their sample indicated they were more likely to buy on impulse if they were in a positive rather than a negative mood. Pleasure was the most frequently reported mood state preceding impulse buying. Not coincidentally, it has been found that a pleasant mood state can bias evaluations and judgments in a positive direction (Gardner, 1985). By making everything look better, pleasure and other positive moods may increase impulse buying by enhancing desire. People in pleasant moods also want to extend this desirable feeling (Rook & Gardner, 1993) and this motivation may also serve to increase the desire to buy.

Although negative mood states lead to impulse buying less frequently than do positive moods, the effects of negative emotions are not negligible: over one-third of the Rook and Gardner (1993) sample indicated they had made impulse purchases when in a negative mood. These respondents indicated that impulsive purchases are often made with the hope of alleviating the unpleasant mood. In this situation, consumers may be making a deliberate decision not to exert self-regulation in one area (spending) in order to achieve another goal (a more positive mood state; see Tice, Bratslavsky, & Baumeister, 2001). In this case, the effort to exert control is diminished, and impulse buying results from this change in willpower. This notion that people make a conscious decision to reduce self-control is supported by the fact that respondents state that they spend less money on impulse purchases in negative mood states than in positive ones (Rook & Gardner, 1993). This may indicate that consumers have made a conscious decision to permit a small lapse in self-control to achieve the greater good of balancing mood state. Similar findings of reduced self-control during negative mood states have been found for other self-regulatory behaviors (Baumeister, Vohs, DeWall, & Zhang, 2007).

The previous example may be labeled as a self-regulatory failure that occurs through acquiescence (Baumeister, Heatherton, & Tice, 1994) because the person chooses to give up self-regulation. Similar acquiescence failures occur when people are tired from either physical exertion or, more directly, recent use of self-regulatory resources. The ability to command self-regulation successfully has been conceptualized as a finite resource that can be depleted by situational demands (Baumeister, 2002; Bauer & Baumeister, Chapter 4, this volume; Vohs & Heatherton, 2000). Both exerting self-control and making decisions (Bruyneel, Dewitte, Vohs, & Warlop, 2006; Vohs et al., 2008) have been shown to deplete this resource. Thus, use of self-regulatory resources leaves an individual with a lowered ability to maintain self-control soon thereafter. This model suggests that impulse buying may be more common at the end of a shopping trip or after a long day of decision making.

One series of studies has tested the effect of depletion of self-regulatory resources on impulse buying (Vohs & Faber, 2007). In the first study, participants were randomly assigned to either a resource depletion or a no-depletion condition. In the resource depletion condition, participants were instructed to watch a silent video but avoid looking at part of the content on the screen. Control (no-depletion) participants viewed the same tape but with no instructions to avoid looking at any of the content. This manipulation had previously been found to manipulate self-regulatory resources successfully (Schmeichel, Vohs, & Baumeister, 2003).

Following exposure to the video, participants completed a modified version of the Buying Impulsiveness Scale (BIS; Rook & Fisher, 1995). The BIS was initially designed to assess trait impulse buying, but here it was reworded to pertain just to the participants' desires, urges, and inhibitions for buying in the current situation. The results of this study indicated that participants in the resource depletion condition scored significantly higher on the modified (State) BIS scale than did the no-depletion participants. Thus, reducing self-regulatory resources seemed to increase the propensity for impulse buying.

In a second study, self-regulatory resources were similarly manipulated with an attention control task, after which participants were shown pictures of 18 high-priced items (e.g., expensive watches, cars). Participants were asked to indicate how much they would be willing to pay for each item. The results showed that resource-depleted participants reported that they would pay significantly more for the items than the no-depletion participants.

Finally, a third study used a different manipulation of self-regulatory resources to examine actual impulse buying. In this study, resource-depleted participants were asked to read aloud a series of boring historical biographies while exaggerating their hand gestures, facial expressions, and emotionality. This task required self-control because it involved amplifying and creating an emotional reaction while reading dull biographies that lacked emotional content. Participants in the no-depletion condition read aloud the same information but were not asked to change their reading style. After the manipulation, participants were given the opportunity to buy at a discounted price items commonly found in a college bookstore or a supermarket. Participants who experienced resource depletion chose to buy more items and spend more total dollars than those whose regulatory resources were not depleted. This finding was especially strong for participants who scored high in trait impulsive buying (as measured by the original BIS scale; Rook and Fisher, 1995), suggesting that among people for whom impulsive purchasing is a problem, having few regulatory resources available considerably increases the prospect of spending impulsively.

A more recent study (Ackerman, Goldstein, Shapiro, & Bargh, 2009) found that merely imagining having to engage in self-regulation (in this case, not eating tempting food) led people to say they would pay more for products in a procedure similar to the Vohs and Faber (2007) Study 2. Together, these studies suggest that people are more likely to acquiesce to an impulse buying urge when self-regulatory resources are diminished.

COMPULSIVE BUYING

While impulse buying is a behavior in which almost everyone engages one time or another, compulsive buying is a far more serious problem that affects only a small percentage of people. A general population prevalence study has indicated that about 5.8% of the population may be compulsive buyers (Koran, Faber, Aboujaoude, Large, & Serpe, 2006).

Compulsive buyers often have a history of other disorders, such as alcoholism and substance abuse (McElroy, Keck, Pope, Smith, & Strakowski, 1994; Schlosser, Black, Repertinger, & Freet, 1994), bulimia (Christenson et al., 1994; Faber, Christenson, de Zwaan, & Mitchell, 1995), and depression (Lejoyeux, Tassain, Solomon, & Ades, 1997).

Compulsive buying is defined as chronic, repetitive purchasing that becomes an overlearned and automatic way to cope with negative feelings (Faber, 2000b; Faber & O'Guinn, 2008; O'Guinn & Faber, 1989). Buying provides short-term gratification but ultimately causes harm for the individual and/or others. These negative consequences may range from interpersonal conflicts and financial difficulties to more extreme outcomes, such as divorce, jail sentences for writing bad checks, embezzlement or theft of funds to enable buying, and suicide attempts (Faber, 2004; O'Conner, 2001). In one particularly tragic case, a woman was found dead after being buried under a mountain of items she had compulsively bought and hoarded. It took policeman 2 days to find her body under all of her purchases (Tozer, 2009).

Compulsive buying is a psychiatric disorder that appears to be related to obsessive–compulsive disorder (Frost et al., 1998), impulse control disorder (Christenson et al., 1994; Koran, Bullock, Hartson, Elliott, & D'Andrea, 2002), or both (Hollander & Allen, 2006; Schlosser et al., 1994; Swan-Kremeir, Mitchell, & Faber, 2005). Inconsistent results with a range of different pharmacological treatments have contributed to the confusion regarding the underlying basis of this disorder (Grant, 2003; Koran et al., 2002; McElroy et al., 1994). Perhaps because compulsive buying is often classified as an impulse control disorder, some authors seem to confuse compulsive and impulsive buying. While both may be viewed as stemming from self-regulatory failure, they differ in terms of the cause of the failure and the form it takes.

One distinction in self-regulation failure is between an initial violation and a complete breakdown of self-regulation (Baumeister et al., 1994). Initial violations are cases that involve a single instance of failing to maintain a goal-directed behavior, but control can be quickly reestablished afterwards. Alternatively, when there is a complete breakdown in self-regulation, an initial failure can lead to a major binge in the prohibited behavior. Baumeister and colleagues (1994) refer to this effect as *snowballing*.

A second distinction in different types of failure is based on the underlying cause. Most research in self-regulation failure has focused on *underregulation*, which is the failure to exert sufficient self-control. An alternative cause, *misregulation*, occurs when people attempt to exert regulation but do so using unproductive or counterproductive strategies.

Impulsive buying might best be characterized as a type of initial violation failure that generally results from underregulation. Conversely, compulsive buying appears to be a chronic failure, attributable more to misregulation.

Compulsive buyers often report a repetitive pattern of feeling bad, buying to achieve short-term relief from these feelings, but this is quickly replaced with guilt and further bad self-feelings, leading to an ongoing repetitive cycle. Misregulation occurs because buying is used temporarily to reduce negative feelings. A complete breakdown of the regulatory system can be seen in the reports of many compulsive buyers who purchase multiple, similar items in a shopping trip, such as several T-shirts, sweaters, raincoats, or even cartons of milk (Christenson et al., 1994; O'Guinn & Faber, 1989).

Researchers have found that the primary motivation behind compulsive buying is actually not the desire for the object purchased but rather a temporary improvement in mood or self-esteem (Faber 2000a; O'Guinn & Faber, 1989). Notably, desire for an object as the motivation for purchasing was actually found to be higher among general consumers than among compulsive buyers (O'Guinn & Faber, 1989). In-depth interviews support this notion by demonstrating that many compulsive buyers report that they never use products they purchased. Instead, months or years later, many of these items remain in their original packages or with sales tags still attached. As one compulsive buyer stated, "It's not that I want it, because sometimes I'll just buy it and I'll think, 'Ugh, another sweatshirt'" (O'Guinn & Faber, 1989, p. 154).

Rather than buying to obtain a desired item, compulsive buyers more likely buy to alter their mood state or arousal level (Elliott, 1994; Faber, 2000b; Faber & Christenson, 1996). A study of compulsive buyers examined over 400 possible triggers of compulsive buying episodes and found two primary categories of antecedents. One comprised stimuli associated with buying (e.g., money, sales, department stores) and the other included negative affective states and behaviors that caused them (Faber, Ristvedt, Mackenzie, & Christenson, 1996). Compared to other consumers, compulsive shoppers report experiencing negative mood states more often prior to shopping, and positive mood states more frequently during shopping (Faber & Christenson, 1996). Although virtually all compulsive buyers indicated that buying changes their mood state, this was true for only about one-fourth of the comparison (general shopper) sample. Compulsive buyers were also more likely to state that this change in mood was typically in a positive direction.

Changes in arousal level may also be an important motivating factor behind compulsive buying. Compulsive buyers tend to describe their buying experiences as highly arousing, using terms like feeling such as "high," "a rush," "powerful," "excited," "elated," or "out of control" (Faber, 2000a; Faber & Christenson, 1996; McElroy, Keck, & Phillips, 1995). Several compulsive buyers have reported that their buying occurs in response to feeling bored and when they want something exciting to provide a temporary lift. As one compulsive buyer put it:

> "There's times when I'm depressed or bored or something. I just want something new and I'll just go and feel like buying and it makes me feel good. I feel different, excited, happy and I'm ready to go on with other boring things." (in Faber, 2000a, p. 41)

The impact of mood and arousal fits with research on self-regulation failure. People attempt to alter or prolong emotional states via affect regulation. Probably the most common attempt at affect regulation is to overcome a bad mood (Baumeister, Vohs, DeWall, et al., 2007). Consumption behaviors, such as eating (see Herman & Polivy, Chapter 28, this volume), drinking alcohol, or taking drugs (see Sayette & Griffin, Chapter 27, this volume), represent other types of affect regulation strategy. Importantly, people believe that these behaviors have the ability to alter mood states but, in actuality, they often fail to relieve a bad mood and may in fact eventually worsen it (see Baumeister, Vohs, DeWall, et al., 2007, for a review). It would appear that buying is also a way to regulate affect. Indeed, phrases like "When the going gets tough, the tough go shopping" illustrate a societal view that buying can improve one's emotional state.

For compulsive buyers, attempts at affect regulation through buying may lead to a pattern of misregulation (see Rawn & Vohs, Chapter 20, this volume). The consumer may attempt to overcome a negative mood state by buying, which serves temporarily to improve mood. However, soon after buying, a feeling of guilt sets in when the person is reminded that he or she wasted money or failed at the goal of not buying. This negative state can lead to depression and low self-esteem. Consequently, the person feels a strong need to overcome negative self-evaluations, and this need can lead to buying again (to boost positive affect), and so on. This becomes a vicious cycle that is increasingly difficult to break.

Compulsive buyers may be particularly susceptible to this pattern of attempting to cure negative affect with buying because they often experience painful self-awareness. Self-awareness is an important determinant of maintaining self-regulation. To self-regulate, a person must monitor his or her current circumstances, including progression through the environment, tracking progress to and from the goal, and reevaluating desired outcomes. All of these tasks require a certain degree of self-awareness. Reductions in self-awareness are linked to disinhibition, which in turn leads to self-regulation failure (e.g., Heatherton & Baumeister, 1991; see Carver & Scheier, Chapter 1, this volume).

The need to avoid self-awareness often starts with the presence of exceptionally high standards or expectations for oneself (Duval & Wicklund, 1972). Compulsive buyers have been reported to be perfectionists (DeSarbo & Edwards, 1996; Faber, 2000a; O'Guinn & Faber, 1989). They often report that they tried hard to please their parents during childhood, but generally felt as if they failed (Faber & O'Guinn, 1988). This can clearly be seen in a quotation from one compulsive buyer:

> "Because you are the oldest you're suppose to be the good little person. I was always trying to win their [parents'] approval but couldn't. You know you could have stood on your head and turned blue and it wouldn't matter. I got straight A's and all kinds of honors and it never mattered." (in Faber & O'Guinn, 1988, p. 10)

The perception of being unable to please parents, feelings of inadequacy, and failure to receive recognition for diligent efforts leads many compulsive buyers to develop low self-esteem. Numerous studies have found that compulsive buyers have low self-esteem compared to other consumers (Elliott, 1994; O'Guinn & Faber, 1989; Scherhorn, Reisch, & Raab, 1990). The relationship between low self-esteem and having a high standard of comparison (e.g., being perfectionistic) is particularly apparent in interviews in which compulsive buyers compare themselves with their siblings. The following two examples illustrate this:

> "I have a brother who is now a dentist, who is everything Mother and Dad ever wanted without question. He was bright and he was very engaging and he is very well to do and all of that. And then there is (informant's name) and my mother did my schoolwork ever since I was in fifth grade. She did all of my schoolwork, even my college papers. It's not much to be proud of." (in O'Guinn & Faber, 1989, p. 153)

> "Right now my brothers are both millionaires. My father's a millionaire. I was not poor, but I was not very rich." (in Faber & O'Guinn, 1988, p. 9)

Moreover, aversive self-awareness can lead to depression and anxiety (Ingram, 1990). Not surprisingly, compulsive buyers have higher than average levels of depression (McElroy et al., 1994; Schlosser et al., 1994) and anxiety (Christenson et al., 1994; Scherhorn et al., 1990). Not only do compulsive buyers experience these negative feelings more often, but the intensity may also be more extreme. Researchers report that between 25 and 50% of compulsive buyers have clinical histories of major depressive disorder (Christenson et al., 1994; McElroy et al., 1994; Schlosser et al., 1994). These negative self-appraisals may impel people to try to escape from self-awareness. One way to do this is to focus on an immediate, concrete, low-level task, such as shopping or buying. This phenomenon, referred to as *cognitive narrowing*, is a form of misregulation (see Rawn & Vohs, Chapter 20, this volume). Cognitive narrowing creates disinhibition and prevents consideration of the longer-term consequences of an action (Heatherton & Baumeister, 1991). In self-regulation terms, this is referred to as *transcendence failure*.

Research on compulsive buying matches the predictions generated from self-regulation and escape theory. If compulsive buying occurs in an effort to cope with adverse self-awareness, it should follow as a direct response to such negative moods. Several studies have shown this to be the case. Compulsive buyers were asked to complete the sentence fragment "I am most likely to buy myself something when. . . . " Almost three-fourths finished the sentence by including some mention of a negative emotion, such as "I'm depressed" or "I feel bad about myself" (Faber, O'Guinn, & Krych, 1987). In a different study, compulsive buyers were asked to nominate from a list of over 400 items factors associated with a worsening of their compulsive buying. A factor analysis of commonly mentioned items indicated that the two things that led to compulsive buying urges were shopping-related stimuli (e.g., being around malls or stores; having money or credit cards) and experiencing negative emotions related to the self (e.g., feeling fat, bored, stressed, depressed, angry, hurt, or irritable). Finally, some compulsive buying informants have stated that the only time they escape negative feelings is when they are shopping (Elliott, 1994).

Compulsive buyers may be particularly susceptible to cognitive narrowing when shopping. They frequently mention noticing stimuli such as colors, textures, sounds, and smells while shopping (Schlosser et al., 1994). The concept of *absorption*, which is the tendency to become immersed in self-involving experiences triggered by engagement in external stimuli, has been applied to compulsive shoppers. Individuals high in absorption (1) are emotionally responsive and readily captured by engaging sights and sounds; (2) become absorbed in vivid and compelling recollections and imaginings; and (3) experience episodes of altered states. Perhaps not surprisingly, people who are prone to compulsive buying score higher on the personality trait of absorption than other consumers (Faber, Peterson, & Christenson, 1994). This aspect of shopping was captured by one compulsive buyer's description of a particular episode:

> "But it was like, it was almost like my heart was palpitating, I couldn't wait to get in to see what was there. It was such a sensation. In the store, the lights, the people; they were playing Christmas music. I was hyperventilating and my hands were starting to sweat, and all of the sudden I was touching sweaters and the whole of it was just beckoning to me." (in O'Guinn & Faber, 1989, p. 154)

The intense level of cognitive narrowing that can accompany compulsive buying episodes is viewed as desirable by these shoppers. It may well be that this phenomenological experience is why many compulsive buyers consider sales people to be an unwanted intrusion in their shopping, and why most prefer to go shopping by themselves rather than with others (Elliott, 1994; Schlosser et al., 1994).

Another consequence of cognitive narrowing is the failure to recognize the implausibility of beliefs, allowing noncritical, irrational thoughts to emerge that produce magical or fanciful thinking (Heatherton & Baumeister, 1991). Fantasies are common among compulsive buyers. Many report that during buying episodes they imagine themselves as being more powerful or admired. Their buying is accompanied by self-perceptions of being more fashionable, more admired, or being part of an exclusive and desirable group (Krueger, 2000; Scherhorn et al., 1990). Some researchers have found that compulsive buyers are more prone to fantasizing than other consumers (Elliott, 1994; O'Guinn & Faber, 1989).

Cognitive narrowing and fantasizing keep compulsive buyers from focusing their attention on the goal of not spending money. Thus, although the behavior creates a temporary boost in self-esteem, arousal, and mood, it soon turns to feelings of guilt, regret, and despair. This creates a lapse-activated pattern of spiraling distress that is common among people suffering from behavioral and impulse control problems (Baumeister et al., 1994).

CONCLUSION

An understanding of both buying behavior and the self-regulation process can benefit from greater collaboration and cross-fertilization. In this chapter we have attempted to show how the self-regulation literature can be used to better understand impulsive and compulsive buying behaviors. In doing so, we demonstrated how, when, and why buying may result from self-regulatory failure. Although much of the work has focused on personality factors (i.e., trait characteristics) that can help to explain which people are more prone to engage in these behaviors, the self-regulation literature may be particularly beneficial in explaining situational effects (i.e., state effects), such as why a particular episode of impulsive or compulsive buying may take place.

Self-regulatory research also helps to explain how several commonalities found in descriptions of compulsive buyers work together to cause this behavior. Research regarding cognitive narrowing and misregulation is particularly valuable in explaining compulsive buying behavior. Findings regarding the primacy of emotional regulation over other areas of self-regulation help to explain why compulsive buyers may continue to engage in this behavior despite serious consequences for them and their families. The application of self-regulatory failure to other behaviors, such as eating disorders along with compulsive buying, is potentially helpful in explaining the comorbidity among these disorders.

Self-regulation research may also be helpful in distinguishing between different buying behaviors. A good deal of controversy has emerged in the buying behavior literature over whether impulsive and compulsive buying are qualitatively different behaviors, or whether they simply differ as a matter of degree. Work on self-regulatory failure helps to identify their similarities, as well as their differences. Regarding similarities, both disorders may be forms of self-regulatory failure. Regarding differences, however, they may represent different types of failure and stem from different underlying causes. Impulse buying is primarily concerned with single instances or initial violations of self-regulation. Generally, people set a goal and purchase mainly what they intended to purchase. From time to time, however, people may experience a violation of this goal. Typically, this type of lapse is due to underregulation caused by resource depletion. Following this temporary lapse, people are again able to establish control over purchasing.

Although compulsive buying also represents a form of self-regulatory failure, it is chronic and consistent rather than occasional. As a result, it leads to a complete breakdown of the self-regulatory system. The cause of this problem may more likely be a problem of conflicting goals or ineffective monitoring than one of resource depletion. Repeated buying occurs because emotional goals consistently overpower purchasing goals. Additionally, binge buying and multiple-item purchases common in compulsive buying may stem primarily from an inability to monitor behavior resulting from cognitive narrowing. Thus, the problem of compulsive buying is one of misregulation rather than underregulation (Rawn & Vohs, Chapter 20, this volume).

Research in consumer behavior may also help to extend our understanding of the process of self-regulation. Whereas buying is an everyday activity that can offer much opportunity to those interested in the naturalistic study of self-regulation, self-regulation is a critical component in purchasing behavior. As a result, research at the intersection of these areas seems to represent a perfect partnership to enhance our knowledge of both domains.

REFERENCES

Ackerman, J. M., Goldstein, N. J., Shapiro, J. R., & Bargh, J. A. (2009). You wear me out: The vicarious depletion of self-control. *Psychological Science, 20*, 326–332.

Baumeister, R. F. (2002). Yielding to temptation: Self-control failure, impulsive purchasing, and consumer behavior. *Journal of Consumer Research, 28*, 670–676.

Baumeister, R. F., & Heatherton, T. F. (1996). Self-regulation failure: An overview. *Psychological Inquiry, 7*, 1–15.

Baumeister, R. F., Heatherton, T. F., & Tice, D. M. (1994). *Losing control: How and why people fail at self-regulation.* San Diego, CA: Academic Press.

Baumeister, R. F., & Vohs, K. D. (2003). Self-regulation and the executive function of the self. In M. R. Lear & J. P. Tangney (Eds.), *Handbook of self and identity* (pp. 197–217). New York: Guilford Press.

Baumeister, R. F., Vohs, K. D., DeWall, N., & Zhang, L. (2007). How emotion shapes behavior: Feedback, anticipation, and reflection, rather than direct causation. *Personality and Social Psychology Review, 11*, 167–203.

Baumeister, R. F., Vohs, K. D., & Tice, D. M. (2007). The strength model of self-control. *Current Directions in Psychological Science, 16*, 351–355.

Beatty, S. E., & Ferrell, M. E. (1998). Impulse buying: Modeling its precursors. *Journal of Retailing, 74*, 169–191.

Bellenger, D. N., Robertson, D. H., & Hirschman, E. C. (1978). Impulse buying varies by product. *Journal of Advertising Research, 18*, 15–18.

Bruyneel, S., Dewitte, S., Vohs, K. D., & Warlop, L. (2006). Sweet instigator: Choosing increases susceptibility to affective product features. *International Journal of Research in Marketing, 23*, 215–225.

Christenson, G. A., Faber, R. J., de Zwaan, M., Raymond, N., Specker, S., Eckert, M. D., et al. (1994). Compulsive buying: Descriptive characteristics and psychiatric comorbidity. *Journal of Clinical Psychiatry, 55*, 5–11.

DeSarbo, W. S., & Edwards, E. A. (1996). Typologies of compulsive buying behavior:

A constrained clusterwise regression approach. *Journal of Consumer Psychology, 5*, 231–262.

Duval, S., & Wicklund, R. A. (1972). *A theory of objective self-awareness*. San Diego, CA: Academic Press.

Elliott, R. (1994). Addictive consumption: Function and fragmentation in postmodernity. *Journal of Consumer Policy, 17*, 159–179.

Faber, R. J. (2000a). A systematic investigation into compulsive buying. In A. L. Benson (Ed.), *I shop, therefore I am: Compulsive buying and the search for self* (pp. 27–54). Northvale, NJ: Aronson Press.

Faber, R. J. (2000b). The urge to buy: A uses and gratifications perspective. In S. Ratneshwar, D. G. Mick, & C. Huffman (Eds.), *The why of consumption: Contemporary perspectives on consumer motives, goals, and desires* (pp. 177–196). London: Routledge.

Faber, R. J. (2004). Self-control and compulsive buying. In T. Kasser & A. Kanner (Eds.), *Psychology and the culture of consumption* (pp. 169–187). Washington, DC: American Psychological Association.

Faber, R. J., & Christenson, G. A. (1996). In the mood to buy: Differences in the mood states experienced by compulsive buyers and other consumers. *Psychology and Marketing, 13*, 803–820.

Faber, R. J., Christenson, G. A., de Zwaan, M., & Mitchell, J. E. (1995). Two forms of compulsive consumption: Comorbidity of compulsive buying and binge eating. *Journal of Consumer Research, 22*, 296–304.

Faber, R. J., & O'Guinn, T. C. (1988). Dysfunctional consumer socialization: A search for the roots of compulsive buying. In P. Vanden Abeele (Ed.), *Psychology in micro and macro economics*. Leuven, Belgium: International Association for Research in Economic Psychology.

Faber, R. J., & O'Guinn, T. C. (2008). Compulsive buying: Review and reflection. In C. P. Haugtvedt, P. M. Herr, & F. R. Kardes (Eds.), *Handbook of consumer psychology* (pp. 1039–1056). New York: Taylor & Francis.

Faber, R. J., O'Guinn, T. C., & Krych, R. (1987). Compulsive consumption. In M. Wallendorf & P. Anderson (Eds.), *Advances in consumer research* (pp. 132–135). Provo, UT: Association for Consumer Research.

Faber, R. J., Peterson, C., & Christenson, G. A. (1994, August). *Characteristics of compulsive buyers: An examination of stress reaction and absorption*. Paper presented at the annual conference of the American Psychological Association, Los Angeles.

Faber, R. J., Ristvedt, S. L., Mackenzie, T. B., & Christenson, G. A. (1996, October). *Cues that trigger compulsive buying*. Paper presented at the annual conference of the Association for Consumer Research, Tucson, AZ.

Frost, R. O., Kim, H., Morris, C., Bloss, C., Murray-Close, M., & Steketee, G. (1998). Hoarding, compulsive buying and reasons for savings. *Behaviour Research and Therapy, 36*, 657–664.

Gardner, M. P. (1985). Mood states and consumer behavior: A critical review. *Journal of Consumer Research, 12*, 281–300.

Grant, J. E. (2003). Three cases of compulsive buying treated with naltrexone. *International Journal of Psychiatry in Clinical Practice, 7*, 223–225.

Heatherton, T. F., & Baumeister, R. F. (1991). Binge eating as escape from self-awareness. *Psychological Bulletin, 110*, 86–108.

Higgins, E. T. (1996). Knowledge and activation: Accessibility, applicability, and salience. In E. T. Higgins & A. W. Kruglanski (Eds.) *Social psychology: Handbook of basic principles* (pp. 133–168). New York: Guilford Press.

Hoch, S. J., & Loewenstein, G. F. (1991). Time inconsistent preferences and consumer self-control. *Journal of Consumer Research, 18*, 492–507.

Hollander, E., & Allen, A. (2006). Is compulsive buying a real disorder, and is it really compulsive? *American Journal of Psychiatry, 163*, 1670–1672.

Ingram, R. E. (1990). Self-focused attention in clinical disorders: Review and a conceptual model. *Psychological Bulletin, 107*, 156–176.

Kacen, J. J., & Lee, J. A. (2002). The influence of culture on consumer impulsive buying behavior. *Journal of Consumer Psychology, 12*, 163–176.

Koran, L. M., Bullock, K. D., Hartson, H. J., Elliott, M. A., & D'Andrea, V. (2002). Citalopram treatment of compulsive shopping: An open-label study. *Journal of Clinical Psychiatry, 63*, 704–708.

Koran, L. M., Faber, R. J., Aboujaoude, E., Large, M. D., & Serpe, R. T. (2006). Estimated prevalence of compulsive buying in the United States. *American Journal of Psychiatry, 163*, 1806–1812.

Krueger, D. (2000). The use of money as an action symptom. In A. L. Benson (Ed.), *I shop, therefore I am: Compulsive buying and the search for self* (pp. 288–310). Northvale, NJ: Aronson Press.

Lejoyeux, M., Tassain, V., Solomon, J., & Ades, J. (1997). Study of compulsive buying in depressed patients. *Journal of Clinical Psychiatry, 58*, 169–173.

McElroy, S. L., Keck, P. E., Jr., & Phillips, K. A. (1995). Kleptomania, compulsive buying and binge-eating disorder. *Journal of Clinical Psychiatry, 56*, 14–26.

McElroy, S. L., Keck, P. E., Jr., Pope, H. J., Jr., Smith, J. M., & Strakowski, S. M. (1994). Compulsive buying: A report of 20 cases. *Journal of Clinical Psychiatry, 55*, 242–248.

Mischel, W., & Ebbesen, E. B. (1970). Attention in delay of gratification. *Journal of Personality and Social Psychology, 16*, 329–337.

Mogelonsky, M. (1998). Keep candy in the aisles. *American Demographics, 20*, 32.

O'Conner, M. (2001, May 24). Judge buys shopaholic defense in embezzling. *Chicago Tribune*, p. 1.

O'Guinn, T. C., & Faber, R. J. (1989). Compulsive buying: A phenomenological exploration. *Journal of Consumer Research, 16*, 147–157.

Puri, R. (1996). Measuring and modifying consumer impulsiveness: A cost–benefit accessibility framework. *Journal of Consumer Psychology, 5*, 87–113.

Rook, D. W. (1987). The buying impulse. *Journal of Consumer Research, 14*, 189–199.

Rook, D. W., & Fisher, R. J. (1995). Normative influences on impulsive buying behavior. *Journal of Consumer Research, 22*, 305–313.

Rook, D. W., & Gardner, M. P. (1993). In the mood: Impulse buying's affective antecedents. *Research in Consumer Behavior, 6*, 1–28.

Rook, D. W., & Hoch, S. J. (1985). Consuming impulses. *Advances in Consumer Research, 12*, 23–27.

Scherhorn, G., Reisch, L. A., & Raab, G. (1990). Addictive buying in West Germany: An empirical study. *Journal of Consumer Policy, 13*, 355–387.

Schlosser, S., Black, D. W., Repertinger, S., & Freet, D. (1994). Compulsive buying: Demography, phenomenology, and comorbidity in 46 subjects. *General Hospital Psychiatry, 16*, 205–212.

Schmeichel, B. J., Vohs, K. D., & Baumeister, R. F. (2003). Intellectual performance and ego depletion: Role of the self in logical reasoning and other information processing. *Journal of Personality and Social Psychology, 85*, 33–46.

Swan-Kremeir, L. A., Mitchell, J. E., & Faber, R. J. (2005). Compulsive buying: A disorder of compulsivity or impulsivity? In J. S. Abramowitz & A. D. Houts (Eds.), *Concepts and controversies in obsessive–compulsive disorder* (pp. 185–190). New York: Springer-Verlag.

Tice, D. M., Bratslavsky, E., & Baumeister, R. F. (2001). Emotional distress regulation takes precedence over impulse control: If you feel bad, do it! *Journal of Personality and Social Psychology, 80*, 53–67.

Tozer, J. (2009, January 9). Shopaholic spinster found dead under 3 ft of unopened goods. *Daily Mail Online*. Retrieved August 4, 2009, from *www.dailymail.co.uk/news/article-1109168*.

Vohs, K. D., Baumeister, R. F., Schmeichel, B. J., Twenge, J. M., Nelson, N. M., & Tice, D. M. (2008). Making choices impairs subsequent self-control: A limited resource account of decision making, self-regulation, and active initiative. *Journal of Personality and Social Psychology, 94*, 883–898.

Vohs, K. D., & Faber, R. J. (2007). Spent resources: Self-regulatory resource availability affects impulse buying. *Journal of Consumer Research, 33*, 537–547.

Vohs, K. D., & Heatherton, T. F. (2000). Self-regulatory failure: A resource-depletion approach. *Psychological Science, 11*, 249–254.

Weinberg, P., & Gottwald, W. (1982). Impulsive consumer buying as a result of emotions. *Journal of Business Research, 10*, 43–57.

CHAPTER 30

Attention-Deficit/Hyperactivity Disorder, Self-Regulation, and Executive Functioning

RUSSELL A. BARKLEY

Current psychiatric taxonomy describes attention-deficit/hyperactivity disorder, or ADHD, as involving developmentally inappropriate degrees of inattention and hyperactive–impulsive behavior. These symptoms frequently arise in early childhood, are relatively pervasive or cross-situational in nature, may persist into adolescence and even adulthood in the majority of clinically diagnosed cases, and result in impairment in major life activities, such as family functioning, peer relations, and educational and occupational functioning, among others (American Psychiatric Association, 2001; Barkley, 2006; Barkley, Murphy, & Fischer, 2008). This perspective emphasizes problems in the realms of attention, impulsiveness, and activity level as being central to a conceptualization of the disorder. But children and adults with ADHD often demonstrate deficiencies in many other motor, cognitive, and emotion regulation abilities (for reviews, see Barkley, 2006, 2010).

Many of these disabilities fall within the domain of "executive functions" (EFs) in neuropsychology (Barkley, 1997a, 1997b; Denckla, 1996) or "metacognition" in developmental psychology (Welsh, Pennington, & Grossier, 1991), or are affected by these functions. All seem to be mediated, at least in part, by the frontal cortex, and particularly the prefrontal lobes and at least three or more neural networks that are implicated in the neuropsychology of ADHD (Castellanos, Sonuga-Barke, Milham, & Tannock, 2006; Fuster, 1997; Nigg & Casey, 2005; Sagvolden, Johansen, Aase, & Russell, 2005). Theorists have long speculated that problems with executive functioning specifically and self-regulation more generally are at the heart of this disorder, and give rise to the more superficial and surface symptoms represented in clinical diagnostic criteria (Barkley, 1997b; Pontius, 1973).

551

But viewing ADHD as a disorder of executive functioning and self-regulation necessitates that (1) one operationally define these terms, (2) give a reasonable account of how normal self-regulation develops in children, and (3) explain just how ADHD acts to disrupt that normal developmental process. For 15 years, I have tried to do so in constructing and researching a theory of ADHD (Barkley, 1997a, 2001; Barkley & Murphy, in press; Barkley et al., 2008).

DEFINING INHIBITION, SELF-CONTROL, AND EXECUTIVE FUNCTIONING

Behavioral inhibition, self-control, and executive functioning are overlapping and interacting human abilities in this account. The overarching purpose of self-control and EFs is viewed here as an inherently social one: Humans engage in reciprocal social exchanges as a means to their survival and must both track such prior exchanges with others, and anticipate and prepare for such future interactions with others. That purpose probably arose out of the group living niche that humans occupy—one of social groups that comprise genetically unrelated or distantly related individuals who came to depend on forms of reciprocal exchange or selfish altruism and the formation of cooperative coalitions for orchestrating non-zero-sum activities on which their survival depended. Such coalitions attain economic and other survival benefits that cannot be achieved by the individual acting alone or purely selfishly, as in zero-sum interactions (Wright, 2000). From this perspective, nonsocial organisms that live relatively independently of other members of their species (other than for mating/reproductive activities) do not need self-control or the EFs that permit it.

Response inhibition here refers to three overlapping yet somewhat distinct and separately measurable processes:

1. Inhibiting the initial prepotent (dominant) response to an event so as to create a delay in responding; the response is now temporarily decoupled from the stimulus that served to elicit it.
2. Interrupting an ongoing response that is proving ineffective, thereby permitting a delay in and reevaluation of the decision to continue responding (a sensitivity to error).
3. Protecting the self-directed (executive) responses that occur within these delays, as well as the goal-directed behavior they generate from disruption by competing events and responses (interference control or resistance to distraction) (Barkley, 1997a, 1997b; Fuster, 1997).

The first is the most important. Without a delay in the prepotent response (self-stopping), any thinking and related goal-directed actions pertinent to that situation are impossible and pointless (Barkley, 1997a; Bronowski, 1967/1977). It is not just the response that is delayed, but the decision about a response (Bronowski, 1967/1977). The prepotent response is that response for which immediate reinforcement (positive or negative) is available within a particular context, or which has previously been associated with that response in that context (Barkley, 1997b).

Self-control is a response (or series of responses) by the individual that functions to alter the probability of subsequent response to an event, and in so doing thereby changes the likelihood of a *later* consequence related to that event (Barkley, 1997a, 1997b; Kanfer & Karoly, 1972; Mischel, 1983; Mischel, Shoda, & Rodriguez, 1989; Skinner, 1953). It is any action directed by someone toward the self so as to change behavior and therein alter future rather than merely immediate consequences. It involves the choice of a delayed, larger reward over a more immediate, smaller one (Ainslie, 1974; Burns & Powers, 1975; Logue, 1988; Mischel, 1983; Mischel & Ayduk, Chapter 5, this volume; Navarick, 1986). But this ignores the self-directed actions in which the individual must engage so as to value the delayed over the immediate reward, then pursue that delayed consequence. Self-control seems to involve four minimum steps: (1) the inhibition of the prepotent response directed toward some environmental event, (2) the direction of actions (both cognitive and motoric) toward oneself that (3) result in the alteration of the subsequent response from what it would have been had none of these self-directed actions been enacted [a different response is enacted as a consequence of these self-directed actions that replaces the originally prepotent response], and (4) change in the likelihood of a delayed (future) consequence that arises as a function of this change in the behavior employed.

What, then, is executive functioning? Neuropsychology seems to view it as being comprised largely of unobservable "cognitive" or mentalistic events accomplished chiefly by the prefrontal cortex. That literature is typified by descriptions of various other constructs thought to be included under the meta-construct of executive functioning, while the meta-construct itself goes undefined. For instance, literature reviews, executive functioning scale developers, and research papers may define executive functioning by listing its component features, such as inhibition, working memory, planning, emotional or motivational regulation, strategy development and use, flexible sequencing of actions, maintenance of behavioral set, resistance to interference, and so forth (i.e., Denckla, 1996; Frazier, Demareem, & Youngstrom, 2004; Gioia, Isquith, Guy, & Kenworthy, 2000; Hervey, Epstein, & Curry, 2004; Thorell & Nyberg, 2008), or by just listing measures believed to reflect executive functioning (Biederman et al., 2007; Huizinga, Dolan, & van der Molen, 2006). Lezak (1995) describes EFs as "those capacities that enable a person to engage successfully in independent, purposive, self-serving behavior" (p. 42). Others simply conclude that EF encompasses all future-directed behavior (Huizinga et al., 2006) and is what the frontal lobes do (Stuss & Benson, 1986). The underlying theme of the EFs seems to be this future orientation, as conjectured by Denckla (1996) and which the philosopher Daniel Dennett (1995) has called "the intentional stance." Just what specifically makes a cognitive or behavioral action executive in nature?

To answer this question, consider that all goal-directed behavior requires a capacity for understanding time and the temporal ordering of events, holding such information actively in mind, and using it to order and execute timely responses to events (Shimamura, Janowsky, & Squire, 1990). To do so, behavior must be hierarchically organized, nesting smaller units within larger goals that are themselves nested within even larger goals (Badre, 2008; Goel & Grafman, 1995; Sirigu et al., 1995) that seems to map onto a rostrocaudal organization of the frontal cortex (Badre, 2008). In my theory of executive functioning and self-regulation, *EFs comprise the principal classes of behavior that we use toward our selves for purposes of self-regulation (changing our future)*. An *executive act* is any action directed toward oneself that functions to modify one's own behavior so as to change future outcomes for that individual. Doing so achieves the requirements for self-stopping, self-management within time, self-organization and problem solving across time, self-activation to initiate outcomes, and self-motivation to sustain action toward the goal (Barkley & Murphy, in press). Such actions may be covert but need not be so to be classified as "executive" actions here. The term *covert* merely means that the outward, publicly observable (musculoskeletal) manifestations of such behavior are being inhibited and made very difficult to detect by others over the course of human evolution (and human development). But the central neural equivalents of those actions still occur in the brain and can be thought of as forms of behavior, albeit behavior-to-the-self. They are volitional, effortful, conscious, and self-initiated actions.

Developments in the technology of neuroimaging and the fine-grained recording of shifts in muscle potential now suggest that this covert behavior-to-the-self is capable of being measured (D'Esposito et al., 1997; Livesay, Liebke, Samaras, & Stanley, 1996; Livesay & Samaras, 1998; Ryding, Bradvik, & Ingvar, 1996). As these studies suggest, when we engage in verbal thought (covert self-speech) and imagined actions, the peripheral muscles and brain substrates ordinarily associated with the outward or public display of these same actions continue to be activated. But the movements of the peripheral muscles are being centrally suppressed, making them largely imperceptible to others. Yet these actions-to-the-self may still be detected through small changes in muscle electrical potentials at those peripheral muscle sites. In short, executive functioning is viewed here as behavior-to-the-self developing in such a way that by adulthood the peripheral musculoskeletal apparatus associated with such actions is being largely inhibited so as to create a private form of behavior.

The conceptual linkage of inhibition with self-regulation and EFs is now obvious. Response inhibition is a prerequisite to self-regulation because one cannot direct actions or behavior toward oneself if one has already responded impulsively to an immediate event. They are mutually exclusive acts. The EFs are the general forms or classes of self-directed actions that humans use in self-regulation following the delay in the immediate response. I have identified at least four such classes besides inhibition below.

Often unstated in discussions of self-control or EFs is that they make little or no sense if there is not some means by which the individual is capable of perceiving and valuing future over immediate outcomes. In short, if there is no sense of the future, there is no self-control. A longer-term outcome may have greater reward value than a shorter-term reward if the two are compared to each other without regard to time. But arranged temporally as they are, the reward value of the longer-term outcome will be discounted by all organisms as a function of the length of the temporal delay involved to get it (Mazur, 1993). Humans demonstrate a remarkable shift over the first three decades of life toward a greater preference for larger, delayed rewards over smaller, more immediate ones (Green, Myerson, Lichtman, Rosen, & Fry, 1996). They discount future outcomes less steeply with age in comparison to younger individuals or other species. As noted earlier, this requires some neuropsychological capacity to sense the future, that is, the ability to construct hypothetical futures, particularly for social consequences. It also simultaneously involves the weighing of alternative responses and their temporally proximal and distal outcomes—a calculation of risk–benefit ratios over time. Some neuropsychological mechanism(s) must have evolved that permitted this relatively rapid construction of hypothetical social futures, while engaging in an economic analysis of immediate versus delayed outcomes. Without such an evolved mental mechanism, self-control would not occur. As I show below, the first EFs to develop in children provide the capacity for just such a cross-temporal economic spreadsheet—they are inhibition coupled with visual imagery. Imagery offers a means of iconically representing past transactions and recalling them as needed in evaluating the ongoing stream of social interactions in which an individual participates. But seeing to one's self (visual imagery) will not arise or be effective in informing the choice of a response if the ongoing stream of behavior is not interrupted by inhibition.

CONSTRUCTING A THEORY OF THE EFs AND SELF-CONTROL

I have suggested that humans have at least five means of self-control—that is, five classes of action that they direct toward themselves to change themselves to improve their future. They are self-stopping (volitional inhibition), sensing to the self, self-speech, emoting and motivating to the self, and self-play. The details of this model of EFs can be found in previous publications (Barkley, 1997a, 1997b, 2001, 2006), along with the evidence that seems to support their existence. I then extend this theory to an understanding of ADHD, a disorder of inhibition and executive functioning that originates in the prefrontal–striatal–cerebellar networks (Bush, Valera, & Seidman, 2005; Hutchinson, Mathias, & Banich, 2008; Mackie et al., 2007; Paloyelis, Mehta, Kuntsi, & Asherson, 2007; Valera, Faraone, Murray, & Seidman, 2007).

The initial structure of this model is taken from Bronowski (1967/1977), who first proposed it in his discussion of the unique properties of human language that he attributed to the prefrontal cortex. I further elaborated this framework by drawing heavily from Fuster's (1977) insights into the functioning of the prefrontal cortex. To this, I added the findings of Goldman-Rakic (1995) and others on working memory, and also those of Damasio (1994, 1995) on the somatic marker system and the rapid economic (motivational) analysis of hypothetical outcomes it affords. This model of EFs is thereby a hybrid one.

In this model, inhibition sets the occasion for the occurrence of the EFs and provides the protection from interference those EFs will require so as to construct hypothetical futures and direct behavior toward them. The EFs are interactive and share a common purpose: to "internalize" or make private certain self-directed behavior so as to anticipate and prepare for the social future to maximize net long-term versus short-term social outcomes.

I view inhibition and the other four EFs as developing by a common process. I have borrowed Vygotsky's theory for the internalization of speech (Diaz & Berk, 1992; Vygotsky, 1978; Vygotsky & Luria, 1994), which I propose as being the basis for the verbal working memory system of EF, and extended it to the other EFs, which can now be seen as forms of behavior that become self-directed and eventually covert or internalized. All five EFs represent private, covert forms of behavior that at one time in early child development (and in human evolution) were entirely publicly observable and directed toward others and the external world at large. With maturation, this outer-directed behavior becomes turned on the self as a means to control one's own behavior. Such self-behaving then becomes increasingly less observable to others as the suppression of the public musculoskeletal aspects of the behavior progresses. This progressively greater capacity to suppress the publicly observable aspects of behavior is what is meant here by the terms *covert, privatized,* or *internalized.*

Sensing to the Self (Nonverbal Working Memory)

The first EF has been called by others nonverbal working memory, or the visuospatial sketchpad (Baddeley, 1986; Baddeley & Hitch, 1994). In my theory it is the privatization of sensorimotor actions—sensing to the self (literally, re-sensing to the self). The most important of the senses to humans are vision and hearing, so this EF chiefly comprises visual imagery and covert audition—re-seeing and re-hearing to the self. This EF has both retrospective (sensory or re-sensing) and prospective (preparatory motor) elements (Fuster, 1997; Goldman-Rakic, 1995). They require interference control (resistance to distraction) for their effective performance. Here then arises the mental module for sensing the hypothetical future from the experienced past. This serves to generate the private or mental representations (images, auditions, etc.) that bridge the cross-temporal elements within a contingency arrangement (event–response–outcome) that is so crucial for self-control across time toward the future. This unit grants individuals the capacity to manage themselves relative to time (or *time management*). It may also be the prerequisite to symbolization (Deacon, 1997; Donald, 1991, 1993; Pierce, 1897/1955).

Speech to the Self (Verbal Working Memory)

The second EF is verbal working memory (Baddeley, 1986). I think it can be better understood, however, using Vygotsky's model of the developmental internalization of speech. The individual is capable of activating the central or cortical aspects of speech without engaging the actual peripheral motor execution of that speech. One can literally talk to oneself without moving the face or activating the larynx to any appreciable degree. Such self-speech permits self-description and reflection, self-instruction, self-questioning and problem solving, as well as the invention of rules and meta-rules to be applied to oneself (Diaz & Berk, 1992). It contributes to a major form of self-control via language and provides the basis for private verbal reasoning, strategy (rule) development, and verbal problem solving, not to mention moral conduct (internalizing socially prescribed rules of conduct). It also makes possible reading comprehension through silent reading (self-speech) that must be held in mind for the extraction of its semantic (nonverbal) content.

Emotion to the Self (Self-Regulation of Affect–Motivation–Arousal Emotion)

This EF may occur initially as a mere consequence of the first three (inhibition, private sensing, and self-speech). These mentally represented events have associated affective and motivational properties or valences that Damasio (1994, 1995) called *somatic markers*. Initially those affective valences have publicly visible counterparts—emotional displays, such as when we laugh out loud in response to a mentally visualized incident. Eventually they are kept private or covert in form. Here originates, I believe, the next EF of private, self-directed affect and its motivational properties—feeling (emoting/motivating) to the self. It is the wellspring of intrinsic motivation (willpower) so necessary to support future-directed behavior, especially across large delays in schedules of reinforcement or when external consequences for such future-directed action are otherwise not available in the immediate context. It provides the motivational basis for persistence (sustained attention) toward future goals.

Self-Play (Reconstitution)

The last EF is self-directed private (covert) play, or reconstitution. *Fluency, flexibililty*, and *generativity* are other terms by which this EF is known in neuropsychology. This EF serves to generate a diversity of new combinations of behavioral units out of old ones and so is the source of self-organization and innovation (problem solving) during goal-directed actions. It occurs, I believe, through a two-step process: analysis and synthesis. Both are applied to the mental contents being held in the working memory systems (self-sensing and self-speech systems). In analysis, old behavior sequences are broken down into smaller units. These units are then recombined (synthesized) into new sequences that can be tested against the requirements of the problem to be solved (Corballis, 1989; Fuster, 1997). It is hypothesized here to arise from the internalization of play (both sensorimotor and symbolic) and serves to create novel, future-directed actions. Such novel actions will be needed when one encounters obstacles to a goal (problems) in order to overcome them and successfully attain the goal. The generation of such novel responses is especially problematic for patients with frontal lobe injuries (Godefroy & Rosseaux, 1997). It has been blamed on their inability to form and sustain mental referents from instructions so as to manipulate them to discover a means to achieve a goal. And that, as I have argued, is simply covert play to oneself.

This EF may be subdivided further into verbal and nonverbal components (fluencies) comparable to the working memory subsystem (verbal or nonverbal) on which it acts. Neuroimaging studies suggest that verbal and nonverbal (design) fluency are mediated by separate (left vs. right) regions of the dorsolateral frontal cortex (Lee et al., 1997; Stuss et al., 1998). However, prior factor-analytic studies of EF measures have found only a single dimension representing both verbal and nonverbal fluency (Levin et al., 1996).

Further Implications of the Theory

Each executive function is also hypothesized to contribute to the following developmental shifts in the sources of control over human behavior:

- From external events to mental representations related to those events.
- From control by others to control by the self.
- From immediate reinforcement to delayed gratification.
- From the temporal now to the conjectured social future.

With maturation, the individual progressively comes to be guided more by covert representations that permit self-control, deferred gratification, and goal-directed actions toward conjectured social futures.

Briefly put, the privatization (internalization) of self-directed sensorimotor action, speech, emotion–motivation, and play (reconstitution) provide an exceptionally powerful set of mind tools that greatly facilitate adaptive functioning in anticipation of the future. In a sense, these EFs permit the private simulation of actions within specific settings that can be tested out mentally for their probable consequences (somatic markers) before a response is selected for eventual public execution. This, as Karl Popper noted, allows our ideas to die in our place should they prove not to be correct or suitable in such mental simulations (see Dennett, 1995). It constitutes a form of mental trial-and-error learning that is devoid of real-world consequences for one's mistakes.

When extrapolated into daily life activities, these EFs have been found to contribute to the following dimensions as manifested in behavior over time as seen in natural settings: (1) self-inhibition (of cognition, motor behavior, verbal behavior, and emotion); (2) self-management to time and the future; (3) self-organization and problem solving; (4) self-motivation; and (5) self-regulation of emotion (Barkley, in press).

THE IMPACT OF ADHD ON SELF-CONTROL

A central problem in those with ADHD is the capacity for behavioral inhibition (Barkley, 1997a, 2006; Nigg, 2001; Quay, 1997). In my theory, a deficit in inhibition will result in a cascade of secondary deficits into the remaining four EFs. Behavioral disinhibition leads to deficiencies in nonverbal working memory, resulting in (1) particular forms of forgetfulness (forgetting to do things at certain critical points in time); (2) impaired ability to organize and execute actions relative to time (e.g., time management); (3) reduced hindsight and forethought; (4) a reduction in the creation of anticipatory action toward future events. Consequently, the capacity for the cross-temporal organization of behavior in those with ADHD is diminished, disrupting the ability to string together complex chains of actions directed, over time, to a future goal. The greater the degree to which time separates the components of the behavioral contingency (event, response, consequence), the more difficult the task will prove for those with ADHD who cannot bind the contingency together across time so as to use it to govern their own behavior. Working memory, especially nonverbal, may be as much a primary deficit in ADHD as a secondary one that arises from poor inhibition (Rapport et al., 2008, 2009). Nonetheless, inhibition and working memory are interactive, and deficits in each are likely to affect the other adversely. Researchers find that nonverbal working memory, timing, and forethought are deficient in ADHD (Barkley, 1997a; Barkley & Murphy, in press; Barkley et al., 2008; Frazier et al., 2004; Hervey et al., 2004; Rapport et al., 2008).

In ADHD, the privatization of speech should also be delayed, resulting in greater public speech (excessive talking), less verbal reflection before acting, less organized and rule-oriented self-speech, diminished influence of self-directed speech in organizing and controlling one's own behavior, and difficulties following rules and instructions given by others. Researchers find this to be the case (Berk & Potts, 1991; Landau, Berk, & Mangione, 1996; Winsler, 1998; Winsler, Diaz, Atencio, McCarthy, & Chabay, 2000). Those with ADHD have difficulties with verbal working memory tasks, such as digit span backwards, mental arithmetic, paced auditory serial addition, paired associated learning, and other tasks believed to reflect verbal working memory (Barkley, 1997a; Frazier et al., 2004; Hervey et al., 2004; Kuntsi, Oosterlaan, & Stevenson, 2001).

These deficits lead to a third problem—impaired emotional–motivational self-regulation. Children with ADHD display (1) greater impulsive emotional expressions in their reactions to events; (2) less objectivity in the selection of a response to an event; (3) diminished social perspective taking because the child does not delay his or her initial emotional reaction long enough to take the view of others and their own needs into account; (4) greater difficulties in self-soothing the initially strong emotional reaction; (5) greater problems with self-distracting and otherwise modifying attention to the emotionally provocative event so as to diminish its ongoing impact; and (6) a diminished ability to construct in place of the original emotion more socially appropriate and moderate emotions that are more supportive of long-term welfare or social interests. ADHD also impairs the capacity to induce drive and motivational states in the service of goal-directed behavior. Those with ADHD remain more dependent than others upon the environmental contingencies within a situation or task to determine their motivation (Barkley, 1997a; Barkley, 2010; Barkley & Murphy, in press).

The model further predicts ADHD's associating with impaired reconstitution, or self-directed play, evident in a diminished use of analysis and synthesis in the formation of both verbal and nonverbal responses to events. The capacity to visualize or verbalize mentally, manipulate, then generate multiple plans of action (options) in the service of goal-directed behavior, and to select from among them those with the greatest likelihood of succeeding, should therefore be reduced. This impairment in reconstitution will be evident in everyday verbal fluency when the person with ADHD is required by a task or situation to assemble rapidly, accurately, and efficiently the parts of speech into messages (sentences) so as to accomplish the goal or requirements of the task. It will also be evident in tasks where visual information must be held in mind and manipulated to generate diverse scenarios to help solve problems (Barkley, 1997a). In general it should result in poorer self-organization and problem solving in support of one's goals or assigned tasks. Evidence for a deficiency in verbal and nonverbal fluency, planning, problem solving, and strategy development more generally in ADHD is limited, but what exists is consistent with the theory (Barkley, 1997a; Barkley & Murphy, in press; Clark, Prior, & Kinsella, 2000; Klorman et al., 1999).

In general, ADHD is predicted to disrupt the four transitions noted earlier in the source of control over behavior. Those having ADHD will be more under the control of external events than of mental representations about time and the future, under the influence of others rather than acting to control oneself, in pursuit of immediate gratification over deferred gratification, and under the influence of the temporal now more than of the probable social futures that lie before them. From this vantage point, ADHD is not a disorder of attention, at least not to the moment or to the external environment, but is more a disorder of intention—that is, attention to the future and what one needs to do to prepare for its arrival. It is also a disorder of time—time management specifically—in that individuals manifest an inability to regulate their behavior relative to time as well as to others at their developmental level. This creates a sort of temporal myopia in which the individual responds to or prepares only for events that are relatively imminent rather than ones that lie further ahead in time to which others their age are preparing to be ready for their eventual arrival (Barkley, 1997a).

CONCLUSIONS

There is much promise in viewing ADHD as a disorder of self-regulation (and its underlying executive functioning). It encourages psychopathologists more fully to develop models of how normal self-control arises across childhood and even into adulthood, and to examine where in these models disorders such as ADHD disrupt the normal structure and processes of self-regulation to produce what is known about the disorder. Moreover, such model building also suggests new hypotheses that can be pursued not only in testing the models but also in providing a greater understanding of what is disrupted by the disorder (see Barkley, 2006, Ch. 7). Self-control may have arisen by evolution for a set of largely social functions, such as reciprocal exchange, cooperative coalitions, and vicarious learning (Barkley, 2001). This perspective gives further grounds for the development of testable hypotheses about not only self-control but also the social deficiencies that arise in disorders of self-regulation such as ADHD.

REFERENCES

Ainslie, G. (1974). Impulse control in pigeons. *Journal of the Experimental Analysis of Behavior, 21*, 485–489.

American Psychiatric Association. (2001). *Diagnostic and statistical manual of mental disorders* (4th ed., text revision). Washington, DC: Author.

Baddeley, A. D. (1986). *Working memory*. London: Clarendon Press.

Baddeley, A. D., & Hitch, G. J. (1994). Developments in the concept of working memory. *Neuropsychology, 8*, 1485–493.

Badre, D. (2008). Cognitive control, hierarchy, and the rostro-caudal organization of the frontal lobes. *Trends in Cognitive Science, 12*, 193–200.

Barkley, R. A. (1997a). *ADHD and the nature of self-control*. New York: Guilford Press.

Barkley, R. A. (1997b). Behavioral inhibition, sustained attention, and executive functions: Constructing a unifying theory of ADHD. *Psychological Bulletin, 121*, 65–94.

Barkley, R. A. (2001). The executive functions and self-regulation: An evolutionary neuropsychological perspective. *Neuropsychology Review, 11*, 1–29.

Barkley, R. A. (2006). *Attention-deficit/hyperactivity disorder: A handbook for diagnosis and treatment* (3rd ed.). New York: Guilford Press.

Barkley, R. A. (2010). Deficient emotional self-regulation is a core component of attention-deficit/hyperactivity disorder. *Journal of ADHD and Related Disorders, 1*, 5–37.

Barkley, R. A. (in press). *Executive Functioning Scale: Assessing difficulties in executive functioning in daily life activities*. New York: Guilford Press.

Barkley, R. A., & Murphy, K. R. (in press). Executive function (EF) deficits in adults with ADHD: Comparing EF in daily life activities vs. performance in EF tests. *Journal of ADHD and Related Disorders*.

Barkley, R. A., Murphy, K. R., & Fischer, M. (2008). *ADHD in adults: What the science says*. New York: Guilford Press.

Berk, L. E., & Potts, M. K. (1991). Development and functional significance of private speech among attention-deficit hyperactivity disorder and normal boys. *Journal of Abnormal Child Psychology, 19*, 357–377.

Biederman, J., Petty, C. R., Fried, R., Doyle, A. E., Spencer, T., Seidman, L. J., et al. (2007). Stability of executive function deficits into young adult years: A prospective longitudinal follow-up study of grown up males with ADHD. *Acta Psychiatrica Scandinavica, 116*, 129–136.

Bronowski, J. (1977). Human and animal languages. *A sense of the future* (pp. 104–131). Cambridge, MA: MIT Press. (Original work published 1967)

Burns, D. J., & Powers, R. B. (1975). Choice and self-control in children: A test of Rachlin's model. *Bulletin of the Psychonomic Society, 5*, 156–158.

Bush, G., Valera, E. M., & Seidman, L. J. (2005). Functional neuroimaging of attention-deficit/

hyperactivity disorder: A review and suggested future directions. *Biological Psychiatry, 57,* 1273–1296.

Castellanos, X., Sonuga-Barke, E., Milham, M., & Tannock, R. (2006). Characterizing cognition in ADHD: Beyond executive dysfunction. *Trends in Cognitive Sciences, 10,* 117–123.

Clark, C., Prior, M., & Kinsella, G. J. (2000). Do executive function deficits differentiate between adolescents with ADHD and oppositional defiant/conduct disorder?: A neuropsychological study using the Six Elements Test and Hayling Sentence Completion Test. *Journal of Abnormal Child Psychology, 28,* 405–414.

Corballis, M. C. (1989). Laterality and human evolution. *Psychological Review, 96,* 492–505.

Damasio, A. R. (1994). *Descartes' error: Emotion, reason, and the human brain.* New York: Putnam.

Damasio, A. R. (1995). On some functions of the human prefrontal cortex. *Annals of the New York Academy of Sciences, 769,* 241–251.

Deacon, T. W. (1997). *The symbolic species: The co-evolution of language and the brain.* New York: Norton.

Denckla, M. B. (1996). A theory and model of executive function: A neuropsychological perspective. In G. R. Lyon & N. A. Krasnegor (Eds.), *Attention, memory, and executive function* (pp. 263–277). Baltimore: Brookes.

Dennett, D. (1995). *Darwin's dangerous idea: Evolution and the meanings of life.* New York: Simon & Schuster.

D'Esposito, M., Detre, J. A., Aguirre, G. K., Stallcup, M., Alsop, D. C., Tippet, L. J., et al. (1997). A functional MRI study of mental image generation. *Neuropsychologia, 35,* 725–730.

Diaz, R. M., & Berk, L. E. (1992). *Private speech: From social interaction to self-regulation.* Mahwah, NJ: Erlbaum.

Donald, M. (1991). *Origins of the modern mind: Three stages in the evolution of culture and cognition.* Cambridge, MA: Harvard University Press.

Donald, M. (1993). Precis of origins of the modern mind: Three stages in the evolution of culture and cognition. *Behavioral and Brain Sciences, 16,* 737–791.

Frazier, T. W., Demareem H. A., & Youngstrom, E. A. (2004). Meta-analysis of intellectual and neuropsychological test performance in attention-deficit/hyperactivity disorder. *Neuropsychology, 18,* 543–555.

Fuster, J. M. (1997). *The prefrontal cortex: Anatomy, physiology, and neuropsychology of the frontal lobe* (3rd ed.). Philadelphia: Lippincott-Raven.

Gioia, G. A., Isquith, P. K., Guy, S. C., & Kenworthy, L. (2000). *BRIEF: Behavior Rating Inventory of Executive Function professional manual.* Odessa, FL: Psychological Assessment Resources.

Godefroy, O., & Rosseaux, M. (1997). Novel decision making in patients with prefrontal or posterior brain damage. *Neurology, 49,* 695–701.

Goel, V., & Grafman, J. (1995). Are the frontal lobes implicated in "planning" functions?: Interpreting data from the Tower of Hanoi. *Neuropsychologia, 33,* 623–642.

Goldman-Rakic, P. S. (1995). Architecture of the prefrontal cortex and the central executive. *Annals of the New York Academy of Sciences, 769,* 71–83.

Green, L., Myerson, J., Lichtman, D., Rosen, S., & Fry, A. (1996). Temporal discounting in choice between delayed rewards: The role of age and income. *Psychology and Aging, 11,* 79–84.

Hervey, A. S., Epstein, J. N., & Curry, J. F. (2004). Neuropsychology of adults with attention-deficit/hyperactivity disorder: A meta-analytic review. *Neuropsychology, 18,* 495–503.

Huizinga, M., Dolan, C. V., & van der Molen, M. W. (2006). Age-related change in executive function: Developmental trends and a latent variable analysis. *Neuropsychologia, 44,* 2017–2036.

Hutchinson, A. D., Mathias, J. L., & Banich, M. T. (2008). Corpus callosum morphology in children and adolescents with attention deficit hyperactivity disorder: A meta-analytic review. *Neuropsychology, 22*, 341–349.

Kanfer, F. H., & Karoly, P. (1972). Self-control: A behavioristic excursion into the lion's den. *Behavior Therapy, 3*, 398–416.

Klorman, R., Hazel-Fernandez, H., Shaywitz, S. E., Fletcher, J. M., Marchione, K. E., Holahan, J. M., et al. (1999). Executive functioning deficits in attention-deficit/hyperactivity disorder are independent of oppositional defiant or reading disorder. *Journal of the American Academy of Child and Adolescent Psychiatry, 38*, 1148–1155.

Kuntsi, J., Oosterlaan, J., & Stevenson, J. (2001). Psychological mechanisms in hyperactivity: I. Response inhibition deficit, working memory impairment, delay aversion, or something else? *Journal of Child Psychology and Psychiatry, 42*, 199–210.

Landau, S., Berk, L. E., & Mangione, C. (1996, March). *Private speech as a problem-solving strategy in the face of academic challenge: The failure of impulsive children to get their act together.* Paper presented at the annual meeting of the National Association of School Psychologists, Atlanta, GA.

Lee, G. P., Strauss, E., Loring, D. W., McCloskey, L., Haworth, J. M., & Lehman, R. A. W. (1997). Sensitivity of figural fluency on the Five-Point Test to focal neurological dysfunction. *Clinical Neuropsychologist, 11*, 59–68.

Levin, H. S., Fletcher, J. M., Kufera, J. A., Harward, H., Lilly, M. A., Mendelsohn, D., et al. (1996). Dimensions of cognition measured by the Tower of London and other cognitive tasks in head-injured children and adolescents. *Developmental Neuropsychology, 12*, 17–34.

Lezak, M. D. (1995). *Neuropsychological assessment* (3rd ed.). New York: Oxford University Press.

Livesay, J. R., Liebke, A. W., Samaras, M. R., & Stanley, S. A. (1996). Covert speech behavior during a silent language recitation task. *Perceptual and Motor Skills, 83*, 1355–1362.

Livesay, J. R., & Samaras, M. R. (1998). Covert neuromuscular activity of the dominant forearm during visualization of a motor task. *Perceptual and Motor Skills, 86*, 371–374.

Logue, A. W. (1988). Research on self-control: An integrating framework. *Behavioral and Brain Sciences, 11*, 665–709.

Mackie, S., Shaw, P., Lenroot, R., Greenstein, D. K., Nugent, T. F., III, Sharp, W. S., et al. (2007). Cerebellar development and clinical outcome in attention deficit hyperactivity disorder. *American Journal of Psychiatry, 76*, 647–655.

Mazur, J. E. (1993). Predicting the strength of a conditioned reinforcer: Effects of delay and uncertainty. *Current Directions in Psychological Science, 2*, 70–74.

Mischel, W. (1983). Delay of gratification as process and as person variable in development. In D. Magnusson & U. L. Allen (Eds.), *Human development: An interactional perspective* (pp. 149–166). New York: Academic Press.

Mischel, W., Shoda, Y., & Rodriguez, M. I. (1989). Delay of gratification in children. *Science, 244*, 933–938.

Navarick, D. J. (1986). Human impulsivity and choice: A challenge to traditional operant methodology. *Psychological Record, 36*, 343–356.

Nigg, J. T. (2001). Is ADHD an inhibitory disorder? *Psychological Bulletin, 125*, 571–596.

Nigg, J. T., & Casey, B. J. (2005). An integrative theory of attention-deficit/hyperactivity disorder based on the cognitive and affective neurosciences. *Development and Psychopathology, 17*, 765–806.

Paloyelis, Y., Mehta, M. A., Kuntsi, J., & Asherson, P. (2007). Functional MRI in ADHD: A systematic literature review. *Expert Reviews in Neurotherapeutics, 7*, 1337–1356.

Pierce, C. S. (1955). Logic as semiotic: The theory of signs. In J. Buchler (Ed.), *The philosophical writings of Peirce* (pp. 98–119). New York: Dover. (Original work published 1897)

Pontius, A. A. (1973). Dysfunction patterns analogous to frontal lobe system and caudate nucleus syndromes in some groups of minimal brain dysfunction. *Journal of the American Medical Women's Association, 26*, 285–292.

Quay, H. C. (1997). Inhibition and attention deficit hyperactivity disorder. *Journal of Abnormal Child Psychology, 25*, 7–13.

Rapport, M. D., Alderson, R. M., Kofler, M. J., Sarver, D. E., Bolden, J., & Sims, V. (2008). Working memory deficits in boys with attention-deficit/hyperactivity disorder (ADHD): The contribution of central executive and subsystem processes. *Journal of Abnormal Child Psychology, 36*, 825–837.

Rapport, M. D., Bolden, J., Kofler, M. J., Sarver, D. E., Raiker, J. S., & Alderson, R. M. (2009). Hyperactivity in boys with attention-deficit/hyperactivity disorder (ADHD): A unique core symptom or a manifestation of working memory deficits? *Journal of Abnormal Child Psychology, 37*, 521–534.

Ryding, E., Bradvik, B., & Ingvar, D. H. (1996). Silent speech activates prefrontal cortical regions asymmetrically, as well as speech-related areas in the dominant hemisphere. *Brain and Language, 52*, 435–451.

Sagvolden, T., Johansen, E. B., Aase, H., & Russell, V. A. (2005). A dynamic developmental theory of attention-deficit/hyperactivity disorder (ADHD) predominantly hyperactive/impulsive and combined subtypes. *Behavioral and Brain Sciences, 25*, 397–468.

Shimamura, A. P., Janowsky, J. S., & Squire, L. R. (1990). Memory for the temporal order of events in patients with frontal lobe lesions and amnesic patients. *Neuropsychologia, 28*, 803–813.

Sirigu, A., Zalla, T., Pillon, B., Grafman, J., DuBois, B., & Agid, Y. (1995). Planning and script analysis following prefrontal lobe lesions. In J. Grafman, K. J. Holyoke, & F. Boller (Eds.), Structure and functions of the human prefrontal cortex. *Annals of the New York Academy of Sciences, 769*, 277–288.

Skinner, B. F. (1953). *Science and human behavior.* New York: Macmillan.

Stuss, D. T., Alexander, M. A., Hamer, L., Palumbo, C., Dempster, R., Binns, M., et al. (1998). The effects of focal anterior and posterior brain lesions on verbal fluency. *Journal of the International Neuropsychological Society, 4*, 265–278.

Stuss, D. T., & Benson, D. F. (1986). *The frontal lobes.* New York: Raven.

Thorell, L. B., & Nyberg, L. (2008). The Childhood Executive Functioning Inventory (CHEXI): A new rating instrument for parents and teachers. *Developmental Neuropsychology, 33*, 536–552.

Valera, E. M., Faraone, S. V., Murray, K. E., & Seidman, L. J. (2007). Meta-analysis of structural imaging findings in attention-deficit/hyperactivity disorder. *Biological Psychiatry, 61*, 1361–1369.

Vygotsky, L. S. (1978). *Mind in society.* Cambridge, MA: Harvard University Press.

Vygotsky, L. S. (1987). Thinking and speech. In *The collected works of L. S. Vygotsky: Vol. 1. Problems in general psychology* (N. Minick, Trans.) (pp. 37–285). New York: Plenum Press.

Vygotsky, L. S., & Luria, A. (1994). Tool and symbol in child development. In R. van der Veer & J. Valsiner (Eds.), *The Vygotsky reader* (pp. 99–174). Cambridge, MA: Blackwell Science.

Welsh, M. C., Pennington, B. F., & Grossier, D. B. (1991). A normative-developmental study of executive function: A window on prefrontal function in children. *Developmental Neuropsychology, 7*, 131–149.

Winsler, A. (1998). Parent–child interaction and private speech in boys with ADHD. *Applied Developmental Science, 2*, 17–39.

Winsler, A., Diaz, R. M., Atencio, D. J., McCarthy, E. M., & Chabay, L. A. (2000). Verbal self-regulation over time in preschool children at risk for attention and behavior problems. *Journal of Child Psychology and Psychiatry, 41*, 875–886.

Wright, R. (2001). *Nonzero.* New York: Vintage Books.

Author Index

Author Index

Subject Index